Covid-19 and Diabetes: Associations and Possible Mechanisms

Covid-19 and Diabetes: Associations and Possible Mechanisms

Editor: Brie Madsen

MURPHY & MOORE
www.murphy-moorepublishing.com

www.murphy-moorepublishing.com

MURPHY & MOORE

Cataloging-in-Publication Data

Covid-19 and diabetes : associations and possible mechanisms / edited by Brie Madsen.
p. cm.
Includes bibliographical references and index.
ISBN 978-1-63987-797-3
1. Diabetes. 2. COVID-19 (Disease)--Complications. 3. Diabetics--Health and hygiene. I. Madsen, Brie.
RA644.C67 C68 2023
616.462--dc23

Murphy & Moore Publishing
1 Rockefeller Plaza,
New York City,
NY 10020, USA

ISBN 978-1-63987-797-3 (Hardback)

Contents

Preface

In my initial years as a student, I used to run to the library at every possible instance to grab a book and learn something new. Books were my primary source of knowledge and I would not have come such a long way without all that I learnt from them. Thus, when I was approached to edit this book; I became understandably nostalgic. It was an absolute honor to be considered worthy of guiding the current generation as well as those to come. I put all my knowledge and hard work into making this book most beneficial for its readers.

Coronavirus disease (COVID-19) is a family of viruses which causes illnesses like Middle East respiratory syndrome (MERS), severe acute respiratory syndrome (SARS) and common cold. Diabetes is a complex chronic disease characterized by dysregulation of blood glucose levels in the body. It is caused by a complete deficiency of insulin or body inability to utilize insulin. There are various factors present in diabetes that are likely to increase the risk and contribute to the development of COVID-19. Some of these factors include older age, a hypercoagulable and proinflammatory state, hyperglycemia and underlying comorbidities such as chronic kidney disease hypertension, obesity and cardiovascular disease. The treatment of a severe COVID-19 infection with steroids can lead to the worsening of hyperglycemia through increased insulin resistance and reduced β-cell secretory function. This book provides significant insights into the associations between COVID-19 and diabetes as well as its possible mechanisms. It consists of researches and studies performed by experts across the globe. The book is appropriate for students seeking detailed information in this area of study as well as for experts.

I wish to thank my publisher for supporting me at every step. I would also like to thank all the authors who have contributed their researches in this book. I hope this book will be a valuable contribution to the progress of the field.

Editor

1

Impaired Fasting Glucose and Diabetes are Related to Higher Risks of Complications and Mortality Among Patients with Coronavirus Disease 2019

Jiaoyue Zhang[1,2†], Wen Kong[1,2†], Pengfei Xia[3†], Ying Xu[4], Li Li[5], Qin Li[6], Li Yang[7], Qi Wei[8], Hanyu Wang[1,2], Huiqing Li[1,2], Juan Zheng[1,2], Hui Sun[1,2], Wenfang Xia[1,2], Geng Liu[1,2], Xueyu Zhong[1,2], Kangli Qiu[1,2], Yan Li[5], Han Wang[1,2], Yuxiu Wang[1,2], Xiaoli Song[1,2], Hua Liu[1,2], Si Xiong[4], Yumei Liu[7], Zhenhai Cui[1,2], Yu Hu[9,10], Lulu Chen[1,2], An Pan[3*] and Tianshu Zeng[1,2*]*

[1] Department of Endocrinology, Union Hospital, Tongji Medical College, Huazhong University of Science and Technology, Wuhan, China, [2] Hubei Provincial Clinical Research Center for Diabetes and Metabolic Disorders, Wuhan, China, [3] Department of Epidemiology and Biostatistics, School of Public Health, Tongji Medical College, Huazhong University of Science and Technology, Wuhan, China, [4] Department of Endocrinology, The Fifth Hospital of Wuhan, Wuhan, China, [5] Department of Endocrinology, Wuhan Wuchang Hospital, Wuchang Hospital Affiliated to Wuhan University of Science and Technology, Wuhan, China, [6] Department of Endocrinology, General Hospital of the Yangtze River Shipping, Wuhan, China, [7] Department of Endocrinology, Hankou Hospital of Wuhan City, Wuhan, China, [8] Department of Endocrinology, Red Cross Hospital of Wuhan City, Wuhan, China, [9] Institute of Hematology, Union Hospital, Tongji Medical College, Huazhong University of Science and Technology, Wuhan, China, [10] Hubei Clinical and Research Centre of Thrombosis and Haemostasis, Wuhan, China

***Correspondence:**
Lulu Chen
cheria_chen@126.com
An Pan
panan@hust.edu.cn
Tianshu Zeng
tszeng@126.com

† These authors have contributed equally to this work

Background: Diabetes correlates with poor prognosis in patients with COVID-19, but very few studies have evaluated whether impaired fasting glucose (IFG) is also a risk factor for the poor outcomes of patients with COVID-19. Here we aimed to examine the associations between IFG and diabetes at admission with risks of complications and mortality among patients with COVID-19.

Methods: In this multicenter retrospective cohort study, we enrolled 312 hospitalized patients with COVID-19 from 5 hospitals in Wuhan from Jan 1 to Mar 17, 2020. Clinical information, laboratory findings, complications, treatment regimens, and mortality status were collected. The associations between hyperglycemia and diabetes status at admission with primary composite end-point events (including mechanical ventilation, admission to intensive care unit, or death) were analyzed by Cox proportional hazards regression models.

Results: The median age of the patients was 57 years (interquartile range 38–66), and 172 (55%) were women. At the time of hospital admission, 84 (27%) had diabetes (and 36 were new-diagnosed), 62 (20%) had IFG, and 166 (53%) had normal fasting glucose (NFG) levels. Compared to patients with NFG, patients with IFG and diabetes developed more primary composite end-point events (9 [5%], 11 [18%], 26 [31%]), including receiving mechanical ventilation (5 [3%], 6 [10%], 21 [25%]), and death (4 [2%], 9 [15%], 20 [24%]). Multivariable Cox regression analyses showed diabetes was associated increased risks of primary composite end-point events (hazard ratio 3.53; 95% confidence interval 1.48–8.40) and mortality (6.25; 1.91–20.45), and IFG was associated with an increased risk of mortality (4.11; 1.15–14.74), after adjusting for age, sex, hospitals and comorbidities.

Conclusion: IFG and diabetes at admission were associated with higher risks of adverse outcomes among patients with COVID-19.

Keywords: cohort study, coronavirus, COVID-19, diabetes, hyperglycemia, impaired fasting glucose, severe acute respiratory coronavirus 2 (SARS-CoV-2)

INTRODUCTION

The coronavirus disease 2019 (COVID-19) pandemic, a public health emergency of international concern, had affected more than 8.1 million cases and caused over 440,000 deaths globally by June 18, 2020 (1). People of all ages can be infected, whereas older people and those with underlying diseases were more likely to develop severe illness (2, 3).

The prevalence of diabetes among patients with COVID-19 varied in different studies. Studies in Chinese patients reported prevalence rates ranged from 5.3 to 8.2% (3–5), while a recent study in 5,700 patients with New York reported that 33.8% had diabetes (6). Previous studies have reported that diabetes and uncontrolled glycemia were significant predictors of severity and mortality in patients infected with lower respiratory tract infections (7, 8), 2009 pandemic influenza A (H1N1) (9), severe acute respiratory syndrome coronavirus (SARS-CoV) (10), and Middle East respiratory syndrome coronavirus (MERS-CoV) (11, 12). However, it remains controversial whether diabetes is related to adverse outcomes among patients with COVID-19 (13, 14). Most studies reported that diabetes was associated with higher risks for severe events and mortality (3–5, 15–17), whereas others showed no clear association (18, 19). The inconsistency may be related to the varied sample size, different populations, and different degrees of confounding adjustment. Hyperglycemia has been widely accepted to be harmful to the control of infection. A recent study of 7,337 cases with COVID-19 in China found that well-controlled blood glucose (3.9–10.0 mmol/L) was associated with markedly lower mortality compared to individuals with poorly controlled BG (>10.0 mmol/L) (20). On the other hand, an overly rigid glucose control might also increase the risk of severe hypoglycemia, which can also lead to an increased mortality (21). Nevertheless, no study has specifically examined the prevalence of impaired fasting glucose (IFG) in patients with COVID-19 and whether prediabetes condition was a risk factor.

Many studies have reported the clinical features of patients with COVID-19 in different countries (2, 5, 6, 16, 22–24), while few has specifically compared the clinical characteristics of COVID-19 in patients with and without diabetes. And also, the clinical characteristics of IFG patients with COVID-19 are obscure until now. It is unclear whether the differences in those characteristics including laboratory markers may explain the increased risks of adverse outcomes related to prediabetes and diabetes. Therefore, we analyzed clinical and laboratory characteristics, as well as treatment and prognosis of hospitalized patients with COVID-19 by diabetes and hyperglycemia status at admission in Wuhan city. We hypothesized that diabetes and IFG were related to increased risks of adverse outcomes and differences in clinical features could mediate the associations.

MATERIALS AND METHODS

Study Design and Participants

In this multicenter, retrospective cohort study, we recruited hospitalized patients with COVID-19 from six departments of five hospitals in Wuhan from Jan 1 to Mar 17, 2020. All hospitals were designated to treat patients with COVID-19, including the Department of Infectious Disease and the Department of Oncology of the Union Hospital of Tongji Medical College, Huazhong University of Science and Technology, the Departments of Endocrinology in the following four hospitals: Fifth Hospital of Wuhan, Wuhan Wuchang Hospital Affiliated to Wuhan University of Science and Technology, General Hospital of the Yangtze River Shipping, and Wuhan Hankou Hospital. Those six departments were temporarily converted into isolated wards for patients with COVID-19. We only had access to the data of the six departments that the investigators were in charge of, and thus data from other departments in the five hospitals were not available.

COVID-19 was diagnosed according to the Diagnosis and Treatment Scheme for the Novel Coronavirus Pneumonia released by the National Health Commission of China [**Supplementary Table 1**; (3)], and the severity status of the patients were classified as non-severe and severe types [**Supplementary Table 2**; (25)]. We only included cases with positive results for severe acute respiratory coronavirus 2 (SARS-CoV-2) virus by real-time reverse transcriptase-polymerase chain reaction (RT-PCR) assay of nasal and pharyngeal swab specimens, or positive serum specific IgM and IgG antibody.

The study was approved by the Ethics Committee of the Union Hospital, Tongji Medical College, Huazhong University of Science and Technology. Informed consent was waived by using anonymous clinical data in this retrospective study.

Data Collection

We extracted data from electronic medical records for demographics, clinical, laboratory, and radiological characteristics, treatment, and outcomes for all patients with COVID-19. Two researchers independently reviewed and double checked the data collection forms.

General characteristics (age, sex, and comorbidities) and clinical symptoms and signs at admission were recorded. Vital signs (respiratory rate, blood pressure) were measured, height and weight were self-reported. Comprehensive laboratory test results were compiled within 3 days of admission and before steroid therapy. If fasting glucose concentrations were measured multiple times after admission, we only used the first one to represent the glycemic status at the time of admission. The treatment regimens for COVID-19 and other comorbidities were also extracted from the medical records.

Diabetes was diagnosed as fasting plasma glucose ≥7.0 mmol/L, or self-reported physician-diagnosed diabetes or anti-diabetic medication use; IFG was defined as glucose levels between 5.6 and 6.9 mmol/L. Patients with fasting glucose levels below 5.6 mmol/L were considered as having normal fasting glucose (NFG). Patients without previous diagnosis of diabetes while presenting with plasma fasting glucose ≥7.0 mmol/L at hospital admission was considered as new-diagnosed diabetes.

The primary composite endpoints included mechanical ventilation, admission to intensive care unit (ICU), or death. Other endpoints were also recorded, including acute respiratory distress syndrome (ARDS), septic shock, acute kidney injury, cardiac injury, rhabdomyolysis, diabetic ketoacidosis, hyperosmolar hyperglycemic state, and hypoglycemic coma. Details of the definitions of the outcomes are provided in the **Supplementary Material.**

Laboratory test results were compiled including standard blood counts, blood biochemistry [including renal and liver function, creatine kinase, fasting plasma glucose, lactate dehydrogenase (LDH), and lipid profiles], urine routine test, coagulation profile, procalcitonin, C-reactive protein (CRP), erythrocyte sedimentation rate (ESR), myocardial enzyme spectrum and routine bacterial, fungal, and viral examinations. Additional data were collected including medical imaging, treatment regimens [e.g., antiviral and antibacterial drugs, systemic corticosteroid, immunoglobulin G, respiratory support (e.g., nasal tube, high-flow nasal cannula, non-invasive, and invasive mechanical ventilation)], and prognosis (discharged or death). Anti-diabetic agents during hospitalization were recorded.

Statistical Analysis

Descriptive statistics included counts and proportions for categorical variables and median (IQR) for continuous variables. Comparisons across the three categories (diabetes, IFG, NFG) were performed using Kruskal Wallis test for continuous variables and chi-square or Fisher's exact test for categorical variables as appropriate. Logistical regression was performed to evaluate the association between diabetes status and severity of COVID-19 with adjustment for age, sex, hospitals and other comorbidities. Time to a composite endpoint was investigated using survival analysis by a Kaplan- Meier plot and compared by the log-rank test. Furthermore, Cox proportional hazards regression models were used to evaluate the association between glycemic status and outcomes with adjustment for age, sex, hospitals and other comorbidities. To further investigate whether the associations were mediated by certain laboratory markers, we classified the markers into different categories (such as blood biochemistry, inflammatory markers, metabolic markers) and chose a marker with the strongest association with the outcomes as a representative of the category and included in the final model. This was used to avoid over-adjustment for many markers with collinearity in the model with limited sample size. There were missing values for some laboratory tests and were treated as missing indicators in the regression models to retain maximum sample size. Sensitivity analysis was performed by removing patients with new-diagnosed diabetes to exclude the possibility of stress induced hyperglycemia. Statistical analyses were performed with SAS 9.4, and statistical significance was set at 2-tailed $p < 0.05$.

RESULTS

General Information

By Mar 17, 2020, 729 patients with pneumonia were admitted to the six departments of five hospitals. Among them, the following patients were excluded from the analyses: 316 suspected cases without positive RT-RCP tests, 80 patients who were still in hospital until Mar 17, 2020, 21 patients without intact information of clinical outcomes because of transferring to other hospitals. Therefore, 312 patients were included in the final analysis. Among them, 84 (27%) had diabetes, 62 (20%) had IFG, and 166 (53%) had NFG. Among the 84 patients with diabetes, 57 had fasting glucose levels ≥7.0 mmol/L, including 30 without and 27 with a known history of diabetes.

The median age of the 312 patients was 57 years (interquartile range 38–66), and 172 (55%) were female (**Table 1**). Comparing to patients with NFG, patients with IFG and diabetes were older and more likely to be men. As expected, patients with IFG and diabetes were more likely to have other comorbidities, including hypertension, coronary heart diseases, chronic kidney disease, and cerebrovascular disease.

Clinical Symptoms and Signs

The common symptoms at hospital admission included fever (268 [86%]), cough (264 [85%]), fatigue (181 [58%]), loss of appetite (179 [57%]), dyspnea (145 [46%]), and chest pain 139 (45%; **Table 1**). Among the symptoms, patients with diabetes were more likely to have dyspnea (67 vs. 33%), appetite loss (76 vs. 51%), and polypnea (15 vs. 5%) compared to those with NFG. The median time from onset of symptoms to hospital admission was 8 days (5–11 days), and no significant differences were found across the three groups (**Table 1**).

Laboratory Tests and Imaging Examinations

At admission, patients with diabetes and IFG had higher neutrophils, while lower lymphocytes, eosinophils, and platelets compared with patients with NFG; thus the proportions of lymphocytopenia, eosinopenia, and thrombocytopenia were higher among patients with diabetes and IFG (**Table 2**). No significant differences were found in the levels of leucocyte, monocytes, basophils, and hemoglobin (**Table 2**).

TABLE 1 | Demographics and clinical symptoms of patients with COVID-19 according to diabetes status.

	All patients (n = 312)	Diabetes (n = 84)	IFG (n = 62)	NFG (n = 166)	P-value
Age	57 (38-66)	62 (55-70)	62 (43-66)	46 (34-64)	<0.001
Sex, females	172 (55%)	34 (40%)	28 (45%)	110 (66%)	<0.001
Any comorbidities	115 (37%)	45 (54%)	28 (45%)	42 (25%)	<0.001
Hypertension	89 (29%)	42 (50%)	22 (35%)	25 (15%)	<0.001
Coronary heart disease	22 (7%)	13 (15%)	4 (6%)	5 (3%)	0.002
Chronic lung disease	12 (4%)	3 (4%)	2 (3%)	7 (4%)	>0.99
Chronic liver disease	6 (2%)	0 (0%)	2 (3%)	4 (2%)	0.24
Chronic kidney disease	8 (3%)	4 (5%)	3 (5%)	1 (1%)	0.04
Cerebrovascular disease	15 (5%)	8 (10%)	4 (6%)	3 (2%)	0.01
Cancer	12 (4%)	2 (2%)	4 (6%)	6 (4%)	0.45
Signs and symptoms at admission					
Fever	268 (86%)	75 (89%)	57 (92%)	136 (82%)	0.09
Fatigue	181 (58%)	53 (63%)	31 (50%)	97 (58%)	0.28
Cough	264 (85%)	75 (89%)	51 (82%)	138 (83%)	0.38
Myalgia	70 (22%)	17 (20%)	13 (21%)	40 (24%)	0.75
Redness of the eyes	0 (0%)	0 (0%)	0 (0%)	0 (0%)	NA
Dyspnea	145 (46%)	56 (67%)	34 (55%)	55 (33%)	<0.001
Headache	37 (12%)	8 (10%)	6 (10%)	23 (14%)	0.51
Rhinorrhea	5 (2%)	1 (1%)	0 (0%)	4 (2%)	0.60
Chest pain	139 (45%)	46 (55%)	26 (42%)	67 (40%)	0.09
Diarrhea	78 (25%)	27 (32%)	17 (27%)	34 (20%)	0.12
Nausea and vomiting	41 (13%)	13 (15%)	9 (15%)	19 (11%)	0.63
Palpitation	34 (11%)	8 (10%)	8 (13%)	18 (11%)	0.81
Loss of appetite	179 (57%)	64 (76%)	30 (48%)	85 (51%)	<0.001
polypnea	30 (10%)	13 (15%)	8 (13%)	9 (5%)	0.02
Hypoxemia	120 (38%)	50 (60%)	30 (48%)	40 (24%)	<0.001

Data are shown as median (IQR) and n (%).
P-values were derived from χ^2 test, Fisher's exact test, Kruskal Wallis test when appropriate.
COVID-19, 2019 novel coronavirus; IFG, impaired fasting glucose; NFG, normal fasting glucose.

Compared with those with NFG, patients with IFG and diabetes were more likely to have abnormal levels of laboratory markers, including increased liver enzymes, decreased albumin and estimated glomerular filtration rate (eGFR), elevated cystatin C, creatine kinase, d-dimer and fibrinogen, positive urine protein, higher levels of inflammatory markers (CRP, ESR, procalcitonin, LDH, and neutrophil-to-lymphocyte ratio) and systolic blood pressure (**Table 2**). No significant differences were found in BMI, lipid profiles, uric acid and diastolic blood pressure across the groups (**Table 2**).

Patient with diabetes and IFG were more frequently infected with bacteria than those with NFG (11, 8, and 1%, respectively; **Supplementary Table 3**). No significant differences were found in the chest CT findings among the three groups (**Supplementary Table 3**).

Clinical Severity, Complications, and Treatment Regimens

The proportion of severe cases was higher in patients with diabetes (36 [43%]) and IFG (20 [32%]), compared with those with NFG (19 [11%]), and the corresponding odds ratio (OR) and 95% confidence interval (CI) was 4.04 (1.87–8.75) for diabetes and 2.86 (1.19–6.83) for IFG compared to NFG (**Supplementary Table 4**). The association remained significant even after adjustment for laboratory markers.

Compared with patients with NFG, patients with IFG and diabetes were more likely to develop ARDS (3 [2%], 2 [3%], and 7 [8%]), acute kidney injury (0 [0%], 1 [2%], and 4 [5%]), and septic shock (3 [2%], 5 [8%], and 15 [18%]). Among patients with diabetes, 2 had diabetic ketoacidosis and 1 had drug-induced hypoglycemic coma during follow-up, while none developed hyperosmolar hyperglycemic state (**Table 3**).

The treatment regimens are shown in the **Table 3**. Patients with diabetes and IFG, compared with patients with NFG, were more likely to receive the treatment of ganciclovir (34 [40%], 25 [40%] vs. 39 [23%]), intravenous antibacterial agents (74 [88%], 52 [84%] vs. 116 [70%]), glucocorticoids (43 [51%], 36 [59%] vs. 50 [30%]), and intravenous immunoglobulin therapy (47 [56%], 31 [51%] vs. 53 [32%]), while were less likely to be treated with arbidol hydrochloride (52 [62%], 45 [73%] vs. 130 [78%]; **Table 3**).

TABLE 2 | Laboratory results and radiologic findings of patients with COVID-19 according to diabetes status.

	All patients (n = 312)	Diabetes (n = 84)	IFG (n = 62)	NFG (n = 166)	P-value
Blood routine					
Leucocytes (×10^9 per L)	4.8 (3.5–6.5)	5.0 (3.6–6.9)	4.6 (3.4–6.6)	4.6 (3.5–6.1)	0.34
Neutrophils (×10^9 per L)	3.0 (2.1–4.6)	3.6 (2.4–5.7)	3.1 (2.1–4.8)	2.7 (2.0–3.7)	0.005
Increased (>6.3)	30 (11%)	14 (18%)	7 (11%)	9 (6%)	0.047
Decreased (<1.8)	43 (15%)	7 (9%)	11 (18%)	25 (17%)	
Lymphocytes (×10^9 per L)	1.1 (0.8–1.4)	0.8 (0.6–1.2)	1.0 (0.7–1.5)	1.2 (0.9–1.6)	<0.001
Increased (>3.2)	2 (1%)	0 (0%)	0 (0%)	2 (1%)	<0.001
Decreased (<1.1)	146 (51%)	56 (72%)	35 (57%)	55 (38%)	
Eosinophils (×10^9 per L)	0.01 (0–0.06)	0 (0–0.03)	0.01 (0–0.03)	0.03 (0–0.08)	<0.001
Decreased (<0.02)	152 (53%)	54 (68%)	38 (62%)	60 (41%)	<0.001
Basophils (×10^9 per L)	0.01 (0–0.02)	0.01 (0–0.03)	0.01 (0–0.01)	0.01 (0.01–0.02)	0.013
Hemoglobin (g/L)	126 (116–136)	128 (116–139)	128 (114–137)	124 (116–135)	0.44
Platelets (×10^9 per L)	175 (129–234)	161 (113–200)	161 (129–203)	199 (144–247)	<0.001
Increased (>350)	13 (5%)	2 (3%)	2 (4%)	9 (6%)	0.02
Decreased (<120)	51 (19%)	22 (29%)	13 (23%)	16 (12%)	
Blood biochemistry					
Alanine aminotransferase (U/L)	23 (16-35)	28 (19-39)	26 (18-43)	21 (15-30)	0.002
Increased (>35.0)	70 (25%)	24 (30%)	21 (34%)	25 (17%)	0.01
Aspartate aminotransferase (U/L)	27 (20-40)	34 (20-47)	33 (23-46)	23 (19-32)	<0.001
Increased (>40.0)	69 (24%)	26 (33%)	21 (35%)	22 (15%)	0.002
Glutamate transpeptidase (U/L)	23 (16-39)	25 (17-40)	36 (17.0–55.0)	20 (14-32)	<0.001
Albumin (g/L)	36.5 (33.1–40.8)	35.7 (33.0–38.7)	35.6 (33.1–40.5)	37.8 (34.2–41.1)	0.03
Decreased (<35.0)	103 (36%)	33 (42%)	28 (46%)	42 (29%)	0.04
eGFR (mL/min/1.73m^2)	95.3 (82.2–108.6)	91.7 (70.9–99.8)	91.4 (78.7–101.5)	99.6 (90.5–114.5)	<0.001
Decreased (<90)	100 (36%)	38 (49%)	28 (47%)	34 (24%)	<0.001
Cystatin C (mg/L)	0.9 (0.8–1.1)	1.1 (0.9–1.4)	0.9 (0.8–1.3)	0.8 (0.7–1.1)	<0.001
Increased (>1.15)	52 (24%)	19 (33%)	14 (30%)	19 (17%)	0.03
Creatine kinase (U/L)	69.9 (45.5–127)	90 (49–160)	93 (50–179)	59 (43–100)	0.002
Increased (>140.0)	52 (22%)	19 (31%)	15 (28%)	18 (15%)	0.007
Decreased (<26.0)	4 (2%)	0 (0%)	3 (6%)	1 (1%)	
Troponin I (ng/L)	5.35 (2.6–10.0)	10 (2.6–10.0)	10 (3.3–19.4)	4.55 (1.2–10.0)	0.03
Increased (>26.2)	11 (10%)	4 (14%)	4 (19%)	3 (5%)	0.15
CKMB (ng/ml)	2.0 (0.6–2.9)	2.0 (1.4–2.6)	1.5 (0.8–2.9)	2.0 (0.5–3.2)	0.88
Increased (≥6.6)	6 (4%)	2 (5%)	0 (0%)	4 (4%)	0.64
Brain natriuretic peptide (pg/mL)	42.8 (10.0–92.2)	82.0 (14.1–91.6)	202.8 (68.4–327.3)	11.9 (10.0–49.4)	0.10
Increased (≥27.5)	8 (50%)	3 (60%)	3 (100%)	2 (25%)	0.16
Total carbon dioxide (mmol/L)	23.6 (21.2–25.5)	23.4 (19.7–25.3)	22.0 (19.9–24.5)	23.9 (22.0–25.8)	0.004
Decreased (<21.0)	53 (24%)	18 (32%)	17 (40%)	18 (15%)	0.001
Coagulation function					
D-dimer (mg/L)	0.44 (0.22–0.97)	0.78 (0.34–1.38)	0.55 (0.22–1.31)	0.33 (0.22–0.59)	<0.001
Increased (≥0.5)	86 (28%)	40 (48%)	17 (27%)	29 (17%)	<0.001
Prothrombin time (second)	12.9 (12.0–13.8)	12.7 (12.0–14.4)	12.8 (11.7–14.4)	12.9 (12.3–13.6)	0.99
Activated partial thromboplastin time (second)	36.8 (32.65–41.1)	35.3 (32.5–41.2)	34.8 (29.7–40.3)	38.0 (35.0–41.4)	0.04
Fibrinogen (g/L)	3.92 (3.05–4.93)	4.34 (3.30–5.24)	4.43 (3.44–5.48)	3.42 (2.82–4.47)	<0.001
Increased (>4.0)	103 (48%)	34 (52%)	32 (68%)	37 (37%)	0.004
Decreased (<2.0)	9 (4%)	4 (6%)	1 (2%)	4 (4%)	
Urine routine					
Positive protein	44 (28%)	17 (40%)	13 (37%)	14 (17%)	0.009
Positive ketones	28 (17%)	11 (24%)	5 (13%)	12 (15%)	0.31

(Continued)

TABLE 2 | Continued

	All patients (n = 312)	Diabetes (n = 84)	IFG (n = 62)	NFG (n = 166)	P-value
Inflammatory markers					
C-reactive protein (mg/L)	17.6 (3.8–41.3)	28.1 (13.0–76.7)	34.9 (8.1–67.8)	8.0 (3.1–30.2)	<0.001
Increased (>8.0)	166 (65%)	61 (85%)	39 (78%)	66 (50%)	<0.001
Erythrocyte sedimentation rate (mm/h)	21 (9-38)	31 (10-59)	25 (12-40)	16 (8-33)	0.03
Procalcitonin (μg/L)	0.10 (0.06–0.16)	0.13 (0.07–0.30)	0.10 (0.09–0.25)	0.08 (0.04–0.10)	<0.001
Increased (>0.5)	11 (8%)	7 (13%)	3 (10%)	1 (2%)	0.002
Lactate dehydrogenase (g/L)	225 (180–291)	264 (225–373)	258 (198–336)	195 (167–244)	<0.001
Increased (>245.0)	99 (41%)	41 (64%)	28 (51%)	30 (25%)	<0.001
Decreased (<109.0)	1 (0.4%)	0 (0%)	0 (0%)	1 (0.8%)	
Neutrophil-to-lymphocyte ratio	2.65 (1.73–4.95)	4.07 (2.20–7.68)	3.00 (1.74–4.75)	2.19 (1.50–3.46)	<0.001
Platelet-to-lymphocyte ratio	163 (116–236)	177 (136–295)	154 (100–229)	156 (117–219)	0.08
Metabolic variables					
BMI (kg/m^2)	23.5 (21.1–25.2)	23.6 (22.7–26.1)	24.2 (21.2–25.5)	22.8 (20.8–24.9)	0.21
Fasting plasma glucose (mmol/L)	5.62 (5.07–6.88)	8.35 (6.91–11.69)	6.11 (5.82–6.54)	5.04 (4.72–5.26)	<0.001
Total cholesterol (mmol/L)	3.68 (3.27–4.47)	3.57 (3.13–4.00)	3.74 (3.30–4.38)	3.80 (3.41–4.60)	0.08
Triglyceride (mmol/L)	1.11 (0.84–1.53)	1.29 (0.85–1.68)	1.14 (0.86–1.49)	1.05 (0.82–1.44)	0.10
HDL-C (mmol/L)	1.12 (0.89–1.37)	1.03 (0.87–1.32)	1.02 (0.89–1.37)	1.17 (0.94–1.43)	0.09
LDL-C (mmol/L)	2.19 (1.77–2.72)	1.99 (1.60–2.56)	2.21 (1.79–2.71)	2.24 (1.91–2.88)	0.054
Uric acid (μmol/L)	250 (192–328)	265 (186–328)	252 (203–337)	244 (192–321)	0.61
Systolic blood pressure (mmHg)	125 (119–134)	130 (120–142)	126 (120–133)	123 (118–130)	0.003
Diastolic blood pressure (mmHg)	76 (70–83)	77 (70–85)	78 (70–87)	75 (70–82)	0.44

Data are shown as median (IQR) and n (%).

P-values were derived from χ^2-test, Fisher's exact test, or Kruskal Wallis test when appropriate.

COVID-19, 2019 novel coronavirus; IFG, impaired fasting glucose; NFG, normal fasting glucose; eGFR, estimated glomerular filtration rate; CKMB, creatine kinase MB; HDL-C, high density lipoprotein cholesterol; LDL-C, low density lipoprotein cholesterol.

Primary Endpoints and Mortality of the Patients

Primary composite endpoints occurred in 46 (15%) patients, including 32 (10%) who underwent mechanical ventilation, 9 (3%) who were admitted to the ICU, and 33 (11%) who died. Among the 33 deaths, majority were respiratory failure (27 [81.8%]), and the rest were multiorgan failure (5 [15.2%]) and cardiovascular event (1 [3.0%]; **Supplementary Table 5**).

Compared with patients with NFG, patients with IFG and diabetes were more likely to develop primary composite events (9 [5%], 11 [18%], and 26 [31%]; **Supplementary Table 5**), including more receiving mechanical ventilation (5 [3%], 6 [10%], and 21 [25%]), more deaths (4 [2%], 9 [15%], and 20 [24%]), but similar admission rate to ICU (3 [2%], 2 [3%], and 4 [5%]).

Patients with IFG and diabetes had significantly escalated risks of reaching to the composite endpoint or death compared with those with NFG (all $P < 0.05$; **Supplementary Figure 1**). After adjustment for age, sex, hospitals and other comorbidities, diabetes remained as a significant predictor for the composite endpoints (HR 3.53, 95% CI 1.48–8.40; **Table 4**), while the association with IFG was not statistically significant (HR 1.42, 95% CI 0.53–3.81). Per-SD increment of fasting glucose levels was associated with 25% (2–53%) higher risk of composite endpoints. Both IFG and diabetes were associated with higher risk of mortality among patients with COVID-19, and the HR (95% CI) was 4.11 (1.15–14.74) and 6.25 (1.91–20.45), respectively, and per-SD increment of fasting glucose levels was associated with 31% (4–65%) higher risk of mortality (**Table 4**; **Figure 1**).

In the model adjusted for age, sex, and hospital, the following laboratory variables were found to be associated with increased risks of the primary endpoints: decreased eGFR, increased aspartate aminotransferase (AST), cystatin C, creatine kinase MB (CKMB), prothrombin time (PT), procalcitonin, LDH, and neutrophil-to-lymphocyte ratio (**Supplementary Table 6**). We selected decreased eGFR, increased AST, PT, and procalcitonin in the final multivariate model, and found that further adjustment for those variables did not materially alter the associations between diabetes and mortality, whereas the associations between diabetes and composite outcome were attenuated to insignificance, as well as the association between IFG and mortality (Model 3, **Table 4**).

In the sensitivity analysis of excluding the new-diagnosed diabetes (**Supplementary Table 7**), the above associations remained unchanged.

We further compared the anti-diabetic drugs among patients with diabetes stratified by the status of primary endpoints. Among the 26 patients with diabetes and experienced the primary endpoints, 1 patient used only metformin, while 19 out of 58 patients with diabetes and who did not experience the primary endpoints used metformin (4 vs. 33%, $P = 0.004$; **Supplementary Table 8**). No dramatic differences

TABLE 3 | Complications and treatment regimens of patients with COVID-19 according to diabetes status.

	All patients (n = 312)	Diabetes (n = 84)	IFG (n = 62)	NFG (n = 166)	P-value
Any complications	47 (15%)	23 (27%)	11 (17%)	13 (8%)	<0.001
ARDS	12 (4%)	7 (8%)	2 (3%)	3 (2%)	0.04
Acute kidney injury	5 (2.0%)	4 (5%)	1 (2%)	0 (0%)	0.01
Cardiac injury	18 (6%)	7 (8%)	3 (5%)	8 (5%)	0.49
Rhabdomyolysis	1 (0.3%)	0 (0%)	1 (2%)	0 (0%)	0.20
Septic shock	23 (7%)	15 (18%)	5 (8%)	3 (2%)	<0.001
Diabetic ketoacidosis	2 (1%)	2 (2%)	0 (0%)	0 (0%)	0.11
Hyperosmolar hyperglycemic state	0 (0%)	0 (0%)	0 (0%)	0 (0%)	NA
Hypoglycemic coma	1 (0.3%)	1 (1%)	0 (0%)	0 (0%)	0.47
Treatment					
Oxygen therapy	231 (74%)	70 (83%)	53 (85%)	108 (65%)	<0.001
Nasal tube	190 (61%)	45 (54%)	43 (69%)	102 (61%)	<0.001
High-flow nasal cannula	9 (3%)	4 (5%)	4 (6%)	1 (1%)	
Non-invasive ventilator	25 (8%)	18 (21%)	4 (6%)	3 (2%)	
Invasive ventilator	7 (2%)	3 (4%)	2 (3%)	2 (1%)	
Antiviral treatment					
Oseltamivir	186 (60%)	52 (62%)	33 (53%)	101 (61%)	0.51
Ganciclovir	98 (31%)	34 (40%)	25 (40%)	39 (23%)	0.006
Lopinavir and ritonavir	39 (13%)	13 (15%)	8 (13%)	18 (11%)	0.58
Arbidol hydrochloride	227 (73%)	52 (62%)	45 (73%)	130 (78%)	0.02
Ribavirin	46 (15%)	11 (13%)	13 (21%)	22 (13%)	0.30
Interferon	140 (45%)	32 (38%)	28 (45%)	80 (48%)	0.32
>2 antiviral agents	138 (44%)	34 (40%)	31 (50%)	73 (44%)	0.52
Antibacterial treatment					
Intravenous antibiotics	242 (78%)	74 (88%)	52 (84%)	116 (70%)	0.002
Numbers of antibiotics	3 (2-4)	3 (2-4)	3 (2-4)	3 (2-4)	0.55
>2 antibacterial agents	34 (11%)	15 (18%)	5 (8%)	14 (8%)	0.06
Antifungal treatment	22 (7%)	9 (11%)	6 (10%)	7 (4%)	0.08
Glucocorticoids	129 (41%)	43 (51%)	36 (59%)	50 (30%)	<0.001
Intravenous immunoglobulin therapy	131 (42%)	47 (56%)	31 (51%)	53 (32%)	<0.001
Thymosin	92 (30%)	24 (29%)	24 (39%)	44 (27%)	0.17

Data are shown as median (IQR) and n (%).
P-values were derived from χ^2-test, Fisher's exact test, or Kruskal Wallis test when appropriate.
COVID-19, 2019 novel coronavirus; IFG, impaired fasting glucose; NFG, normal fasting glucose; ARDS, acute respiratory distress syndrome coronavirus.

were observed for other anti-diabetic drugs between the two groups.

DISCUSSIONS

In this multicenter retrospective cohort study among 312 patients with COVID-19 from Wuhan, China, we found that diabetes and IFG were associated with higher risks of primary adverse endpoints and mortality. In addition, dose-response association was also found between fasting plasma glucose levels on hospital admission and risk of adverse prognosis for patients with COVID-19. The associations were independent of other comorbidities, but the association between diabetes and IFG and primary endpoints was partially explained by some laboratory markers.

A number of studies have reported that diabetes was a risk factor for severity and poor prognosis of influenza and other pneumonia diseases. For example, a study among 239 patients with influenza A in Canada reported that diabetes tripled the risk of hospitalization and quadrupled the risk of ICU admission once hospitalized (9); a study among 144 patients with SARS in Canada reported that diabetes was independently associated with poor primary endpoints (death, ICU admission or mechanical ventilation) (26). In another retrospective analysis of 520 patients with SARS in Hong Kong, a known history of diabetes was associated with 3-fold risk of mortality and fasting plasma glucose levels were negatively associated with mortality and hypoxia (10). The risk of developing severe or lethal disease following MERS-CoV infection was increased by 2.47 to 7.24-folds when the patient had comorbid diabetes (11, 12). However, it is still controversial whether diabetes is a major risk factor for severity and poor prognosis of COVID-19 (13, 14). And no study emphasizes on the relationship between prediabetes and severity of COVID-19 until now.

TABLE 4 | Association between diabetes status and risk of adverse outcomes among patients with COVID-19.

	Diabetes	IFG	NFG	*P*-value for trend	Per SD increase in plasma fasting glucose levels
Primary composite outcomes					
Cases/person-days	26/1,875	11/1,455	9/4,419		
Model 1	2.76 (1.22–6.24)	1.61 (0.63–4.11)	1.00	0.001	1.20 (1.00–1.44)
Model 2	3.53 (1.48–8.40)	1.42 (0.53–3.81)	1.00	0.002	1.25 (1.02–1.53)
Model 3	2.18 (0.89–5.31)	1.21 (0.43–3.39)	1.00	0.045	1.21 (0.98–1.50)
Mortality					
Cases/person-days	20/2,059	9/1,516	4/4,521		
Model 1	6.36 (2.10–19.30)	4.02 (1.18–13.64)	1.00	0.001	1.31 (1.07–1.60)
Model 2	6.25 (1.91–20.45)	4.11 (1.15–14.74)	1.00	0.002	1.31 (1.04–1.65)
Model 3	6.87 (1.92–24.58)	4.06 (1.00–16.42)	1.00	0.002	1.37 (1.05–1.79)
Mechanical ventilation					
Cases/person-days	21/1,868	6/1,453	5/4,415		
Model 1	3.21 (1.12–9.23)	1.34 (0.39–4.69)	1.00	0.01	1.19 (0.95–1.50)
Model 2	6.33 (1.87–21.48)	1.66 (0.42–6.54)	1.00	0.001	1.22 (0.96–1.55)
Model 3	2.31 (0.76–7.03)	0.95 (0.25–3.66)	1.00	0.047	1.32 (1.01–1.74)

Model 1, adjusted for age, sex, and hospital.
Model 2, adjusted for age, sex, hospital, and comorbidities.
Model 3, adjusted for age, sex, hospital, aspartate aminotransferase, estimated glomerular filtration rate, prothrombin time, and procalcitonin.

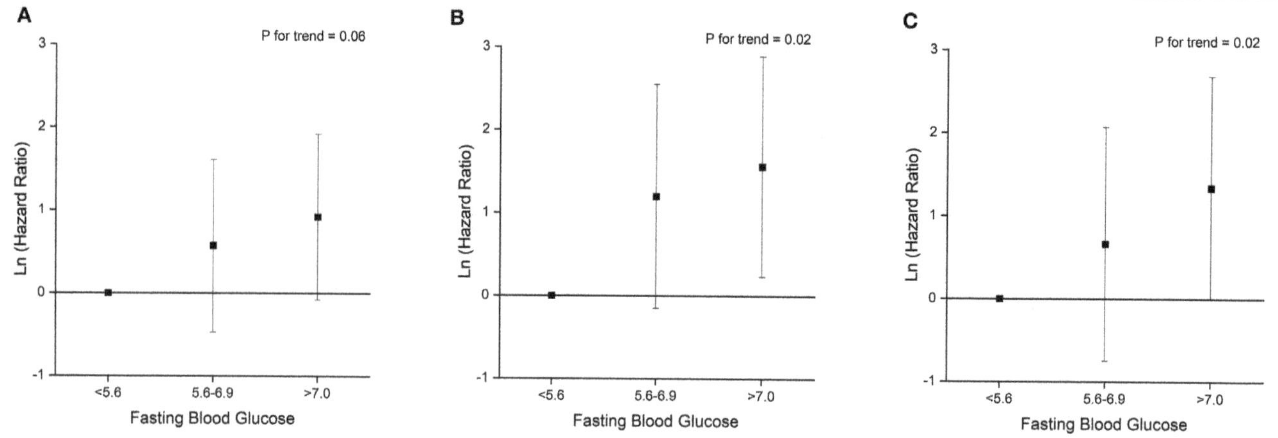

FIGURE 1 | Associations between fasting blood glucose levels and primary composite endpoint **(A)**, mortality **(B)**, and mechanical ventilation **(C)**.

In our study, we observed that patients with hyperglycemia were more likely to be severe cases at the time of hospital admission with an odds ratio of 3.14 for diabetes and 2.36 for IFG compared to NFG. This is consistent with a recent meta-analysis of 31 reports with varied sample sizes (ranged from 21 to 1099) which found that patients with diabetes had a significantly increased odds (OR 2.61; 95% CI 2.05–3.33) of developing severe COVID-19 compared with patients free of diabetes (15). Among 1,590 patients with COVID-19 across China, severe cases were found in 34.6% of patients with diabetes (45/130) and 14.3% of patients without diabetes (209/1,460) (4). However, many of the studies were either preprint reports or did not control for important confounders, such as age, sex and other comorbidities.

A few studies have evaluated the association between comorbid diabetes and poor prognosis among patients with COVID-19. The study by Guan et al. (4) reported that diabetes was associated with a higher risk of composite endpoints (HR 1.59; 95% CI 1.03–2.45) in 1,590 patients with COVID-19 across China; Zhou et al. (27) reported that diabetes was associated with a higher odds of in-hospital death (OR 2.85; 95% CI 1.35–6.05) in the univariable analysis of 191 patients with COVID-19 from two hospitals in Wuhan; a large-scale report among 44,672 confirmed cases of COVID-19 across China found that the crude case fatality rate was 7.3% among patients with diabetes compared to 2.3% in the total samples (28); another research among 7,337 cases with COVID-19 reported recently found that subjects with type 2 diabetes required more medical interventions and had a significantly higher mortality (7.8 vs. 2.7%) than the non-diabetic individuals (20). Therefore, our results are largely consistent with those studies but with additional advantages: we adjusted for some confounding factors, including age, sex, hospital, and comorbidities, and also showed that diabetes and IFG was risk factors for in-hospital death.

Although the relationship between diabetes and COVID-19 has been currently extensively explored, less research has paid attention to the relationship between IFG and worse COVID-19 prognosis. Whether diabetes patients need a rigid glucose control when affected with COVID-19 is still unknown. Previous clinical trials examining the effects of glucose control on mortality have yielded conflicting results (20, 21, 29). Zhu et al. reported well-controlled blood glucose (3.9–10.0 mmol/L) was associated with markedly lower mortality compared to individuals with poorly controlled BG (>10.0 mmol/L) (20). Plasma glucose concentrations with 4–8 mmol/L was recommended as therapeutic aim in the practical recommendations for the management of diabetes patients with COVID-19 (30). In our study, even mild elevated fasting glucose level (5.6–6.9 mmol/L) was associated with increased in-hospital death.

Two small studies (a total of 102 and 138 patients, and 11 and 14 patients had diabetes, respectively) described that patients admitted to ICU had higher prevalence of diabetes compared to those who did not receive ICU care (22, 31); Wu et al. (32) reported that the prevalence of diabetes was higher among patients who developed ARDS (16/84) compared to those with ARDS (6/117) among 201 patients from a hospital in Wuhan. In our study, 9 patients received ICU care, 4 (5%) in patients with diabetes, 2 (3%) in patients with IFG and 3 (2%) in patients with NFG; only 12 patients developed ARDS, 7 [8%] in patients with diabetes, 2 [3%] in patients with IFG and 3 (2%) in patients with NFG. Furthermore, acute kidney injury (5, 2, and 0%) and septic shock (18, 8, and 2%) were also higher in patients with diabetes and IFG compared to patients with NFG. However, we did not perform multivariate analysis because of limited sample size.

Several factors may contribute to the increased risks of severity and poor prognosis of COVID-19 related to hyperglycemia. First, patients with diabetes were more likely to have other comorbidities, such as hypertension, cardiovascular disease, and kidney injuries, and studies have demonstrated that multiple comorbidities increased risk of composite endpoints and mortality among patients with COVID-19 (4, 6, 15, 33, 34). However, we have adjusted for a number of comorbidities in the multivariate models and the associations with diabetes remained significant. Second, patients with diabetes and IFG had a number of worse laboratory markers, including dysregulated immune response, increased proinflammatory reactions, metabolic abnormalities, procoagulant, or impaired fibrinolytic states and which could be related to adverse prognosis for patients with COVID-19 (2, 22, 23, 27, 35). When adjusted for several markers, the association between diabetes and primary endpoints were no long statistically significant, which indicated that the association might be partly explained by those factors, but sample size could also be a factor for the insignificant results. The association between diabetes and mortality was not altered. Third, individuals with diabetes and IFG were at increased risk for bacterial co-infection and septic shock in our study, and bacterial infections have been found to be related to higher risk of mortality in patients with COVID-19 (36).

To the best of our knowledge, our study is the first to classify glycemic status into three different groups (NFG, IFG, and diabetes) and also investigate the relations between fasting glucose levels at admission and adverse prognosis among patients with COVID-19. We have controlled for a number of covariates and tried to evaluate the laboratory markers in the pathway of the associations. Nevertheless, out study also has several limitations. First, we did not know the exact type of diabetes and assumed that majority, if not all, should be type 2 diabetes. Second, HbA1c was not routinely measured at the time of hospital admission, particularly for those without diabetes, therefore, we could not evaluate the association between HbA1c and risk of adverse outcomes because of lack of data. Third, we did not have information on some confounding factors such as socioeconomic status and lifestyle factors, and residual confounding was possible as in any observational studies. Besides, only 30% (93 out of 312) of the participants had data available on BMI, and thus we could not adjust for BMI in the multivariable models. Fourth, although we have retrieved medication information, we still could not evaluate the impact of different types or combinations of anti-diabetic drugs on the prognosis, which would require a much larger sample size. Fifth, we did not have information on glycemic control measures, kinetics of viral load and antibody titers during the follow-up, and more studies are still needed to understand the impact of those factors in the development of adverse outcomes. Finally, our study had limited sample size and all patients were Chinese recruited from 5 hospitals in Wuhan city by convenience sampling; furthermore, the prevalence rates of diabetes and IFG were higher than the rates in the general population or in patients with COVID-19 from national surveys of Chinese. However, representativeness was not strictly required in cohort studies to generalize the observed associations (37). Nevertheless, studies in other populations are needed to further validate our findings.

CONCLUSIONS

In this retrospective cohort of 312 Chinese patients with COVID-19, we found that diabetes was associated with higher risks of composite adverse endpoints (mechanical ventilation, admission to ICU, or death) and mortality, and IFG was also associated with higher risk of mortality. The associations appeared to be dose-dependent and were not explained by other comorbidities. Given the global high prevalence of diabetes in adults and the current COVID-19 pandemic, many patients with diabetes are infected with SARS-COV-2; therefore, the knowledge provided in this study could be useful for understanding the clinical characteristics of patients with diabetes and COVID-19, and to help develop more targeted and effective management strategies for those patients to reduce the poor prognosis. More studies are still warranted to validate our findings and further understand the potential mechanisms.

AUTHOR CONTRIBUTIONS

JZha, WK, TZ, LC, and AP co-conceived the study. YX, LL, QL, LY, QW, HanyW, GL, XZ, KQ, YLi, HanW, YW, XS, HLiu, SX, YLiu, and ZC collected the epidemiological and clinical data. HanyW, KQ, HanW, YW, GL, and XZ summarized all data. PX did the analysis. JZha, WK, KQ, and YW drafted the manuscript. HLi, JZhe, HS, WX, and YH contributed to the discussion. LC, AP, and TZ revised the final manuscript. TZ was guarantor of this work and, as such, had full access to all the data in the study and takes responsibility for the integrity of the data and the accuracy of the data analysis. All authors contributed to the article and approved the submitted version.

ACKNOWLEDGMENTS

The authors are grateful to all health-care workers who were involved in caring for patients with COVID-19 and collected data for the study.

REFERENCES

1. World Health Organization. *Disease Outbreak News*. (2020). Available online at: https://www.who.int/csr/don/en/ (accessed May 27, 2020).
2. Huang C, Wang Y, Li X, Ren L, Zhao J, Hu Y, et al. Clinical features of patients infected with 2019 novel coronavirus in Wuhan, China. *Lancet*. (2020) 395:497–506. doi: 10.1016/S0140-6736(20)30183-5
3. Wu Z, McGoogan JM. Characteristics of and important lessons from the coronavirus disease 2019 (COVID-19) outbreak in China: summary of a Report of 72314 cases from the chinese center for disease control and prevention. *JAMA*. (2020) 323:1239–42. doi: 10.1001/jama.2020.2648
4. Guan WJ, Liang WH, Zhao Y, Liang HR, Chen ZS, Li YM, et al. Comorbidity and its impact on 1590 patients with COVID-19 in China: a nationwide analysis. *Eur Respir J*. (2020) 55:2000547. doi: 10.1183/13993003.01227-2020
5. Guan WJ, Ni ZY, Hu Y, Liang WH, Ou CQ, He JX, et al. Clinical characteristics of coronavirus disease 2019 in China. *N Engl J Med*. (2020) 382:1708–20. doi: 10.1056/NEJMoa2002032
6. Richardson S, Hirsch JS, Narasimhan M, Crawford JM, McGinn T, Davidson KW, et al. Presenting characteristics, comorbidities, and outcomes among 5700 patients hospitalized with COVID-19 in the New York City Area. *JAMA*. (2020) 323:2052–59. doi: 10.1001/jama.2020.6775
7. Lopez-de-Andres A, Perez-Farinos N, de Miguel-Diez J, Hernandez-Barrera V, Jimenez-Trujillo I, Mendez-Bailon M, et al. Type 2 diabetes and postoperative pneumonia: an observational, population-based study using the Spanish Hospital Discharge Database, 2001-2015. *PLoS ONE*. (2019) 14:e0211230. doi: 10.1371/journal.pone.0211230
8. Klekotka RB, Mizgala E, Krol W. The etiology of lower respiratory tract infections in people with diabetes. *Pneumonol Alergol Pol*. (2015) 83:401–8. doi: 10.5603/PiAP.2015.0065
9. Allard R, Leclerc P, Tremblay C, Tannenbaum TN. Diabetes and the severity of pandemic influenza A (H1N1) infection. *Diabetes Care*. (2010) 33:1491–3. doi: 10.2337/dc09-2215
10. Yang JK, Feng Y, Yuan MY, Yuan SY, Fu HJ, Wu BY, et al. Plasma glucose levels and diabetes are independent predictors for mortality and morbidity in patients with SARS. *Diabet Med*. (2006) 23:623–8. doi: 10.1111/j.1464-5491.2006.01861.x
11. Garbati MA, Fagbo SF, Fang VJ, Skakni L, Joseph M, Wani TA, et al. A comparative study of clinical presentation and risk factors for adverse outcome in patients hospitalised with acute respiratory disease due to MERS Coronavirus or other causes. *PLoS ONE*. (2016) 11:e0165978. doi: 10.1371/journal.pone.0165978
12. Kulcsar KA, Coleman CM, Beck SE, Frieman MB. Comorbid diabetes results in immune dysregulation and enhanced disease severity following MERS-CoV infection. *JCI Insight*. (2019) 4:e131774. doi: 10.1172/jci.insight.131774
13. Hussain A, Bhowmik B, do Vale Moreira NC. COVID-19 and diabetes: knowledge in progress. *Diabetes Res Clin Pract*. (2020) 162:108142. doi: 10.1016/j.diabres.2020.108142
14. Hill MA, Mantzoros C, Sowers JR. Commentary: COVID-19 in patients with diabetes. *Metabolism*. (2020) 107:154217. doi: 10.1016/j.metabol.2020.154217
15. Wang X, Fang X, Cai Z, Wu X, Gao X, Min J, et al. Comorbid chronic diseases and acute organ injuries are strongly correlated with disease severity and mortality among COVID-19 patients: a systemic review and meta-analysis. *Research*. (2020) 2020:2402961. doi: 10.34133/2020/2402961
16. Onder G, Rezza G, Brusaferro S. Case-fatality rate and characteristics of patients dying in relation to COVID-19 in Italy. *JAMA*. (2020) 323:1775–76. doi: 10.1001/jama.2020.4683
17. Guo W, Li M, Dong Y, Zhou H, Zhang Z, Tian C, et al. Diabetes is a risk factor for the progression and prognosis of COVID-19. *Diabetes Metab Res Rev*. (2020) e3319. doi: 10.1002/dmrr.3319. [Epub ahead of print].
18. Zhang JJ, Dong X, Cao YY, Yuan YD, Yang YB, Yan YQ, et al. Clinical characteristics of 140 patients infected with SARS-CoV-2 in Wuhan, China. *Allergy*. (2020). doi: 10.1111/all.14238. [Epub ahead of print].
19. Lippi G, Plebani M. Laboratory abnormalities in patients with COVID-2019 infection. *Clin Chem Lab Med*. (2020) 58:1131–4. doi: 10.1515/cclm-2020-0198
20. Zhu L, She ZG, Cheng X, Qin JJ, Zhang XJ, Cai J, et al. Association of blood glucose control and outcomes in patients with COVID-19 and pre-existing Type 2 diabetes. *Cell Metab*. (2020) 31:1068–77.e3. doi: 10.1016/j.cmet.2020.04.021
21. Rodriguez-Gutierrez R, Gonzalez-Gonzalez JG, Zuniga-Hernandez JA, McCoy RG. Benefits and harms of intensive glycemic control in patients with type 2 diabetes. *BMJ*. (2019) 367:l5887. doi: 10.1136/bmj.l5887
22. Wang D, Hu B, Hu C, Zhu F, Liu X, Zhang J, et al. Clinical characteristics of 138 hospitalized patients with 2019 novel coronavirus-infected pneumonia in Wuhan, China. *JAMA*. (2020) 323:1061–9. doi: 10.1001/jama.2020.1585
23. Chen N, Zhou M, Dong X, Qu J, Gong F, Han Y, et al. Epidemiological and clinical characteristics of 99 cases of 2019 novel coronavirus pneumonia in Wuhan, China: a descriptive study. *Lancet*. (2020) 395:507–13. doi: 10.1016/S0140-6736(20)30211-7
24. Young BE, Ong SWX, Kalimuddin S, Low JG, Tan SY, Loh J, et al. Epidemiologic features and clinical course of patients infected with SARS-CoV-2 in Singapore. *JAMA*. (2020) 323:1488–94. doi: 10.1001/jama.2020.3204
25. Metlay JP, Waterer GW, Long AC, Anzueto A, Brozek J, Crothers K, et al. Diagnosis and treatment of adults with community-acquired Pneumonia. An official clinical practice guideline of the American thoracic society and infectious diseases society of America. *Am J Respir Crit Care Med*. (2019) 200:e45–67. doi: 10.1164/rccm.201908-1581ST
26. Booth CM, Matukas LM, Tomlinson GA, Rachlis AR, Rose DB, Dwosh HA, et al. Clinical features and short-term outcomes of 144 patients with SARS in the greater Toronto area. *JAMA*. (2003) 289:2801–9. doi: 10.1001/jama.289.21.JOC30885
27. Zhou F, Yu T, Du R, Fan G, Liu Y, Liu Z, et al. Clinical course and risk factors for mortality of adult inpatients with COVID-19 in Wuhan, China: a retrospective cohort study. *Lancet*. (2020) 395:1054–62. doi: 10.1016/S0140-6736(20)30566-3
28. Epidemiology Working Group for NCIP Epidemic Response, Chinese Center for Disease Control and Prevention. The epidemiological characteristics of an outbreak of 2019 novel coronavirus diseases (COVID-19) in China. *Zhonghua Liu Xing Bing Xue Za Zhi*. (2020) 41:145–51. doi: 10.3760/cma.j.issn.0254-6450.2020.02.003
29. Forbes A, Murrells T, Mulnier H, Sinclair AJ. Mean HbA1c, HbA1c variability, and mortality in people with diabetes aged 70 years and older: a retrospective cohort study. *Lancet Diabetes Endocrinol*. (2018) 6:476–86. doi: 10.1016/S2213-8587(18)30048-2
30. Bornstein SR, Rubino F, Khunti K, Mingrone G, Hopkins D, Birkenfeld AL, et al. Practical recommendations for the management of diabetes

in patients with COVID-19. *Lancet Diabetes Endocrinol.* (2020) 8:546–50. doi: 10.1016/S2213-8587(20)30152-2

31. Cao J, Hu X, Cheng W, Yu L, Tu W-J, Liu Q. Clinical features and short-term outcomes of 18 patients with corona virus disease 2019 in intensive care unit. *Intensive Care Med.* (2020) 46:851–3. doi: 10.1007/s00134-020-05987-7
32. Wu C, Chen X, Cai Y, Xia Ja, Zhou X, Xu S, et al. Risk factors associated with acute respiratory distress syndrome and death in patients with coronavirus disease 2019 Pneumonia in Wuhan, China. *JAMA Int Med.* (2020) 13:e200994. doi: 10.1001/jamainternmed.2020.0994
33. Li B, Yang J, Zhao F, Zhi L, Wang X, Liu L, et al. Prevalence and impact of cardiovascular metabolic diseases on COVID-19 in China. *Clin Res Cardiol.* (2020) 109:531–8. doi: 10.1007/s00392-020-01626-9
34. Wang B, Li R, Lu Z, Huang Y. Does comorbidity increase the risk of patients with COVID-19: evidence from meta-analysis. *Aging.* (2020) 12:6049–57. doi: 10.18632/aging.103000
35. Stegenga ME, van der Crabben SN, Levi M, de Vos AF, Tanck MW, Sauerwein HP, et al. Hyperglycemia stimulates coagulation, whereas hyperinsulinemia impairs fibrinolysis in healthy humans. *Diabetes.* (2006) 55:1807–12. doi: 10.2337/db05-1543
36. Li X, Wang L, Yan S, Yang F, Xiang L, Zhu J, et al. Clinical characteristics of 25 death cases with COVID-19: a retrospective review of medical records in a single medical center, Wuhan, China. *Int J Infect Dis.* (2020) 94:128–32. doi: 10.1016/j.ijid.2020.03.053
37. Rothman KJ. Six persistent research misconceptions. *J Gen Intern Med.* (2014) 29:1060–4. doi: 10.1007/s11606-013-2755-z

2

Metformin use is Associated with Reduced Mortality in a Diverse Population With COVID-19 and Diabetes

Andrew B. Crouse[1], Tiffany Grimes[2], Peng Li[3], Matthew Might[1], Fernando Ovalle[2] and Anath Shalev[2]*

[1] Hugh Kaul Precision Medicine Institute, University of Alabama at Birmingham, Birmingham, AL, United States, [2] Comprehensive Diabetes Center, Department of Medicine, Division of Endocrinology, Diabetes and Metabolism, University of Alabama at Birmingham, Birmingham, AL, United States, [3] School of Nursing, University of Alabama at Birmingham, Birmingham, AL, United States

***Correspondence:**
Anath Shalev
shalev@uab.edu

Background: Coronavirus disease-2019 (COVID-19) is a growing pandemic with an increasing death toll that has been linked to various comorbidities as well as racial disparity. However, the specific characteristics of these at-risk populations are still not known and approaches to lower mortality are lacking.

Methods: We conducted a retrospective electronic health record data analysis of 25,326 subjects tested for COVID-19 between 2/25/20 and 6/22/20 at the University of Alabama at Birmingham Hospital, a tertiary health care center in the racially diverse Southern U.S. The primary outcome was mortality in COVID-19-positive subjects and the association with subject characteristics and comorbidities was analyzed using simple and multiple linear logistic regression.

Results: The odds ratio of contracting COVID-19 was disproportionately high in Blacks/African-Americans (OR 2.6; 95% CI 2.19–3.10; p<0.0001) and in subjects with obesity (OR 1.93; 95% CI 1.64–2.28; p<0.0001), hypertension (OR 2.46; 95% CI 2.07–2.93; p<0.0001), and diabetes (OR 2.11; 95% CI 1.78–2.48; p<0.0001). Diabetes was also associated with a dramatic increase in mortality (OR 3.62; 95% CI 2.11–6.2; p<0.0001) and emerged as an independent risk factor in this diverse population even after correcting for age, race, sex, obesity, and hypertension. Interestingly, we found that metformin treatment prior to diagnosis of COVID-19 was independently associated with a significant reduction in mortality in subjects with diabetes and COVID-19 (OR 0.33; 95% CI 0.13–0.84; p=0.0210).

Conclusion: Thus, these results suggest that while diabetes is an independent risk factor for COVID-19-related mortality, this risk is dramatically reduced in subjects taking metformin prior to diagnosis of COVID-19, raising the possibility that metformin may provide a protective approach in this high risk population.

Keywords: African-American, coronavirus disease-2019, diabetes, metformin, mortality

INTRODUCTION

Coronavirus disease-2019 (COVID-19) caused by the severe acute respiratory syndrome-coronavirus-2 (SARS-CoV-2) is a growing global pandemic that has devastated Asia, Europe, and now the United States. Its increasing death toll has been linked to higher age and a number of comorbidities including hypertension, obesity, and diabetes (1, 2), but approaches to counteract this trend are still lacking. Being a new disease, the specific patient characteristics of these at risk populations are also only starting to emerge with studies reported from China (3–5), Europe (6, 7) and more recently New York (1, 2).

However, currently still very little is known about patient characteristics in the U.S., particularly in more diverse communities with a large proportion of Blacks/African-Americans such as in the South. This information is especially relevant as African-Americans have been disproportionally affected by this pandemic across the nation (8–10) and the prevalence of comorbidities including diabetes is very high in these communities (11). We therefore conducted a retrospective observational study of subjects diagnosed with COVID-19 at the University of Alabama at Birmingham (UAB) Hospital, a tertiary health care center in the South, aimed at identifying the patient characteristics and factors affecting mortality especially in the context of diabetes in this diverse cohort.

METHODS

Study Design and Participants

We conducted a retrospective analysis of de-identified electronic health record data (EHR). The sampling method consisted of including subjects consecutively tested for COVID-19 between February 25, 2020 and June 22, 2020 at UAB (Institutional Review Board protocol E160105006). To make the results as generalizable as possible and minimize any selection bias, completed testing within that time frame was also the only inclusion criteria and lack of outcome data in terms of survival was the only exclusion criteria. Subjects were categorized as confirmed COVID-19 positive or negative based on RT-PCR results from SARS-CoV-2 viral nucleic acid testing in respiratory specimens. The primary outcome was mortality and the effects of patient characteristics and comorbidities as documented in the EHR data (including 12 months before COVID-19 diagnosis) were analyzed. EHR data definitions for obesity included a body mass index (BMI) of ≥30 kg/m^2 and for hypertension a systolic blood pressure of ≥140 mmHg and/or a diastolic blood pressure of ≥90 mmHg. HbA1C was analyzed as a continuous variable. In terms of treatment, we focused on metformin and insulin as they were the two most common used drugs for diabetes and reliable electronic health record data were available. The number of subjects on other antidiabetic medications such as sodium-glucose cotransporter 2 (SGLT2) inhibitors or dipeptidyl peptidase IV (DPPIV) inhibitors was too small to allow for meaningful statistical analysis. This may have been due to the much higher costs of these newer medications and our cohort that included underserved communities.

Statistical Analysis

Patient characteristics and comorbidities were summarized as mean and standard deviation (SD) for continuous variables and frequency and proportion for categorical variables. In analysis, age was categorized into three groups: <50, 50–70, and >70 years old. The association with COVID-19 diagnosis was explored utilizing a simple linear logistic regression for each of the potential risk factors and the raw odds ratio (OR) and the 95% confidence interval (95% CI) were calculated for the strength of association. The associations with COVID-19 mortality for the potential risk factors were explored with both simple linear logistic regression for raw ORs and multiple linear logistic regression for adjusted ORs. Potential interactions were evaluated and removed from the multiple logistic regression model if not significant. The sample size of this study was determined by the available and eligible cases from EHR between February 25, 2020 and June 22, 2020 at UAB, including 24,722 COVID-19 negative and 604 COVID-19 positive subjects. This large sample size achieved >80% power to detect even a very small effect (e.g., OR=1.25) in the association of potential risk factors and contracting COVID-19. Among COVID-19 positive subjects 67 were identified as deceased during the study period and this sample size achieved >80% power to detect a medium effect size (e.g., OR=2.4 or smaller depending on the distribution of risk factors) for the association of subject characteristics and mortality. The power analyses were conducted with a two-sided test in a logistic regression under the significance level of 0.05, using PASS 14 Power Analysis and Sample Size Software (NCSS, LLC. Kaysville, Utah). The statistical analyses were conducted using SAS 9.4 (Cary, NC).

RESULTS

Subject Characteristics and Coronavirus 2019 Diagnosis

The characteristics of the 24,722 subjects who tested negative for COVID-19 and 604 subjects who had a confirmed positive COVID-19 test are listed in **Table 1**. This low positivity rate of 2.4% is most likely due to the fact that asymptomatic hospital staff and patients coming for elective procedures were included in this screening. To explore the association between COVID-19 diagnosis and potential risk factors, a simple logistic regression was used. Notably, despite only representing 26% of the population in Alabama, the number of African-Americans who tested positive for COVID-19 was disproportionally high as African-Americans represented 52% of those who tested positive while accounting for only 30% of those who tested negative. This resulted in a highly significant odds ratio (OR 2.6, 95% CI 2.19–3.10; p<0.0001) (**Table 1**). In contrast, only 36% of COVID-19 positive subjects were Whites, whereas Whites made

TABLE 1 | Subject characteristics and COVID-19 diagnosis.

Subject characteristics	Covid-19		Comparison	OR (95%CI)	P-value
	Negative(n = 24,722)	Positive(n = 604)			
Age Group					
<50 years	10626 (43.0%)	239 (39.6%)			
50–70 years	9862 (39.9%)	245 (40.6%)	50–70 vs <50	1.10 (0.92, 1.32)	0.2798
>70 years	4234 (17.1%)	120 (19.9%)	>70 vs 50–70	1.14 (0.91, 1.42)	0.2432
Race					
African-American (AA)	7498 (30.3%)	311 (51.5%)	AA vs White	2.61 (2.19, 3.10)	<0.0001
White	13821 (55.9%)	220 (36.4%)			
Other	3403 (13.8%)	73 (12.1%)			
Sex					
Male	10671 (43.2%)	272 (45.0%)	M vs F	1.06 (0.90, 1.25)	0.4629
Female	13841 (56.0%)	332 (55.0%)			
Unidentified	210 (0.8%)				
Obesity					
Yes	11167 (45.2%)	371 (61.4%)	Y vs N	1.93 (1.64, 2.28)	<0.0001
No	13555 (54.8%)	233 (38.6%)			
Hypertension					
Yes	11891 (48.1%)	420 (69.5%)	Y vs N	2.46 (2.07, 2.93)	<0.0001
No	12831 (51.9%)	184 (30.5%)			
Diabetes					
Yes	5865 (23.7%)	239 (39.6%)	Y vs N	2.11 (1.78, 2.48)	<0.0001
No	18857 (76.3%)	365 (60.4%)			

up 56% of those who tested negative, further underlining the racial disparity. Interestingly, 70% of all subjects diagnosed with COVID-19 had pre-existing hypertension, 61% had obesity and 40% had diabetes and the risk of being diagnosed with COVID-19 while suffering from any one of these comorbidities was significantly elevated (p<0.0001) (**Table 1**). In the case of diabetes, 92% of subjects also had hypertension and 74% were obese, which may have further contributed to the increased risk observed in this population. Overall, these results are very much in line with global observations and suggested that our cohort provided a representative sample.

Characteristics and Mortality of Coronavirus 2019 Positive Subjects

Overall mortality in COVID-19 positive individuals was 11%, but varied a lot depending on a number of subject characteristics. Ninety three percent of deaths occurred in subjects over the age of 50 and male sex as well as hypertension were associated with a

TABLE 2 | Characteristics and mortality of COVID-19 positive subjects.

Subject characteristics	Mortality		Comparison	OR (95%CI)	P-value
	Alive (n = 537)	Deceased (n = 67)			
Age Group					
<50 years	234 (43.6%)	5 (7.5%)			
50–70 years	216 (40.2%)	29 (43.3%)	50–70 vs <50	6.28 (2.39, 16.5)	0.0002
>70 years	87 (16.2%)	33 (49.2%)	>70 vs 50–70	2.83 (1.62, 4.93)	0.0003
Race					
African-American (AA)	277 (51.6%)	34 (50.8%)	AA vs White	0.84 (0.49, 1.43)	0.5262
White	192 (35.7%)	28 (41.8%)			
Other	68 (12.7%)	5 (7.5%)			
Sex					
Male	231 (43.0%)	41 (61.2%)	M vs F	1.52 (1.19, 1.72)	0.0055
Female	306 (57.0%)	26 (38.8%)			
Obesity					
Yes	328 (61.1%)	43 (64.2%)	Y vs N	1.14 (0.67, 1.94)	0.6234
No	209 (38.9%)	24 (35.8%)			
Hypertension					
Yes	361 (67.2%)	59 (88.1%)	Y vs N	3.60 (1.68, 7.69)	0.001
No	176 (32.8%)	8 (11.9%)			
Diabetes					
Yes	194 (36.1%)	45 (67.2%)	Y vs N	3.62 (2.11, 6.20)	<0.0001
No	343 (63.9%)	22 (32.8%)			

significantly elevated risk of death as assessed by bivariate logistic regression analysis (**Table 2**). In addition, diabetes was associated with a dramatic increase in mortality (OR 3.62; 95% CI 2.11–6.2; p<0.0001). In fact, 67% of deaths occurred in subjects with diabetes.

We also conducted multiple logistic regression analysis with age, race, sex, obese status, hypertension status, and diabetes status as covariates and the adjusted odds ratios and 95% CIs are illustrated in **Figure 1**. Specifically, after controlling for these other covariates, age, sex, and diabetes emerged as the major factors significantly associated with COVID-19 related mortality, suggesting that they are independent risk factors.

Characteristics and Mortality of Coronavirus 2019 Positive Subjects With Diabetes

Based on the identification of diabetes as an independent risk factor for mortality in COVID-19 positive subjects, we explored potential additional risk factors within this diabetic subgroup. Notably, higher

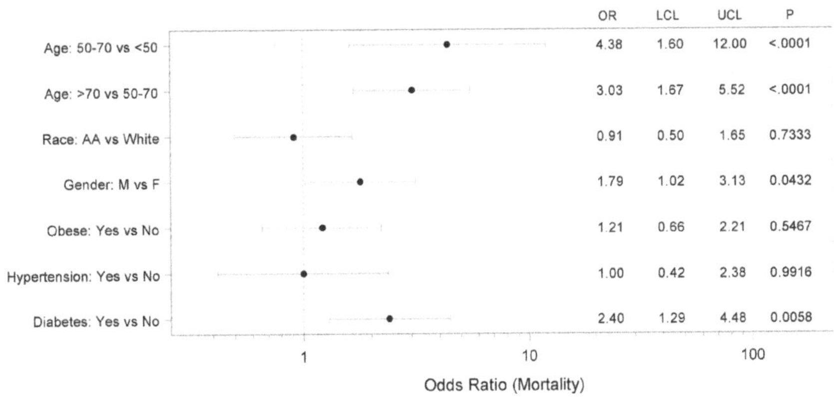

FIGURE 1 | Forest plot showing adjusted mortality risk in subjects with coronavirus 2019 (COVID-19). Multiple logistic regression analysis with age, race, sex, obese status, hypertension status, and diabetes status as covariates was performed. The regression yielded a significant model (p<0.0001) with AUC of 0.79 (95% CI 0.74–0.85) and the adjusted odds ratios (OR), 95% confidence intervals (LCL-UCL) and corresponding P-values are shown.

TABLE 3 | Characteristics and mortality of COVID-19 positive subjects with diabetes.

Subject characteristics	Mortality		Comparison	OR (95%CI)	P-value
	Alive (n = 194)	Deceased (n = 45)			
Age Group					
<50 years	50 (25.8%)	2 (4.4%)			
50–70 years	104 (53.6%)	20 (44.4%)	50–70 vs <50	4.81 (1.08, 21.4)	0.0392
>70 years	40 (20.6%)	23 (51.1%)	>70 vs 50–70	2.99 (1.48, 6.03)	0.0022
Race					
African-American (AA)	127 (65.5%)	28 (62.2%)	AA vs White	0.82 (0.40, 1.68)	0.5855
White	52 (26.8%)	14 (31.1%)			
Other	15 (7.7%)	3 (6.7%)			
Sex					
Male	91 (46.9%)	30 (66.7%)	M vs F	2.26 (1.15, 4.47)	0.0187
Female	103 (53.1%)	15 (33.3%)			
Obesity					
Yes	144 (74.2%)	34 (75.6%)	Y vs N	1.07 (0.51, 2.28)	0.8539
No	50 (25.8%)	11 (24.4%)			
Hypertension					
Yes	176 (90.7%)	43 (95.6%)	Y vs N	2.20 (0.49, 9.84)	0.3027
No	18 (9.3%)	2 (4.4%)			
Diabetes					
Type 1 (T1D)	16 (8.2%)	3 (6.7%)	T1D vs T2D	0.79 (0.22, 2.85)	0.7245
Type 2 (T2D)	178 (91.8%)	42 (93.3%)			
Insulin in T2D					
Yes	72 (40.5%)	15 (35.7%)	Y vs N	0.82 (0.41, 1.64)	0.5728
No	106 (59.5%)	27 (64.3%)			
Metformin in T2D					
Yes	68 (38.2%)	8 (19.1%)	Y vs N	0.38 (0.17, 0.87)	0.0221
No	110 (61.8%)	34 (81.0%)			

age and male sex continued to be associated with increased mortality in the context of diabetes, while no significant difference between type 1 (T1D) and type 2 diabetes (T2D) was observed (**Table 3**). Next, we investigated the effects of diabetes treatment on adverse COVID-19 outcome. We focused on insulin and metformin as the two most common medications prescribed for T2D. To avoid confounding effects from insulin being initiated for stress hyperglycemia and from metformin being discontinued in hospitalized patients, only medications used prior to the diagnosis of COVID-19 were considered. Interestingly, while prior insulin use did not seem to affect mortality risk, metformin use significantly reduced the odds of dying (OR 0.38; 95% CI 0.17–0.87; p=0.0221). In fact, with 11% the mortality of metformin users was comparable to that of the general COVID-19-positive population and dramatically lower than the 24% mortality observed in subjects with diabetes and not on metformin. Of note, this beneficial effect of metformin use on adverse outcome remained even when subjects with chronic kidney disease or chronic heart failure, classical contraindications for metformin, were excluded from the analysis (OR 0.17; 95% CI 0.04–0.79; p=0.0231). This makes any potential confounding effects from skewing metformin users toward healthier subjects without these additional comorbidities, very unlikely. To further determine whether the effect might be just driven by female sex, as one report proposed that women particularly benefit from metformin (12), we also analyzed males separately. Interestingly, the odds ratio of dying remained significantly lower in male subjects on metformin (OR 0.28; 95% CI 0.09–0.88; p=0.0286).

Moreover, we again performed multiple logistic regression analysis with metformin use, insulin use, age, race, sex, obese status, and hypertension status as covariates and the adjusted odds ratios and 95% CIs are shown in **Figure 2**. Specifically, after controlling for other covariates, age, sex, and metformin use emerged as independent factors affecting COVID-19 related mortality. Interestingly, even after controlling for all these other covariates, the likelihood of death for subjects taking metformin for their T2D was significantly less than for those who did not take metformin (OR 0.33; 95% CI 0.13–0.84; p=0.0210). In this regard it is also important to note that subjects not taking metformin did not have more severe metabolic disease or diabetes than those on metformin as demonstrated by comparable or even lower body mass index (BMI) and hemoglobin A1C (HbA1C) values (**Table 4**).

Still, since metformin is known and used for its weight neutral or even weight lowering properties, while improving glycemic

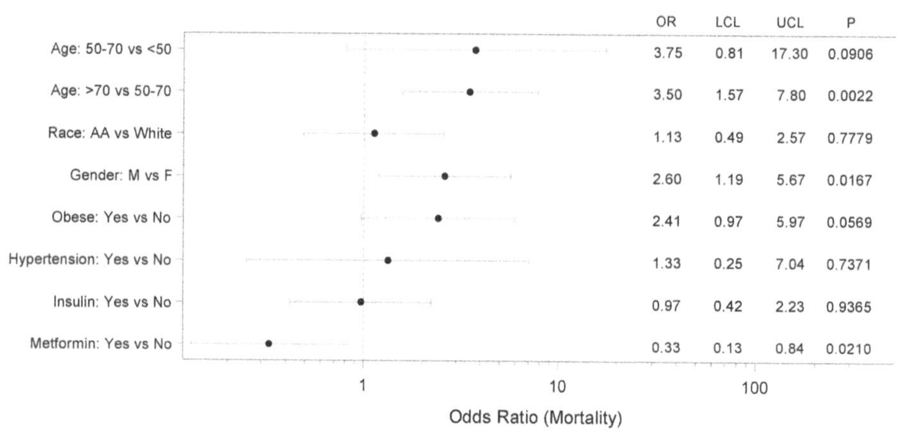

FIGURE 2 | Forest plot showing adjusted mortality risk in subjects with coronavirus 2019 (COVID-19) and T2D. Multiple logistic regression analysis with metformin use, insulin use, age, race, sex, obese status, and hypertension status as covariates was performed and yielded a significant model (p=0.0001) with AUC of 0.77 (0.69, 0.85). The adjusted odds ratios (OR), 95% confidence intervals (LCL-UCL), and corresponding P-values are shown.

TABLE 4 | BMI, BG, and HbA1C of subjects with COVID-19 and T2D treated with/without metformin.

		Alive		Deceased		P-value
		Mean	***SD***	**Mean**	***SD***	**t-test**
BMI (kg/m2)	Metformin use - Yes	35.2	*9.4*	30.9	*6.9*	0.2406
	Metformin use - No	33.6	*8.7*	32.4	*9.8*	0.6039
HbA1C (%)	Metformin use - Yes	8.0	*2.6*	7.3	*1.3*	0.4627
	Metformin use - No	7.0	*1.8*	6.6	*2.1*	0.4428
BG-diagnosis (mg/dL)	Metformin use - Yes	181.4	*84.6*	207.3	*81.0*	0.5166
	Metformin use - No	148.6	*58.2*	156.2	*60.2*	0.5799
BG-illness (mg/dL)	Metformin use - Yes	156.6	*48.4*	173.7	*53.9*	0.4713
	Metformin use - No	143.0	*33.1*	147.8	*51.7*	0.6466

control in T2D (13), we wondered whether these effects might contribute to the reduced risk of COVID-19 related mortality. However, neither BMI nor HbA1C were lower in metformin users who survived as compared to those who died (**Table 4**). While surprising, this is consistent with the notion that long-term glycemic control does not affect COVID-19 outcome, as recently reported (6). Also, only one subject in our cohort experienced a hyperosmolar hyperglycemic state and ended up surviving and there were no subjects with diabetic ketoacidosis (DKA). Moreover, blood glucose at diagnosis and during the illness were not significantly different in metformin-users who survived as compared to those who died (**Table 4**). This further suggests that other factors may play a more important role in terms of the metformin effects on outcome in the context of COVID-19 and T2D.

DISCUSSION

In summary, the findings of this study in a racially diverse population demonstrate that diabetes is an independent risk factor associated with increased mortality in individuals with COVID-19, whereas metformin treatment is associated with dramatically reduced mortality in subjects with T2D even after correcting for multiple covariates.

Most strikingly, we found that metformin use prior to the diagnosis of COVID-19 was associated with a ~3-fold decrease in mortality and significantly lower unadjusted and adjusted odds ratios in subjects with diabetes. Of note, this effect remained even after correcting for age, sex, race, obesity, and hypertension or chronic kidney disease and heart failure. Interestingly and in alignment with this finding, an early report from Wuhan, China also suggested that metformin was associated with decreased mortality in hospitalized COVID-19 patients with diabetes in (14). Metformin was also found to be associated with reduced risk of early death in the French CORONADO study (6) and most recently, it was suggested to be associated with decreased mortality in women with COVID-19 based on a UnitedHealth data analysis (12). The fact that such similar results were obtained in different populations from around the world suggests that the observed reduction in mortality risk, associated with metformin use in subjects with T2D and COVID-19, might be generalizable. In fact, a very recent meta-analysis of this collective work concluded that metformin has benefits in reducing the mortality rate from COVID-19 (15). Furthermore, these findings underline the importance of following general diabetes treatment and prevention guidelines and not delaying or discontinuing any metformin treatment. Especially during this pandemic that puts subjects with diabetes at particularly high risk, this treatment might not only help with diabetes management, but also reduce the risk of adverse outcome in case of a COVID-19 infection.

At this point, the mechanisms by which metformin might improve prognosis in the context of COVID-19 are not known. Our findings suggest that they go beyond any expected improvement in glycemic control or obesity as blood glucose, HbA1C, or BMI were not lower in COVID-19 survivors on metformin. Interestingly, metformin has previously been shown to also have anti-inflammatory (16, 17) and anti-thrombotic effects (18, 19) and excessive inflammatory responses, e.g., cytokine storm as well as disseminated thromboembolic events have been recognized as deadly complications of COVID-19 infection (20–22). It is therefore tempting to speculate that by exerting some of its anti-fibrinolytic activities (18) and inhibiting inflammatory cytokines such as tumor necrosis factor alpha or interleukin-6 (16, 17), suspected to play a role in the immune response to COVID-19 (12), metformin might improve outcome. In fact, even prior to the COVID-19 pandemic, preadmission metformin use was found to be associated with reduced mortality in medical and surgical intensive care patients with T2D (23).

While diabetes has been recognized universally as one of the major comorbidities adversely affecting COVID-19 outcome, the factors responsible for this phenomenon are not well understood. Of note, we found that the increased mortality risk of subjects with diabetes persisted even after correcting for covariates such as age, race, obesity, and hypertension, suggesting that while these factors might contribute to a worse outcome, they cannot fully account for it. In the CORONADO study higher glucose levels at admission were associated with a trend toward increased mortality (6) and in-hospital hyperglycemia contributed to worse prognosis in a large multicenter study of patients with COVID-19 from Wuhan (24). Consistently, we found in general slightly higher glucose levels in subjects who died. However, neither blood glucose levels at diagnosis nor during the illness were lower in metformin-users, making it very unlikely that better control of blood glucose was responsible for the improved outcome observed in subjects taking metformin. Also, long-term glycemic control as assessed by HbA1C did not affect mortality in our study, in alignment with previous reports (6). Similar to the issue with metformin, other factors such as diabetes-associated inflammation (25) and coagulopathy (26) may therefore play a more prominent role in this regard. In addition, a recent report also demonstrated that pancreatic beta cells can get infected and damaged by SARS-CoV-2 (27) providing a potential explanation for the extremely high insulin requirements seen in some subject with COVID-19 as well as the development of diabetic ketoacidosis and possibly new onset diabetes (28, 29).

Higher age and male sex were the other independent risk factors associated with increased mortality that we found consistently across subjects with and without diabetes. In fact, the mortality rate in males was more than two-fold higher than in females, which is in line with previous studies (30). Many theories have been proposed for why this might be, including the different concentrations of sex steroids, different fat distribution, different level of circulating pro-inflammatory cytokines, and different innate and adaptive immune response to viral infections (30, 31). In fact, due to this striking sexual dimorphism, studies using anti-androgens in COVID-19 positive men are currently ongoing. In any case, it is encouraging that the beneficial effects of metformin remained strong in the male subjects of our study.

In our cohort being African-American appeared to be primarily a risk factor for contracting COVID-19 rather than for mortality. These findings are supported by a recent study using an integrated-delivery health system cohort with similar demographics (~30% Blacks/African-American), which found that Black race was not associated with higher in-hospital mortality than White race. This suggests that any racial disparity observed may be more likely due to exposure risk and external, socioeconomic factors than to biological differences. The fact that other geographic areas (mostly with a smaller proportion of African-Americans), did see a difference in mortality (10), might be related to issues with healthcare access.

Limitations of the study include the size that did not allow for any separate analyses of additional subgroups such as T1D or subjects on other anti-diabetic drugs besides metformin. On the other hand, the diverse community comprising a large proportion of African-American men and women represents a unique feature of our study. Also, the fact that in our study metformin-users did not have lower blood glucose levels than non-users, suggested that better metabolic control was unlikely to be responsible for the improved outcome observed in these subjects.

Taken together, our study reaffirmed the role of the major comorbidities associated with COVID-19 in a more diverse population with a higher proportion of African-Americans, demonstrated the prominence of diabetes as an independent risk factor associated with higher mortality and revealed that metformin use prior to a diagnosis of COVID-19 was associated with a consistent and robust decrease in mortality in subjects with diabetes. Future studies will have to explore how metformin might confer these protective effects, provide a careful risk benefit assessment and determine whether the indications for metformin treatment should be broadened in the face of the ongoing COVID-19 pandemic.

AUTHOR CONTRIBUTIONS

AC and TG were responsible for data acquisition and analysis. PL performed all the statistical analyses. MM and FO helped with the approach and interpretation. AS conceived the study and wrote the manuscript. All authors contributed to the article and approved the submitted version.

ACKNOWLEDGMENTS

AS is supported by National Institutes of Health grants R01DK078752 and U01DK120379 and the UAB Center for Clinical and Translational Science (CCTS) by UL1TR001417. This manuscript has been released as a pre-print at medRxiv https://www.medrxiv.org/content/10.1101/2020.07.29.20164020v1 (32).

REFERENCES

1. Richardson S, Hirsch JS, Narasimhan M, Crawford JM, McGinn T, Davidson KW, et al. Presenting Characteristics, Comorbidities, and Outcomes Among 5700 Patients Hospitalized With COVID-19 in the New York City Area. *Jama* (2020) 323(20):2052–9. doi: 10.1001/jama.2020.6775
2. Palaiodimos L, Kokkinidis DG, Li W, Karamanis D, Ognibene J, Arora S, et al. Severe obesity, increasing age and male sex are independently associated with worse in-hospital outcomes, and higher in-hospital mortality, in a cohort of patients with COVID-19 in the Bronx, New York. *Metabol: Clin Experiment* (2020) 108:154262. doi: 10.1016/j.metabol.2020.154262
3. Cai Q, Chen F, Wang T, Luo F, Liu X, Wu Q, et al. Obesity and COVID-19 Severity in a Designated Hospital in Shenzhen, China. *Diabetes Care* (2020) 43(7):1392–8. doi: 10.2337/dc20-0576
4. Chen Q, Zheng Z, Zhang C, Zhang X, Wu H, Wang J, et al. Clinical characteristics of 145 patients with corona virus disease 2019 (COVID-19) in Taizhou, Zhejiang, China. *Infection* (2020) 48(4):543–51. doi: 10.1007/s15010-020-01432-5
5. Wang D, Hu B, Hu C, Zhu F, Liu X, Zhang J, et al. Clinical Characteristics of 138 Hospitalized Patients With 2019 Novel Coronavirus-Infected Pneumonia in Wuhan, China. *Jama* (2020) 323(11):1061–9. doi: 10.1001/jama.2020.1585
6. Cariou B, Hadjadj S, Wargny M, Pichelin M, Al-Salameh A, Allix I, et al. Phenotypic characteristics and prognosis of inpatients with COVID-19 and diabetes: the CORONADO study. *Diabetologia* (2020) 63(8):1500–15. doi: 10.1007/s00125-020-05180-x
7. Scheen AJ, Marre M, Thivolet C. Prognostic factors in patients with diabetes hospitalized for COVID-19: Findings from the CORONADO study and other recent reports. *Diabetes Metab* (2020) 46(4):265–71. doi: 10.1016/j.diabet.2020.05.008
8. Price-Haywood EG, Burton J, Fort D, Seoane L. Hospitalization and Mortality among Black Patients and White Patients with Covid-19. *New Engl J Med* (2020) 382(26):2534–43. doi: 10.1056/NEJMsa2011686
9. Tai DBG, Shah A, Doubeni CA, Sia IG, Wieland ML. The Disproportionate Impact of COVID-19 on Racial and Ethnic Minorities in the United States. *Clin Infect Dis Off Publ Infect Dis Soc A* (2020). doi: 10.1093/cid/ciaa815
10. Holmes L Jr, Enwere M, Williams J, Ogundele B, Chavan P, Piccoli T, et al. Black-White Risk Differentials in COVID-19 (SARS-COV2) Transmission, Mortality and Case Fatality in the United States: Translational Epidemiologic Perspective and Challenges. *Int J Environ Res Public Health* (2020) 17 (12):4322. doi: 10.3390/ijerph17124322
11. Golden SH, Yajnik C, Phatak S, Hanson RL, Knowler WC. Racial/ethnic differences in the burden of type 2 diabetes over the life course: a focus on the USA and India. *Diabetologia* (2019) 62(10):1751–60. doi: 10.1007/s00125-019-4968-0
12. Bramante C, Ingraham N, Murray T, Marmor S, Hoversten S, Gronski J, et al. Observational Study of Metformin and Risk of Mortality in Patients Hospitalized with Covid-19. *MedRxiv Prepr Server Health Sci* (2020). doi: 10.1101/2020.06.19.20135095
13. Tan MH, Alquraini H, Mizokami-Stout K, MacEachern M. Metformin: From Research to Clinical Practice. *Endocrinol Metab Clinics North A* (2016) 45 (4):819–43. doi: 10.1016/j.ecl.2016.06.008
14. Luo P, Qiu L, Liu Y, Liu XL, Zheng JL, Xue HY, et al. Metformin Treatment Was Associated with Decreased Mortality in COVID-19 Patients with Diabetes in a Retrospective Analysis. *Am J Trop Med Hygiene* (2020) 103 (1):69–72. doi: 10.4269/ajtmh.20-0375
15. Hariyanto TI, Kurniawan A. Metformin use is associated with reduced mortality rate from coronavirus disease 2019 (COVID-19) infection. *Obes Med* (2020) 19:100290. doi: 10.1016/j.obmed.2020.100290
16. Cameron AR, Morrison VL, Levin D, Mohan M, Forteath C, Beall C, et al. Anti-Inflammatory Effects of Metformin Irrespective of Diabetes Status. *Circ Res* (2016) 119(5):652–65. doi: 10.1161/CIRCRESAHA.116.308445
17. Tsoyi K, Jang HJ, Nizamutdinova IT, Kim YM, Lee YS, Kim HJ, et al. Metformin inhibits HMGB1 release in LPS-treated RAW 264.7 cells and increases survival rate of endotoxaemic mice. *Br J Pharmacol* (2011) 162 (7):1498–508. doi: 10.1111/j.1476-5381.2010.01126.x

18. Grant PJ. The effects of metformin on the fibrinolytic system in diabetic and non-diabetic subjects. *Diabete Metabol* (1991) 17(1 Pt 2):168–73.
19. Xin G, Wei Z, Ji C, Zheng H, Gu J, Ma L, et al. Metformin Uniquely Prevents Thrombosis by Inhibiting Platelet Activation and mtDNA Release. *Sci Rep* (2016) 6:36222. doi: 10.1038/srep36222
20. McFadyen JD, Stevens H, Peter K. The Emerging Threat of (Micro) Thrombosis in COVID-19 and Its Therapeutic Implications. *Circ Res* (2020) 127(4):571–87. doi: 10.1161/CIRCRESAHA.120.317447
21. Connors JM, Levy JH. COVID-19 and its implications for thrombosis and anticoagulation. *Blood* (2020) 135(23):2033–40. doi: 10.1182/blood.2020006000
22. Khan IH, Savarimuthu S, Leung MST, Harky A. The need to manage the risk of thromboembolism in COVID-19 patients. *J Vasc Surg* (2020) 72(3):799–804. doi: 10.1016/j.jvs.2020.05.015
23. Christiansen C, Johansen M, Christensen S, O'Brien JM, Tonnesen E, Sorensen H. Preadmission metformin use and mortality among intensive care patients with diabetes: a cohort study. *Crit Care* (2013) 17(5):R192. doi: 10.1186/cc12886
24. Zhu L, She ZG, Cheng X, Qin JJ, Zhang XJ, Cai J, et al. Association of Blood Glucose Control and Outcomes in Patients with COVID-19 and Pre-existing Type 2 Diabetes. *Cell Metab* (2020) 31(6):1068–77 e3. doi: 10.1016/j.cmet.2020.04.021
25. Mugabo Y, Li L, Renier G. The connection between C-reactive protein (CRP) and diabetic vasculopathy. Focus on preclinical findings. *Curr Diabetes Rev* (2010) 6(1):27–34. doi: 10.2174/157339910790442628
26. Nogami K, Muraki I, Imano H, Iso H. Risk of disseminated intravascular coagulation in patients with type 2 diabetes mellitus: retrospective cohort study. *BMJ Open* (2017) 7(1):e013894. doi: 10.1136/bmjopen-2016-013894
27. Yang L, Han Y, Nilsson-Payant BE, Gupta V, Wang P, Duan X, et al. A Human Pluripotent Stem Cell-based Platform to Study SARS-CoV-2 Tropism and Model Virus Infection in Human Cells and Organoids. *Cell Stem Cell* (2020) 27(1):125–36 e7. doi: 10.1016/j.stem.2020.06.015
28. Apicella M, Campopiano MC, Mantuano M, Mazoni L, Coppelli A, Del Prato S. COVID-19 in people with diabetes: understanding the reasons for worse outcomes. *Lancet Diabetes Endocrinol* (2020) 8(9):782–92. doi: 10.1016/S2213-8587(20)30238-2
29. Li J, Wang X, Chen J, Zuo X, Zhang H, Deng A. COVID-19 infection may cause ketosis and ketoacidosis. *Diabetes Obes Metab* (2020) 22(10):1935–41. doi: 10.1111/dom.14057
30. Mauvais-Jarvis F. Aging, Male Sex, Obesity, and Metabolic Inflammation Create the Perfect Storm for COVID-19. *Diabetes* (2020) 69(9):1857–63. doi: 10.2337/dbi19-0023
31. Klein SL, Flanagan KL. Sex differences in immune responses. *Nat Rev Immunol* (2016) 16(10):626–38. doi: 10.1038/nri.2016.90
32. Crouse A, Grimes T, Li P, Might M, Ovalle F, Shalev A. Metformin Use Is Associated with Reduced Mortality in a Diverse Population with Covid-19 and Diabetes. *MedRxiv Prepr Server Health Sci* (2020). doi: 10.1101/2020.07.29.20164020

3

Risk Factors for Poor Outcomes of Diabetes Patients with COVID-19: A Single-Center, Retrospective Study in Early Outbreak

Nan Zhang[1†]*, Cheng Wang*[2†]*, Feng Zhu*[2]*, Hong Mao*[3]*, Peng Bai*[4]*, Lu-Lu Chen*[1]*, Tianshu Zeng*[1]*, Miao-Miao Peng*[1]*, Kang Li Qiu*[1]*, Yixuan Wang*[4]*, Muqing Yu*[5,6]*, Shuyun Xu*[5,6]*, Jianping Zhao*[5,6]*, Na Li*[3*] *and Min Zhou*[5,6*]

[1] *Department of Endocrinology, Union Hospital, Tongji Medical College, Huazhong University of Science and Technology, Wuhan, China,* [2] *Department of Cardiology, Union Hospital, Tongji Medical College, Huazhong University of Science and Technology, Wuhan, China,* [3] *Department of Endocrinology, Tongji Medical College, Central Hospital of Wuhan, Huazhong University of Science and Technology, Wuhan, China,* [4] *Department of Cardiovascular Surgery, Union Hospital, Tongji Medical College, Huazhong University of Science and Technology, Wuhan, China,* [5] *Department of Pulmonary and Critical Care Medicine, Tongji Hospital, Tongji Medical College, Huazhong University of Science and Technology, Wuhan, China,* [6] *Key Laboratory of Respiratory Diseases, National Ministry of Health of the People's Republic of China and National Clinical Research Center for Respiratory Disease, Wuhan, China*

***Correspondence:**
Na Li
3979841@qq.com
Min Zhou
minzhou@tjh.tjmu.edu.cn

† *These authors have contributed equally to this work*

Background: Diabetes has been found to increase severity and mortality under the current pandemic of coronavirus disease of 2019 (COVID-19). Up to date, the clinical characteristics of diabetes patients with COVID-19 and the risk factors for poor clinical outcomes are not clearly understood.

Methods: The study was retrospectively carried out on enrolled diabetes patients with laboratory confirmed COVID-19 infection from a designated medical center for COVID-19 from January 25th, 2020 to February 14th, 2020 in Wuhan, China. The medical record was collected and reviewed. Univariate and multivariate analyses were performed to assess the risk factors associated with the severe events which were defined as a composite endpoint of admission to intensive care unit, the use of mechanical ventilation, or death.

Results: A total of 52 diabetes patients with COVID-19 were finally included in the study. 21 (40.4%) patients had developed severe events in 27.50 (IQR 12.25–35.75) days follow-up, 15 (28.8%) patients experienced life-threatening complications and 8 patients died with a recorded mortality rate of 15.4%. Only 13 patients (41.9%) were in optimal glycemic control with HbA1c value of < 7.0%. In addition to general clinical characteristics of COVID-19, the severe events diabetes patients showed higher counts of white blood cells and neutrophil, lower lymphocytes (40, 76.9%), high levels of hs-CRP, erythrocyte sedimentation rate (ESR) and procalcitonin (PCT) as compared to the non-severe diabetes patients. Mild higher level of cardiac troponin I (cTNI) (32.0 pg/ml; IQR 16.80–55.00) and D-dimer (1.70 μg/L, IQR 0.70–2.40) were found in diabetes patients with severe events as compared to the non-severe patients (cTNI:20.00 pg/ml, IQR5.38–30.00, $p = 0.019$; D-dimer: 0.70 μg/L, IQR 0.30–2.40, $p = 0.037$). After adjusting age and sex, increased level of cTNI was found to significantly associate with the incidence of severe events (HR: 1.007; 95% CI: 1.000–1.013; $p = 0.048$), Furthermore, using of α-glucosidase inhibitors was found to be the potential protectant for severe events (HR: 0.227; 95% CI: 0.057–0.904; $p = 0.035$).

Conclusion: Diabetes patients with COVID-19 showed poor clinical outcomes. Vigorous monitoring of cTNI should be recommended for the diabetes patients with COVID-19. Usage of α-glucosidase inhibitors could be a potential protectant for the diabetes patients with COVID-19.

Keywords: SARS-CoV-2, COVID-19, Diabetes Mellitus, risk factors, severe clinical events

INTRODUCTION

Since late December 2019, a number of pneumonia cases caused by a novel coronavirus named Severe Acute Respiratory Syndrome Coronavirus 2 (SARS-CoV-2) has been reported in Wuhan, China. The resultant disease from SARS-CoV-2 infection is named as Coronavirus Disease of 2019 (COVID-19) by the World Health Organization (WHO) (1). The COVID-19 pandemic has so far spread to all continents. By April 10th, the COVID-19 had caused over 1,521,252 infections with over 92,798 deaths globally (2).

Studies have shown that patients with Diabetes Mellitus (DM) are more susceptible to infectious diseases, including pneumonia (3). Indeed, in human Severe Acute Respiratory Syndrome (SARS) and Middle East Respiratory Syndrome (MERS) patients, diabetic groups were associated with higher mortality than their other counterparts (4, 5). Furthermore, SARS-CoV-2 was found to be a clade from the betacoronaviruses associated with the SARS and MERS-CoV (6).

Previous studies have reported increased severity and mortality on COVID-19 patients with diabetic history (7, 8). However, up to now, only a few studies have focused on the risk factors affecting the prognosis of diabetes patients with COVID-19. Zhu et al. found that a well-controlled blood glucose level (3.9–10.0 mmol/L) was associated with lower mortality as compared to individuals with poorly controlled blood glucose level (>10.0 mmol/L) in patients with COVID-19 and those with pre-existing type 2 Diabetes (9). However, the critical issues concerning treatment principles have remained unclear. Indeed, what risk factors are specific for diabetes patients with COVID-19 infection indicating their clinical progression and outcome, and whether the different anti diabetic therapies potentially affected the clinical course of the COVID-19 patients are still unclear (10). In this regard, this study was aimed at describing the clinical features of diabetes patients with COVID-19 infection and investigating the risk factors influencing the prognosis, especially the impact of different anti-diabetic drugs, through a mono-centered retrospective cohort study.

METHODS

Study Design

A retrospective cohort study was undertaken on diabetic patients with COVID-19 infection in Central Hospital of Wuhan, a designated medical institution in SARS-CoV-2 infection. We reviewed the medical records of 563 patients with COVID-19 who were admitted in the general ward between January 25th, 2020 and February 14th, 2020, early in this outbreak. After excluding the non-diabetic patients ($n = 496$) as well as those lacking the required important clinical data ($n = 15$), 52 patients were included in the study. The following clinical retrospective data was retrieved from the medical records; demographic features, clinical evaluation, laboratory tests, chest CT, therapies and outcomes. Additionally, composite endpoint for severe clinical events such as admission to Intensive Care Unit (ICU), the need for mechanical ventilation, or death, were followed-up to April 1st 2020. Two physicians (N.L. and M.Z.) independently collected and reviewed the data. The included patients were classified into severe group and non-severe group, based on whether the individuals experienced the severe clinical events. The risk factors associated with the incidence of severe events were analyzed within the study cohort.

This study was approved by the Ethics Committee of Central Hospital of Wuhan and written informed consent was waived due to the rapid spread and the emergency status of this infectious disease.

Study Definition

COVID-19 was diagnosed based on the criteria of WHO with a confirmed SARS-CoV-2 RNA detection in nasopharyngeal swabs (7). The diagnosis of DM was according to the criteria of the 2020 American Diabetes Association (11). Acute Respiratory Distress Syndrome (ARDS) were diagnosed according to the interim guidance of WHO for COVID-19 (12). Chronic Kidney Disease (CKD) and Acute Renal Injury (AKI) were diagnosed based on the 2012 Kidney Disease Improving Global Outcomes (KDIGO) guideline (13). Acute Myocardial Infarction (AMI) were defined based on the 2017 European Society of Cardiology (ESC) clinical guidelines (14).

Laboratory Procedures and Chest CT

Laboratory confirmation method for SARS-CoV-2 infection followed the WHO guidelines (1). Nasopharyngeal swabs were tested for SARS-CoV-2 RNA on admission and throughout the clinical course. Laboratory detection of the viral RNA in the swabs was determined by Real-Time reverse-transcriptase Polymerase-Chain-Reaction (RT-PCR) assay as previously described (7). Laboratory tests to evaluate the status of DM included the Fasting Plasma Glucose (FPG), 2 h Post-challenge Glucose (2 h-PG), Hemoglobin A1c(HbA1c), blood Total

Cholesterol (TC), High-Density Lipoprotein Cholesterol (HDL-C), Low-Density Lipoprotein Cholesterol (LDL-C) and Triglycerides Levels (TG). Plasma glucose was measured by hexokinase enzymatic method. Blood samples were drawn before breakfast after an overnight fasting of at least 10 h for FPG and 120 min after breakfast for 2 h-PG. HbA1c was performed by using an ultra-high performance liquid chromatograph (UHPLC Nexera X2, Kyoto, Japan). The other routine blood tests performed on admission included; complete blood count, arterial blood gas analysis, serum biochemical tests [renal and liver function, Creatine Kinase (CK), Lactate Dehydrogenase (LDH)], inflammatory biomarkers [high sensitive C Reaction Protein (hsCRP), PCT and Interleukin-6 (IL-6)], cardiac troponin I(cTnI) and D-dimer. To evaluate the COVID-19 pneumonia, chest CT was acquired for all patients following local protocols.

Statistical Analysis

Continuous and categorical variables were presented as median Interquartile Range (IQR) and *N* (%), respectively. Mann Whitney U-test, χ^2 test, or Fisher's exact test was applied to compare, where appropriate, the differences between the severe group and the non-severe group. Survival curve on severe event-free survival was presented. Cox proportional-hazard models were used to estimate the Hazard Ratios (HR) and the associated 95% confidence interval (95%CI) for both the univariate and multivariate analysis. In multivariate analysis, White Blood cell (WBC) counts, hs-CRP, CK, LDH, and ESR were excluded for collinearity. Eventually, age, gender, Fasting Plasma Glucose (FPG) levels, cTnI and using of α-GI were included as covariates in the Cox proportional-hazard models of α-GI for severe events, respectively. Interactions with prognostic factors were also examined with the COX proportional-hazards model. All tests were two-sided, and differences with a $p < 0.05$ were considered statistically significant. All analyses were performed using SPSS version 22.0 software, EmpowerStats (R) (X&Y solutions, Inc., Boston, MA) and R (http://www.R-project.org).

RESULTS

Demographic and Clinical Characteristics of Severe and Non-severe DM Patients With COVID-19

Five hundred and sixty three patients with COVID-19 were admitted in general ward of Central Hospital of Wuhan between January 25th, 2020 and February 14th, 2020. After excluding the non-diabetic patients ($n = 496$) as well as those lacking the required important clinical data ($n = 15$), 52 patients were included in the final analysis.

According to the level of occurred severe clinical events, the patients were divided into severe group ($n = 21$) and non-severe group ($n = 31$).

Baseline characteristics of the 52 diabetic patients with COVID-19 are present in **Table 1**. The diabetic patients (9.2%) were from the 563 COVID-19 patients admitted in Central Hospital of Wuhan between January 25th, 2020 and February 14th, 2020. 33 (63.5%) patients were males with median age of 65.50 years (IQR 61.00–72.75). All the patients were diagnosed with type 2 DM and median duration for the disease occurrence on the studied diabetic patients was 10.00 years (IQR 1.25–15.00). In addition to DM, 36 (69.2%) patients had at least one or more other coexisting chronic diseases (**Table 1**). Thirty four patients (65.4%) and 14 patients (26.9%) had history of essential hypertension and coronary artery disease (CHD), respectively. Furthermore, there was a borderline significant difference in a comorbidity of CHD between two groups (42.9% in severe group vs. 16.1% in non-severe group, $p = 0.055$). It was also found that 22 (42.3%) patients had developed at least one long-term complication of DM prior to the COVID-19 infection. Among the complications, the most common complication was arteriosclerosis (18, 34.6%), followed by diabetic nephropathy (12, 23.1%), then diabetic retinopathy (3, 5.8%) and lastly diabetic foot (1, 1.9%). In the studied cohort, the most common symptoms of the DM patients with COVID-19 on admission were fever 45 (86.5%), dry cough 41 (78.8%), fatigue 32 (61.5%) and dyspnea 22 (42.3%). During the hospitalization time, FPG was monitored in each patient and median value of 8.88 mmol/L (IQR 7.31–11.51) was recorded. HbA1c test was available on 31 patients (59.6%) and median value of 7.2% (IQR 6.5–8.0%) was recorded. Among the patients with HbA1c test, 13 patients (13/31, 41.9%) were in optimal glycemic control with HbA1c at 6–7%, while 18 patients (18/31, 58.1%) were in poor control with HbA1c of above 7% (**Table 1**). 2 h-PG was tested in 20 patients (38.4%) and median level of 14.80 mmol/L (IQR 11.34–16.38) was recorded. A borderline difference in 2 h-PG was found between two groups (15.20 mmol/L [13.30–18.60] in non-severe group vs. 11.46 mmol/L [10.39–15.65] in severe group, $p = 0.053$). No significant differences occurred in gender, age, disease course of DM, FPG, HbA1c and blood lipid levels between the two groups.

Laboratory Findings

Laboratory results for the admitted diabetic patients with COVID-19 infection are shown in **Supplementary Table 1**. The blood counts showed higher counts of leukocytes 7.25 × 10^9/L (IQR 4.87–8.99) and neutrophil counts 6.68 × 10^9/L (IQR 4.73–8.34) within the severe events diabetic patients with COVID-19 infection as compared to the values of non-severe group (leukocytes 5.26 × 10^9/L [IQR 3.24–7.18]; neutrophil counts 3.93 × 10^9/L, [IQR 1.98–6.08]), the difference was statistically significant ($p < 0.05$). Specifically, the neutrophil counts of the severe patients (6.68 × 10^9/L, IQR 4.73–8.34) was higher than the expected normal range. Lymphopenia was frequently found in the diabetic patients with COVID-19 infection (40, 76.9%), without a different between severe and non-severe diabetic patients with COVID-19. There were numerous abnormal infection-related biomarkers in sera of the diabetic patients, hs-CRP, ESR, PCT, and IL-6 were beyond the normal range. Furthermore, the value of hs-CRP, ESR and PCT in the severe patients were significantly higher than those value in non-severe patients ($p < 0.05$). The difference in IL-6 values between the severe and non-severe patients was borderline significant ($p = 0.067$).

TABLE 1 | Demographic and clinical characteristics of severe and non-severe diabetic patients with COVID-19.

	Total (n = 52)	Severe (n = 21)	Non-severe (n = 31)	p-value
Male, n (%)	33 (63.5)	14 (66.7)	19 (61.3)	0.774
Age (years)	65.50 (61.00-72.75)	70.00 (62.50–75.50)	65.00 (59.00–71.00)	0.164
BMI (Kg/m^2)	24.67 (22.35–26.56)	24.34 (22.85–27.03)	24.67 (21.48–26.34)	0.995
Smokers, n (%)	15 (28.8)	5 (23.8)	10 (32.3)	1.000
DM history (years)	10.00 (1.25–15.00)	5.00 (1.00–15.00)	10.00 (5.00–15.00)	0.136
Comorbidities, n (%)	36 (69.2)	14 (66.7)	22 (71.0)	0.768
EH	34 (65.4)	14 (66.7)	20 (64.5)	1.000
CHD	14 (26.9)	9 (42.9)	5 (16.1)	0.055
CKD	3 (5.8)	2 (9.5)	1 (3.2)	0.558
Complications of DM, n (%)	22 (42.3)	11 (52.4)	11 (35.5)	0.263
ASCVD	18 (34.6)	9 (42.9)	9 (29.0)	0.217
Diabetic nephropathy	12 (23.1)	5 (23.8)	7 (22.6)	1.000
Diabetic retinopathy	3 (5.8)	0	3 (9.7)	0.271
Diabetic foot	1 (1.9)	1 (4.8)	0	0.392
Clinical features				
Fever, n (%)	45 (86.5)	18 (85.7)	27 (87.1)	1.000
Cough, n (%)	41 (78.8)	18 (85.7)	23 (74.2)	0.491
Dyspnea, n (%)	22 (42.3)	12 (57.1)	10 (32.3)	0.093
Nausea or vomiting, n (%)	19 (36.5)	5 (23.8)	14 (45.2)	0.149
Days from onset to Hospital admission	7.00 (6.00–13.25)	7.00 (5.00–17.00)	8.00 (6.00–14.00)	0.587
SBP (mmHg)	128.00 (120.00–142.00)	130.00 (120.00–145.75)	126.00 (120.00–135.00)	0.339
DBP (mmHg)	78.00 (70.00–85.00)	77.50 (70.00–85.00)	78.00 (72.00–85.00)	1.000
HbA1c (%)[a]	7.20 (6.50–8.00)	6.75 (6.30–7.63)	7.20 (6.55–9.25)	0.263
HbA1c ≥ 7%, n (%)	18 (34.6)	4 (19.0)	14 (45.2)	0.247
FPG (mmol/L, 3.9–6.1*)	8.88 (7.31–11.51)	8.20 (6.77–11.00)	9.00 (7.26–11.03)	0.424
2 h-PG (mmol/L, <7.8*)[b]	14.80 (11.34–16.38)	11.46 (10.39–15.65)	15.20 (13.30–18.60)	0.053
TC (mmol/L; <5.18*)	3.71 (3.26–4.59)	3.92 (2.82–4.62)	3.71 (3.29–4.66)	0.733
TG (mmol/L; <1.7*)	1.15 (0.88–1.68)	1.26 (0.83–1.71)	1.11 (0.87–1.64)	0.655
HDL-C (mmol/L; >1.04*)	0.95 (0.75–1.21)	0.82 (0.58–1.21)	1.01 (0.80–1.26)	0.436
LDL-C (mmol/L; <3.37*)	2.14 (1.63–2.80)	1.95 (1.54–2.82)	2.17 (1.76–2.78)	0.524
eGFR (ml/min/1.73 m^2; 90–120*)	116.44 (75.53–140.91)	112.77 (57.86–170.35)	118.08 (77.07–138.02)	0.861
Proteinuria, n (%)[c]	9 (17.3)	5 (23.8)	4 (12.9)	0.457

eGFR, estimated glomerular filtration rate; ASCVD, atherosclerotic cardiovascular disease.
Proteinuria defined as the urine protein qualitative test showed positive in the urine routine examination.
*[a] data available in 31 patients; [b] data available in 20 patients; [c] data available in 29 patients; * Normal range.*

Moderately higher level of cTnI (32.0 pg/ml; IQR 16.80–55.00) was found in patients with severe events as compared to the non-severe patients (20.00 pg/ml, IQR5.38–30.00, p = 0.019). Mild increased D-dimer (1.00 μg/L, IQR 0.50–2.40) was also found in the diabetic patients with COVID-19 co-infection, with significantly higher level in the severe patients (1.70 μg/L, IQR 0.70–2.40) as compared to the non-severe patients (0.70 μg/L, IQR 0.30–2.40, $p < 0.05$). Urine routine test was available on 29 patients (55.8%) and 9 (17.3%) patients was positive for proteinuria. The arterial blood gas analysis showed significantly lower PaO_2 values (61.50 mmHg, IQR 52.8–77.8) in the severe patients than value in the non-severe patients (88.50 mmHg, IQR: 66.80-123.50, $p < 0.05$).

Radiology findings of chest CT for diabetic patients with COVID-19 on admission are similar to the previous report (7), shown in **Supplementary Table 1**. There was no difference in CT imaging patterns between the severe and the non-severe cases. Bilateral involvement in lungs (47, 90.4%) was more common than unilateral involvement (5, 9.6%). Ground-glass opacities (45, 86.5%) and patchy consolidation (25, 48.1%) were the common CT imaging pattern on the studied patients.

Treatment, Complications, and Outcome of Severe and Non-severe Diabetic Patients With COVID-19

Treatment and clinical outcome of diabetic patients with COVID-19 are shown in **Table 2**. In total, 8 (15.4%) patients were put on non-invasive mechanical ventilation and 5 (9.6%) patients had endotracheal intubation and invasive ventilation under progressive hypoxia. 12 (23.1%) of the patients were admitted to ICU as the disease progressed. As of 1st April 2020,

TABLE 2 | Treatment and clinical outcomes of severe and non-severe diabetic patients with COVID-19.

	Total ($n = 52$)	Severe ($n = 21$)	Non-severe ($n = 31$)	p-value
Treatment	23 (44.2)	13 (61.9)	10 (32.3)	0.002
Oxygen therapy, *n* (%)				
Non-invasive	8 (15.4)	8 (38.1)	0	<0.001
Invasive	5 (9.6)	5 (23.8)	0	<0.001
ECMO	0	0	0	
Admission to ICU, *n* (%)	12 (23.1)	12 (57.1)	0	<0.001
DM therapy, *n* (%)				
Insulin	24 (46.2)	7 (33.3)	17 (54.8)	0.159
α-GI	24 (46.2)	5 (23.8)	19 (61.3)	0.021
Metformin	15 (28.8)	5 (23.8)	10 (32.3)	0.754
DPP4 inhibitor	4 (7.7)	1 (4.8)	3 (9.77)	1.000
Thiazolidinedione	2 (3.8)	2 (9.5)	0	0.149
Sulfonylurea secretagogue	2 (3.8)	0	2 (6.5)	0.514
Non-sulfonylurea secretagogue	2 (3.8)	1 (4.8)	1 (3.2)	1.000
Complications, *n* (%)	15 (28.8)			
ARDS	11 (21.2)	9 (42.9)	2 (6.5)	0.002
Septic shock[a]	5 (9.6)	5 (23.8)	0	0.008
Acute kidney injury[b]	4 (7.7)	4 (19.0)	0	0.022
AMI[c]	1 (1.9)	1 (4.8)	0	0.404
days form onset to severe event	11.00 (8.50-16.50)	11.00 (8.50-16.50)	NA.	NA.
Death	8 (15.4)	8 (38.1)	0	<0.001

ECMO, extracorporeal membrane oxygenation; α-GI, α-Glucosidase inhibitor; DPP4, dipeptidyl peptidase-4; ARDS, acute respiratory distress syndrome; AMI, acute myocardial infarction; NA, not available.

[a] Three patients had ARDS by co-incidence.

[b] Two patients had ARDS by co-incidence.

[c] One patient had ARDS by co-incidence.

21 (40.4%) of the patients had developed severe clinical events, 23.1% were admitted to ICU, 28.8% experienced life-threatening complications and 8 patients died, with the recorded mortality rate of 15.4%.

49 (94.2%) diabetic patients had at least one antiviral agent subscription, such as arbidol (21, 40.4%), ribavirin (29, 51.9%), and ganciclovir (4, 7.7%). Empirical antibiotic was given to most of the patients (47, 90.4%). Systemic corticosteroid (34, 65.4%) and intravenous immunoglobin (20, 38.5%) were also given to the patients. There was no difference in all the medicines provided to the both the severe and the non-severe cases.

Treatment information for DM are also shown in **Table 2.** 42 (80.8%) patients received hypoglycemic therapy, 8 (15.4%) patients used insulin only, 17 (32.7%) patients used one or more types of oral hypoglycemic drugs while 17 (32.7%) patients used oral hypoglycemic drug combined with insulin. Oral hypoglycemic drugs used included α-glucosidase inhibitors (α-GIs) (24, 46.2%), metformin (15, 28.8%), sulfonylurea secretagogues (2, 3.8%), non-sulfonylurea secretagogues (2, 3.8%), dipeptidyl peptidase 4 (DPP4) inhibitors (4, 7.7%) and thiazolidinediones (2, 3.8%). The proportion of α-GI was significantly higher in the non-severe cases as compared to the severe cases (61.3%vs23.8%, $p = 0.021$).

The most common complication on diabetic patients with COVID-19 was ARDS (11, 21.2%), followed by septic shock (5, 9.6%), then acute kidney injury (4, 7.7%) and lastly AMI (1, 1.9%). From the 52 diabetic patients, 8 (15.4%) patients died within a median time of 10.5 days (IQR 9.0–13.0) from the admission day to the day of death. The cause of death included ARDS (8, 15.4%), followed by septic shock (2, 3.8%) and lastly AMI (1, 1.9%).

Risk Factors for Developing Severe Event by Univariate and Multivariate Analysis

Results of univariate analysis are shown in **Table 3.** In univariate analysis, Cox proportional hazards model was used to access the association between the clinical factors and the severe clinical events. The WBC counts, neutrophil counts, LDH levels, creatine kinase levels, hsCRP levels, ESR levels, IL-6 levels and use of α-GI were all significantly associated with severe events ($p < 0.05$). The cTnI levels had a higher association risk of developing severe events with a borderline statistical significance ($p = 0.097$).

Results of multivariate analysis on the risk of severe clinical events are shown on **Table 4.** After being adjusted in regard to age and gender in the multivariate adjusted Cox proportional hazards model, cTnI and α-GI were observed to be meaningful factors associated with the occurrence of severe events. Diabetic patients with COVID-19 who had elevated levels of cTnI had a significant increased risk of developing severe events (HR = 1.01, 95%CI: 1.0–1.01, $p = 0.048$). Diabetic patients with COVID-19 infection who were using α-GIs had 72% lower risk (HR: 0.23; 95% CI: 0.06–0.90; $p = 0.035$) of severe clinical events than those not using α-GIs. The survival curve for severe clinical events based on α-GIs usage are shown in **Figure 1.**

DISCUSSION

In the present study, the clinical characteristics of 52 diabetic patients with COVID-19 from a designated hospital in Wuhan, China are described, and the risk factors associated with severe clinical events which were defined as the patients' admission to ICU, the use of mechanical ventilation, or death are investigated. At the follow-up endpoint, 40.4% of the patients developed severe events, 23.1% were admitted to ICU, 28.8% had life-threatening complications, and 8 patients finally died with a recorded mortality rate of 15.4%.

Diabetic patients with COVID-19 infection in the studied cohort were found to partly share similar clinical features with the general population such as; typical symptoms of fever, dry cough, fatigue and dyspnea, along with lymphopenia and high level of infection biomarkers, including hs-CRP and IL-6 (7). However, diabetic patients presented character of higher leucocyte and neutrophil counts, especially in the severe events patients, which were different with the leukopenia frequently found in the general population (7). In addition, for infection-related biomarkers, especially for PCT, the severe events cases had significantly higher

TABLE 3 | Univariate analysis of the severe events in diabetic patients with COVID-19.

Variables	Univariate analysis		
	HR	95% CI	*p*-value
Gender (female vs. male)	0.86	0.35–2.14	0.748
Age (years)	1.03	0.98–1.08	0.202
DM history (years)	0.96	0.90–1.03	0.289
FPG (mmol/L)	0.98	0.84–1.14	0.761
HbA1c (%)	0.70	0.42–1.16	0.169
BMI (Kg/m^2)	0.99	0.83–1.18	0.936
HDL-C (mmol/L)	0.43	0.08–2.21	0.31
LDL-C (mmol/L)	0.93	0.48–1.80	0.826
TC (mmol/L)	0.87	0.58–1.30	0.485
TG (mmol/L)	0.97	0.71–1.32	0.829
Comorbidity			
EH	0.93	0.37–2.31	0.876
CHD	2.20	0.92–5.23	0.075
CKD	1.94	0.45–8.38	0.373
DM therapy			
Insulin	0.50	0.20–1.25	0.138
Metformin	0.73	0.26–2.00	0.537
Thiazolidinedione	5.00	1.14–21.93	0.033
α-GI	0.28	0.10–0.76	0.013
Non-sulfonylurea secretagogue	1.26	0.17–9.41	0.824
DPP4 inhibitors	0.61	0.08–4.59	0.635
Complications			
ASCVD	1.30	0.54–3.14	0.558
Diabetic nephropathy	1.11	0.40–3.05	0.845
Diabetic foot	3.47	0.45–26.55	0.231
Laboratory findings of COVID-19			
WBC ($\times 10^9$/L)	1.14	1.01–1.27	0.029
LYM ($\times 10^9$/L)	1.08	0.75–1.56	0.677
NEU ($\times 10^9$/L)	1.02	1.00–1.04	0.030
TBil (μmol/L)	1.07	0.98–1.18	0.132
DBil (μmol/L)	1.16	0.97–1.39	0.101
LDH (U/L)	1.00	1.00–1.01	0.006
CK (U/L)	1.01	1.00–1.01	0.048
D-Dimer (μg/L)	1.02	0.97–1.08	0.413
hsCRP (mg/L)	1.01	1–1.02	0.006
PCT (ng/mL)	1.60	0.37–6.96	0.531
cTnI (pg/mL)	1.005	0.999–1.011	0.097
ESR (mm/h)	1.03	1–1.06	0.026
IL-6 (pg/mL)	1.01	1–1.01	0.022

TABLE 4 | Multivariate analysis for the risk of severe events in DM patients with COVID-19 co-infection.

Clinical factors	Multivariate analysis		
	HR	95% CI	*p*-value
Gender	1.930	0.546–6.819	0.307
Age	1.016	0.962–1.074	0.568
FPG	1.005	0.855–1.181	0.953
cTnI	1.007	1.000–1.013	0.048
α-GI	0.227	0.057–0.904	0.035

levels than those of non-severe cases. Combined with the features of higher leucocyte and neutrophil counts, the higher PCT indicated elevated risks of systemic infection and sepsis in the diabetic patients with COVID-19 infection in the studied cohort.

Furthermore, a recent comparative study had showed that even the diabetic patients with optimal control (HbA1c 6–7%) had an elevated risk of serious infection as compared to patients without diabetes, and the risks rose with increasing HbA1c (15). Majority of the diabetic patients were considered to experience relatively poor glycemic control in the studied cohort. Among the patients with HbA1c test, 58.1% were in poor control with HbA1c of above 7%, which would increase the baseline infection risk as well as the incidence of sepsis.

In the studied cohort, increasing cTnI level was significantly associated with the occurrence of severe clinical events. cTnI is a sensitive biomarker of cardiac injury in variety situation, and was discovered as an important prognostic factor for the patients with COVID-19 infection (16). The mechanism of cardiac injury in COVID-19 was not fully understood, and may be though to be probably related to the presence of underlying CHD, hypoxemia, myocarditis, AMI or septic shock (17). It was noted that 26.9% of the diabetic patients in the studied cohort had a comorbidity of CHD, and the severe events cases had a borderline of higher proportion as compared to the non-severe cases. Endothelial injury is the pathophysiological basis of diabetic vascular disease, and oxidative stress and inflammatory injury play an important role in it. SARS-CoV-2 infects the host through the angiotensin converting enzyme 2 (ACE2) receptor, which is expressed in several organs, including the lung, heart and kidney. ACE2 receptors are also expressed by endothelial cells. Varga et al. (18) indicated the evidence of direct infection of the endothelial cell by the SARS-CoV-2. For the patients with pre-existing endothelial dysfunction and with cardiac dysfunction, which were common in diabetic condition, the cardiac injuries were more severe and the prognosis was worse.

Due to lack of effective therapy for the pandemic, there has been an urgent need for potential agents that can act against the deadly and infectious SARS-CoV-2. The investigation provided interesting information that α-GI could be an independent protector for clinical outcome in diabetic patients with COVID-19 infection. Moreover, the protecting effect is obvious even though only a small portion of α-glucosidase inhibitor is absorbed into circulation (19) Both the SARS-CoV-2 and the Severe Acute Respiratory Syndrome Coronavirus (SARS-CoV) use ACE2 for entry into host cells. Previous studies have found that the N-linked glycan structure of the ACE2 could be altered by glucosidase inhibitors (20). Moreover, inhibition of glucosidases has also been found to impair SARS-CoV and human coronavirus nl63 spike protein-mediated entry into the host cells by altering the N-linked glycan structure (21). Since SARS-CoV-2 also uses ACE2 for entry into host cells, we hypothesized that α-GIs may interfere with SARS-CoV-2 by

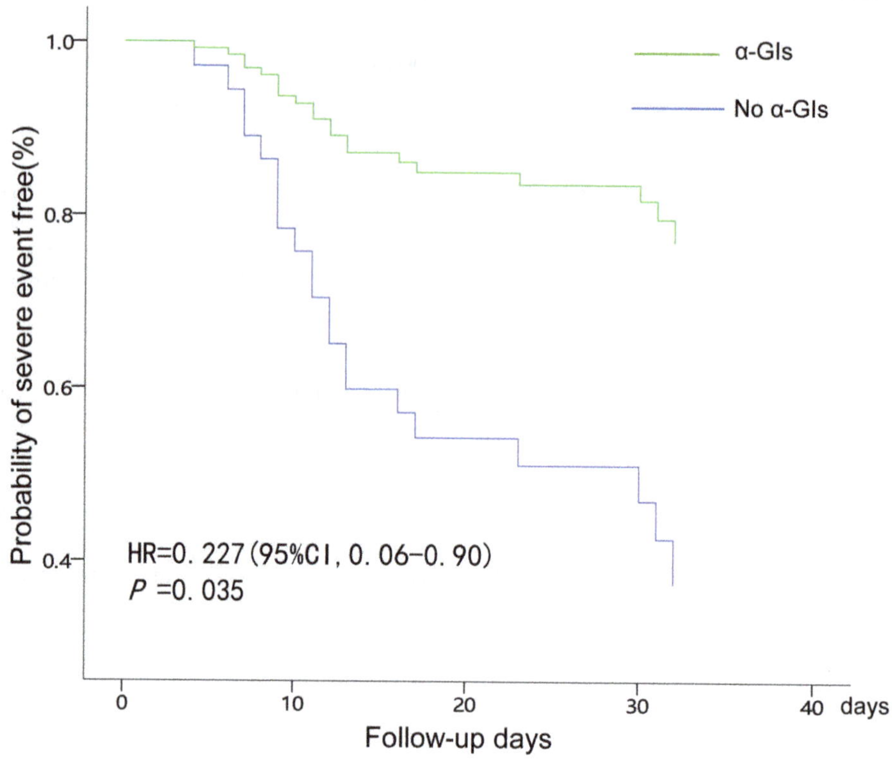

FIGURE 1 | COX regression analysis of administration of α-GIs for developing severe events in diabetes patients with COVID-19.

altering the glycan structure of ACE2 and thus disrupt the entry of the SARS-CoV-2 to the body cells. In addition, inhibition of α-glucosidase has been found to work as antiviral agents for many enveloped RNA viruses, such as the human immunodeficiency virus and hepatitis C virus (22). Both SARS-CoV and SARS-CoV-2 are enveloped RNA viruses which contain N-linked glycans. Treatment with the glucosidase inhibitor N-butyl-deoxynojirimycin inhibits N-glycan processing in SARS-CoV. Therefore, it indicates the potential role of glucosidase inhibitors in the treatment of SARS-CoV-2 infections (23) by disrupting the proper folding and function of the glycoproteins on the SARS-CoV-2 envelope. However, molecular data demonstrating direct antiviral effects of α-glucosidase inhibitors, as well as data on the plasma concentrations of these largely intestinally active and non-absorbed drugs are needed in future studies.

There has been much concern about the pharmacological therapy for diabetic patients with COVID-19. Current recommendations for anti-diabetic drugs for diabetic patients with COVID-19 mainly include maintaining previous medication for the mild cases and changing to insulin for regular and severe cases (10). The present study indicates that α-GIs are independent protective factor for incidence of severe clinical events in COVID-19 infection. Of course, replications in large cohorts are needs to confirm our results.

Even though the study has provided interesting findings, it had some few limitations. First, the study was retrospectively designed from a single center and based on a relatively small sample size, therefore, the roles of the study confounders predicting the severe events might be underestimated. Moreover, it might have unavoidable selection bias as well as heterogeneity. Second, some important confounders were not able to be included in the multivariate analyses, such as the IL-6 and hs-CRP. Although the univariable analyses showed statistically significant association, the study could not include them in the multivariable Cox analysis due to the relatively small sample sizes. Third, since comorbidity of diabetes has been previously reported to lead to more severe and more deadly COVID-19, it would be urgent and to see what risk factors are specific for diabetes patients predicting to the severe course of COVID-19. We only reported and analyzed the outcome and mortality in diabetes patients with COVID-19. The comparisons between diabetes and non-diabetes patients with COVID-19 could reveal more useful information, as would comparisons of less severe cases not included in our study population. Lastly, the present study indicates that using α-GI might have a lower risk of endpoint of severe outcomes, but further randomized control studies with larger sample size are required to ascertain this. Thus, future studies with larger sample sizes and prospective study designs are warranted to further explore the risk factors and potential therapeutic effect of α-GIs in diabetic patients with COVID-19.

In summary, the current study described the detailed clinical features and poor outcome of diabetic patients with COVID-19 in early outbreak of China. The study found increased level of cTnI was a risk factor predicting the incidence of clinical outcome. It is therefore recommend that diabetic patients with COVID-19 infection should have vigorous monitoring of the cTnI. Even more important, we found, α-GIs might have a potential protective effect from severe clinical events for those patients and need to be studied more for clear understanding.

AUTHOR CONTRIBUTIONS

MZ, NL, NZ, CW, FZ, HM, PB, L-LC, TZ, M-MP, KQ, YW, MY, SX, and JZ implemented the study and collected the data. NZ, CW, FZ, MZ, and NL wrote the manuscript. CW and NZ analyzed the data. All authors participated in the design and interpretation of the studies, analysis of the data and review of the manuscript.

ACKNOWLEDGMENTS

We would like to thank the members of information department and medical ethics committee of Wuhan Central Hospital for their helpful data and critical reading and review of the manuscript.

REFERENCES

1. WHO. *Director-General's Remarks at the Media Briefing on 2019-nCoV on 11 February 2020.* World Health Organization (2020). Available online at: https://www.who.int/dg/speeches/detail/who-director-general-s-remarks-at-the-media-briefing-on-2019-ncov-on-11-february-2020
2. Coronavirus disease 2019. *(COVID-19) Situation Report-81.* Available online at: https://www.who.int/docs/default-source/coronaviruse/situation-reports/20200410-sitrep-81-covid-19.pdf?sfvrsn=ca96eb84_2 (accessed April 10, 2020).
3. Schuetz P, Castro P, Shapiro NI. Diabetes and sepsis: preclinical findings and clinical relevance. *Diabetes Care.* (2011) 34:771–8. doi: 10.2337/dc10-1185
4. Yang JK, Feng Y, Yuan MY, Yuan SY, Fu HJ, Wu BY, et al. Plasma glucose levels and diabetes are independent predictors for mortality and morbidity in patients with SARS. *Diabet Med.* (2006) 23:623–8. doi: 10.1111/j.1464-5491.2006.01861.x
5. Alqahtani FY, Aleanizy FS, Ali El Hadi Mohamed R, Alanazi MS, Mohamed N, Alrasheed MM, et al. Prevalence of comorbidities in cases of Middle East respiratory syndrome coronavirus: a retrospective study. *Epidemiol Infect.* (2018) 147:1–5. doi: 10.1017/S0950268818002923
6. Zhu N, Zhang D, Wang W, Li X, Yang B, Song J, et al. A novel coronavirus from patients with pneumonia in China, 2019. *N Engl J Med.* (2020) 382:727–33. doi: 10.1056/NEJMoa2001017
7. Huang C, Wang Y, Li X, Ren L, Zhao J, Hu Y, et al. Clinical features of patients infected with 2019 novel coronavirus in Wuhan, China. *Lancet.* (2020) 395:497–506. doi: 10.1016/S0140-6736(20)30183-5
8. Guan W, Ni Z, Hu Y, Liang W, Ou C, He J, et al. Clinical characteristics of coronavirus disease 2019 in China. *N Engl J Med.* (2020) 382:1708–20. doi: 10.1056/NEJMoa2002032
9. Zhu L, She Z-G, Cheng X, Qin J-J, Zhang X-J, Cai J, et al. Association of blood glucose control and outcomes in patients with COVID-19 and pre-existing type 2 diabetes. *Cell Metab.* (2020) 31:1068–77.e3. doi: 10.1016/j.cmet.2020.04.021
10. Bornstein SR, Rubino F, Khunti K, Mingrone G, Hopkins D, Birkenfeld AL, et al. Practical recommendations for the management of diabetes in patients with COVID-19. *Lancet Diabetes Endocrinol.* (2020) 8:546–50. doi: 10.1016/S2213-8587(20)30152-2
11. American Diabetes Association. 2. Classification and diagnosis of diabetes: standards of medical care in diabetes-2020. *Diabetes Care.* (2020) 43(Suppl. 1):S14–31. doi: 10.2337/dc20-S002
12. World Health Organization. *Clinical Management of Severe Acute Respiratory Infection When Novel Coronavirus (nCoV) Infection is Suspected.* Interim Guidance. Available online at https://www.who.int/publications-detail/clinical-management-of-severe-acute-respiratory-infection-when-novel-coronavirus-(ncov)-infection-is-suspected (accessed April 4, 2020).
13. Palevsky PM, Liu KD, Brophy PD, Chawla LS, Parikh CR, Thakar CV, et al. KDOQI US commentary on the 2012 KDIGO clinical practice guideline for acute kidney injury. *Am J Kidney Dis.* (2013) 61:649–72. doi: 10.1053/j.ajkd.2013.02.349
14. Ibánez B, James S, Agewall S, Antunes MJ, Bucciarelli-Ducci C, Bueno H, et al. 2017 ESC guidelines for the management of acute myocardial infarction in patients presenting with ST-segment elevation. *Rev Esp Cardiol.* (2017) 70:1082. doi: 10.1016/j.rec.2017.11.010
15. Critchley JA, Carey IM, Harris T, deWilde S, Hosking FJ, Cook DG. Glycemic control and risk of infections among people with type 1 or type 2 diabetes in a large primary care cohort study. *Diabetes Care.* (2018) 41:2127–35. doi: 10.2337/dc18-0287
16. Shi S, Qin M, Shen B, Cai Y, Liu T, Yang F, et al. Association of cardiac injury with mortality in hospitalized patients with COVID-19 in Wuhan, China. *JAMA Cardiol.* (2020) 5:802–10. doi: 10.1001/jamacardio.2020.0950
17. Emami A, Javanmardi F, Pirbonyeh N, Akbari A. Prevalence of underlying diseases in hospitalized patients with covid-19: a systematic review and meta-analysis. *Arch Acad Emerg Med.* (2020) 8:e35.
18. Varga Z, Flammer AJ, Steiger P, Haberecker M, Andermatt R, Zinkernagel AS, et al. Endothelial cell infection and endotheliitis in COVID-19. *Lancet.* (2020) 395:1417–8. doi: 10.1016/S0140-6736(20)30937-5
19. Fernandez E, Ross C, Liang H, Javors M, Tardif S, Salmon AB. Evaluation of the pharmacokinetics of metformin and acarbose in the common marmoset. *Pathobiol Aging Age Relat Dis.* (2019) 9:1657756. doi: 10.1080/20010001.2019.1657756
20. Zhang H, Penninger JM, Li Y, Zhong N, Slutsky AS. Angiotensin-converting enzyme 2 (ACE2) as a SARS-CoV-2 receptor: molecular mechanisms and potential therapeutic target. *Intensive Care Med.* (2020) 46:586–90. doi: 10.1007/s00134-020-05985-9
21. Wrapp D, Wang N, Corbett KS, Goldsmith JA, Hsieh C-L, Abiona O, et al. Cryo-EM structure of the 2019-nCoV spike in the prefusion conformation. *Science.* (2020) 367:1260–3. doi: 10.1126/science.abb2507
22. Zhao X, Guo F, Comunale MA, Mehta A, Sehgal M, Jain P, et al. Inhibition of endoplasmic reticulum-resident glucosidases impairs severe acute respiratory syndrome coronavirus and human coronavirus NL63 spike protein-mediated entry by altering the glycan processing of angiotensin I-converting enzyme 2. *Antimicrob Agents Chemother.* (2015) 59:206–16. doi: 10.1128/AAC.03999-14
23. Chang J, Block TM, Guo J-T. Antiviral therapies targeting host ER alpha-glucosidases: current status and future directions. *Antiviral Res.* (2013) 99:251–60. doi: 10.1016/j.antiviral.2013.06.011

4

COVID-19 and Undiagnosed Pre-Diabetes or Diabetes Mellitus Among International Migrant Workers

*Louis Y. Tee [1], Sharifah Munirah Alhamid [1], Jeriel L. Tan [1], Theik Di Oo [1], Jaime Chien [2], Primavera Galinato [1], Seow Yen Tan [2], Shafi Humaira [2], Raymond Kok Choon Fong [2], Troy H. Puar [3], Wann Jia Loh [3], Anindita Santosa [4], Joan Khoo [3] and Barbara Helen Rosario [1]**

[1] Department of Geriatric Medicine, Changi General Hospital, Singapore, Singapore, [2] Department of Infectious Diseases, Changi General Hospital, Singapore, Singapore, [3] Department of Endocrinology, Changi General Hospital, Singapore, Singapore, [4] Department of Rheumatology, Changi General Hospital, Singapore, Singapore

***Correspondence:**
Barbara Helen Rosario
rosario.barbara.helen@singhealth.com.sg

Objective: Migrant workers, a marginalized and under-resourced population, are vulnerable to coronavirus disease 2019 (COVID-19) due to limited healthcare access. Moreover, metabolic diseases—such as diabetes mellitus (DM), hypertension, and hyperlipidemia—predispose to severe complications and mortality from COVID-19. We investigate the prevalence and consequences of undiagnosed metabolic illnesses, particularly DM and pre-diabetes, in international migrant workers with COVID-19.

Methods: In this retrospective analysis, we analyzed the medical records of international migrant workers with laboratory-confirmed COVID-19 hospitalized at a tertiary hospital in Singapore from April 21 to June 1, 2020. We determined the prevalence of DM and pre-diabetes, and analyzed the risk of developing complications, such as pneumonia and electrolyte abnormalities, based on age and diagnosis of DM, and pre-diabetes.

Results: Two hundred and fouty male migrant workers, with mean age of 44.2 years [standard deviation (SD), 8.5years], were included. Twenty one patients (8.8%) were diagnosed with pre-diabetes, and 19 (7.9%) with DM. DM was poorly controlled with a mean HbA1c of 9.9% (SD, 2.4%). 73.7% of the patients with DM and all the patients with pre-diabetes were previously undiagnosed. Pre-diabetes was associated with higher risk of pneumonia [odds ratio (OR), 10.8, 95% confidence interval (CI), 3.65–32.1; $P < 0.0001$], hyponatremia (OR, 8.83; 95% CI, 1.17–66.6; $P = 0.0342$), and hypokalemia (OR, 4.58; 95% CI, 1.52–13.82; $P = 0.0069$). Moreover, patients with DM or pre-diabetes developed COVID-19 infection with lower viral RNA levels.

Conclusions: The high prevalence of undiagnosed pre-diabetes among international migrant workers increases their risk of pneumonia and electrolyte abnormalities from COVID-19.

Keywords: COVID-19, diabetes mellitus, impaired glucose tolerance (IGT), international migrant worker, pre-diabetes (pre-DM)

INTRODUCTION

There are 164 million international migrant workers globally, making them the world's largest transnational migrant population (1). Migrant workers face systemic injustices that lead to limited access to healthcare, such as segregated housing, inadequate education, and socioeconomic deprivation (1–4). Moreover, effective healthcare policies designed to protect this vulnerable patient group are challenging to formulate because data regarding the health outcomes of this neglected population are scarce and fragmented (1). Therefore, migrant workers are at a heightened risk of transmission of coronavirus 2019 (COVID-19) (5).

Indeed, as of July 2, 2020, there were 41,646 migrant workers living in dormitories diagnosed with COVID-19 in Singapore, making up 94.4% of the 44,122 cases of COVID-19 in the country (6). As of December 2019, there were 1.4 million international migrant workers in Singapore (7). Close to 1 million entered on work permits for low-wage jobs, such as 293,300 male construction workers who live in dormitories (7), and previous studies have found that these migrant workers are especially susceptible to outbreaks of infectious diseases such as malaria, enteric fevers, viral hepatitis, and tuberculosis compared to residents (4). With large numbers of migrant workers admitted to the healthcare system for COVID-19, this situation has provided a unique opportunity to evaluate the general health of this hidden population. In the course of caring for these migrant workers, physicians searched for potential complications of COVID-19 infections, and screened for common chronic diseases, such as diabetes mellitus, which may exacerbate COVID-19 infections.

Emerging evidence from the COVID-19 pandemic have demonstrated that hyperglycemia on admission to a hospital portends increased severity of disease and higher mortality (8, 9). While diabetes mellitus (DM) is a risk factor for severe COVID-19 (10–13), hyperglycemia itself, and not just a known history of DM, have been shown to be associated with worse prognosis (8, 9). It has been proposed that this is because glycosylation of the spike protein of severe acute respiratory syndrome coronavirus 2 (SARS-CoV-2), the virus that causes COVID-19, modulates its binding to the angiotensin converting enzyme receptor 2 (ACE2) on host tissue (14). Since increased glycosylation of SARS-CoV-2 and ACE2 promotes the entry of SARS-CoV-2 into host cells, it has been postulated that higher blood glucose levels would lead to greater susceptibility to COVID-19 infection and amplified disease severity (15). Moreover, SARS-CoV-2 binds to tissues with high ACE2 expression, such as the lungs, liver, kidneys and blood (16), and in addition to pneumonia, COVID-19 has been reported to cause systemic complications such as electrolyte abnormalities (17), thrombocytopenia (18), anemia (19), leukopenia (20), and transaminitis (21). In fact, it has been proposed that screening for hyperglycemia and prompt blood glucose control should be mandatory for all COVID-19 cases to improve prognosis (22). Even though current guidelines suggest routine screening for DM and pre-diabetes (also known as impaired glucose tolerance) for adults aged 40 years and older (23), underdiagnosis is common among Singapore residents (24). Among Singapore residents, the prevalence of DM is 8.6%, of which a third are unaware they have the disease (25). We hypothesized that the prevalence of undiagnosed DM and pre-diabetes will be higher among international migrant workers compared to Singapore residents due to their limited access to health care, and that this will lead to more complications of COVID-19.

METHODS

Inclusion Criteria

This retrospective cohort study was performed in a cohort of adult migrant workers diagnosed with COVID-19. The patients were admitted to one of the three COVID-19 cohort wards available in Changi General Hospital, a tertiary hospital in Singapore, from April 21 to June 1, 2020. Patients admitted to this ward were cared for by physicians from the Department of Geriatric Medicine with regular advice from the Department of Infectious Diseases and were selected for admission based on male sex, hemodynamic stability, and no requirement for supplemental oxygen. Inclusion criteria for the analysis were age of 21 years old and above, a confirmed laboratory diagnosis of COVID-19 infection using SARS-CoV-2 reverse-transcriptase polymerase-chain reactions (RT-PCR) from nasopharyngeal swabs and employment outside the country of origin. The demographic data collected from their electronic medical records were age, sex, ethnicities, and past medical histories. Additionally, hemodynamic parameters (blood pressure, BP; and heart rate, HR) on admission and discharge; new diagnoses of chronic diseases made during hospitalization (such as hypertension, diabetes mellitus, and hyperlipidemia); and hematological, biochemical, and radiological abnormalities were extracted from the medical records.

Diagnosis and Treatment of Chronic Diseases

Patients were screened for diabetes mellitus with HbA1c or OGTT if random blood glucose was elevated. Diagnosis of diabetes mellitus and pre-diabetes was based on the American Diabetic Association 2019 guidelines (23). BP was monitored closely throughout admission. The diagnostic criterion for hypertension was based on the Eighth Joint National Committee (JNC 8) guidelines (26). Screening for hyperlipidemia was done if there were clinical risk factors or presence of other cardiovascular risk factors (27). Patients were deemed tachycardic if HR was more than 100 beats per minute (beats/min). Hyperlipidemia was diagnosed according to the American Heart Association guidelines (27). Appropriate and prompt treatment was started for newly diagnosed DM, such as metformin, glipizide and/or linagliptin; and pre-meal capillary blood glucose measurements with subcutaneous sliding-scale insulin.

Statistics

Statistical analysis was performed using SPSS 25 software. Statistical significance, determined with two-tailed, unpaired testing, was evaluated at the 0.05 level. For continuous variables (such as age, Ct values, blood pressures, and heart rates), two-tailed t-tests were used to compare the means of two groups, and single-factor ANOVA was used to compare the means of three or more groups. For categorical variables (such as the proportion of patients with complications like pneumonia), the chi-square test was used to compare the proportions between groups. Odds ratios were calculated using binomial logistic regression. There was no funding obtained specifically for this study. Ethics review was overseen by the Singapore Heath System (SingHealth) Centralized Institutional Review Board (CIRB). All data was anonymized and irreversibly de-identified to protect patient privacy.

RESULTS

Patient Characteristics

Two hundred and fouty four patients' electronic medical records were reviewed. Three patients were Singapore residents and one patient was younger than 21 years old, and their records were excluded from the analysis. The medical records of 240 patients were included in our study. The demographic data were collated and analyzed based on age (**Table 1**) and diagnosis of DM or pre-diabetes (**Table 2**). All the patients were male, and the mean age was 44.2 years [standard deviation (SD), 8.5 years]. Our population consists of the following ethnicities: Bangladeshi ($n =$ 86, 35.8%), Indian ($n = 70$, 29.2%), Chinese ($n = 66$, 27.5%), Thai ($n = 12$, 5.0%), and other ethnicities ($n = 6$, 2.5%). The mean cycle threshold (Ct) value for the N gene was 23.9 (SD, 8.3), and the mean Ct value for the E gene was 23.6 (SD, 8.1). The Ct value was significantly higher in patients with DM (N gene Ct value, 30.7; SD, 4.9 and E gene Ct value, 30.8; SD, 5.1) and pre-diabetes (N gene Ct value, 25.8; SD, 7.5 and E gene Ct value, 26.8; SD, 7.5), suggesting that lower viral RNA levels resulted in COVID-19 infection. On admission, 23 patients (9.6%) were asymptomatic, while the rest had symptoms of rhinorrhea, sore throat, cough, dyspnea, pleuritic chest pain, diarrhea, lethargy, and myalgia.

Screening for DM and Pre-diabetes

The prevalence of DM in our cohort is 7.9% (19 of 240 patients), of which 73.7% (14 of 19 patients with diabetes) were newly diagnosed. The mean serum glucose on admission, measured in 201 patients, was 7.5 mmol/L (SD, 3.0 mmol/L). Random plasma glucose was >7.8 mmol/L in 64 patients (31.8%), of which 59 (24.5%) were not previously known to have DM. Thirty two patients underwent OGTT, and HbA1c levels were measured in 45 patients. From the OGTT and/or HbA1c results, 14 patients (5.8%) were newly diagnosed to have DM. All the patients with DM had an HbA1c >7.0%, with a mean HbA1c of 9.9% (SD, 2.4%). Patients diagnosed with DM were started on appropriate oral hypoglycemic agents such as metformin, glipizide and/or linagliptin, as well as pre-meal capillary blood glucose monitoring with subcutaneous sliding-scale insulin injections. Additionally, 21 patients (8.8%) were newly diagnosed with pre-diabetes, defined as an HbA1c between 5.7 and 6.4% and/or a 2 h serum glucose for the OGTT between 7.8 and 11.0 mmol/L, and they were counseled on lifestyle modifications and advised to follow up with a primary-care physician for development of diabetes or resolution of pre-diabetes. Patients with DM or pre-diabetes were older (DM, 47.3 years; SD, 4.7 vs. pre-diabetes, 47.7 years; SD, 7.8 vs. normal glucose control, 44.2 years; SD, 8.5; $P =$ 0.0248), and had a higher prevalence of hyperlipidemia (DM, 15.8% vs. pre-diabetes, 19.0% vs. normal glucose control, 2.0%; $P = 0.0005$; **Table 2**).

Hypertension

The prevalence of hypertension in our cohort was 7.5% (18 of 240 patients), of which 61.1% (8 of 18 patients with hypertension) were newly diagnosed. Eighty two patients (34.2%) were hypertensive on admission, with a mean systolic BP of 149 mmHg (SD, 10 mmHg) and a mean diastolic BP of 93 mmHg (SD, 9 mmHg). No patients were in hypertensive urgency, defined as a systolic BP >180 mHg and/or a diastolic BP >120 mmHg. Eleven patients (4.6%) were diagnosed with hypertension because they were persistently hypertensive over 2 to 3 days and were started on anti-hypertensive medications such as amlodipine, atenolol or enalapril. Twenty seven patients (11.3%) were hypertensive on discharge, with a mean systolic BP of 138 mmHg (SD, 10 mmHg) and a mean diastolic BP of 92 mmHg (SD, 4 mmHg). Patients who had transient BP readings above 140/90 mmHg were advised to follow up with a family physician to monitor their BP on discharge. Patients with DM and pre-diabetes had higher systolic (DM; 147 mmHg; SD, 21 vs. pre-diabetes; 134 mmHg; SD, 17 vs. normal glucose control; 129 mmHg; SD, 16; $P < 0.0001$) and diastolic (DM, 93 mmHg; SD, 9 vs. pre-diabetes; 85mmHg; SD 8 vs. normal glucose control; 83 mmHg; SD, 10 mmHg; $P < 0.0001$) blood pressures and heart rates (DM; 97 beats/min; SD, 14 vs. pre-diabetes; 92 beats/min; SD 16 vs. normal glucose control; 86 beats/min; SD, 13; $P = 0.0017$) on admission, but not on discharge (**Table 2**).

Hepatic, Electrolyte, and Hematological Abnormalities

Serum sampling was undertaken in 201 patients and the results were analyzed based on age (**Table 3**) and diagnosis of DM/pre-diabetes (**Table 4**), and the association of hepatic, electrolyte, and hematological complications with age and/or DM/pre-diabetes was assessed (**Table 5**). The most common abnormal blood result was deranged liver enzymes with 46 patients (23.4%) affected, of which six (3.6%) had alanine aminotransferase levels >two times the upper limit of normal. The incidence of severe transaminitis was higher in patients with DM (15.8 vs. 1.5%, $P = 0.0238$; **Table 4**).

Hematological abnormalities were also common, and six abnormalities were observed in 44 individual patients (17.9%). Microcytosis was found in 15 patients (7.5%); thrombocytopenia in eight (4.0%); leukopenia in eight (4.0%); anemia in eight (4.0%); polycythemia in four (1.99%); and macrocytosis in one (0.5%). Of the eight patients who were anemic, five had normocytic anemia, two had microcytic anemia, and one had macrocytic anemia. Of the five patients who had the anemia work-up completed, three cases were iron-deficient, one was vitamin-B12 deficient, and one was both iron and vitamin-B12 deficient. One patient had macrocytosis without anemia and was found to be vitamin-B12 deficient.

Lastly, the renal panels revealed electrolyte disturbances, such as hypokalemia in 20 patients (10.0%) with a mean serum

TABLE 1 | Demographics and clinical characteristics, stratified by age.

	All ages (*n* = 240)	20 to 29 years (*n* = 20)	30 to 39 years (*n* = 39)	40 to 49 years (*n* = 120)	≥ 50 years (*n* = 61)	P value
Age, mean (SD), years	44.2 (8.5)	26.2 (2.1)	33.6 (2.8)	46.4 (2.1)	52.7 (2.8)	<0.0001
Ethnicity						
Bangladeshi, *n* (%)	86 (35.8)	16 (80.0)	23 (59.0)	38 (31.7)	9 (14.8)	0.0115
Indian, *n* (%)	70 (29.2)	4 (20.0)	14 (36.0)	33 (27.5)	19 (31.2)	
Chinese, *n* (%)	66 (27.5)	0 (0.0)	2 (5.1)	43 (35.8)	21 (34.4)	
Thai, *n* (%)	12 (5.0)	0 (0.0)	0 (0.0)	3 (2.5)	9 (14.8)	
Others, *n* (%)	6 (2.5)	0 (0.0)	0 (0.0)	3 (2.5)	3 (4.9)	
Co-morbidity						
Diabetes mellitus, *n* (%)	19 (7.9)	0 (0.0)	1 (2.6)	12 (10.0)	6 (9.8)	0.0057
Hypertension, *n* (%)	18 (7.5)	0 (0.0)	3 (7.7)	7 (5.8)	8 (13.1)	0.0071
Hyperlipidemia, *n* (%)	11 (4.6)	0 (0.0)	2 (5.1)	4 (3.3)	5 (8.2)	0.0495
SARS-CoV-2 RT-PCR statistics						
N gene Ct value, mean (SD)	23.9 (8.3)	17.7 (7.3)	19.0 (8.0)	25.8 (7.7)	27.2 (6.8)	<0.0001
E gene Ct value, mean (SD)	23.6 (8.1)	17.5 (6.7)	19.2 (8.5)	25.4 (7.5)	26.8 (6.6)	<0.0001
Hemodynamic parameters on admission						
Systolic BP, mean (SD), mmHg	131 (17)	122 (11)	128 (16)	130 (15)	138 (20)	0.0004
Diastolic BP, mean (SD), mmHg	84 (10)	79 (8)	80 (11)	84 (9)	87 (9)	0.0009
Heart rate, mean (SD), beats/min	88 (13)	87 (14)	84 (11)	88 (13)	89 (14)	0.2920
Hemodynamic parameters on discharge						
Systolic BP, mean (SD), mmHg	121 (12)	115 (9)	119 (12)	122 (12)	121 (13)	0.8375
Diastolic BP, mean (SD), mmHg	80 (9)	78 (8)	77 (8)	80 (9)	79 (8)	0.3944
Heart rate, mean (SD), beats/min	82 (12)	79 (13	80 (12)	83 (12)	82 (12)	0.3303
Serum glucose, mean (SD), mmol/L	7.5 (3.0)	6.4 (1.7)	6.6 (2.6)	7.7 (3.5)	7.4 (2.2)	0.3877
Length of stay, mean (SD), days	5.3 (2.9)	4.3 (1.8)	5.2 (4.0)	5.5 (3.0)	5.3 (2.1)	0.4353
Discharge destination						
Home, *n* (%)	47 (19.6)	1 (5.0)	4 (10.3)	31 (25.8)	11 (18.0)	0.1835
Isolation facility, *n* (%)	167 (69.6)	19 (95.0)	35 (89.7)	71 (59.2)	42 (68.9)	
Subacute hospital, *n* (%)	27 (11.2)	0 (0.0)	0 (0.0)	18 (15.0)	9 (14.8)	
Re-admission to hospital, *n* (%)	7 (2.92)	0 (0.0)	2 (5.13)	4 (3.33)	1 (1.64)	0.1569

Data are mean (standard deviations) and number of patients (percentage of total number of patients in each age group). P-values are calculated using single-factor ANOVA and chi-square tests. RT-PCR, reverse-transcriptase polymerase-chain reaction; Ct, cycle threshold; BP, blood pressure.

potassium of 3.3 mmol/L (SD, 0.2 mmol/L), and hyponatremia in 5 patients (2.5%), with a mean serum sodium of 130 mmol/L (SD, 4 mmol/L). Pre-diabetes was associated with higher risk of hyponatremia [odds ratio (OR), 8.83; 95% confidence interval (CI), 1.17–66.6; $P = 0.0342$] and hypokalemia (OR, 4.58; 95% CI, 1.52–13.8; $P = 0.0069$; **Table 5**).

Radiographical Abnormalities

Two hundred and twenty six patients (94.2%) had chest X-rays performed. Twenty patients (8.8%) were found to have infective changes consistent with pneumonia, and six patients (2.7%) had atelectasis. Five patients (2.2%) had lung nodules suggestive of past or active tuberculosis. Further sputum examination did not yield evidence of tuberculosis. Pleural thickening was found in three patients (1.3%), and the patients reported either a significant smoking history or previous occupational exposure to asbestos, albeit while wearing protective equipment. Higher risk of pneumonia was linked to pre-diabetes (OR, 10.8; 95% CI, 3.65–32.1; $P < 0.0001$) and age 50 years or older (OR, 3.13; 95% CI, 1.31–8.41; $P = 0.0116$; **Table 5**).

Antibiotics and Hydroxychloroquine

Of the 34 patients with abnormalities on chest X-ray, 15 patients (44.1%) did not receive antibiotics. Eleven patients (32.4%) received oral amoxicillin/clavulanic acid 1 g twice a day for 7 days and azithromycin 500 mg once a day for 3 days. Five patients (14.7%) received amoxicillin/clavulanic acid 1 g twice a day for 5 days and azithromycin 500 mg once a day for 3 days; 2 (5.9%) received amoxicillin/clavulanic acid 1 g twice a day for 7 days and doxycycline 100 mg twice a day for 7 days; and 1 (2.9%) received amoxicillin/clavulanic acid 1 g twice a day for 7 days. Of the 20 patients that had infective changes on their X-rays, 18 (90.0%) received empirical antibiotics, which was indicated for bacterial co-infection.

Of the 240 patients in the cohort, two patients (0.8%) were transferred to another ward due to worsening laboratory and radiological results, where they received oral hydroxychloroquine

TABLE 2 | Demographics and clinical characteristics, stratified by diagnosis of diabetes mellitus, and pre-diabetes.

	All ($n = 240$)	Diabetes mellitus ($n = 19$)	Pre-diabetes ($n = 21$)	Normal glucose control ($n = 200$)	*P*-value
Age, mean (SD), years	44.2 (8.5)	47.3 (4.7)	47.7 (7.8)	43.5 (8.7)	0.0248
Ethnicity					
Bangladeshi, *n* (%)	86 (35.8)	7 (36.8)	2 (9.5)	77 (38.5)	1.0000
Indian, *n* (%)	70 (29.2)	9 (47.4)	6 (28.6)	55 (27.5)	
Chinese, *n* (%)	66 (27.5)	2 (10.5)	12 (57.1)	52 (26.0)	
Thai, *n* (%)	12 (5.0)	1 (5.3)	1 (4.8)	10 (5.0)	
Others, *n* (%)	6 (2.5)	0 (0.0)	0 (0.0)	6 (3.0)	
Co-morbidity					
Hypertension, *n* (%)	18 (7.5)	2 (10.5)	3 (14.3)	13 (6.5)	0.1058
Hyperlipidemia, *n* (%)	11 (4.6)	3 (15.8)	4 (19.0)	4 (2.0)	0.0005
SARS-CoV-2 RT-PCR statistics					
N gene Ct value, mean (SD)	23.9 (8.3)	30.7 (4.9)	25.8 (7.5)	23.2 (8.3)	0.0062
E gene Ct value, mean (SD)	23.6 (8.1)	30.8 (5.1)	26.8 (7.5)	22.6 (8.0)	0.0006
Hemodynamic parameters on admission					
Systolic BP, mean (SD), mmHg	131 (17)	147 (21)	134 (8)	129 (16)	<0.0001
Diastolic BP, mean (SD), mmHg	84 (10)	92 (9)	85 (8)	83 (10)	<0.0001
Heart rate, mean (SD), beats/min	88 (13)	97 (14)	91 (16)	86 (13)	0.0017
Hemodynamic parameters on discharge					
Systolic BP, mean (SD), mmHg	121 (12)	127 (14)	120 (9)	120 (13)	0.0678
Diastolic BP, mean (SD), mmHg	80 (9)	82 (8)	81 (7)	78 (9)	0.1131
Heart rate, mean (SD), beats/min	82 (12)	86 (11)	84 (11)	82 (12)	0.3197
Serum glucose, mean (SD), mmol/L	7.5 (3.0)	13.8 (5.0)	9.6 (1.5)	6.4 (1.4)	<0.0001
Length of stay, mean (SD), days	5.3 (2.9)	6.3 (2.3)	6.0 (3.1)	5.1 (2.9)	0.1340
Discharge destination					
Home, *n* (%)	47 (19.6)	4 (21.1)	4 (19.0)	39 (19.4)	0.9594
Isolation facility, *n* (%)	167 (69.6)	14 (73.7)	14 (66.7)	139 (69.2)	
Subacute hospital, *n* (%)	27 (11.2)	1 (5.3)	3 (14.3)	23 (11.4)	
Re-admission to hospital, *n* (%)	7 (2.92)	1 (5.3)	0 (0.0)	6 (3.0)	0.5768

Data are mean (standard deviations) and number of patients (percentage of total number of patients in each group). P-values are calculated by comparing three groups (diabetes mellitus, pre-diabetes, and normal glucose control) using single-factor ANOVA and chi–square tests. RT-PCR, reverse-transcriptase polymerase-chain reaction; Ct, cycle threshold; BP, blood pressure.

400 mg twice a day for 1 day then 200 mg twice a day for 4 days. They did not require supplemental oxygen nor intensive care during their admission and were discharged home. One of the patients had pre-diabetes and the other was not diagnosed with pre-diabetes/DM.

Lengths of Stay, Discharge Destinations, and Re-admissions

The mean length of stay (LOS) in the acute hospital ward was 5.3 days (SD, 2.9 days), and patients with DM and pre-diabetes were on average hospitalized for 1 day longer (6.1 days; SD, 2.7 days vs. 5.1 days; SD, 2.9 days; $P = 0.0379$). Seven patients (2.9%) were re-admitted to an acute hospital within 30 days of discharge. Two cases (0.8%) were re-admitted for complications of COVID-19, both of whom were not diagnosed with DM or pre-diabetes, while five cases (2.1%) were re-admitted for other reasons. Fouty seven patients (19.6%) were discharged after testing negative for SARS-CoV-2 on two consecutive days. For the rest of the patients, who tested SARS-CoV-2 PCR positive during their admissions, 166 patients (69.2%) were sent to an isolation facility within the community, and 27 patients (11.3%) were transferred to a subacute community hospital, where they were monitored more closely compared to isolation facilities. There were no mortalities at 30 days. Patients with DM and pre-diabetes did not have a significant difference in re-admission rates at 30 days and discharge destination.

Newly Diagnosed Diseases

Thirteen patients (5.4%) reported that they had a known past medical history on admission. Nine patients reported one co-morbidity and four patients reported multiple co-morbidities, which included type 2 diabetes mellitus in five patients (2.1%), hypertension in seven patients (2.9%), and hyperlipidemia in three patients (1.3%). Other notable past medical issues included work-related injuries (such as hand laceration, blunt trauma to upper limb, and vehicular trauma to knee) in three patients, asthma and ischemic heart disease.

TABLE 3 | Incidence of laboratory and radiographical abnormalities, stratified by age.

	All ages	20 to 29 years	30 to 39 years	40 to 49 years	≥50 years	P-value
Renal panel (*n* = 201)						
Hyponatremia, *n* (%)	5 (2.5)	0 (0.0)	0 (0.0)	2 (1.74)	3 (4.9)	0.0557
Hypokalemia, *n* (%)	20 (10.0)	0 (0.0)	2 (10.0)	10 (8.7)	8 (13.1)	0.0111
Liver function test (*n* = 197)						
Transaminitis, *n* (%)	46 (23.4)	3 (75.0)	5 (27.8)	22 (19.3)	16 (26.2)	<0.0001
ALT >2 times ULN, *n* (%)	7 (3.6)	0 (0.0)	0 (0.0)	4 (3.5)	3 (5.0)	0.0527
Full blood count (*n* = 201)						
All disorders, *n* (%)	44 (21.9)	0 (0.0)	3 (15.0)	29 (25.2)	12 (19.6)	<0.0001
Thrombocytopenia, *n* (%)	8 (4.0)	0 (0.0)	0 (0.0)	7 (6.1)	1 (1.6)	0.0151
Leukopenia, *n* (%)	8 (4.0)	0 (0.0)	0 (0.0)	7 (6.1)	1 (1.6)	0.0151
Anemia, *n* (%)	8 (4.0)	0 (0.0)	0 (0.0)	5 (4.4)	3 (4.9)	0.0418
Polycythemia, *n* (%)	4 (2.0)	0 (0.0)	0 (0.0)	2 (1.7)	2 (3.3)	0.1834
Microcytosis, *n* (%)	15 (7.5)	0 (0.0)	3 (15.0)	7 (6.1)	5 (8.2)	0.0015
Macrocytosis, *n* (%)	1 (0.5)	0 (0.0)	0 (0.0)	1 (0.9)	0 (0.0)	0.6213
Chest X-ray (*n* = 226)						
Infective changes, *n* (%)	20 (8.9)	0 (0.0)	2 (6.9)	8 (6.7)	10 (16.4)	0.0010
Atelectasis, *n* (%)	6 (2.7)	0 (0.0)	0 (0.0)	1 (0.8)	5 (8.2)	0.0004
Nodules, granulomata, *n* (%)	5 (2.2)	0 (0.0)	0 (0.0)	5 (4.2)	0 (0.0)	0.0391
Pleural thickening/scarring, *n* (%)	3 (1.3)	0 (0.0)	0 (0.0)	1 (0.8)	2 (3.3)	0.1268

Data are number of patients (percentage of the total number of patients tested in each group). P-values are calculated by comparing all four age groups using chi-square tests. ALT, alanine aminotransferase; ULN, upper limit of normal.

TABLE 4 | Incidence of laboratory and radiographical abnormalities stratified by diagnosis of diabetes mellitus and pre-diabetes.

	All	Diabetes mellitus	Pre-diabetes	Normal glucose control	P-value
Renal panel (*n* = 201)					
Hyponatremia, *n* (%)	5 (2.5)	1 (5.2)	2 (9.5)	2 (1.2)	0.1119
Hypokalemia, *n* (%)	20 (10.0)	1 (5.3)	6 (28.6)	13 (8.0)	0.0236
Liver function test (*n* = 197)					
Transaminitis, *n* (%)	46 (23.4)	7 (36.8)	2 (9.5)	37 (18.5)	0.0631
ALT >2 times ULN, *n* (%)	7 (3.6)	3 (15.8)	1 (4.8)	3 (1.5)	0.0238
Full blood count (*n* = 201)					
Thrombocytopenia, *n* (%)	8 (4.0)	1 (5.3)	2 (9.5)	5 (3.1)	0.2685
Leukopenia, *n* (%)	8 (4.0)	0 (0.0)	3 (14.3)	5 (3.1)	0.0988
Anemia, *n* (%)	8 (4.0)	0 (0.0)	2 (9.5)	6 (3.7)	0.3680
Chest X-ray (*n* = 226)					
Infective changes, *n* (%)	20 (8.9)	2 (10.5)	8 (38.1)	10 (5.4)	0.0001
Atelectasis, *n* (%)	6 (2.7)	0 (0.0)	1 (4.8)	5 (2.7)	0.6604

Data are number of patients (percentage of the total number of patients tested in each group). P-values are calculated by comparing three groups (diabetes mellitus, pre-diabetes and normal glucose control) using chi-square tests. ALT, alanine aminotransferase; ULN, upper limit of normal.

TABLE 5 | Association between age, diabetes mellitus, and pre-diabetes with complications of COVID-19.

	Diabetes mellitus	P-value	Pre-diabetes	P-value	Age ≥50 years	P-value
Pneumonia, OR (95% CI)	2.07 (0.42–10.2)	0.3783	10.8 (3.65–32.1)	<0.0001	3.13 (1.31–8.41)	0.0116
Hyponatremia, OR (95% CI)	4.67 (0.40–54.3)	0.2194	8.83 (1.17–66.6)	0.0342	3.57 (0.58–21.9)	0.1703
Hypokalemia, OR (95% CI)	0.64 (0.07–5.16)	1.2571	4.58 (1.52–13.82)	0.0069	1.62 (0.63–4.20)	0.3227
Transaminitis, OR (95% CI)	1.88 (0.69–5.11)	0.2206	0.339 (0.08–1.52)	1.2006	1.24 (0.62–2.50)	0.5516

Data are odds ratios (95% confidence intervals), calculated using binomial logistic regression. Diabetes mellitus and pre-diabetes are compared to normal glucose control (OR = 1). Age 50 and greater is compared to age <50 (OR = 1). OR, odds ratio; CI, confidence interval.

In total, 70 patients (29.2%) in the cohort were diagnosed with either a chronic disease or another concomitant disease during their hospitalization (**Supplementary Table 1**). Newly diagnosed metabolic diseases include pre-diabetes in 21 patients (8.8%), type 2 diabetes mellitus in 14 patients (5.8%), hypertension in eleven patients (4.6%) and hyperlipidemia in eight patients (2.9%). The majority of the patients with chronic diseases were previously unaware of their diagnoses: 73.7% for diabetes mellitus, 61.1% for hypertension and 72.7% for hyperlipidemia (**Table 6**).

DISCUSSION

To our knowledge, this is the first analysis that investigated the clinical complications of COVID-19 and the associated burden of undiagnosed chronic disease among international migrant workers. Notably the prevalence of previously undiagnosed DM among international migrant workers is 5.8%, which is two times higher than the prevalence of undiagnosed DM among Singapore residents (2.9%) (24, 25). Even though the prevalence of hyperlipidemia (7.5 vs. 33.6%) and hypertension (5.8 vs. 21.5%) are lower in our cohort of migrant workers compared to Singapore residents, the unawareness rates are higher among migrant workers: 72.7 vs. 40.9% for hyperlipidemia, and 61.1 vs. 43.9% for hypertension (24, 25). Interestingly, our analysis shows that pre-diabetes, which is more prevalent than DM in Singapore (14.4 vs. 8.6%) (25), increases the risk of pneumonia and electrolyte abnormalities with COVID-19, indicative of more severe lung and kidney involvement. Pre-diabetes might have conferred a greater risk for pneumonia and electrolyte abnormalities than DM because, unlike patients with DM, patients with pre-diabetes were not started on pre-meal capillary blood glucose monitoring, subcutaneous sliding-scale insulin or oral hypoglycemic agents to control their blood glucose levels during their hospitalizations. Furthermore, patients with DM or pre-diabetes contract COVID-19 with lower viral RNA levels, which suggests a lower threshold for infection for both DM and pre-diabetes.

Therefore, clinicians should be encouraged to screen migrant workers for chronic diseases, in particular for DM, which increases the risk of developing severe infections, and has devastating systemic complications if not adequately treated at an early stage. Moreover, public health policies targeting migrant workers should encompass metabolic diseases, which we found to be largely undiagnosed in the migrant community compared to the resident population. For instance, most migrant workers in Singapore already incur considerable debt due to expensive fees charged by employment agencies in their home countries and are not entitled to health care subsidies afforded to Singapore residents (4). While employers of migrant workers in Singapore are required to maintain medical insurance coverage of at least $15,000 for hospitalization and day surgery costs (28), healthcare accessibility, and affordability may be improved through the extension of the mandatory insurance scheme to include preventative, primary, and outpatient care. Accessible, affordable, and appropriate heath care and insurance coverage would ensure that both chronic and acute diseases are detected and treated adequately.

Even though serious complications of COVID-19 were less prevalent in our cohort, possibly due in part to the younger demographic profile, we found significant incidental findings such as pulmonary tuberculosis, lung nodules, and pleural thickening on chest X-rays. As occupational respiratory illnesses and pulmonary tuberculosis were more prevalent among migrant workers, contributed by crowded living conditions, high stress levels, long working hours, and occupational exposure to hazardous substances (1, 4), our review suggests that screening chest X-rays might be relevant for this vulnerable population. Moreover, the COVID-19 outbreak among migrant workers also highlights the importance of improving the living and working conditions of migrant workers, to reduce the incidence of infective and occupational lung disease.

Antibiotic use was also appropriate in our study. In total, 19 of 240 (7.9%) hospitalized patients in our cohort received antibiotics for superimposed bacterial infections, which is similar to the prevalence of bacterial coinfection among hospitalized COVID-19 patients worldwide (29). Notably, a literature review of studies of hospitalized COVID-19 patients determined that while 72% of hospitalized patients received antibiotics, only 8% had evidence of superimposed bacterial or fungal coinfection (29). Responsible antimicrobial stewardship would prevent the emergence of untreatable drug-resistant pathogens that could lead to another public health emergency (30), and prompt control of blood glucose levels may prevent overuse of antibiotics by attenuating the effects of hyperglycemia on the severity of COVID-19.

This review has a number of limitations. First, our cohort of 240 migrant workers is a small subset of the population of international migrant workers in Singapore who developed COVID-19, and its demographics are limited to male migrant workers aged from 21 to 65 years with mild to moderate COVID-19 on admission. To our knowledge, this is the first analysis of COVID-19 among hospitalized international migrant workers. Hence, we are unable to compare our cohort to other cohorts of international migrant workers in Singapore or in other countries. Second, some demographic data, such as body mass index (BMI) and length of DM in patients diagnosed before admission, are not available from our data set. Third, another limitation is the lack of a similar-sized comparison group consisting of patients in the resident population. Therefore, we had to use previously published reports to compare the prevalence of chronic diseases. Fourth, since this is a retrospective review based on a brief stay in an acute hospital, and the vast majority of the patients do not have past medical records in the Singapore health system, we are unable to ascertain if some of the laboratory abnormalities are due to COVID-19 itself or an underlying chronic condition (such as thalassemia trait causing microcytosis or chronic liver disease causing transaminitis). Moving forward, a prospective cohort study that follows up on these patients' laboratory abnormalities would enable us to better understand these abnormalities. More ambitiously, a national or international database comprising both resident and migrant

TABLE 6 | Prevalence of chronic diseases.

	All ages (*n* = 240)	20 to 29 years (*n* = 20)	30 to 39 years (*n* = 39)	40 to 49 years (*n* = 120)	≥ 50 years (*n* = 61)	*P*-value
Pre-diabetes						
Total, *n* (%)	21 (8.8)	1 (5.0)	2 (5.1)	9 (7.5)	9 (14.8)	0.0601
Previously known, *n* (%)	0 (0.0)	0 (0.0)	0 (0.0)	0 (0.0)	0 (0.0)	Not applicable
Newly diagnosed, *n* (%)	21 (8.8)	1 (5.0)	2 (5.1)	9 (7.5)	9 (14.8)	0.0601
Diabetes mellitus						
Total, *n* (%)	19 (7.9)	0 (0.0)	1 (2.6)	12 (10.0)	6 (9.8)	0.0057
Previously known, *n* (%)	5 (2.1)	0 (0.0)	0 (0.0)	4 (3.3)	1 (1.6)	0.1710
Newly diagnosed, *n* (%)	14 (5.8)	0 (0.0)	1 (2.6)	8 (6.7)	5 (8.2)	0.0329
Hypertension						
Total, *n* (%)	18 (7.5)	0 (0.0)	3 (7.7)	7 (5.8)	8 (13.1)	0.0071
Previously known, *n* (%)	7 (2.9)	0 (0.0)	0 (0.0)	4 (3.3)	3 (4.9)	0.0639
Newly diagnosed, *n* (%)	11 (4.6)	0 (0.0)	3 (7.7)	3 (2.5)	5 (8.2)	0.0148
Hyperlipidemia						
Total, *n* (%)	11 (4.6)	0 (0.0)	2 (5.1)	4 (3.3)	5 (8.2)	0.0495
Previously known, *n* (%)	3 (1.3)	0 (0.0)	0 (0.0)	2 (1.7)	1 (1.6)	0.4301
Newly diagnosed, *n* (%)	8 (3.3)	0 (0.0)	2 (5.1)	2 (1.7)	4 (6.6)	0.0411

Data are number of patients (percentage of total number of patients in each age group). P-values are calculated using chi–squared tests.

COVID-19 cases would enable us to determine which factors and treatments may affect health outcomes in migrant workers with COVID-19 infections.

In conclusion, this retrospective review demonstrates that there is a significant burden of undiagnosed chronic diseases, in particular metabolic diseases such as pre-diabetes and diabetes mellitus, in migrant populations. Since many of these chronic diseases benefit from early treatment, screening of asymptomatic individuals should be extended to migrant populations. Moreover, our analysis suggests that migrant workers with DM and pre-diabetes are at a higher risk of developing complications of COVID-19 despite having lower viral RNA levels, alerting clinicians to consider screening for pneumonia and electrolyte abnormalities in this vulnerable group. Importantly, this report reinforces the public health axiom that "a community is only as strong as its weakest link," and public health policies should advocate for improved living and working conditions for neglected groups such as migrant workers, to protect the health and well-being of all.

AUTHOR CONTRIBUTIONS

BR, LT, SA, JT, and TO conceived and designed the study. BR, LT, SA, JT, TO, and PG collected the data. BR, LT, and SA did the data and statistical analyses. BR, LT, SA, JC, ST, AS, SH, RF, JK, TP, and WL did the data interpretation. LT and BR wrote the manuscript. All authors contributed to the article and approved the submitted version.

REFERENCES

1. Hargreaves S, Rustage K, Nellums LB, McAlpine A, Pocock N, Devakumar D, et al. Occupational health outcomes among international migrant workers: a systematic review and meta-analysis. *Lancet Glob Health.* (2019) 7:e872–82. doi: 10.1016/S2214-109X(19)30204-9
2. Ang JW, Koh CJ, Chua BWB, Narayanaswamy S, Wijaya L, Chan LG, et al. Are migrant workers in Singapore receiving adequate healthcare? A survey of doctors working in public tertiary healthcare institutions. *Singapore Med J.* (2019) 61:540–7. doi: 10.11622/smedj.2019101
3. Ang JW, Chia C, Koh CJ, Chua BWB, Narayanaswamy S, Wijaya L, et al. Healthcare-seeking behaviour, barriers and mental health of non-domestic migrant workers in Singapore. *BMJ Glob Health.* (2017) 2:e000213. doi: 10.1136/bmjgh-2016-000213
4. Sadarangani SP, Lim PL, Vasoo S. Infectious diseases and migrant worker health in singapore: a receiving country's perspective. *J Travel Med.* (2017) 24:1–9. doi: 10.1093/jtm/tax014
5. Wang P, Lu JA, Jin Y, Zhu M, Wang L, Chen S. Statistical and network analysis of 1212 COVID-19 patients in Henan, China. *Int J Infect Dis.* (2020) 95:391–8. doi: 10.1016/j.ijid.2020.04.051
6. Ministry of Health, Singapore. *COVID-19 Situation Report.* (2020). Available online at: https://covidsitrep.moh.gov.sg (accessed July 2, 2020).
7. Ministry of Manpower, Singapore. *Foreign Workforce Numbers.* (2020). Available online at: https://www.mom.gov.sg/documents-and-publications/foreign-workforce-numbers (accessed July 2, 2020).
8. Bode B, Garett V, Messler J, McFarland R, Crowe J, Booth R, et al. Glycemic characteristics and clinical outcomes of COVID-19 patients hospitalized in the United States. *J Diabetes Sci Technol.* (2020) 14:813–21. doi: 10.1177/1932296820924469
9. Iacobellis G, Penaherrera CA, Bermudez LE, Mizrachi EB. Admission hyperglycemia and radiological findings of SARS-CoV2 in patients with and without diabetes. *Diabetes Res Clin Pract.* (2020) 164:108185. doi: 10.1016/j.diabres.2020.108185
10. Guan W, Ni Z, Hu Y, Liang W, Ou C, He J, et al. Clinical characteristics of coronavirus disease 2019 in China. *N Engl J Med.* (2020) 382:1708–20. doi: 10.1101/2020.02.06.20020974
11. Wang D, Hu B, Hu C, Zhu F, Liu X, Zhang J, et al. Clinical characteristics of 138 hospitalized patients with 2019 novel coronavirus–infected pneumonia in Wuhan, China. *JAMA.* (2020) 323:1061–9. doi: 10.1001/jama.2020.1585

12. Bhatraju PK, Ghassemieh BJ, Nichols M, Kim R, Jerone KR, Nalla AK, et al. Covid-19 in critically ill patients in the Seattle region—case series. *N Engl J Med.* (2020) 382:2012–22. doi: 10.1056/NEJMoa2004500
13. Zhou F, Yu T, Du R, Fan G, Liu Y, Liu Z, et al. Clinical course and risk factors for mortality of adult inpatients with COVID-19 in Wuhan, China: a retrospective cohort study. *Lancet.* (2020) 395:1054–62. doi: 10.1016/S0140-6736(20)30566-3
14. Walls AC, Park YJ, Tortorici MA, Wall A, McGuire AT, Veesler D. Structure, function, and antigenicity of the SARS-CoV-2 spike glycoprotein. *Cell.* (2020) 181:281–92.e6. doi: 10.1101/2020.02.19.956581
15. Brufsky A. Hyperglycemia, hydroxychloroquine, and the COVID-19 pandemic. *J Med Virol.* (2020) 92:770–5. doi: 10.1002/jmv.25887
16. Puelles VG, Lütgehetmann M, Lindenmeyer MT, Sperhake, JP, Wong MN, et al. Multiorgan and renal tropism of SARS-CoV-2. *N Engl J Med.* (2020) 383:590–2. doi: 10.1056/NEJMc2011400
17. Lippi G, South AM, Henry BM. Electrolyte imbalances in patients with severe coronavirus disease 2019 (COVID-19). *Ann Clin Biochem.* (2020) 57:262–5. doi: 10.1177/0004563220922255
18. Ahmed MZ, Khakwani M, Venkatadasari I, Horgan C, Giles H, Jobanputra S, et al. Thrombocytopenia as an initial manifestation of COVID-19; case series and literature review. *Br J Haematol.* (2020) 189:1057–8. doi: 10.1111/bjh.16769
19. Lazarian G, Quinquenel A, Bellal M, Siavellis J, Jacquy C, Re D, et al. Autoimmune hemolytic anemia associated with covid-19 infection. *Br J Haematol.* (2020) 190:24–39. doi: 10.1111/bjh.16794
20. Terpos E, Ntanasis-Stathopoulos I, Elalamy I, Kastritis E, Sergentanis TN, Politou M, et al. Hematological findings and complications of COVID-19. *Am J Hematol.* (2020) 95:834–47. doi: 10.1002/ajh.25829
21. Feng G, Zheng KI, Yan QQ, Rios RS, Targher G, Byrne CD, et al. COVID-19 and liver dysfunction: current insights and emergent therapeutic strategies. *J Clin Transl Hepatol.* (2020) 8:18–24. doi: 10.14218/JCTH.2020.00018
22. Ceriello A. Hyperglycemia and the worse prognosis of COVID-19. Why a fast blood glucose control should be mandatory. *Diabetes Res Clin Pract.* (2020) 163:108186. doi: 10.1016/j.diabres.2020.108186
23. American Diabetes Association. Classification and diagnosis of diabetes: standards of medical care in diabetes-2019. *Diabetes Care.* (2019) 42(Suppl. 1):S13–28. doi: 10.2337/dc19-S002
24. Man REK, Gan AHW, Fenwick EK, Gan ATL, Gupta P, Sabanayagam C, et al. Prevalence, determinants and association of unawareness of diabetes, hypertension and hypercholesterolemia with poor disease control in a multi-ethnic Asian population without cardiovascular disease. *Popul Health Metr.* (2019) 17:17. doi: 10.1186/s12963-019-0197-5
25. Ministry of Health, Singapore. *National Population Health Survey 2016/17.* Singapore: Ministry of Health (2018).
26. James PA, Oparil S, Carter BL, Cushman WC, Dennison-Himmelfarb C, Handler J, et al. 2014 evidence-based guideline for the management of high blood pressure in adults: report from the panel members appointed to the eighth joint national committee (JNC 8). *JAMA.* (2014) 311:507–20. doi: 10.1001/jama.2013.284427
27. Arnett DK, Blumenthal RS, Albert MA, Buroker AB, Goldberger ZD, Hahn EJ, et al. 2019 ACC/AHA guideline on the primary prevention of cardiovascular disease: a report of the American college of cardiology/American heart association task force on clinical practice guidelines. *Circulation.* (2019) 140:e596–646. doi: 10.1161/CIR.0000000000000725
28. Ministry of Manpower, Singapore. *Medical Insurance Requirements for Foreign Workers.* (2020). Available online at: https://www.mom.gov.sg/passes-and-permits/work-permit-for-foreign-worker/sector-specific-rules/medical-insurance (accessed July 2, 2020).
29. Rawson TM, Moore LSP, Zhu N, Ranganathan N, Skolimowska K, Gilchrist M, et al. Bacterial and fungal co-infection in individuals with coronavirus: a rapid review to support COVID-19 antimicrobial prescribing. *Clin Infect Dis.* (2020) 530:1–10. doi: 10.1093/cid/ciaa530
30. Getahun H, Smith I, Trivedi K, Paulin S, Balkhy HH. Tackling antimicrobial resistance in the COVID-19 pandemic. *Bull World Health Organ.* (2020) 98:4442–2A. doi: 10.2471/BLT.20.268573

5

Physiological and Immunological Causes of the Susceptibility of Chronic Inflammatory Patients to COVID-19 Infection: Focus on Diabetes

Nasim Rahmani-Kukia[1] *and Ardeshir Abbasi*[2*]

[1] Department of Biochemistry, School of Medicine, Shiraz University of Medical Sciences, Shiraz, Iran, [2] Department of Immunology, Faculty of Medical Sciences, Tarbiat Modares University, Tehran, Iran

Correspondence:
Ardeshir Abbasi
Ardeshir.abbasi66@gmail.com

The coronavirus disease 2019 (COVID-19) pandemic has recently emerged, which was then spread rapidly in more than 190 countries worldwide so far. According to the World Health Organization, 3,232,062 global cases of COVID-19 were confirmed on April 30th with a mortality rate of 3.4%. Notably, the symptoms are almost similar to those of flu such as fever, cough, and fatigue. Unfortunately, the global rates of morbidity and mortality caused by this disease are more and still increasing on a daily basis. The rates for patients suffering from inflammatory diseases like diabetes, is even further, due to their susceptibility to the pathogenesis of COVID-19. In this review, we attempted to focus on diabetes to clarify the physiological and immunological characteristics of diabetics before and after the infection with COVID-19. We hope these conceptions could provide a better understanding of the mechanisms involved in COVID-19 susceptibility and increase the awareness of risk to motivate behavior changes in vulnerable people for enhancing the prevention. Up to now, the important role of immune responses, especially the innate ones, in the development of the worst signs in COVID-19 infection have been confirmed. Therefore, to better control patients with COVID-19, it is recommended to consider a history of chronic inflammatory diseases as well as the way of controlling immune response in these patients.

Keywords: COVID-19, diabetes, ACE2, chronic inflammatory disease, immune responses

INTRODUCTION AND EPIDEMIOLOGY OF COVID-19

In December 2019, an unknown pneumonia was identified in Wuhan, China. In past years, two pneumonia-related to coronaviruses have been appeared with the name of severe acute respiratory syndrome coronavirus (SARS-CoV) in 2002 and as Middle East respiratory syndrome coronavirus (MERS-CoV) in 2012, which infected nearly 8,422 and 1,600 people and resulted in 916 and 574 individuals' death, respectively (1, 2). Chinese scientists identified new coronavirus on January 7th as

SARS-CoV-2 (3). Afterward, the World Health Organization (WHO) in February 2020 named it coronavirus disease 2019 (COVID-19) (4). The clinical spectrum of SARS-CoV-2 is similar to SARS, which includes systemic infection, respiratory tract involvement, and pneumonia associated with respiratory failure and eventually death (5). Moreover, the most important symptoms of this infection are fever, cough, and fatigue. COVID-19 has been rapidly spread in more than 200 countries worldwide and the rates of its morbidity and mortality are globally increasing on a daily basis. In this regard, WHO has reported 3,232,062 cases of COVID-19 up to April 30th 2020 and confirmed 3.4% mortality rate worldwide. These mortality rates vary due to geographical location, age, and other factors in different countries (6). The comorbidity of chronic diseases such as hypertension, diabetes, and cardiovascular and respiratory diseases can increase the risk of severity and mortality in a way that these susceptibilities can be associated with the pathogenesis of COVID-19 infection. Notably, chronic diseases have several common features such as inflammatory state, immune response complications, and a higher susceptibility to infectious diseases. In a systematic study performed in February 25, 2020 on 46,248 patients, the average age to be affected by COVID-19 was shown 48 years old with the clinical symptoms of cough (86–97%), fever (59–76%), fatigue (34–68%), and shortness of breath (21–40%). Moreover, in terms of comorbidity, the prevalence rates for severe COVID-19 were as follows: hypertension (22–24%), diabetes (6–11%), cardiovascular disease (4–7%), and respiratory system diseases (1–3%), which are higher compared to non-severe patients (7). In another study conducted on 1,527 COVID-19 patients with chronic diseases, the comorbid conditions were hypertension (17.1%), cardiovascular disease (16.4%), and diabetes (9.7%) (8). In addition, on 637 MERS-CoV patients, a 50% prevalence rate for both diabetes and hypertension was verified (9). Out of 41 cases of COVID-19 in Wuhan-China, 20% of patients had diabetes comorbidity (10). Therefore, comorbidity of diabetes mellitus is one of the most common COVID-19-related death responsiveness. Since understanding the causes of high susceptibility to COVID-19 can guide the vulnerable population to evaluate the infection risk and sever outcomes, the aim of this study is to review the role of diabetes in facilitating the improvement of COVID-19.

DIABETES AND COVID-19

Diabetes as a complex metabolic and maybe an inflammatory disorder is characterized by hyperglycemia. If hyperglycemia prolongs for a long time, pro-inflammatory responses can be triggered, especially in macrophages. This can enhance the risk of diabetes-associated complications (such as cardiovascular and heart diseases), and being infected and seriously ill from infections (11). Diabetes is pathologically classified into type 1 (T1D) and type 2 (T2D). However, regardless of the type of diabetes, the severity of illness differs according to the age, complications, and how well it is controlled. It has been documented that old aged patients with pre-existing comorbidities (obesity, hypertension, heart disease, etc.), uncontrolled diabetes, and high inflammatory factors are more disposed to severe illness from COVID-19 and even display a high mortality rate from it (12). However, the interaction between diabetes and COVID-19 is reciprocal. As people with diabetes are more susceptible to COVID-19, infection with SARS-CoV-2 also can exacerbate the dysglycemia, inflammatory responses, and diabetic complications such as diabetic ketoacidosis (13) and hypokalemia, which increase the risk of being critically ill (14).

On the other hand, obesity as a general comorbidity with diabetes, improves the systemic chronic inflammation by affecting the both innate and adaptive immune systems as well as the level of IL-6 and even TNF-α (15). It has been indicated that both diabetes and obesity can prompt the cytokine storm (16) and also impair the coagulation system and thrombotic mechanisms (17), which are also identified in COVID-19 (18). Therefore, infection with SARS-CoV-2 in these patients can exacerbate the pre-existent pro-inflammatory condition, which in turn can improve the cytokine storm as well as several organ dysfunctions. Therefore, the following guidelines (**Table 1**) are recommended to be considered in patients:

TABLE 1 | Regarding for Diabetics and people with chronic diseases before and during comorbidity with COVID-19.

Subject	Description Subject	Reference
Hyperglycemia	Hyperglycemia can increase the risk of severe outcomes resulting from COVID-19, the length of hospitalization, and even the risk of death, which can be reduced by glycemic control.	(19, 20)
Nutrition	Due to the same nutrition of comorbidity diabetic patients with COVID-19 and other COVID-19 patients, careful attention should be paid to nutrition, minerals, proteins, and vitamins in these patients.	(21)
Exercise	Lack of exercise can reduce the immune response of these patients; therefore, a proper indoor exercise is needed to regulate and strengthen the immune system in the patients affected by COVID-19.	(22)
Vaccination	Because of similarities in the functional mechanism of both flu and COVID-19 infections, vaccination may reduce the risk of COVID-19. This suggestion is supported by a study performed on 91,605 diabetics after the flu vaccination, and reported a reduction in the prevalence rate of pneumonia by 55% in patients over the age of 65 years old and by 43% in those under the age of 65 years old. COVID-19 also has some flu-like complications (such as fever, cough, and fatigue), which may be reduced to some extent by flu vaccination.	(23–25)
Stress	Stress in comorbidity diabetic patients with COVID-19 increases blood sugar level and exacerbates mortality in these patients. Therefore, anxiety and stress should be controlled and also reduced.	(26–28)
Pancreatic tissue	Pancreatic tissue is known as a potential target for viral in patients, leading to the impaired glucose metabolism. In COVID-19, damage to this tissue is better to be considered.	(29, 30)

ASSOCIATION BETWEEN ANGIOTENSIN-CONVERTING ENZYME 2 AND COVID-19

Angiotensin-converting enzyme 2 (ACE2) is a membrane aminopeptidase presented on the surface of cardiovascular, kidney, intestinal, immune, and lung endothelial cells. ACE2 can degrade angiotensin II and produce angiotensin 1-7. Angiotensin 1-7 unlike angiotensin II has anti-oxidant, anti-fibrotic, and anti-inflammatory properties as well as vasodilatory activity. Therefore, ACE2 can protect the lung from severe respiratory injuries like acute respiratory distress syndrome (ARDS) caused by COVID-19. ACE2 is also identified as a functional receptor and target for SARS-CoV and SARS-CoV-2 (31, 32). Correspondingly, the molecular modeling has revealed some similarities between these two coronavirus receptors (33). Thus, one way of viral infection is the pneumonia caused by the binding of virus to ACE2 on the surface of lung epithelial cells (18). Throughout SARS-CoV-2 entrance, ACE2 becomes downregulated, which consequently results in a high ACE/ACE2 ratio contributing to the progression of pre-exciting pro-inflammatory responses and subsequently worsen outcomes from COVID-19 (34). Indeed, the expression of ACE2 becomes down regulated in diabetics as a consequence of the glycosylation process, which might be considered as a contributory factor for the severity of lung complications in comorbidity with SARS-CoV-2 invasion (35). Likewise, the ratio of ACE/ACE2 is found to be significantly higher in diabetics compared to healthy controls. Moreover, the relationship among ACE/ACE2 level and the increased blood pressure, fasting blood glucose, serum creatinine, and hemoglobin A1c (HbA1c) has also been demonstrated (36). As a result, it seems that there is a correlation between ACE2 level and susceptibility to COVID-19 in diabetic, which is highly debatable, so it should be considered in these patients.

IMMUNE CELLS IN DIABETIC PATIENTS

The balance among immune cells is essential for preserving homeostasis and the best performance of immune responses, however this balance can be impaired in diabetics. Several studies have revealed the increased pathological function of TCD4 cells in obesity, insulin resistance, and diabetes. TCD4 effector cells can be divided into inflammatory [T helper1 (Th1) and Th17) and anti-inflammatory (Th2 and regulatory Th (Treg)] cells with their specific cytokine secretions (37). It has been demonstrated that in adipose tissue and peripheral blood of diabetic patients, CD4 cells tend to be polarized into Th1 and Th17 inflammatory cells. However, the anti-inflammatory polarization of Th2 and its secreted cytokines (IL-4, IL-5, and IL-13) is reduced (37, 38). Moreover, in diabetes, it has been found that the Th1/Th2 ratio and the level of the related cytokines (IL-4, IL-10, IL-13, and IFN-γ) become remarkably high, whereas the anti-oxidant level decreases (39). On the other hand, it has been proved that the increased cytokine production by Th1 (IFN-γ, IL-2, TNF-α, and TNF-β) and Th17 (IL-6, IL-17A, and IL-17F) in diabetics can affect the HbA1c level (40).

Treg as a regulator of immune responses, constitutes about 5–20% of overall CD4 cells which is characterized by CD4, CD25, and Foxp3. Moreover, Treg plays a very essential role in suppressing T effector cells, inflammatory responses, and protecting against autoimmunity (41, 42). The activation of these cells leads to the secretion of IL-10, and TGF-β as well as the expression of co-inhibitory molecule cytotoxic T lymphocyte antigen-4 (CTLA-4) on their surface in order to inactivate the T effector cells. It has been shown that Treg is decreased in diabetes (43). Furthermore, the balance between Treg and Th1 or Th17 is very important in diabetic patients. Because, the balance between Treg/Th17 and Treg/Th1 ratio decrease in patients suffering from T2D (44). T $CD8^+$ is also activated against infection and by releasing IFN-γ and TNF-α cytokines, which consequently increases the antiviral responses. However, an elevation in the level of T $CD8^+$ has been verified in diabetes (45).

Gamma delta T (Tγδ) cells also play an important role in generating chronic inflammation by secreting cytokines (like IFN-γ and TNF-α) and affecting the function of other immune cells such as macrophages, cytotoxic T lymphocytes, Th1, Th2, Treg, and Th17 cells in the diabetics (46). It has been proved that natural killer t (NKT) cells which produce some cytokines such as IL-4 and IFN-γ are decreased in diabetic patients. Reduction of NKT cells leads to increase in the level of M1 macrophages, insulin resistance, and glucose intolerance (47). In addition, the enhancement of B cells, which play key roles in the development of insulin resistance following the production of IgG, activations of macrophages and T cells have been demonstrated in diabetes (48). NK cells, as a type of immune cells are divided into the following two subsets based on CD56 marker: dim and bright. $CD56^{dim}$ NK cells have cytotoxic effects, while, $CD56^{bright}$ ones are more likely to produce pro-inflammatory cytokines. In chronic inflammatory diseases like diabetes, $CD56^{bright}$ NK cells are dominant which, release more inflammatory cytokines (49).

Changes in the myeloid cells such as macrophages, monocytes, neutrophils, eosinophils, and basophils happen in diabetic patients as well. It has been revealed that most macrophages in the adipose tissue of diabetics are M1 macrophages, which play key functions during the pathological processes by secreting TNF-α and triggering chronic inflammation in these patients (50). Additionally, the elevation of monocytes, as effective cells on the reduction of neutrophils and eosinophils numbers as well as on the development of inflammation is perceived in diabetics (51, 52). This imbalance in the immune system of diabetics increases their susceptibility to viral pneumonia as shown in **Figure 1**. An obvious pro-inflammatory Th1 and Th17 responses was detected in the cytokine profile of SARS patients with diabetes. Similarly a significant increase has been identified in IFN-γ and IL-17A level in the lungs of patients infected with MERS-CoV and diabetes (53, 54). Therefore, it seems that any imbalance in the immune responses can increase people's susceptibility to viral infections.

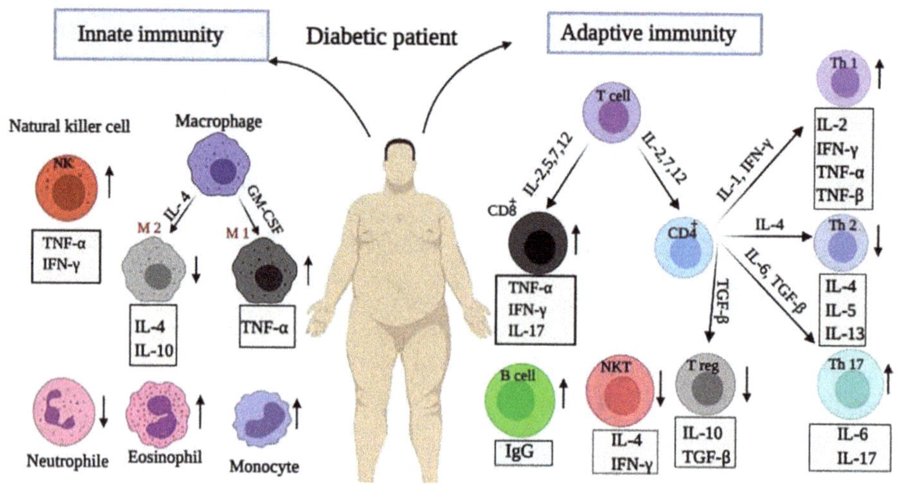

FIGURE 1 | Immunological alteration in diabetic patients. Immune responses change during diabetices. Changes in innate immunity include: increase in the plasma levels of macrophages, NK cells and eosinophils, as well as their secreted cytokines with a reduction in the number of neutrophils. Moreover, adaptive immunity changes included: enhancement in Th1, Th17, $TCD8^{+}$ cells, and released cytokines whereas reduction in Th2, Treg, and NKT cells.

IMMUNE RESPONSE IN COVID-19 INFECTION

Immune responses to COVID-19 can be divided into two phases as follows: non-severe and severe. At non-sever response, immune system tries to eliminate the virus by IFN-I (α/β) and avoids the stage's progression to the severe phase. At severe response, inflammation arises in the lung, which may be due to impaired IFN-I regulation. Overproduction of IFN-I increases the penetration of neutrophils, macrophages, and inflammatory factors into the lung, which is then followed by cytokine storm syndrome, as well (**Figure 2**). Since chronic inflammation is generated in the body of patients with chronic diseases like diabetes, the balance of the immune system becomes dis-regulated and the inflammatory state potentially perseveres. In this situation, the numbers of Th1, Th17, M1 macrophage, NK cells (most in the affected area are probably $CD56^{bright}$) and their secreted inflammatory cytokines increase. Moreover, the negative regulation of Treg and its secreted cytokines is decreased, which result in the loss of control and homeostasis of immune responses. All of these can heighten the diabetic patients' susceptibility to severe COVID-19. On the other hand, SARS-CoV-2 invasion to lung enhances the influx of activated neutrophils and macrophages. An increase in the content of activated immune cells at the site of infection and their released inflammatory cytokines triggers cytokine storm. Subsequently, serious pathological complications induced in the patients' lung can worsen the illness from COVID-19 and even terminate the life. This phenomenon is supported by some clinical studies. Accordingly, experimental findings of a study on patients with severe COVID-19 infection in China showed an elevation in neutrophils level and reduction in lymphocytes, monocytes, eosinophils, and basophils, which are followed by a sharp increase in the pro-inflammatory cytokines profile. Besides, the B, T, NK cells, and Treg depletion have been observed in patients compared to normal cases (55). Moreover, there was an increase in the plasma levels of IL-2, IL-7, IL-10, GCSF, interferon gamma-induced protein 10 (IP-10), monocyte chemoattractant protein-1 (MCP-1), macrophage inflammatory protein 1-alpha (MIP1-α), and TNFα in ICU patients (10). High concentrations of IL-1β, IFN-γ, IP-10, and MCP-1 in COVID-19 patients have also been detected (10, 56). Notably, patients who were in the ICU had higher inflammatory factors (that can be associated with cytokine storm in severe patients) compared to other patients. These clinical findings indicated that lymphocytopenia in COVID-19 patients may be due to cytokine storm (IL-1, IL-6, and TNF-α) as well as pathological effects of leukocytes and macrophages. Overall, it can be suggested that innate immune responses are extremely involved in COVID-19 infection and these points can be considered for the treatment of COVID-19 patients with co-existence of other diseases to better control the innate immune responses.

THE EFFECTS OF SOME ANTIDIABETIC DRUGS ON COVID-19

Considering the above-mentioned main points stating that the immune cells pattern changes to pro-inflammatory one with high level of IL-1 and TNF-α during a long-term hyperglycemia and regarding amplified immune responses to SARS-CoV-2 invasion in the lung of COVID-19 patients, this question arises that whether antidiabetic drugs with anti-inflammatory, anti-fibrotic, and anti-oxidant effects can be beneficial on prevention from infection with SARS-CoV-2 and even suffering from severe consequence of COVID-19.

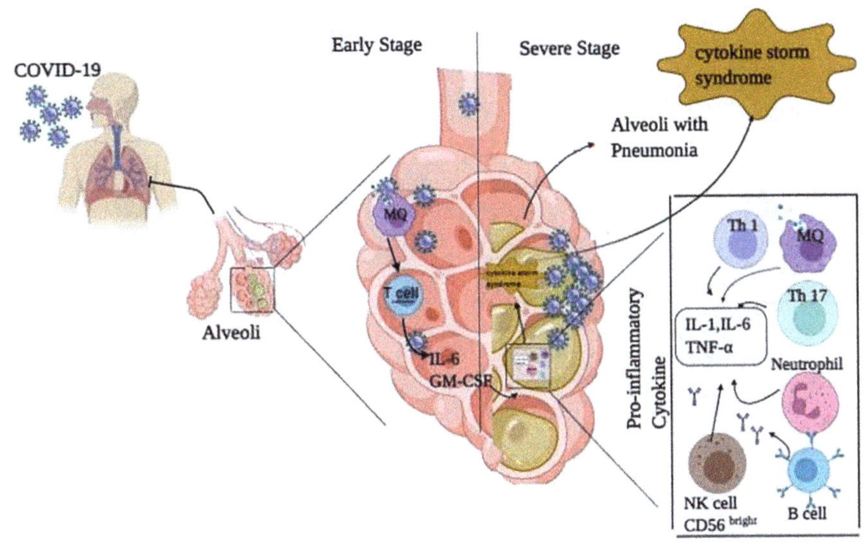

FIGURE 2 | Immune response in COVID-19 infected people. The immune responses against COVID-19 infection are divided into two phases: non-severe and severe ones. In the non-sever stage response, activated T cells and macrophages release IFN-I (α, β) to remove the virus and prevent entry to severe phase. In the severe stage of infection, inflammation occurs in the lung which may increase the penetration of neutrophils, macrophages, Th1, Th17, B cells, and NK (CD56^{bright}) cells with their secreted pro-inflammatory cytokines (IL-1, IL-6, and TNF-α) into the lung. This is followed by cytokine release syndrome and pneumonia in the lung.

In this regard, several considerable theories are proposed for ACE inhibitors (ACEIs), angiotensin II Type-I receptor blockers (ARBs), and dipeptidyl peptidase 4 (DPP4) inhibitors (57). Accordingly, ACEIs and ARBs are used in patients with diabetes to prevent the risks of developing diabetes and organ failure. As a result of taking, ACE2 becomes over-expressed in these patients (58). Therefore, due to anti-inflammatory/anti-oxidant/anti-fibrotic and other promising effects of ACE2, it is suggested that the increased ACE2 may preserve them from sever outcomes of COVID-19 infection. However, there is a fear from their unfavorable impacts as well. Because, over-expressed ACE2 may also facilitate infection with SARS-CoV-2 (due to its receptor role), as displayed in **Figure 3** (13).

On the other hand, DPP4 inhibitors, as effective hyperglycemic drugs, are frequently used in diabetes. Their biological effects is not only limited to glucose metabolism, but also the anti-inflammatory and anti-fibrotic, impacts of DPP4 inhibitors on various cells have also been proved (59). DPP4 is highly expressed on lung mesothelium and various lung cells (such as alveolar cells, resident macrophages) as well as multiple immune cell types (such as macrophages, T cells, B/NK, and dendritic cells) (60). Thus, it is logical to assume DPP4 effect on their functions (57). In addition, DPP4 possesses a pro-inflammatory function by stimulating monocytes to produce IL-6 and TNF-α. Therefore, DPP4 inhibitors can also be verified as anti-inflammatory agents (60). Accordingly, their anti-inflammatory and protective impacts have been confirmed in mice and human lung injuries (61). Moreover, it is demonstrated that DPP4 inhibitors display their positive anti-inflammatory effects by reducing the high level of pro-inflammatory factors such as TNF-α, as well as elevating anti-inflammatory IL-10 in T2D patients (**Figure 3**) (62). Therefore, DPP4 inhibitors exert their anti-inflammatory functions on different cell types such as macrophages, T cells, and lung cells. In addition, it seems that DPP4 inhibitors have some anti-fibrotic effects on the lung by affecting the proliferative and inflammatory-signaling-pathways of human pulmonary arterial smooth muscle cells and fibroblasts (63).

As a result, considering the promising inflammatory and immunological impacts of DPP4 inhibitors, they might be beneficial on modulating immune and inflammatory responses in the respiratory system of COVID-19, which are abnormally amplified to minimize the severity of illness and its mortality rate. On the other hand, it is suggested that DDP4 4 inhibitors could reduce the SARS-CoV-2 internalization/replication within the airway due to the estimated co-receptor role of DPP4 (64). In this regard, more clinical data are required to confirm these findings.

CONCLUSION

In chronic inflammatory diseases like diabetes, the proliferation, differentiation, distribution, and function of both the innate and adaptive immunities become dysregulated and the immune homeostatic balance becomes disrupted. Accordingly, these in turn make patients more susceptible to be infected with SARS-CoV-2, severe outcomes, and the increased mortality rate resulted from it compared to people without it. Since the activation of innate and adaptive immune responses plays an essential role in severity of symptoms and the risk of mortality from COVID-19, all efforts attempt to reduce the incidence and

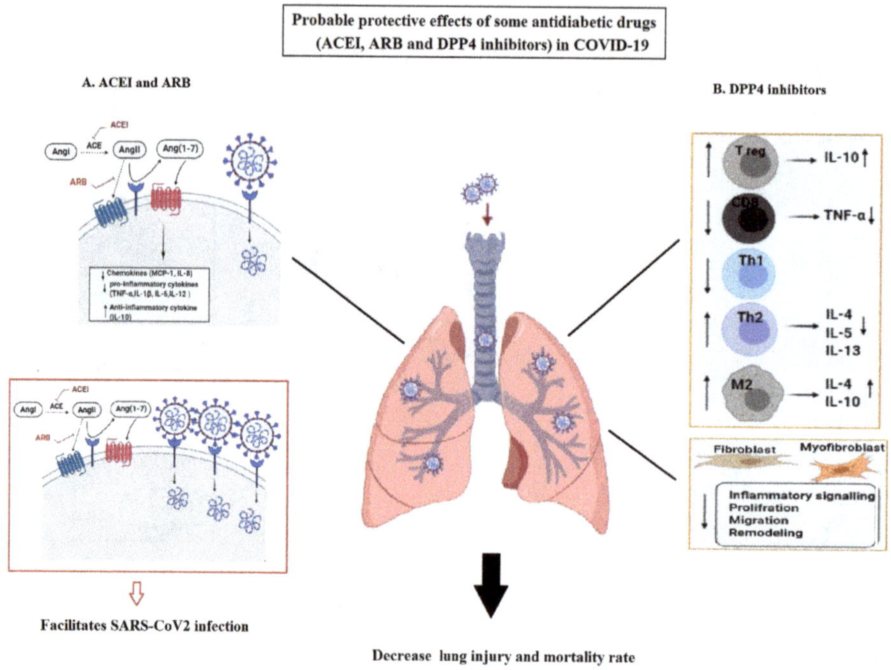

FIGURE 3 | The possible protective effects of angiotensin-converting enzyme inhibitors (ACEIs), angiotensin II Type-I receptor blockers (ARBs), and also dipeptidyl peptidase 4 (DPP4) inhibitors as antidiabetic drugs in COVID-19. **(A)** Usage of ACEIs and ARB lead to over expression of ACE2. Overexpressed ACE2 can degrade angiotensin II and lead to the production of angiotensin 1-7 with favorable (anti-oxidant, anti-fibrotic, anti-inflammatory, and vasodilatory) effects in COVID-19. Its anti-inflammatory function can be related to the reduction in chemokines (MCP-1 and IL-8) and pro-inflammatory cytokines (TNF-α, IL-1β, IL-6, and IL-12) as well as increase in anti-inflammatory cytokines (IL-10) in the lung. However, the increased ACE2 can facilitate infection with SARS-CoV-2. **(B)** DPP4 inhibitors exert their anti-inflammatory impacts in the lung through regulating multiple immune cells function and anti-fibrotic effects by influencing fibroblasts and myofibroblasts activities. These effects may result in the decreased lung injury and mortality rate in COVID-19.

death rates. In this regard, we tried to focus on diabetes to clarify the physiological and immunological characteristics of diabetic patients once before and once after infecting with COVID-19. We hope it could provide better understanding on inflammatory mechanisms to better control the immune responses and its consequences in COVID-19.

AUTHOR CONTRIBUTIONS

AA: the original draft preparation, writing, editing, and graphic design. NR-K: writing, editing, and relevant idea for graphic design. All authors contributed to the article and approved the submitted version.

REFERENCES

1. Badawi A, Ryoo SG. Prevalence of diabetes in the 2009 influenza A (H1N1) and the Middle East respiratory syndrome coronavirus: a systematic review and meta-analysis. *J Public Health Res* (2016) 5(3):130–8. doi: 10.4081/jphr.2016.733
2. Chan K, Zheng J, Mok Y, Li Y, LIU YN, Chu C, et al. SARS: prognosis, outcome and sequelae. *Respirology* (2003) 8:S36–40. doi: 10.1046/j.1440-1843.2003.00522.x
3. Phelan A, Katz R, Gostin L. The novel coronavirus originating in Wuhan. *Challenges Global Health Governance JAMA* (2020) 323(8):709–10. doi: 10.1001/jama.2020.1097
4. Gorbalenya AE. Severe acute respiratory syndrome-related coronavirus–The species and its viruses, a statement of the Coronavirus Study Group. *BioRxiv* (2020) 937862:1–16. doi: 10.1101/2020.02.07.937862v1
5. Bai Y, Yao L, Wei T, Tian F, Jin D-Y, Chen L, et al. Presumed asymptomatic carrier transmission of COVID-19. *Jama* (2020) 323(14):1406–07. doi: 10.1001/jama.2020.2565
6. Guan W-j, Ni Z-y, Hu Y, Liang W-h, Ou C-q, He J-x, et al. Clinical characteristics of coronavirus disease 2019 in China. *New Engl J Med* (2020) 382:1708–20. doi: 10.1101/2020.02.06.20020974
7. Yang J, Zheng Y, Gou X, Pu K, Chen Z, Guo Q, et al. Prevalence of comorbidities in the novel Wuhan coronavirus (COVID-19) infection: a systematic review and meta-analysis. *Int J Infect Dis* (2020) 30136-3:1–14. doi: 10.1016/j.ijid.2020.03.017
8. Li B, Yang J, Zhao F, Zhi L, Wang X, Liu L, et al. Prevalence and impact of cardiovascular metabolic diseases on COVID-19 in China. *Clin Res Cardiol* (2020) 109:1–8. doi: 10.1007/s00392-020-01626-9
9. Badawi A, Ryoo SG. Prevalence of comorbidities in the Middle East respiratory syndrome coronavirus (MERS-CoV): a systematic review and meta-analysis. *Int J Infect Dis* (2016) 49:129–33. doi: 10.1016/j.ijid.2016.06.015
10. Huang C, Wang Y, Li X, Ren L, Zhao J, Hu Y, et al. Clinical features of patients infected with 2019 novel coronavirus in Wuhan, China. *Lancet* (2020) 395 (10223):497–506. doi: 10.1016/S0140-6736(20)30183-5
11. Peric S, Stulnig TM. Diabetes and COVID-19: Disease—Management—People. *Wiener Klinische Wochenschrift* (2020) 1:356–61. doi: 10.1007/s00508-020-01672-3
12. Guo W, Li M, Dong Y, Zhou H, Zhang Z, Tian C, et al. Diabetes is a risk factor for the progression and prognosis of COVID-19. *Diabetes/Metabol Res Rev* (2020) 36(7):e3319. doi: 10.1002/dmrr.3319

13. Pal R, Bhadada SK. COVID-19 and diabetes mellitus: An unholy interaction of two pandemics. *Diabetes Metab Syndrome: Clin Res Rev* (2020) 14:513–7. doi: 10.1016/j.dsx.2020.04.049
14. Li X, Hu C, Su F, Dai J. Hypokalemia and clinical implications in patients with coronavirus disease 2019 (COVID-19). *MedRxiv* (2020) 20028530:1–22. doi: 10.1101/2020.02.27.20028530
15. Coelho M, Oliveira T, Fernandes R. Biochemistry of adipose tissue: an endocrine organ. *Arch Med Sci: AMS* (2013) 9(2):191. doi: 10.5114/aoms.2013.33181
16. Papadokostaki E, Tentolouris N, Liberopoulos E. COVID-19 and diabetes: What does the clinician need to know? *Primary Care Diabetes* (2020) 14:558–63. doi: 10.1016/j.pcd.2020.06.010
17. Kaye SM, Pietiläinen KH, Kotronen A, Joutsi-Korhonen L, Kaprio J, Yki-Järvinen H, et al. Obesity-related derangements of coagulation and fibrinolysis: a study of obesity-discordant monozygotic twin pairs. *Obesity* (2012) 20(1):88–94. doi: 10.1038/oby.2011.287
18. Magro C, Mulvey JJ, Berlin D, Nuovo G, Salvatore S, Harp J, et al. Complement associated microvascular injury and thrombosis in the pathogenesis of severe COVID-19 infection: a report of five cases. *Trans Res* (2020) 220:1–13. doi: 10.1016/j.trsl.2020.04.007
19. Sardu C, D'Onofrio N, Balestrieri ML, Barbieri M, Rizzo MR, Messina V, et al. Outcomes in Patients With Hyperglycemia Affected by Covid-19: Can We Do More on Glycemic Control? *Diabetes Care* (2020) 43:1408–15. doi: 10.2337/figshare.12275516.v1
20. Zhou J, Tan J. Diabetes patients with COVID-19 need better blood glucose management in Wuhan, China. *Metabolism* (2020) 107:154216. doi: 10.1016/j.metabol.2020.154216
21. Li T, Zhang Y, Gong C, Wang J, Liu B, Shi L, et al. Prevalence of malnutrition and analysis of related factors in elderly patients with COVID-19 in Wuhan, China. *Eur J Clin Nutr* (2020) 74:1–5. doi: 10.1038/s41430-020-0642-3
22. Banerjee M, Chakraborty S, Pal R. Diabetes self-management amid COVID-19 pandemic. *Diabetes Metab Syndrome: Clin Res Rev* (2020) 14:351–4. doi: 10.1016/j.dsx.2020.04.013
23. Patel A, Jernigan DB. Initial public health response and interim clinical guidance for the 2019 novel coronavirus outbreak—United States, December 31, 2019–February 4, 2020. *Morbid Mortal Weekly Rep* (2020) 69(5):140. doi: 10.15585/mmwr.mm6908e1
24. Lau D, Eurich DT, Majumdar SR, Katz A, Johnson JA. Effectiveness of influenza vaccination in working-age adults with diabetes: a population-based cohort study. *Thorax* (2013) 68(7):658–63. doi: 10.1136/thoraxjnl-2012-203109
25. Goeijenbier M, Van Sloten TT, Slobbe L, Mathieu C, Van Genderen P, Beyer WE, et al. Benefits of flu vaccination for persons with diabetes mellitus: a review. *Vaccine* (2017) 35(38):5095–101. doi: 10.1016/j.vaccine.2017.07.095
26. Qiu J, Shen B, Zhao M, Wang Z, Xie B, Xu Y. A nationwide survey of psychological distress among Chinese people in the COVID-19 epidemic: implications and policy recommendations. *Gen Psychiatry* (2020) 33(2):1–3. doi: 10.1136/gpsych-2020-100213
27. Hartmann-Boyce J, Morris E, Goyder C, Kinton J, Perring J, Nunan D, et al. Diabetes and COVID-19: risks, management, and learnings from other national disasters. *Diabetes Care* (2020) 43(8):1695–703. doi: 10.2337/dc20-1192
28. Miazgowski T, Bikowska M, Ogonowski J, Taszarek A. The impact of health locus of control and anxiety on self-monitored blood glucose concentration in women with gestational diabetes mellitus. *J Women's Health* (2018) 27(2):209–15. doi: 10.1089/jwh.2017.6366
29. Cure E, Cure MC. COVID–19 may affect the endocrine pancreas by activating Na+/H+ exchanger 2 and increasing lactate levels. *J Endocrinol Invest* (2020) 43:1167—8. doi: 10.1007/s40618-020-01307-4
30. Wang F, Wang H, Fan J, Zhang Y, Wang H, Zhao Q. Pancreatic injury patterns in patients with COVID-19 pneumonia. *Gastroenterology* (2020) 159:367–70. doi: 10.1053/j.gastro.2020.03.055
31. Li F, Li W, Farzan M, Harrison SC. Structure of SARS coronavirus spike receptor-binding domain complexed with receptor. *Science* (2005) 309(5742):1864–8. doi: 10.1126/science.1116480
32. Turner AJ, Hiscox JA, Hooper NM. ACE2: from vasopeptidase to SARS virus receptor. *Trends Pharmacol Sci* (2004) 25(6):291–4. doi: 10.1016/j.tips.2004.04.001
33. Lu R, Zhao X, Li J, Niu P, Yang B, Wu H, et al. Genomic characterisation and epidemiology of 2019 novel coronavirus: implications for virus origins and receptor binding. *Lancet* (2020) 395(10224):565–74. doi: 10.1016/S0140-6736(20)30251-8
34. Pagliaro P, Penna C. ACE/ACE2 Ratio: A Key Also in 2019 Coronavirus Disease (Covid-19)? *Front Med* (2020) 7:1–5. doi: 10.3389/fmed.2020.00335
35. Pal R, Bhansali A. COVID-19, diabetes mellitus and ACE2: the conundrum. *Diabetes Res Clin Practice* (2020) 162:1–2. doi: 10.1016/j.diabres.2020.108132
36. Mizuiri S, Hemmi H, Arita M, Ohashi Y, Tanaka Y, Miyagi M, et al. Expression of ACE and ACE2 in individuals with diabetic kidney disease and healthy controls. *Am J Kidney Dis* (2008) 51(4):613–23. doi: 10.1053/j.ajkd.2007.11.022
37. Raphael I, Nalawade S, Eagar TN, Forsthuber TG. T cell subsets and their signature cytokines in autoimmune and inflammatory diseases. *Cytokine* (2015) 74(1):5–17. doi: 10.1016/j.cyto.2014.09.011
38. Cortez-Espinosa N, Cortés-Garcia JD, Martínez-Leija E, Rodríguez-Rivera JG, Barajas-López C, González-Amaro R, et al. CD39 expression on Treg and Th17 cells is associated with metabolic factors in patients with type 2 diabetes. *Hum Immunol* (2015) 76(9):622–30. doi: 10.1016/j.humimm.2015.09.007
39. Sireesh D, Dhamodharan U, Ezhilarasi K, Vijay V, Ramkumar KM. Association of NF-E2 related factor 2 (Nrf2) and inflammatory cytokines in recent onset type 2 diabetes mellitus. *Sci Rep* (2018) 8(1):1–10. doi: 10.1038/s41598-018-22913-6
40. Ip B, Cilfone NA, Belkina AC, DeFuria J, Jagannathan-Bogdan M, Zhu M, et al. Th17 cytokines differentiate obesity from obesity-associated type 2 diabetes and promote TNF α production. *Obesity* (2016) 24(1):102–12. doi: 10.1002/oby.21243
41. Dimeloe S, Burgener AV, Grählert J. Hess C. T-cell metabolism governing activation, proliferation and differentiation; a modular view. *Immunology* (2017) 150(1):35–44. doi: 10.1111/imm.12655
42. Zheng Y, Rudensky AY. Foxp3 in control of the regulatory T cell lineage. *Nat Immunol* (2007) 8(5):457–62. doi: 10.1038/ni1455
43. Du X, Liu M, Su J, Zhang P, Tang F, Ye P, et al. Uncoupling therapeutic from immunotherapy-related adverse effects for safer and effective anti-CTLA-4 antibodies in CTLA4 humanized mice. *Cell Res* (2018) 28(4):433–47. doi: 10.1038/s41422-018-0012-z
44. Zeng L, Lu H, Deng H, Mu P, Li X, Wang M. Noninferiority effects on glycemic control and β-cell function improvement in newly diagnosed type 2 diabetes patients: basal insulin monotherapy versus continuous subcutaneous insulin infusion treatment. *Diabetes Technol Ther* (2012) 14(1):35–42. doi: 10.1089/dia.2011.0123
45. Monteiro-Sepulveda M, Touch S, Mendes-Sá C, André S, Poitou C, Allatif O, et al. Jejunal T cell inflammation in human obesity correlates with decreased enterocyte insulin signaling. *Cell Metab* (2015) 22(1):113–24. doi: 10.1016/j.cmet.2015.05.020
46. Rhodes KA, Andrew EM, Newton DJ, Tramonti D. Carding SR. A subset of IL-10-producing γδ T cells protect the liver from Listeria-elicited, CD8+ T cell-mediated injury. *Eur J Immunol* (2008) 38(8):2274–83. doi: 10.1002/eji.200838354
47. Guzik TJ, Skiba DS, Touyz RM, Harrison DG. The role of infiltrating immune cells in dysfunctional adipose tissue. *Cardiovasc Res* (2017) 113(9):1009–23. doi: 10.1093/cvr/cvx108
48. Simar D, Versteyhe S, Donkin I, Liu J, Hesson L, Nylander V, et al. DNA methylation is altered in B and NK lymphocytes in obese and type 2 diabetic human. *Metabolism* (2014) 63(9):1188–97. doi: 10.1016/j.metabol.2014.05.014
49. Carvelli J, Piperoglou C, Bourenne J, Farnarier C, Banzet N, Demerlé C, et al. Imbalance of circulating innate lymphoid cell subpopulations in patients with septic shock. *Front Immunol* (2019) 10:2179. doi: 10.3389/fimmu.2019.02179
50. Kim Y, Bayona PW, Kim M, Chang J, Hong S, Park Y, et al. Macrophage lamin A/C regulates inflammation and the development of obesity-induced insulin resistance. *Front Immunol* (2018) 9:696. doi: 10.3389/fimmu.2018.00696
51. Kawarabayashi R, Motoyama K, Nakamura M, Yamazaki Y, Morioka T, Mori K, et al. The association between monocyte surface CD163 and insulin resistance in patients with type 2 diabetes. *J Diabetes Res* (2017) 2017:1–9. doi: 10.1155/2017/6549242
52. Wu D, Molofsky AB, Liang H-E, Ricardo-Gonzalez RR, Jouihan HA, Bando JK, et al. Eosinophils sustain adipose alternatively activated macrophages associated with glucose homeostasis. *Science* (2011) 332(6026):243–7. doi: 10.1126/science.1201475

53. Mahallawi WH, Khabour OF, Zhang Q, Makhdoum HM, Suliman BA. MERS-CoV infection in humans is associated with a pro-inflammatory Th1 and Th17 cytokine profile. *Cytokine* (2018) 104:8–13. doi: 10.1016/j.cyto.2018.01.025
54. Kulcsar KA, Coleman CM, Beck SE, Frieman MB. Comorbid diabetes results in immune dysregulation and enhanced disease severity following MERS-CoV infection. *JCI Insight* (2019) 4(20):1–18. doi: 10.1172/jci.insight.131774
55. Qin C, Zhou L, Hu Z, Zhang S, Yang S, Tao Y, et al. Dysregulation of immune response in patients with COVID-19 in Wuhan, China. *China (February 17 2020)* (2020) 15:762–8. doi: 10.1093/cid/ciaa248
56. Liu Y, Zhang C, Huang F, Yang Y, Wang F, Yuan J, et al. Elevated plasma level of selective cytokines in COVID-19 patients reflect viral load and lung injury. *Natl Sci Rev* (2020) 109:1–8. doi: 10.1093/nsr/nwaa037
57. Pantanetti P, Cangelosi G, Ambrosio G. Potential role of incretins in diabetes and COVID-19 infection: a hypothesis worth exploring. *Internal Emergency Med* (2020) 15:1–4. doi: 10.1007/s11739-020-02389-x
58. Verma A, Shan Z, Lei B, Yuan L, Liu X, Nakagawa T, et al. ACE2 and Ang-(1-7) confer protection against development of diabetic retinopathy. *Mol Ther* (2012) 20(1):28–36. doi: 10.1038/mt.2011.155
59. Seferović PM, Coats AJ, Ponikowski P, Filippatos G, Huelsmann M, Jhund PS, et al. European Society of Cardiology/Heart Failure Association position paper on the role and safety of new glucose-lowering drugs in patients with heart failure. *Eur J Heart Failure* (2020) 22(2):196–213. doi: 10.1002/ejhf.1673
60. Shao S, Xu Q, Yu X, Pan R, Chen Y. Dipeptidyl peptidase 4 inhibitors and their potential immune modulatory functions. *Pharmacol Ther* (2020) 209:107503. doi: 10.1016/j.pharmthera.2020.107503
61. Kawasaki T, Chen W, Htwe YM, Tatsumi K, Dudek SM. DPP4 inhibition by sitagliptin attenuates LPS-induced lung injury in mice. *Am J Physiol-Lung Cell Mol Physiol* (2018) 315(5):L834–L45. doi: 10.1152/ajplung.00031.2018
62. Satoh-Asahara N, Sasaki Y, Wada H, Tochiya M, Iguchi A, Nakagawachi R, et al. A dipeptidyl peptidase-4 inhibitor, sitagliptin, exerts anti-inflammatory effects in type 2 diabetic patients. *Metabolism* (2013) 62(3):347–51. doi: 10.1016/j.metabol.2012.09.004
63. Smelcerovic A, Kocic G, Gajic M, Tomovic K, Djordjevic V, Stankovic-Djordjevic D, et al. DPP-4 Inhibitors in the Prevention/Treatment of Pulmonary Fibrosis, Heart and Kidney Injury Caused by COVID-19—A Therapeutic Approach of Choice in Type 2 Diabetic Patients? *Front Pharmacol* (2020) 11:1185. doi: 10.3389/fphar.2020.01185
64. Solerte SB, Di Sabatino A, Galli M, Fiorina P. Dipeptidyl peptidase-4 (DPP4) inhibition in COVID-19. *Acta Diabetol* (2020) 57(7):779–83. doi: 10.1007/s00592-020-01539-z

6

Mediterranean Diet and COVID-19: Hypothesizing Potential Benefits in People with Diabetes

Maria Ida Maiorino, Giuseppe Bellastella, Miriam Longo, Paola Caruso and Katherine Esposito*

Department of Advanced Medical and Surgical Sciences, University of Campania "Luigi Vanvitelli", Naples, Italy

Keywords: COVID-19, type 2 diabetes (T2D), mediterranean diet, inflammation, cytokines, glycemic control

***Correspondence:**
Maria Ida Maiorino
mariaida.maiorino@unicampania.it

INTRODUCTION

The outbreak of the Coronavirus Disease 2019 (COVID-19) started in December 2019 in Wuhan (China) and has since spread in more than 200 countries. The pandemic was brought about by a novel virus causing severe acute respiratory syndrome coronavirus 2 (SARS-CoV-2). Among the comorbidities of people suffering from COVID-19, the most prevalent are diabetes, cardiovascular disease, and hypertension, all of which are associated with worse outcomes (1).

People with diabetes are at increased risk of severe viral respiratory tract infections, including the SARS-CoV, H1N1 influenza, and Middle East Respiratory Syndrome (MERS-CoV). The prevalence of diabetes in individuals with COVID-19 has been reported to range between nearly 10% and up to 30%, depending on the location of the study, population, age of participants in the studies, severity of illness, and method of testing (2). Moreover, diabetes has emerged as an important predictor of severity of the SARS-CoV-2, as the risk of fatal outcomes has been reported to be 50% higher in individuals with diabetes than in those without (3). Given the high transmission rate of SARS-CoV-2 and the global prevalence of diabetes, which affects nearly half a billion people worldwide, the coexistence of both COVID-19 and diabetes should be considered alarming, as it represents the combination of two pandemics.

THE HARMFUL TRIO LINKING COVID-19 AND DIABETES: IMPAIRED IMMUNE RESPONSE, INFLAMMATION, PRO-THROMBOTIC STATE

Both COVID-19 and diabetes are responsible for dysfunctional immune responses and generation of a pro-inflammatory and pro-thrombotic status which may lead to disease progression. People with COVID-19 generally present lymphopenia and increased neutrophil–lymphocyte ratio, consequent to the recruitment of immune cells from the blood and the infiltration of lymphocytes into the airways. This phenomenon is induced in the lungs by the release of inflammatory cytokines and chemokines [including Interleukin 6 (IL-6), interferon γ-inducible protein-10, macrophage inflammatory protein 1α (MIPα), MIP1β and monocyte chemoattractant protein-1] from the epithelial and endothelial cells and alveolar macrophage activated by the virus-linked pyroptosis. As a result, monocytes, macrophages and T cells are recruited to the site of infection, promoting further inflammation (together with the IFNγ produced by T cells) and establishing a pro-inflammatory feedback loop (4). It is also known that elevated levels of IL-6 and C-reactive protein (CRP), as well as increased coagulation activity, marked by high d-dimer concentrations, were also associated with varying degrees of severity of the disease.

Diabetes is thought to be a status of chronic inflammation induced by both hyperglycemia and insulin-resistance and characterized by high levels of pro-inflammatory cytokines, oxidative stress, and over-expression of adhesion molecules by endothelial cells (5, 6), which may predispose to an increased risk of infections. Poor glycemic control is also associated with an impaired immune response due to an inhibited lymphocytes ability to counteract different series of pathogenic stimuli and an alteration in monocyte/macrophage functions. Moreover, an imbalance between coagulation and fibrinolysis takes place in diabetes, with enhanced platelet aggregation and activation, favoring the development of a hypercoagulable pro-thrombotic state. Globally, all these alterations may represent the underlying conditions linking diabetes to other chronic conditions, including hypertension and cardiovascular diseases (5).

Ongoing clinical trials are currently evaluating the safety and efficacy of treatment strategies addressing the components of the harmful trio in the context of SARS-CoV-2; until now, however, no drug or vaccine has been officially approved for COVID-19 treatment. On the other hand, evidence from randomized controlled trials evaluating the effect of anti-inflammatory drugs on glycemic control or cardiovascular events in people with type 2 diabetes suggest only a modest effect on HbA1c reduction (5); whether patients with cardiovascular diseases and/or type 2 diabetes may have clinical benefit from marked reductions in circulating inflammatory markers remains also controversial. However, both the maintenance and intensification of the glyco-metabolic control in individuals with diabetes who have not been infected with the SARS-CoV-2 virus has suggested to be a means of primary prevention of COVID-19 disease (3).

THE MEDITERRANEAN DIET: A HEALTHY DIETARY PATTERN FOR PEOPLE WITH DIABETES

Mediterranean diet, which represents the traditional eating habits of populations living around the Mediterranean Sea in the 1960s, including Greece and South Italy, has long been indicated as a dietary pattern able to preserve cardio-metabolic health. The Mediterranean diet is characterized by the high content in plant-based foods, olive oil as the main source of fat, low-to-moderate intake of fish, dairy products, and poultry, low consumption of red or processed meat, and low to moderate consumption of wine with meals (7). This dietary regimen is currently included among the eating patterns recommended by the American Diabetes Association for people with pre-diabetes or diabetes, showing favorable effects on HbA_{1C} reduction, weight, and lipids in a number of randomized controlled trials (RCTs). Moreover, the recent guidelines on diabetes, pre-diabetes, and cardiovascular diseases developed by the European Society of Cardiology in collaboration with the European Association for the Study of Diabetes state that a Mediterranean diet, rich in polyunsaturated and monounsaturated fats, should be considered to reduce cardiovascular events.

THREE HYPOTHETICAL MECHANISMS RESPONSIBLE FOR THE PROTECTIVE EFFECT OF MEDITERRANEAN DIET AGAINST COVID-19 IN DIABETIC PEOPLE

Mediterranean Diet Exerts Anti-inflammatory and Immunomodulatory Effects

Several epidemiological studies confirmed the anti-inflammatory and immunomodulatory effects of a Mediterranean pattern on several diseases associated with chronic low-grade inflammation. These counter the effects of several inflammatory markers and decrease the secretion of circulating and cellular biomarkers involved in the atherosclerotic process (8). A recent meta-analysis of 17 RCTs including 2,300 subjects reported a significant reduction in high-sensitive CRP [weight mean difference (WMD): −0.98 mg/l, 95% CI −1.48 to −0.49, $p < 0.0001$] IL-6 [WMD: −0.42 pg/ml, 95% CI −0.73 to −0.11, $p = 0.008$], and intracellular adhesion molecule-1 [WMD: −23.73 ng/ml, 95% CI −41.24 to −6.22, $p = 0.008$] in individuals assigned to Mediterranean diet, compared with those following a control intervention protocol (9). In two RCTs of people with obesity (10) and metabolic syndrome (11), the consumption of Mediterranean diet for 2 years was associated with a significant reduction of inflammatory markers, including CRP, IL-6, IL-7, and IL-18, as compared with a prudent diet. The MEditerranean DIet and Type 2 diAbetes (MÈDITA) study, provides further evidence of the anti-inflammatory and immunomodulatory effect of Mediterranean dietary pattern in the context of diabetes (12, 13). The MÈDITA trial was a long-term RCT conducted with a Mediterranean diet vs. a low-fat diet for primary prevention of antidiabetic drug need in 215 participants with newly-diagnosed type 2 diabetes. A significant 37% decrease in CPR, associated with a 43% raise in adiponectin was observed in the Mediterranean diet group after 1 year, while remaining unchanged in the low-fat diet group (12). In diabetic people with the highest scores of adherence to Mediterranean dietary pattern, as compared with the diabetic patients who showed the lowest adherence, the lower circulating CRP levels and higher circulating adiponectin concentrations suggested a "dose-dependent" anti-inflammatory effect (12). Moreover, the amelioration of the inflammatory milieu associated with Mediterranean diet was sustained over a 8.1 year-follow up, leading to an improvement of insulin resistance and glucose metabolism as compared with a low-fat diet (13).

Mediterranean Diet Prevents Diabetes and Improves Glucose Control in Diabetic People

The most robust available evidence related to eating patterns for prevention of type 2 diabetes relies to Mediterranean diet, that, in 10 prospective studies, led to a 23% reduced risk of incident diabetes (14). Moreover, meta-analyses of RCTs reported that, compared with control diets, Mediterranean diets reduced HbA_{1c} levels by 0.30–0.47% in type 2 diabetes (7).

Mediterranean Diet Reduces Cardiovascular Risk in Diabetes

In both interventional prospective studies and RCTs, Mediterranean diet has been associated with beneficial effects on weight circumference, blood lipids, and blood pressure. Moreover, in the PREDIMED study, involving people at high cardiovascular risk, of whom 49% had diabetes, a Mediterranean diet supplemented with olive oil or nuts led to a 28% reduction in the incidence of major cardiovascular events (15).

Plausible Mechanisms

As both COVID-19 and diabetes are characterized by increased levels of pro-inflammatory cytokines, including CRP, IL-6 and TNF-α, treatment strategies effective in reducing inflammation may be pursued to prevent the risk of infection or blunt the severity of the disease in diabetic people. Among the components of Mediterranean diet, whole grains, vegetables and fruits, fish and "healthy" fats, including both monounsaturated (MUFA) and polyunsaturated (PUFA), are all associated with lower inflammation; on the other hand, processed red meat and dairy products, processed cheese, which are rich in saturated fatty acids and trans-fatty acids, may have pro-inflammatory properties (16).

The mechanisms by which Mediterranean diet produces its favorable effects in type 2 diabetes may depend mostly on the abundance of anti-inflammatory nutrients (PUFA, fiber, vitamins, minerals, antioxidants, and polyphenols), associated with the lower intake of pro-inflammatory nutrients (refined sugars and starches, trans fatty acids, high-density foods). Among PUFA, the omega-3 free fatty acids exert anti-inflammatory effects via oxygenated metabolites (oxylipins), which are specialized pro-resolving mediators (17). They include α-linolenic acid, derived from various plant sources, as well as eicosapentaenoic acid and docosahexaenoic acid, derived mainly from fish and seafood. Moreover, increased dietary fiber intake has been associated with reduced inflammatory markers (hs-CRP, IL-6, and TNF-α), and modifications in gut microbiota favoring health associated bacteria. There is also evidence supporting the protective role of vitamins against viral infection through different mechanisms (17). Furthermore, vitamin D facilitates the binding of the SARS-CoV-2 cell entry receptor ACE2 (angiotensin converting enzyme 2) to angiotensin II receptor type 1 (AGTR1), minimizing the number of viral particles that could attach to ACE2 and enter the cell, whereas vitamin C and vitamin E are well-known anti-oxidants agents, able to reduce the generation of reactive oxygen (ROS) and reactive nitrogen species (RNS) (17). Finally, polyphenols seem to interact with transcription factors, including NF-kB and Nrf-2, exerting anti-inflammatory and antioxidant effects, respectively (17).

The high content of Mediterranean diet in healthy food, combined with the low content of harmful food may be also responsible for the benefits on cardio-metabolic risk factors (i.e., blood pressure, lipids and lipoprotein, endothelial function, glucose levels) and cardiovascular events (7).

CAN MEDITERRANEAN DIET PROTECT AGAINST INFECTIONS?

An adequate and balanced diet represents an important fundament for an optimal immune response. It helps maintain the antibody production and assure the assumption of nutrients able to modulate inflammatory and oxidative stress processes (17). Despite the proposed mechanisms seem to support the beneficial effects of Mediterranean diet against COVID-19 in people with diabetes, the relationship between this healthy dietary pattern and SARS-CoV-2 remains unexplored. Similarly, literary data linking Mediterranean diet to a reduced risk of infections are scanty. In the REasons for Geographic Differences in Stroke (REGARDS) cohort of 30,239 community-dwelling adults, of whom 20% had diabetes, a high Mediterranean diet-style adherence was associated with 26% lower risk of sepsis (18). Moreover, the only evidence of a favorable effects of Mediterranean diet on respiratory infections derives from a prospective study of 128 boys and girls aged 1–5 years included in a nutritional program aimed at "Learning to eat from the Mediterranean" (19). After 1 year, with the increased Kidmed index, which assessed the quality of the Mediterranean diet, the number of catarrhal episodes, the degree of intensity, the emergency and hospital admissions showed a positive and statistically significant evolution, suggesting that Mediterranean diet could improve outcomes of child with recurring colds and frequent inflammatory complications. On the other hand, several component of food associated with Mediterranean diet, including omega-3 PUFA, polyphenols, flavonoids and vitamin D, have demonstrated to reduce inflammation and improve immune response in both *in vitro* and *in vivo* studies of lung infections (20).

DISCUSSION

Whether the amelioration of the pro-inflammatory milieu associated with Mediterranean diet components may help to prevent or reduce the severity of infections, including COVID-19 diseases, remains unknown. Moreover, there are no studies confirming that, in diabetic people, the improvement of glycemic control associated with a high adherence to the Mediterranean dietary pattern may protect from lung infections or blunt the severity of the disease. However, there is evidence from a large retrospective study of individuals affected by COVID-19, including nearly 1,000 participants with type 2 diabetes, that well-controlled blood glucose was associated with lower mortality compared with individuals with poor glycemic control during hospitalization, supporting the correlation between improved glucose control and better outcomes in SARS-CoV-2 affected-patients with pre-existing diabetes (21). These findings need to be confirmed in prospective studies to validate the importance of a healthy dietary pattern, as Mediterranean diet is thought to be, as a valuable therapeutic strategy to improve the prognosis of diabetic people affected by COVID-19, at least in individuals who do not need to be treated in the context of intensive care units. Currently, the effective behavioral measures able to reduce the risk of COVID-19 remain physical distancing, adequate hygiene and use of mask.

Another crucial point refers to the adherence to the Mediterranean dietary pattern during the COVID-19 pandemic. The lockdown imposed by governments in many countries, including Italy, have profoundly changed the lifestyle habits and everyday behavior of people with and without diabetes. In consequence of the quarantine, the limited access to daily grocery shopping may have reduced the assumption of fruits, vegetables and fish, in favor of processed food. However, a recent survey conducted on 3,533 Italian individuals (age range 12–86 years) suggested that, during the lockdown, Italian people have paid attention to Mediterranean diet, maintaining a high nutritional quality especially in Northern and Central Italy, in which a lower BMI was reported compared with the areas of Southern Italy and the Islands (22). Moreover, subjects falling in the low, medium, and high adherence to the Mediterranean Diet, consumed more than 50% of olive oil, vegetables, and legumes, food highly representative of the Mediterranean dietary pattern, demonstrating that following a healthy diet is feasible even in emergency conditions. The choice of food associated with Mediterranean diet, rich in nutrients with antioxidant and anti-inflammatory activities, may be of paramount importance to reduce the susceptibility to develop viral infections (17).

Diabetes and the associated comorbidities are significant predictors of morbidity and mortality in patients with COVID-19. The prevention of diabetes together with the implementation of glyco-metabolic control in people with diabetes may represent useful strategies to prevent or blunt the severity of the infection in individuals affected by COVID-19. Thanks to its anti-inflammatory and immunomodulatory properties, Mediterranean diet provides a nutritional regimen potentially able to address the common soil of pathogenic factors linking diabetes to COVID-19, offering an opportunity to protect diabetic people from worse outcomes in the context of SARS-CoV-2. However, future studies are warranted to confirm the benefits of these dietary-linked effects on the risk of infections, including COVID-19.

AUTHOR CONTRIBUTIONS

MIM and GB drafted the manuscript. ML and PC contributed to drafting the manuscript and revised it for intellectual content. KE edited the manuscript and revised it for important intellectual content. All authors gave the final approval of the version submitted and agreed to be accountable for all aspects of the work in ensuring that questions related to the accuracy or integrity of any part of the work they have done.

REFERENCES

1. Wu Z, McGoogan JM. Characteristics of and important lessons from the coronavirus disease 2019 (COVID-19) outbreak in china: summary of a report of 72 314 cases from the chinese center for disease control and prevention. *JAMA*. (2020) 323:1239–42. doi: 10.1001/jama.2020.2648
2. Onder G, Rezza G, Brusaferro S. Case-fatality rate and characteristics of patients dying in relation to COVID-19 in Italy. *JAMA*. (2020) 323:1775–6. doi: 10.1001/jama.2020.4683
3. Tay MZ, Poh CM, Rénia L, MacAry PA, Ng LFP. The trinity of COVID-19: immunity, inflammation and intervention. *Nat Rev Immunol*. (2020) 20:36–74. doi: 10.1038/s41577-020-0311-8
4. Maiorino MI, Bellastella G, Giugliano D, Esposito K. Cooling down inflammation in type 2 diabetes: how strong is the evidence for cardiometabolic benefit? *Endocrine*. (2017) 55:360–5. doi: 10.1007/s12020-016-0993-7
5. Esposito K, Giugliano D. The metabolic syndrome and inflammation: association or causation? *Nutr Metab Cardiovasc Dis*. (2004) 14:228–32. doi: 10.1016/S0939-4753(04)80048-6
6. Bornstein SR, Rubino F, Khunti K, Mingrone G, Hopkins D, Birkenfeld AL, et al. Practical recommendations for the management of diabetes in patients with COVID-19. *Lancet Diabetes Endocrinol*. (2020) 8:546–50. doi: 10.1016/S2213-8587(20)30152-2
7. Esposito K, Maiorino MI, Bellastella G, Panagiotakos DB, Giugliano D. Mediterranean diet for type 2 diabetes: cardiometabolic benefits. *Endocrine*. (2017) 56:27–32. doi: 10.1007/s12020-016-1018-2
8. Casas R, Sacanella E, Estruch R. The immune protective effect of the Mediterranean diet against chronic low-grade inflammatory diseases. *Endocr Metab Immune Disord Drug Targets*. (2014) 14:245–54. doi: 10.2174/1871530314666140922153350
9. Schwingshackl L, Hoffmann G. Mediterranean dietary pattern, inflammation and endothelial function: a systematic review and meta-analysis of intervention trials. *Nutr Metab Cardiovasc Dis*. (2014) 24:929–39. doi: 10.1016/j.numecd.2014.03.003
10. Esposito K, Marfella R, Ciotola M, Di Palo C, Giugliano F, Giugliano G, et al. Effect of a mediterranean-style diet on endothelial dysfunction and markers of vascular inflammation in the metabolic syndrome: a randomized trial. *JAMA*. (2004) 292:1440–6. doi: 10.1001/jama.292.12.1440
11. Esposito K, Pontillo A, Di Palo C, Giugliano G, Masella M, Marfella R, et al. Effect of weight loss and lifestyle changes on vascular inflammatory markers in obese women: a randomized trial. *JAMA*. (2003) 289:1799–804. doi: 10.1001/jama.289.14.1799
12. Maiorino MI, Bellastella G, Petrizzo M, Scappaticcio L, Giugliano D, Esposito K. Mediterranean diet cools down the inflammatory milieu in type 2 diabetes: the MÉDITA randomized controlled trial. *Endocrine*. (2016) 54:634–41. doi: 10.1007/s12020-016-0881-1
13. Maiorino MI, Bellastella G, Petrizzo M, Scappaticcio L, Giugliano D, Esposito K. Anti-inflammatory effect of mediterranean diet in type 2 diabetes is durable: 8-year follow-up of a controlled trial. *Diabetes Care*. (2016) 39:e44–5. doi: 10.2337/dc15-2356
14. Maiorino MI, Bellastella G, Giugliano D, Esposito K. Can diet prevent diabetes? *J. Diabetes Complicat*. (2017) 31:288–90. doi: 10.1016/j.jdiacomp.2016.10.009
15. Estruch R, Ros E, Salas-Salvadó J, Covas MI, Corella D, Arós F, et al. Primary prevention of cardiovascular disease with a mediterranean diet supplemented with extra-virgin olive oil or nuts. *N Engl J Med*. (2018) 378:e34. doi: 10.1056/NEJMoa1800389
16. Bellastella G, Scappaticcio L, Esposito K, Giugliano D, Maiorino MI. Metabolic syndrome and cancer: "The common soil hypothesis". *Diabetes Res Clin Pract*. (2018) 143:389–97. doi: 10.1016/j.diabres.2018.05.024
17. Iddir M, Brito A, Dingeo G, Fernandez Del Campo SS, Samouda H, La Frano MR, et al. Strengthening the immune system and reducing inflammation and oxidative stress through diet and nutrition: considerations during the COVID-19 crisis. *Nutrients*. (2020) 12:1562. doi: 10.3390/nu12061562
18. Gray MS, Wang HE, Martin KD, Donnelly JP, Gutiérrez OM, Shikanyet JM, et al. Adherence to Mediterranean-style diet and risk of sepsis in the REasons for geographic and racial differences in stroke (REGARDS) cohort. *Br J Nutr*. (2018) 120:1415–21. doi: 10.1017/S0007114518002866
19. Calatayud FM, Calatayud B, Gallego JG, González-Martín C, Alguacil LF. Effects of Mediterranean diet in patients with recurring colds and frequent complications. *Allergol Immunopathol*. (2017) 45:417–24. doi: 10.1016/j.aller.2016.08.006

20. Messina G, Polito R, Monda V, Cipolloni L, Di Nunno N, Di Mizio G, et al. Functional role of dietary intervention to improve the outcome of COVID-19: a hypothesis of work. *Int J Mol Sci.* (2020) 21:E3104. doi: 10.3390/ijms21093104
21. Zhu L, She ZG, Cheng X, Qin JJ, Zhang XJ, Cai J, et al. Association of blood glucose control and outcomes in patients with COVID-19 and pre-existing type 2 diabetes. *Cell Metab.* (2020) 31:1068–77.e3. doi: 10.1016/j.cmet.2020.04.021
22. Di Renzo L, Gualtieri P, Pivari F, Soldati L, Attinà A, Cinelli G, et al. Eating habits and lifestyle changes during COVID-19 lockdown: an Italian survey. *J Transl Med.* (2020) 18:229. doi: 10.1186/s12967-020-02399-5

7

Under COVID-19 Pandemic: A Quasi-Experimental Trial of Observation on Diabetes Patients' Health Behavior Affected by the Pandemic from a Coaching Intervention Program

Ching-Ling Lin[1,2], *Li-Chi Huang*[1], *Yao-Tsung Chang*[3], *Ruey-Yu Chen*[3*] and *Shwu-Huey Yang*[4,5,6*]

[1] *Department of Endocrinology and Metabolism, Cathay General Hospital, Taipei, Taiwan,* [2] *Department of Internal Medicine, School of Medicine, College of Medicine, Taipei Medical University, Taipei, Taiwan,* [3] *School of Public Health, Taipei Medical University, Taipei, Taiwan,* [4] *School of Nutrition and Health Sciences, Taipei Medical University, Taipei, Taiwan,* [5] *Nutrition Research Center, Taipei Medical University Hospital, Taipei, Taiwan,* [6] *Research Center of Geriatric Nutrition, College of Nutrition, Taipei Medical University, Taipei, Taiwan*

***Correspondence:**
Shwu-Huey Yang
sherry@tmu.edu.tw
Ruey-Yu Chen
rueyyu@tmu.edu.tw

Introduction: The aim of this study was to explore the impact of diabetes self-management and HbA1c affected by the COVID-19 pandemic and the epidemic prevention work.

Methods: This quasi-experimental study collected a pooled data from a randomized-control study between February and May 2020 in which 114 participants who presented type 2 diabetes were recruited. The intervention group had health coaching and usual care, whereas the control had usual care only. The main outcome variables of this observation study were the change of HbA1c, physical activity, and eating out behavior within this time interval.

Results: We found that the eating out behavior of both groups had decreased, and if a health coach helped the patients set physical activity goals in the two groups, the physical activity behavior will not be impacted due to the pandemic.

Conclusions: While every country is focusing on COVID-19 pandemic prevention, especially when strict home quarantine measures and social distancing are adopted, reminding and assisting chronic patients to maintain good self-management behavior may lessen the social and medical system burdens caused by the deterioration of chronic conditions due to the excessive risk prevention behavior and the epidemic prevention work.

Trial Registration: www.isrctn.com, identifier number: ISRCTN14167790, date: 12 July, 2019.

Keywords: COVID-19, pandemic (COVID-19), diabetes, health coaching, health behavior

INTRODUCTION

In December 2019, the new coronavirus disease (COVID-19) first broke out in China and spread around the world quickly in just a few months, killing tens of thousands of people (1, 2). Until now, even though millions of vaccine doses have been administered worldwide, there are still tens of thousands of new cases increasing every day, and many countries are still adopting varying degrees of pandemic prevention measures, such as strict restrictions on people going out and home quarantine (3). Many countries have adopted anti-pandemic measures to close schools and public entertainment venues, and they also encourage people to stay at home as much as possible to reduce the risk of disease transmission. The rapidly spreading and uncontrolled pandemic situation and strong anti-pandemic measures have not only caused huge pressure on medical staff, made people feel anxious and panicked, but also affected people's healthy living habits (4, 5). These changes also impact people with chronic diseases where their original lifestyles and self-management have disrupted.

Taiwan has made quite remarkable pandemic prevention results in this pandemic (6). Until March 2021, there were only about 1,007 confirmed cases and 10 deaths with no new confirmed local cases for over a month (1). As early as January 2020, Taiwan initiated stricter border control measures and put in place quarantine measures, as well as requiring people to wear masks when taking public transportation and control hospital access and visits. Although Taiwan did not implement a lockdown to combat the COVID-19 outbreak, during this period, it still experiences a significant drop in economic activity, with a number of companies allowing employees to work from home, many tourist attractions closed, and people feeling hesitated to go out. This may also affect chronic patients' willingness to have regular visits to the doctor and maintain healthy living habits. In fact, the number of outpatients and inpatients at all levels of hospital has declined significantly, about 14% lower than the same period last year (7).

In October 2019, we launched a diabetes health coaching program at Cathay General Hospital in Taipei, and it ended in August 2020. We tested the effectiveness of coaching on healthy lifestyle habits and mental health of diabetic patients in a randomized controlled trial. However, in the first few months of the COVID-19 pandemic, we found that the behavior of the participants seemed to be affected by the pandemic, such as avoiding going to hospital for regular screening and making regular visits, reducing outdoor physical activity, and changing eating habits, and in turn interfered with the validity of the research. Indeed, other countries also faced similar behavior changes when stricter lockdown measures were imposed (8–11). However, there are not many studies on impact of chronic patients during the pandemic, and most of them are still focused on related studies that chronic diseases increase the mortality and the risk of death from COVID-19 (12–14). Therefore, we intended to probe into the data to determine whether the pandemic would really affect the self-management behavior and health status of chronic patients, and to realize the possible impact of our health coaching program in the first few months of the pandemic. It may be one of the limitations of our original study program.

In this study, our aim was to observe the behavioral impact of the COVID-19 pandemic on diabetes patients and the interference with our original health coaching study. Data were collected for analysis between February and May 2020, when Taiwan was affected by the pandemic the most, and we especially focused on those indicators that might be affected by the pandemic situation and anti-pandemic measures.

Abbreviations: COVID-19, Corona virus disease-2019; ICF, International Coaching Federation; ACC, Associate Certified Coach; HbA1c, Hemoglobin A1c; SMBG, Self-monitoring blood glucose; IRB, Institutional Review Board; SD, Standard deviation; IQR, Inter-Quartile Range; CI, Confidence Interval.

MATERIALS AND METHODS

This quasi-experimental study originated from a 6-month long, single-blinded coaching intervention program. This two-armed, randomized-control trial was endorsed by the Institutional Review Board (IRB) of Cathay General Hospital. The two groups were: (1) coaching intervention every month on top of diabetes shared care or (2) diabetes shared care only. Data were collected at the baseline and at the end of 3- and 6-month intervention.

In this study, we gathered a pooled data between February and May 2020. It meant that the data comprised the 3- and 6-month follow-up patients. This paper was focused on the effect of risk perception behavior under COVID-19 pandemic; in other words, the data were not intended to validate the effectiveness of our intervention. In total, there were 18 patients in the intervention group and 13 in the control group, who had the 6-month follow-up. The period from February to May was chosen since the first confirmed COVID-19 diagnosis occurred in Taiwan on January 21, and various anti-pandemic measures were launched in February. During this period, every hospital had launched numerous anti-pandemic control measures in accordance with government policies, such as access control and limiting inpatient visits. In May, the pandemic prevention measures were gradually relaxed, and on May 10, it had reached a record of no new local cases for a month. Therefore, we believed that the period from February to May was when people in Taiwan began to feel anxious about the COVID-19 pandemic and gradually felt relieved.

Study Procedure

Study Population and Recruitment

Participants were recruited from a medical center—Cathay General Hospital in Taipei, Taiwan, which is one of the highest levels of hospital accreditation in Taiwan. The first author screened potential patients with type 2 diabetes mellitus from the hospital database, randomly assigned them to the intervention group and the control group, and then two physicians who specialize in endocrine and metabolic disorders recruited them separately. To be considered for inclusion, only patients, between 20 and 75 years old, who were diagnosed with type 2 diabetes for at least 1 year and had an HbA1c of 7.0% or greater for the past 6 months, exhibiting no clinically significant depression or cognitive impairment were recruited. Patients in the intervention group were informed of the coaching program whereas the patients in the control group were informed of pre-posted survey. Upon gathering signed informed consent, the health coach then started interviews and data collection. Participant enrolment was carried out from October 2019 to February 2020.

Sample Size

A total of 47 participants in each group was required to establish a clinically meaningful difference in coaching intervention, defined as a 1% between-group difference in HbA1c and standard deviation of 1.7, with a probability of a type I error of 0.05 and a power of 80%. Factoring in a 20% dropout rate, we aimed at recruiting 60 in each study group.

Intervention

A detailed description of our health coaching intervention has previously been published (15). The coaching was provided by a single coach who had over 120 h certified coach training and received the International Coach Federation's (ICF) Associated Certified Coach (ACC) credential and a master's degree in public health. Patients in the intervention group had an initial face-to-face session, together with baseline measurement, and then was offered telephone coaching sessions monthly for 6 months. In the first session, the coach asked each participant to set his or her 6-month HbA1c goal and the first behavior change goal. The behavior goal must be one of the behaviors related to diabetes self-management, including physical activity, healthy diet, medical adherence, and/or regular self-monitoring blood glucose (SMBG). If a patient had more than one behavior change goal, the coach would ask him or her to prioritize the goals. The goal had to be designed to follow the "SMART" rule (i.e., specific, measurable, attainable, realistic, and timely). The coach would then record the goals set by the patient and the content of the coaching for follow-up and analysis. It made us to explore possible clues about patients' health behaviors affected by pandemic from the qualitative record.

Each patient in the control group would only receive a face-to-face coaching session and baseline measurement at the baseline without having any coaching call at all. Coaching also helped patients in the control group set a behavior change goal and encouraged them to carry it out. Both the intervention and control groups received diabetes health education and usual care based on the diabetes shared care network program of Cathay General Hospital. The diabetes health education was conducted by diabetes educators. All participants were allowed to contact diabetes educators to ensure acquiring adequate educational resources.

Outcome Measures

In this study, we collected variables which might be associated with or affected by COVID-19 pandemic and prevention policy. Hence, our outcome variables included HbA1c, physical activity, and eating out behavior.

HbA1c was measured using the patients' blood test when they had regular visits. Physical activity was assessed using the Godin leisure-time physical activity scale (16, 17). It marked the number of days in a week the patients did vigorous, medium and light physical activities. After weighing and summing up each level of physical activity, the higher the figure the more physical activities the patients did. The number of times eating out per week, which also included take-away food, was collected from the coaching record. Physical activity and health diet goal setting were also collected from the coaching record, and both of these two variables were binary variables.

The sociodemographic variables included gender, age, educational level, employment status, diabetes history, and basic SMBG habit (times per week).

Statistical Analysis

Chi-square tests or t-tests were used to assess differences in sociodemographic factors, health behaviors, and HbA1c between the two groups. Paired t-test was used to assess the difference in HbA1c, physical activity, and eating out behavior for each group, and t-test was also used to assess the difference of pre-post differences between the two groups. We used Mann-Whitney U-test and Wilcoxon signed-rank test to assess the sub-group differences in intervention and control group and the pre-post differences under each sub-group.

Fisher's exact test and Mann-Whitney U-test were used to assess difference between those patients dropped from regular visits in the intervention and control groups, and the difference between normal patients and dropped patients within the intervention and control group.

All tests were analyzed at a 95% significance level ($p < 0.05$). The analyses were conducted using PASW 20.0 software for Windows (SPSS, Chicago, IL).

RESULTS

Baseline Data

Between October 2019 and February 2020, two physicians had invited 158 potential patients to participate and eventually a total 114 subjects were enrolled in the study randomly. Between February and May 2020, outcome measures were available for 54 patients (95% of the 57 patients) in the intervention group and for 50 patients (88% of the 57 patients) in the control group (**Figure 1**). In total, nine participants did not return regularly or ask family members to take prescription to avoid coming to the hospital, but no one withdrew from the study.

The demographic characteristics of the study groups are listed in **Table 1**. Of 114 participants, 48.2% were female, mean age was 62.2 years (SD = 8.73), 37.7% had a bachelor's degree or higher, 48.2% was retired, mean years of diagnosed diabetes was 13.5 years (SD = 7.66), mean HbA1c was 8.3% (SD = 1.08), and average 2.2 times of SMBG per week (SD = 2.29). There was no significant difference between these two groups in baseline characteristics, and there was also no significant difference between those patients who skipped their regular visits (gender, $p = 0.667$; age, $p = 0.730$; educational level, $p = 0.217$, employment status, $p = 0.738$, and diabetes history, $p = 0.730$).

Possible Effect of COVID-19 Pandemic

Overall, between February and May, the coaching intervention was associated with a significant decrease of 0.49% (CI = 0.24–0.75, $p < 0.01$), and a non-significant increase of 0.05% (CI =

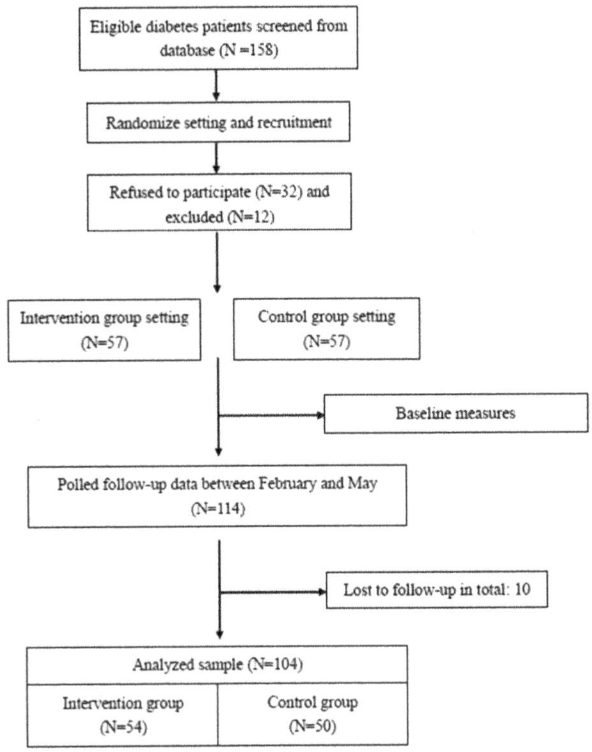

FIGURE 1 | Flow diagram of participants: recruitment, intervention and follow-up.

TABLE 1 | Demographic characteristics and baseline value of study groups.

	Demographic characteristics *N* (%)		***p*-value**
	Intervention group (*n* = 57)	**Control group (*n* = 57)**	
Gender			0.851
Male	30 (52.6)	29 (50.9)	
Female	27 (47.4)	28 (49.1)	
Age, years (mean ± SD)	61.28 ± 9.75	63.22 ± 7.50	0.242
Educational level			0.361
Junior high school or below	11 (19.3)	16 (28.1)	
Senior high school	20 (35.1)	24 (42.1)	
University	19 (33.3)	12 (21.1)	
Master's degree or above	7 (12.3)	5 (8.8)	
Employment status			0.574
Employed	31 (54.4)	28 (49.1)	
Retired	26 (45.6)	29 (50.9)	
Diabetes history (years, mean ± SD)	13.73 ± 7.73	13.16 ± 7.65	0.708
HbA1c (%, mean ± SD)	8.38 ± 1.29	8.14 ± 0.96	0.260
Physical activity points (mean ± SD)	13.42 ± 14.12	9.32 ± 12.80	0.139
SMBG (times per week, mean ± SD)	2.37 ± 2.40	2.04 ± 2.19	0.439

TABLE 2 | Effect of COVID-19 pandemic to diabetes health coaching intervention program and health behaviors according to paired *t*-test and *t*-test.

	Pandemic effect (mean ± SD)		***p*-value**
	Intervention group (*n* = 54)	**Control group (*n* = 50)**	
HbA1c, %			
Pre-test	8.40 ± 1.29	8.19 ± 0.96	0.189
Post-test	7.99 ± 1.00[a,b]	8.24 ± 1.10	0.248
Physical activity points			
Pre-test	13.19 ± 14.10	8.28 ± 9.82	0.048*
Post-test	15.22 ± 11.70	10.30 ± 10.28	0.113
Frequency of eating out in a week, times			
Pre-test	6.26 ± 5.66	5.75 ± 5.74	0.635
Post-test	4.49 ± 4.34[a]	4.10 ± 5.14[a]	0.686

*$p < 0.05$.
[a] Significant difference between pre-post within the same group.
[b] Significant difference in difference between groups.

−1.12 to 0.29, $p = 0.648$) in HbA1c level was observed in the control group (**Table 2**). Both pre-test and post-test in HbA1c level between two groups were non-significant, but the difference of pre-post test was significant different between two groups ($p = 0.002$).

Both the intervention and control groups were associated with a non-significant increase in physical activity, but the intervention group had a significantly more physical activity than the control group at baseline. Then we assessed the difference between different physical activity behavior change in the intervention group and the control group. Those patients with coaching intervention and chose to set physical activity goal had a significant increase in medium of nine points in physical activity indicator (IQR = 18.0, $p = 0.007$) (**Table 3**). On the contrary, patients in the intervention group without setting physical activity goal had a significant decrease (IQR = 3.0, $p = 0.016$). However, the pre-test data also showed those patients who did not make the choice of setting a physical activity goal had a significantly better physical activity habit in both the intervention group and the control group.

In this study, health diet goal setting was about more balanced and healthy diets for the diabetes patients, rather than simply decreasing the number of times to eat out. Both the intervention and control groups had a significant decrease in the number of times of eating out in a week. However, the decrease in the frequency of eating out behavior was associated with the healthy diet goal setting while those without healthy diet goal have non-significant decrease in the number of times.

There were non-significant of the baseline characteristics between follow-up patients and those who skipped hospital visits during the intervention, and it was the same as in the control group.

TABLE 3 | The different between goal setting subgroups and coaching effects under COVID-19 pandemic.

	Physical activity goal setting					
	Intervention group (n = 54)			Control group (n = 50)		
	Yes (n = 22)	No (n = 32)	p-value	Yes (n = 19)	No (n = 31)	p-value
Physical activity points						
Pre-test [MD(IQR)]	0 (10.0)	21.0 (24.0)	<0.001*[a]	0 (10.0)	9.0 (18.0)	<0.001*
Post-test [MD(IQR)]	18.0 (14.0)	18.0 (24.0)	0.451	6.0 (15.0)	12.0 (21.0)	0.451
Pre-post difference [MD(IQR)]	9.0 (18.0)*[b]	0 (3.0)*	<0.001*	0 (7.0)*	0 (8.25)	0.712
	Healthy diet goal setting					
	Yes (n = 38)	No (n = 16)	p-value	Yes (n = 43)	No (n = 7)	p-value
Frequency of eating out in a week, times						
Pre-test [MD(IQR)]	5.0 (10.0)	5.5 (12.0)	0.915	6.0 (12.0)	0 (6.0)	0.094
Post-test [MD(IQR)]	4.0 (8.0)	5.5 (7.0)	0.335	5.0 (10.0)	0 (4.0)	0.070
Pre-post difference [MD(IQR)]	0 (2.25)*	0 (0.0)	0.242	0 (2.0)*	0 (1.0)	0.869

*$p < 0.05$.
[a]Analyzed with Mann-Whitney U-test.
[b]Analyzed with Wilcoxon signed-rank test.

DISCUSSION

In this study, we found that between February and May, the COVID-19 pandemic might cause the decrease in the patients' physical activity and eating out behavior. However, if any patient had set behavior change goal and even had follow-up communication, they were less affected by pandemic. Overall, the intervention group had the decrease in HbA1c by an average of 0.49% in these 3 months. Since the physical activity habit and healthy diet had considerable effect on blood control, helping patients maintain these good habits might be even more important during the COVID-19 pandemic.

In both the intervention and control groups, patients who originally had poorer physical activity habits were more likely to set change goals in coaching during pretest; however, patients with telephone coaching tracking, the effect of the change was significantly better. If the goal of physical activity habit change was not set, those who had better physical activity habits might reduce the amount of physical activity due to the pandemic. It was clear that they might need someone to help them make an appropriate decision to maintain good physical activity habit. Health coaching might have served an effective way to maintain or improve physical activity habit. Some studies have confirmed that health coaching can indeed help diabetes patients improve physical activity habits (18–20).

We also found that during the pandemic, the frequency of eating out was decreased among most of the subjects. Although the difference between the two groups was non-significant, patients who had set diet improvement goals had a significantly lower number of times eating out. Most diabetes health education, nutrition counseling, and health coaches provide guidance on dietary changes for diabetics mainly with dietary choices rather than eating out behavior, and these interventions also seemed to be indirectly affecting eating out habits (21, 22). Reducing the number of eating out means that patients have more chances to prepare their own food, but how to eat healthy is still the main issue.

Since early 2020, only a very small number of studies have specifically focused on the changes in living habits of people with type 2 diabetes during the pandemic, and the results of these studies seem to be inconsistent. A study in Spain found that people with type 2 diabetes have increased their intake of both vegetables and unhealthy snacks and decreased their physical activity during the lockdown (23). However, a study in India found that due to the lockdown policies, work pressure is reduced and it has helped people with type 2 diabetes improve their medication adherence and physical activity at home, thereby improving their blood sugar control (24). It seems that the changes in healthy lifestyle caused by the pandemic are varied in different countries (25), but many scholars still suggest that effective home physical activity and healthy eating strategies should be developed to help chronic patients maintain their health status (26, 27). During this period, telephone coaching or counseling can be a suitable and effective method as well (28, 29), and many studies have even confirmed the effectiveness of telephone coaching before the pandemic (30, 31). Therefore, our study results indeed verify that behavioral coaching should help people with type 2 diabetes maintain a good lifestyle during the pandemic and even continue to improve their blood sugar control.

Health coaching may effectively strengthen communication between doctors and patients, and at the same time strengthen sociopsychological support (32, 33). Of course, it may also help patients reduce unnecessary or excessive risk perception, strengthen their sense of responsibility of self-management, and encourage patients to regular visit the hospital for normal follow-ups to track diabetes and maintain appropriate healthy living habits according to the recommendations of the doctor (34, 35). Because of the lockdown and preventive measures, people's lifestyle and daily habits have changed. For example, instead of swimming and going to the gym people have switched to outdoor sports such as jogging and cycling (36); moreover, people often prepare their own food rather than eating out. However, before the pandemic, making changes in behavior and habits was already quite difficult, and now the imposed restrictions have made effective behavior coaching and guidance even more important. Hence, it is inadequate to rely on normal health education alone (37). Although the COVID-19 pandemic in Taiwan has gradually eased compared with other countries, making the result of this study less clear, we believe that in other countries where the pandemic is more serious, patients with chronic diseases who fail to maintain healthy lifestyle and regular follow-ups will create a huge burden to the society and medical system in the future. Therefore, given that the pandemic is expected to continue for some time, more rigorous interventional studies are still needed.

In this study, of those patients who dropped from regular visits, it seemed that there was no significant difference in patients' characteristics between the two groups. Although this might be because the sample observed in this study was not large enough, it could be interpreted that there were fewer patients in the hospital and more people chose not to visit the hospital during the pandemic. This is consistent with the findings of some studies (11, 38), which means that during the epidemic, it is still important to assist chronic patients to maintain regular visits.

This study has several strengths. First, this is one of the few studies done on health behavior changes in patients with chronic diseases in Taiwan during the pandemic. Although this study is not specifically designed to explore the behavior changes of Taiwanese people under the pandemic and has some limitations due to our statistic method, it can still reflect to a certain degree the effect of the pandemic at that time. Second, this article is specifically for the observation in the early months of the pandemic. Few studies were able to promptly explore the changes in people's living habits at the beginning of the chaos. Therefore, even if the interpretation of the research results is relatively limited, it can still provide valuable observations and discoveries.

Of course, this study has some limitations. First, since we pooled data with two different follow-up periods, it was not possible to accurately compare the pure effect of coaching on the maintenance of diabetes self-management on patients. Hence, detecting the pure difference of HbA1c was also unsuitable. Second, since this study was orientated from a behavior intervention study which focused on patients with type 2 diabetes rather than an observational study; therefore, it had fewer study samples than observational studies and did not compare with a healthy control group. It made the evidence less strong from this quasi-experimental study and had lower reproducibility than normal well-designed observational studies, but we believe it still has considerable reference value when a future outbreak occurs, especially in the early stage of the pandemic, since it can happen too suddenly for people to have a well-designed and rigorous study specifically focusing on the change of the lifestyle of chronic patients under the pandemic, especially at the initial stage.

According to the result of this study, here are some applications. First, during the pandemic prevention period, policy makers should also pay attention to the communication need of chronic patients to lessen excessive risk avoidance by actively offering counseling and intervention programs instead of passively handing out patient guides or providing health education. The pandemic has drastically changed people's lifestyles, so how to assist patients in adjusting and maintaining healthy living habits during the pandemic is still an important issue. People's lifestyles have changed considerably after the outbreak; therefore, assisting people in implementing a healthy lifestyle can reduce the impact of lifestyle changes. For example, we can especially promote some physical activities that are suitable for the home environment, introduce healthy cooking ways, encourage chronic patients for regular screening and visits, or use telemedicine to handle the current status of patients. Second, good communication and establishing a good relationship with patients can encourage patients to use the correct channels to obtain pandemic-related information more effectively and resolve patients' queries; hence, it can avoid risky behaviors, especially skipping regular hospital visits. We believe that if the COVID-19 pandemic does continue to spread for some time, these works may avoid the accidental deterioration of chronic disease control due to pandemic situation and pandemic prevention and will be very pivotal for medical system, government of all countries and the world.

AUTHOR CONTRIBUTIONS

S-HY, C-LL, R-YC, L-CH, and Y-TC participated in the conception, design of the study, performed the statistical analysis, and drafted the manuscript. C-LL screened eligible patients, then C-LL and L-CH recruited patients. Y-TC participated in acquisition of data. All authors contributed to the article and approved the submitted version.

ACKNOWLEDGMENTS

The authors would like to thank the participants of the study for their time and efforts.

REFERENCES

1. Taiwan Center for Disease Control. COVID-19 Global Stastistic (2021). Available online at: https://sites.google.com/cdc.gov.tw/2019ncov/global (accessed March 13, 2021).
2. *Novel Coronavirus (2019-nCoV) Situation Reports.* (2021). Available online at: https://www.who.int/emergencies/diseases/novel-coronavirus-2019/situation-reports (accessed May 04, 2021).
3. Kocak Tufan Z, Kayaaslan B. Crushing the curve, the role of national and international institutions and policy makers in COVID-19 pandemic. *Turk J Med Sci.* (2020) 50:495–508. doi: 10.3906/sag-2004-167
4. Jung SJ, Jun JY. Mental health and psychological intervention amid COVID-19 outbreak: perspectives from South Korea. *Yonsei Med J.* (2020) 61:271–2. doi: 10.3349/ymj.2020.61.4.271
5. Petzold MB, Plag J, Strohle A. *Dealing With Psychological Distress by Healthcare Professionals During the COVID-19 Pandemia.* Nervenarzt (2020).
6. Wang CJ, Ng CY, Brook RH. Response to COVID-19 in Taiwan: big data analytics, new technology, proactive testing. *JAMA.* (2020) 323:1341–2. doi: 10.1001/jama.2020.3151
7. National Health Insurance Administration, Ministry of Health and Welfare Taiwan. *National Health Insurance Medical Declaration Status Statistics.* (2020). Avaliable online at: https://www.nhi.gov.tw/Content_List.aspx?n=D529CAC4D8F8E77B&topn=23C660CAACAA159D,2020.05.21 (accessed May 04, 2021).
8. Mattioli AV, Sciomer S, Cocchi C, Maffei S, Gallina S. Quarantine during COVID-19 outbreak: changes in diet and physical activity increase the risk of cardiovascular disease. *Nutr Metab Cardiovasc Dis.* (2020) 30:1409–17. doi: 10.1016/j.numecd.2020.05.020
9. Robinson E, Boyland E, Chisholm A, Harrold J, Maloney GN, Marty L, et al. Obesity, eating behavior and physical activity during COVID-19 lockdown: a study of UK adults. *Appetite.* (2021) 156:104853. doi: 10.1016/j.appet.2020.104853
10. Werneck AO, Silva DR, Malta DC, Gomes CS, Souza PRB, Azevedo LO, et al. Associations of sedentary behaviours and incidence of unhealthy diet during the COVID-19 quarantine in Brazil. *Public Health Nutr.* (2021) 24:422–6. doi: 10.1017/S1368980020004188
11. Ikesu R, Miyawaki A, Sugiyama T, Nakamura M, Ninomiya H, Kobayashi Y. Trends in diabetes care during the COVID-19 outbreak in Japan: an observational study. *J Gen Int Med.* (2021) 1–3. doi: 10.1007/s11606-020-06413-w
12. Merzon E, Green I, Shpigelman M, Vinker S, Raz I, Golan-Cohen A, et al. Haemoglobin A1c is a predictor of COVID-19 severity in patients with diabetes. *Diabetes Metab Res Rev.* (2020) 37. doi: 10.1002/dmrr.3398
13. Pinto LC, Bertoluci MC. Type 2 diabetes as a major risk factor for COVID-19 severity: a meta-analysis. *Arch Endocrinol Metab.* (2020) 64:199–200. doi: 10.20945/2359-3997000000256
14. McGurnaghan SJ, Weir A, Bishop J, Kennedy S, Blackbourn LAK, McAllister DA, et al. Risks of and risk factors for COVID-19 disease in people with diabetes: a cohort study of the total population of Scotland. *Lancet Diabetes Endocrinol.* (2021) 9:82–93. doi: 10.1016/S2213-8587(20)30405-8
15. Chen R-Y, Huang L-C, Su C-T, Chang Y-T, Chu C-L, Chang C-L, et al. Effectiveness of short-term health coaching on diabetes control and self-management efficacy: a quasi-experimental trial. *Front Public Health.* (2019) 7:314. doi: 10.3389/fpubh.2019.00314
16. Godin G, Shephard R. A simple method to assess exercise behavior in the community. *Can J Appl Sport Sci.* (1985) 10:141–6.
17. Amireault S, Godin G. The Godin-Shephard leisure-time physical activity questionnaire: validity evidence supporting its use for classifying healthy adults into active and insufficiently active categories. *Perceptual motor Skills.* (2015) 120:604–22. doi: 10.2466/03.27.PMS.120v19x7
18. DeJesus RS, Clark MM, Finney Rutten LJ, Jacobson RM, Croghan IT, Wilson PM, et al. A - impact of a 12-week wellness coaching on self-care behaviors among primary care adult patients with prediabetes. *Prev Med Rep.* (2018) 10:100–5. doi: 10.1016/j.pmedr.2018.02.012
19. do Valle Nascimento TM, Resnicow K, Nery M, Brentani A, Kaselitz E, Agrawal P, et al. A pilot study of a community health agent-led type 2 diabetes self-management program using motivational interviewing-based approaches in a public primary care center in São Paulo, Brazil. *BMC Health Serv Res.* (2017) 17:32. doi: 10.1186/s12913-016-1968-3
20. Varney JE, Weiland TJ, Inder WJ, Jelinek GA. Effect of hospital-based telephone coaching on glycaemic control and adherence to management guidelines in type 2 diabetes, a randomised controlled trial. *Int Med J.* (2014) 44:890–7. doi: 10.1111/imj.12515
21. Gilstrap LG, Malhotra R, Peltier-Saxe D, Slicas D, Pineda E, Culhane-Hermann C, et al. Community-based primary prevention programs decrease the rate of metabolic syndrome among socioeconomically disadvantaged women. *J Womens Health.* (2013) 22:322–9. doi: 10.1089/jwh.2012.3854
22. Shawley-Brzoska S, Misra R. Perceived benefits and barriers of a community-based diabetes prevention and management program. *J Clin Med.* (2018) 7:58. doi: 10.3390/jcm7030058
23. Ruiz-Roso MB, Knott-Torcal C, Matilla-Escalante DC, Garcimartin A, Sampedro-Nunez MA, Davalos A, et al. COVID-19 lockdown and changes of the dietary pattern and physical activity habits in a cohort of patients with type 2 diabetes mellitus. *Nutrients.* (2020) 12. doi: 10.3390/nu12082327
24. Rastogi A, Hiteshi P, Bhansali A. Improved glycemic control amongst people with long-standing diabetes during COVID-19 lockdown: a prospective, observational, nested cohort study. *Int J Diabetes Dev Countr.* (2020) 40:476–81. doi: 10.1007/s13410-020-00880-x
25. Murphy B, Benson T, McCloat A, Mooney E, Elliott C, Dean M, et al. Changes in consumers' food practices during the COVID-19 lockdown, implications for diet quality and the food system: a cross-continental comparison. *Nutrients.* (2021) 13. doi: 10.3390/nu13010020
26. Guadalupe-Grau A, Lopez-Torres O, Martos-Bermudez A, Gonzalez-Gross M. Home-based training strategy to maintain muscle function in older adults with diabetes during COVID-19 confinement. *J Diabetes.* (2020) 12:701–2. doi: 10.1111/1753-0407.13051
27. Marcal IR, Fernandes B, Viana AA, Ciolac EG. The urgent need for recommending physical activity for the management of diabetes during and beyond COVID-19 outbreak. *Front Endocrinol.* (2020) 11:584642. doi: 10.3389/fendo.2020.584642
28. Lian X, Dalan R, Seow CJ, Liew H, Jong M, Chew D, et al. Diabetes care during COVID-19 pandemic in Singapore using a telehealth strategy. *Hormone Metab Res.* (2021) 53. doi: 10.1055/a-1352-5023
29. Rachmiel M, Lebenthal Y, Mazor-Aronovitch K, Brener A, Levek N, Levran N, et al. Glycaemic control in the paediatric and young adult population with type 1 diabetes following a single telehealth visit-what have we learned from the COVID-19 lockdown? *Acta Diabetol.* (2021) 1–9. doi: 10.1007/s00592-021-01673-2
30. Miyamoto S, Dharmar M, Fazio S, Tang-Feldman Y, Young HM. mHealth technology and nurse health coaching to improve health in diabetes: protocol for a randomized controlled trial. *JMIR Res Protoc.* (2018) 7:e45. doi: 10.2196/resprot.9168
31. Fazio S, Edwards J, Miyamoto S, Henderson S, Dharmar M, Young HM. More than A1C: types of success among adults with type-2 diabetes participating in a technology-enabled nurse coaching intervention. *Patient Educ Couns.* (2019) 102:106–12. doi: 10.1016/j.pec.2018.08.028
32. Alders I, Smits C, Brand P, van Dulmen S. Does patient coaching make a difference in patient-physician communication during specialist consultations? A systematic review. *Patient Educ Couns.* (2017) 100:882–96. doi: 10.1016/j.pec.2016.12.029
33. Sherifali D, Viscardi V, Bai JW, Ali RMU. Evaluating the effect of a diabetes health coach in individuals with type 2 diabetes. *Can J Diabetes.* (2016) 40:84–94. doi: 10.1016/j.jcjd.2015.10.006
34. Rubak S, Sandbaek A, Lauritzen T, Borch-Johnsen K, Christensen B. General practitioners trained in motivational interviewing can positively affect the attitude to behaviour change in people with type 2 diabetes. One year follow-up of an RCT. ADDITION Denmark. *Scand J Prim Health Care.* (2009) 27:172–9. doi: 10.1080/02813430903072876
35. Miyamoto S, Henderson S, Fazio S, Saconi B, Thiede E, Greenwood DA, et al. Empowering diabetes self-management through technology and nurse health coaching. *Diabetes Educ.* (2019) 45:586–95. doi: 10.1177/0145721719879421

36. Grabia M, Markiewicz-Zukowska R, Puscion-Jakubik A, Bielecka J, Nowakowski P, Gromkowska-Kepka K, et al. The nutritional and health effects of the COVID-19 pandemic on patients with diabetes mellitus. *Nutrients.* (2020) 12. doi: 10.3390/nu12103013

37. Werbrouck A, Swinnen E, Kerckhofs E, Buyl R, Beckwee D, De Wit L. How to empower patients? A systematic review and meta-analysis. *Transl Behav Med.* (2018) 8:660–74. doi: 10.1093/tbm/iby064

38. Fragala MS, Kaufman HW, Meigs JB, Niles JK, McPhaul MJ. Consequences of the COVID-19 pandemic: reduced hemoglobin A1c diabetes monitoring. *Popul Health Manag.* (2021) 24:8–9. doi: 10.1089/pop.2020.0134

8

Immunological Characteristics in Type 2 Diabetes Mellitus Among COVID-19 Patients

Meifang Han[1†], *Ke Ma*[1], *Xiaojing Wang*[1], *Weiming Yan*[1], *Hongwu Wang*[1], *Jie You*[1], *Qiuxia Wang*[2], *Huilong Chen*[1], *Wei Guo*[1], *Tao Chen*[1], *Qin Ning*[1*†] and *Xiaoping Luo*[3*†]

[1] Department and Institute of Infectious Disease, Tongji Hospital of Tongji Medical College, Huazhong University of Science and Technology, Wuhan, China, [2] Department of Radiology, Tongji Hospital, Tongji Medical College, Huazhong University of Science and Technology, Wuhan, China, [3] Department of Pediatrics, Center for the Diagnosis of Genetic Metabolic Diseases, Tongji Hospital, Tongji Medical College, Huazhong University of Science and Technology, Wuhan, China

***Correspondence:**
Xiaoping Luo
xpluo888@sina.com
Qin Ning
qning@vip.sina.com

†ORCID:
Meifang Han
orcid.org/0000-0002-1948-8128
Qin Ning
orcid.org/0000-0002-2027-9593
Xiaoping Luo
orcid.org/0000-0002-3748-4817

Clinical Trial Registration: www.ClinicalTrials.gov, identifier: NCT04365634.

Context: Diabetes mellitus was associated with increased severity and mortality of disease in COVID-19 pneumonia. So far the effect of type 2 diabetes (T2DM) or hyperglycemia on the immune system among COVID-19 disease has remained unclear.

Objective: We aim to explore the clinical and immunological features of type 2 diabetes mellitus (T2DM) among COVID-19 patients.

Design and Methods: In this retrospective study, the clinical and immunological characteristics of 306 hospitalized confirmed COVID-19 patients (including 129 diabetic and 177 non-diabetic patients) were analyzed. The serum concentrations of laboratory parameters including cytokines and numbers of immune cells were measured and compared between diabetic and non-diabetic groups.

Results: Compared with non-diabetic group, diabetic cases more frequently had lymphopenia and hyperglycemia, with higher levels of urea nitrogen, myoglobin, D-dimer and ferritin. Diabetic cases indicated the obviously elevated mortality and the higher levels of cytokines IL-2R, IL-6, IL-8, IL-10, and TNF-α, as well as the distinctly reduced Th1/Th2 cytokines ratios compared with non-diabetic cases. The longitudinal assays showed that compared to that at week 1, the levels of IL-6 and IL-8 were significantly elevated at week 2 after admission in non-survivors of diabetic cases, whereas there were greatly reductions from week 1 to week 2 in survivors of diabetic cases. Compared with survival diabetic patients, non-survival diabetic cases displayed distinct higher serum concentrations of IL-2R, IL-6, IL-8, IL-10, TNF-α, and lower Th1/Th2 cytokines ratios at week 2. Samples from a subset of participants were evaluated by flow cytometry for the immune cells. The counts of peripheral total T lymphocytes, $CD4^+$ T cells, $CD8^+$ T cells and NK cells were markedly lower in diabetic cases than in non-diabetic cases. The non-survivors showed the markedly declined counts of $CD8^+$ T cells and NK cells than survivors.

Conclusion: The elevated cytokines, imbalance of Th1/Th2 cytokines ratios and reduced of peripheral numbers of $CD8^+$ T cells and NK cells might contribute to the pathogenic mechanisms of high mortality of COVID-19 patients with T2DM.

Keywords: type 2 diabetes mellitus, COVID-19, immune cells, cytokines, Th1/Th2 ratio

INTRODUCTION

In late December 2019, a novel viral pneumonia with an acute severe respiratory tract illness developed in Wuhan, China, and spread rapidly worldwide, becoming a public health emergency of international concern (1–5). A previously unknown coronavirus, officially named the severe acute respiratory syndrome coronavirus 2 (SARS-CoV-2), with the genome sequence closely related but distinct to severe acute respiratory syndrome or Middle East respiratory syndrome (MERS) virus, was first isolated as a pathogen of the Novel Coronavirus Disease 2019 (COVID-19) by the Chinese Center for Disease Control and Prevention (2, 6, 7).

Our previous data reported the clinical and immunologic features of severe COVID-19 pneumonia (8), indicating that SARS-CoV-2 may primarily affect T lymphocytes, particularly $CD4^+$ and $CD8^+$ T cells, resulting in a decrease in the number and production of IFN-γ by $CD4^+$ T cells (8, 9). Other studies also showed that T cell counts were significantly reduced in patients with COVID-19, and the surviving T cells appeared functionally exhausted (10). An elevated level of cytokines, such as interleukin (IL)-1, IL-2, IL-6, IL-8, IL-10, TNF-α, and soluble IL-2R, and a sharp inflammatory storm have been reported in patients with severe COVID-19 by our team and other researchers (11–16).

The incidence of type 2 diabetes mellitus (T2DM) is increasing worldwide, and diabetes is one of the leading causes of morbidity and mortality globally among chronic diseases (17). Among chronic comorbidities of COVID-19, diabetes had the second highest incidence rate (7.4%–19.0%), following hypertension (15%–30%) (18, 19). Patients with diabetes were likely at higher risk for severe COVID-19 and mortality (20–25). The IL-6, ferritin, C-reaction protein, and D-dimer levels were significantly increased in patients with diabetes, suggesting that a marked inflammatory cytokine storm was associated with a more pejorative prognosis compared to patients without diabetes (22). To date, the detailed effect of diabetes or hyperglycaemia on the immune cells and immune system in patients with COVID-19 remains unclear.

Based on the retrospective study on 306 patients of COVID-19 disease (129 with diabetes and 177 without diabetes), we first identified that patients with diabetes showed distinct immune characteristics from patients without diabetes, including markedly elevated cytokine level, reduced T-helper type 1 (Th1)/T-helper type 2 (Th2) cytokine ratios, and decreased number of $CD4^+$ T cells, $CD8^+$ T cells, and natural killer (NK) cells. What's more, we found the elevated cytokines and declined immune cells were associated with the mortality of COVID-19 disease with T2DM. These findings may help broaden our understanding of the pathogenesis mechanism and relationship between diabetes and COVID-19.

Abbreviations: PHEIC, Public health emergency of international concern; SARS-CoV-2, Severe acute respiratory syndrome coronavirus 2; COVID-19, Coronavirus Disease 2019; T2DM, Type 2 diabetes mellitus; SOFA, Sepsis-related organ failure assessment; GGO, Ground-glass opacity; Th1, T-helper type 1; Th2, T-helper type 2; RPG, Random plasma glucose; FPG, Fasting plasma glucose; ULN, Upper limit of normal value; LLN, Lower limit of normal value; IQR, Interquartile range.

MATERIALS AND METHODS

Study Design and Participants

This single-centre, retrospective, observational study was conducted in Tongji Hospital (Wuhan, China), which is a designated hospital for patients with severe COVID-19 pneumonia (NTC04365634). All patients were transported from other hospitals. Patients admitted from February 2, 2020, to February 15, 2020, and diagnosed with COVID-19 pneumonia according to the interim guidance of the National Health Commission of the People's Republic of China were enrolled in the study (26). Laboratory-confirmed cases were identified with positive viral RNA by real-time reverse transcription polymerase chain reaction (RT-PCR) detection by the local health authority or our hospital from a specimen obtained from a throat or nasal swab. In the enrolled patients, clinical outcomes were evaluated on March 14, 2020. The ethics committee of Tongji Hospital approved the study (TJ-C20200101). Written informed consent was waived due to the rapid emergence of this fatal disease.

Definitions

Diabetes mellitus was diagnosed according to the standards of the American Diabetes Association (27), which were briefly described as fasting plasma glucose (FPG) level ≥ 7.0 mmol/L (fasting is defined as no caloric intake for at least 8 h) or 2-h plasma glucose level ≥ 11.1 mmol/L during oral glucose tolerance test or with classic symptoms of hyperglycaemia or hyperglycaemic crisis and random plasma glucose (RPG) level ≥11.1 mmol/L. The sepsis-related organ failure assessment (SOFA) and CURB-65 scores are defined or determined using the relative criteria (19, 28, 29). The disease severity of COVID-19 was defined according to the Chinese management guideline for COVID-19 (version 6.0) and described in a previous study (26, 30).

Laboratory Procedures

Clinical laboratory assays were conducted in the Department of Clinical Laboratory of Tongji Hospital with the certificate of laboratory qualification of China for the assay parameters mentioned above in data collection.

Real-Time RT-PCR Assay for SARS-CoV-2

The methods of laboratory confirmation of SARS-CoV-2 infection have been described (5, 31). Briefly, SARS-CoV-2 RNA was extracted from throat or nasal swab samples from suspected patients. The presence of SARS-CoV-2 was detected by real-time RT-PCR assay at the local centres of the Chinese Center for Disease Control and Prevention and Tongji Hospital. The SARS-CoV-2 nucleic acid detection kit was used according to the manufacturer's protocol (DAAN Gene Co., Ltd., of Sun Yat-sen University). These diagnostic methods and criteria were based on the recommendations of the National Institute for Viral Disease Control and Prevention of China.

Measurements of Cytokines

According to hospital's standard procedures, fresh blood samples were centrifuged for 10 min at 2,000g. Serum was collected and tested within 4–6 h. All procedures were performed under level 3 protection. Cytokines including interleukin-2 receptor (sIL-2R), IL-1 β, IL-6, IL-8, IL-10, and TNF-α were assessed in serum samples drawn shortly at each time points by chemiluminescence immunoassay (CLIA) performed on a fully automated analyzer (Immulite 1000, DiaSorin Liaison, Italy or Cobas e602, Roche Diagnostics, Germany) for all patients according to the manufacturer's instructions. IL-2R kit (#LKIP1), IL-1 β kit (#LKL11), IL-8 kit (#LK8P1), IL-10 kit (#LKXP1), and TNF-α kit (#LKNF1) were purchased from DiaSorin (Vercelli, Italy). IL-6 kit (#05109442 190) was purchased from Roche Diagnostics, Germany.

Number of Peripheral Blood Immunological Cells by Flow Cytometry

Samples from a subset of participants were evaluated by flow cytometry for the immune cells. Fresh peripheral blood samples were obtained from nine patients with and 11 patients without diabetes among the patients with COVID-19 after their agreements, and the proportions and numbers of NK, $CD4^+$ T, $CD8^+$ T, and B cells and expression of cell surface markers were studied in these patients in a short time. Flow cytometry antibodies against human surface and intracellular molecules were commercially available. The following antibodies were used: BD Multitest 6-Color TBNK reagent (#644611) and BD Trucount Tubes (#340334). It contains FITC-labeled CD3, clone SK7; PE-labeled CD16, clone B73.1, and CD56, clone NCAM16.2; PerCP-Cy5.5-labeled CD45, clone 2D1; PE-Cy7-labeled CD4, clone SK3; APC-labeled CD19, clone SJ25C1; and APC-Cy7-labeled CD8, clone SK1. The BD Trucount™ Absolute Counting Tubes, which contain a known number of fluorescent beads, were used for quantifying leucocyte populations. After another two washes with PBS, cells were resuspended in 500 µl of PBS. Among all collected events, single events were gated between FSC-A and FSC-H. Cell debris was excluded and intact cells were then gated from single events based on FSC-A and SSC. Each cell population was then detected based on the antibody staining. All reagents were purchased from Becton, Dickinson and Company (BD). All samples were detected using the BD FACSCanto II flow cytometry system and analysed using the BD FACSDiva software.

Chest Computed Tomography (CT) and Evaluation

All chest CT data were acquired using one of the following two commercial multidetector CT scanners: GE Medical Systems/LightSpeed 16 (GE Healthcare, USA) and Siemens/SOMATOM Definition AS (Siemens Healthineers, Germany). Two senior radiologists independently reviewed chest CT images with PACS (Tianjian Health, China). Chest CT images were independently evaluated by two radiologists, and any disagreement in the classification variables was resolved through consultation (32). The distribution of lung abnormalities was mainly subpleural (mainly involving the outer third of the lung), random (subpleural or middle region is not preferred), or diffuse (continuous involvement, not involving the lung segment).

Statistical Analysis

Continuous variables were presented as median and interquartile range (IQR) and compared using the Mann-Whitney U test. Categorical variables were expressed as numbers (%) and compared using χ^2 test. Fisher's exact test was used in the analysis of contingency tables when the sample sizes were small. The Kaplan-Meier method was used for the time-to-event plot in the survival analysis. Comparisons between groups in the survival analysis were conducted using the Cox proportion hazards model. A P-value <0.05 (two-tailed) was considered statistically significant. The data were analysed using SPSS statistical software version 19.0.

RESULTS

Demographic and Clinical Characteristics

From February 2, 2020, to February 15, 2020, 306 patients with COVID-19 pneumonia confirmed by positive nucleotide tests of SARS-CoV-2 were enrolled in this study. According to the T2DM criteria, 129 of 306 (42.2%) patients were diagnosed with T2DM and 177 (57.8%) had no T2DM based on FPG or RPG levels (27). The demographic and clinical characteristics on admission are presented in **Table 1**. SOFA and CURB-65 scores, a clinical predictive score for severity of pneumonia, were significantly higher in patients with diabetes compared with those in patients without diabetes. According to the criteria of disease severity in the Chinese management guideline for COVID-19, the proportion of critical illness cases in the diabetic group was higher than that of the non-diabetic group (10.9% vs. 4.5%, p<0.0001), which, together with the SOFA and CURB-65 scores, strongly demonstrated that patients with T2DM tended to have higher disease severity than patients without diabetes.

TABLE 1 | Comparing demographics, clinical scores, laboratory findings, and CT image features on admission between T2DM and non-T2DM cases among COVID-19 patients.

	Total n = 306	T2DM n = 129	Non-T2DM n = 177	p value
Demographics and clinical scores				
Age, years	60.0(49.0–70.0)	65.0(57.0–73.0)	55.0(43.0–67.0)	<0.0001
Gender, Male	174(56.9%)	81(62.8%)	93(52.5%)	0.08
SOFA score	2.0(0.0–3.0)	2.0(1.0–4.0)	1.0(0.0–2.0)	<0.0001
CURB-65 score	1.0(0.0–1.0)	1.0(0.0–2.0)	0.0(0.0–1.0)	<0.0001
Partial arterial oxygen pressure(mmHg)	63.9(44.7–89.8)	58.6(40.8–74.5)	74.5(48.2–117.5)	0.016
Disease severity status*	.	.	.	<0.0001
Moderate	160(52.3%)	51(39.5%)	109(61.6%)	.
Severe	124(40.5%)	64(49.6%)	60(33.9%)	.
Critical	22(7.2%)	14(10.9%)	8(4.5%)	.
Laboratory findings				
Fasting plasma glucose(mmol/L)	6.3(5.4–8.7)	9.4(7.7–13.6)	5.6(5.1–6.2)	<0.0001
<7.0	174/274(63.5%)	14/110(12.7%)	160/164(97.6%)	<0.0001
7.0–11.1	60/274(21.9)	56/110(50.9%)	4/164(2.4%)	<0.0001
≥11.1	40/274(14.6%)	40/110(36.4%)	0/164(0.0%)	<0.0001
Random plasma glucose(mmol/L)	6.7(5.7–8.9)	8.9(7.2–14.1)	6.0(5.4–6.8)	<0.0001
<7.0	158(53.9%)	27(20.9%)	138(78.0%)	<0.0001
7.0–11.1	94(30.7%)	57(44.2%)	37(20.9%)	<0.0001
≥11.1	47(15.4%)	45(34.9%)	2(1.1%)	<0.0001
White blood cell count(10^9/L)	5.6(4.4–8.0)	6.6(4.7–10.1)	5.1(4.3–7.2)	<0.0001
>10 (ULN)	50(16.3%)	33(25.6%)	17(9.6%)	<0.0001
Lymphocyte count(10^9/L)	0.8(0.6–1.2)	0.7(0.5–0.9)	0.9(0.7–1.3)	<0.0001
<1.1 (LLN)	213(69.6%)	106(82.2%)	107(60.5%)	<0.0001
ALB(g/L)	33.4(30.4–36.6)	32.4(29.6–35.8)	34.2(31.4–37.4)	0.002
≤30 (LLN)	67/303(22.1%)	38/128(29.7%)	29/175(16.6%)	0.007
LDH(U/L)	324.0(246.0–451.0)	361.0(266.3–490.8)	306.0(237.0–414.0)	0.001
>225 (ULN)	249/303(82.2%)	107/128(83.6%)	142/175(81.1%)	0.58
Total cholesterol (mmol/L)	3.5(3.0–4.0)	3.4(3.0–4.1)	3.5(3.0–4.0)	0.67
>5.18 (ULN)	7/303(2.3%)	5/128(3.9%)	2/175(1.1%)	0.11
Triglyceride (mmol/L)	1.3(1.0–1.8)	1.3(1.0–1.9)	1.3(1.0–1.8)	0.55
>1.7 (ULN)	40/139(28.8%)	21/68(30.9%)	19/71(26.8%)	0.59
urea nitrogen (mmol/L)	4.7(3.5–7.0)	5.6(3.9–9.0)	4.3(3.1–5.3)	<0.0001
>8 (ULN)	56/303(18.5%)	39/128(30.5%)	17/175(9.7%)	<0.0001
D-dimer (μg/ml)	1.0(0.5–2.6)	1.6(0.7–7.0)	0.7(0.4–1.6)	<0.0001
≥0.5 (ULN)	215/287(74.9%)	105/124(84.7%)	110/163(67.5%)	0.001
High-sensitivity cardiac troponin I (pg/ml)	7.3(2.8–20.7)	15.6(5.2–41.5)	3.9(2.2–13.3)	<0.0001
>28 (ULN)	45/218(20.6%)	32/99(32.3%)	13/119(10.9%)	<0.0001
Myoglobin (ng/ml)	93.1(34.4–183.1)	128.0(59.5–244.7)	32.0(22.7–104.0)	0.003
>106 (ULN)	21/45(46.7%)	17/29(58.6%)	4/16(25.0%)	0.03
PCT(ng/ml)	0.1(0.04–0.2)	0.1(0.1–0.3)	0.1(0.03–0.2)	<0.0001
≥0.05 (ULN)	186/289(64.4%)	94/120(78.3%)	92/169(54.4%)	<0.0001
CRP (mg/L)	53.0(20.5–101.4)	79.6(35.3–137.5)	44.6(18.2–84.9)	0.002
≥1	301/302(99.7%)	86/86(100.0%)	215/216(99.5%)	1.000
Serum ferritin (μg/L)	885.0(488.5–1566.2)	1086.5(571.3–1809.6)	652.5(380.2–1347.1)	0.002
>300 (ULN)	137/155(88.4%)	79/82(96.3%)	58/73(79.5%)	0.001
Cytokines				
IL-1B (pg/ml)	5.0(5.0–5.0)	5.0(5.0–5.0)	5.0(5.0–5.0)	0.27
≥5 (ULN)	241/242(99.6%)	106/106(100.0%)	135/136(99.3%)	1.00
IL-2R (μ/ml)	740.0(528.3–1063.3)	925.5(567.5–1256.3)	676.0(475.0–911.8)	<0.0001
>710 (ULN) or <223 (LLN)	130/242(53.7%)	67/106(63.2%)	63/136(46.3%)	0.009
IL-6(pg/ml)	16.4(3.9–54.4)	31.5(6.1–79.0)	12.7(2.7–35.5)	0.001
≥7 (ULN)	158/242(65.3%)	78/106(73.6%)	80/136(58.8%)	0.017
IL-8 (pg/ml)	15.1(8.8–24.3)	19.8(10.6–30.4)	12.0(8.2–21.3)	<0.0001
≥62 (ULN)	18/242(7.4%)	13/106(12.3%)	5/136(3.7%)	0.012
IL-10 (pg/ml)	5.3(5.0–10.0)	6.8(5.0–14.8)	5.0(5.0–8.4)	0.001
≥9.1 (ULN)	71/242(29.3%)	42/106(39.6%)	29/136(21.3%)	0.002
TNF-α (pg/ml)	8.4(6.8–10.8)	9.2(7.1–12.5)	8.1(6.2–9.8)	0.001
≥8.1 (ULN)	134/242(55.4%)	66/106(62.3%)	68/136(50.0%)	0.06
CT image features				
Distribution of pulmonary lesions	.	.	.	0.15
Peripheral	42/185(22.7%)	11/67(16.4%)	31/118(26.3%)	.

(Continued)

TABLE 1 | Continued

	Total n = 306	T2DM n = 129	Non-T2DM n = 177	p value
Random	30/185(16.2%)	9/67(13.4%)	21/118(17.8%)	.
Diffuse	113/185(61.1%)	47/67(70.1%)	66/118(55.9%)	.
Bilateral multilobe, n	177,185(95.7%)	66/67(98.5%)	111/118(94.1%)	0.26
Ground-glass opacity (GGO), n	176/185(95.1%)	64/67(95.5%)	112/118(95.1%)	1.00
Crazy-paving pattern, n	106/185(57.3%)	37/67(55.2%)	69/118(58.5%)	0.76
Consolidation, n	152/185(82.2%)	58/67(86.6%)	93/118(78.8%)	0.24

*Data are median (IQR), n (%), or n/N (%). p values were calculated by Mann-Whitney U test, χ^2 test, or Fisher's exact test, as appropriate. T2DM, type 2 diabetes mellitus; ALB, albumin; TBil, Total bilirubin; DBil, Direct bilirubin; LDH, Lactate dehydrogenase; PCT, Procalcitonin; ULN, Upper limit of normal value; LLN, lower limit of normal value. * Disease severity status was evaluated according to interim guidance of National health commission of China.*

Laboratory Parameters and Clinical Outcomes

There were strong differences in laboratory findings on admission between patients with diabetes and those without diabetes (**Table 1**). The FPG and RPG levels were distinctly higher in the diabetes group than in the non-diabetes group. The peripheral lymphocyte count was significantly lower in patients with diabetes than in those without diabetes (p<0.0001), whereas the white and neutral cell counts were higher in patients with diabetes than in those without diabetes, which might be related to the higher risk of infection in patients with diabetes. Laboratory parameters, including the serum urea nitrogen, high-sensitivity cardiac troponin I, myoglobin, D-dimer, lactate dehydrogenase, procalcitonin, C-reactive protein, and ferritin levels, were markedly higher in patients with diabetes than in those without diabetes. However, there was no significant difference in the total cholesterol and triglyceride levels between the diabetes and non-diabetes groups. With regard to the lung CT features, the diabetic group showed no distinct difference from the non-diabetic group.

Our data showed that the mortality on the 28th day after admission in the hospital was much higher in patients with diabetes than in those without diabetes (42.6% vs. 10.7%, p<0.0001). As shown in **Figure 1**, the Kaplan-Meier survival curves were affected by different FPG and RPG levels (**Figures 1A, B**). Patients with FPG level ≥ 11.1 mmol/L (p<0.0001) and FPG level between 7 and 11.1 mmol/L (p=0.0029) showed a greatly decreased survival compared to patients with FPG level < 7.0 mmol/L (separately) (**Figure 1A**). Patients with RPG level ≥ 11.1 mmol/L showed much decreased survival curves than patients with RPG level < 11.1 mmol/L (p<0.0001) (**Figure 1B**). With the increased FPG or RPG levels, the rates of death of patients with COVID-19 were raised accordingly, thus suggesting that hyperglycaemia might be an important risk factor for the mortality of patients with COVID-19.

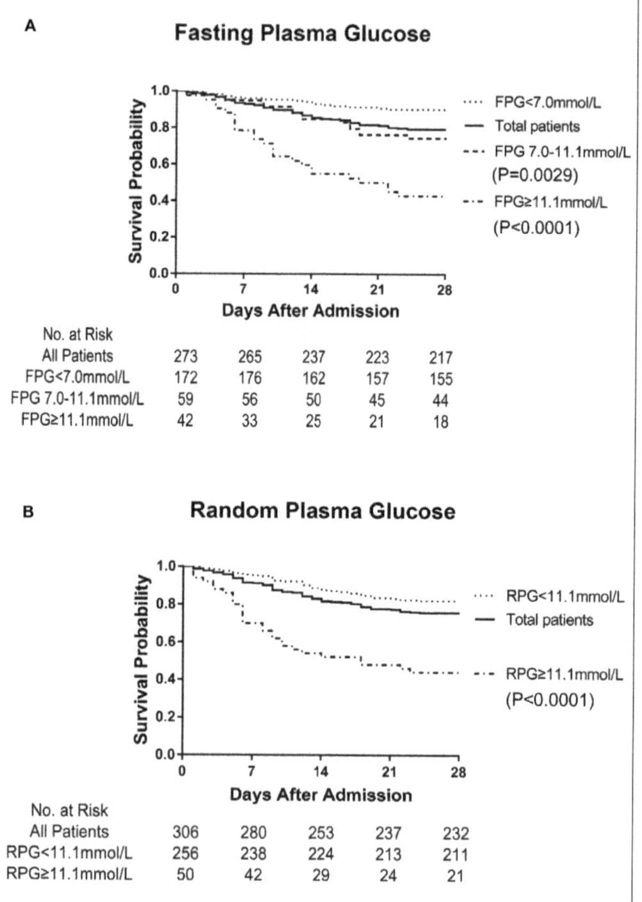

FIGURE 1 | Survival curve of patients with COVID-19 affected by fasting plasma glucose (FPG) and random plasma glucose (RPG) levels on admission. It shows the greatly decreased survival in patients with FPG level ≥ 7.0 mmol/L on admission compared with that in patients with FPG level < 7.0 mmol/L (p < 0.0001) **(A)**. It indicates the obviously decreased survival in patients with RPG level ≥11.1 mmol/L on admission compared with that in patients with RPG level <11.1 mmol/L (p < 0.0001) **(B)**.

Markedly Elevated Cytokine Levels and Decreased Th1/Th2 Cytokine Ratios in Patients With Diabetes

Regarding the Th1 cytokines, patients with diabetes indicated markedly higher IL-2R levels in week 1 and 2 after admission, IL-1β in week 3, and TNF-α in week 1–3 compared to patients without diabetes (**Figure 2**). As for the Th2 cytokines, the IL-6 and IL-10 levels in patients with diabetes in week 1–3, and IL-8 in week 1–3 were significantly higher than those in patients without diabetes. IL-6 and IL-10 levels in the patients without diabetes were observed to be reduced successively from week 1 to 3 and greatly decreased at week 2 and 3 compared to that in week 1,

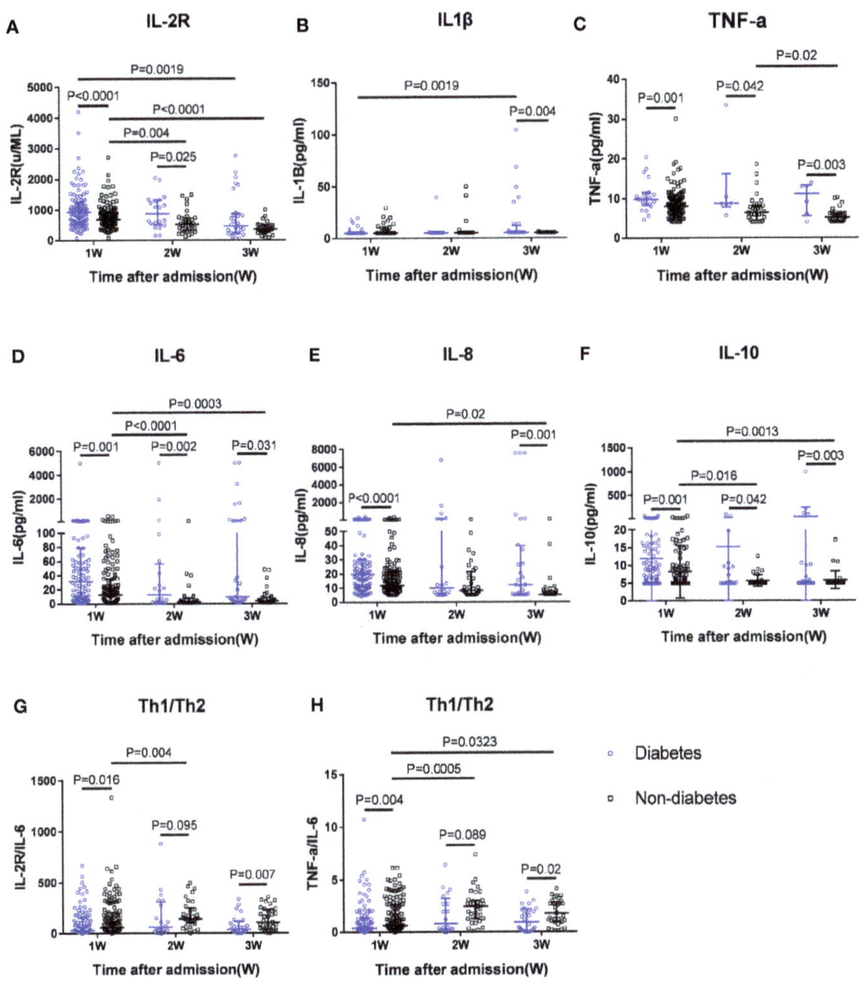

FIGURE 2 | Dynamic serum cytokine levels and Th1/Th2 ratios in diabetic patients and non-diabetic patients. Dynamic changes in Th1 cytokines including IL-2R **(A)**, IL-1β **(B)**, and TNF-α **(C)**; Th2 cytokines, including IL-6 **(D)**, IL-8 **(E)**, and IL-10 **(F)**, and ratios of IL-2R/IL-6 **(G)** and TNF-α/IL-6 **(H)** representing the Th1/Th2 ratios from week 1 to week 3 after admission in patients with T2DM and patients without T2DM with COVID-19 infection.

whereas they were not reduced in patients with diabetes from week 1 to week 3. These results indicated that patients with diabetes had significantly elevated inflammatory cytokine Th1 and Th2 levels, which is known as a cytokine storm.

Furthermore, we used the IL-2R/IL-6 and TNF-α/IL-6 ratios on behalf of the Th1/Th2 ratios to determine which type of T-helper cells was dominant in the progression of COVID-19. The Th1/Th2 ratios in patients with diabetes were much lower than in patients without diabetes through weeks 1–3 after admission, suggesting that Th2 cells were over-activated and the imbalance of Th1/Th2 cytokines in patients with diabetes was much greater than in patients without diabetes. Moreover, in patients without diabetes, the IL-2R/IL-6 and TNF-α/IL-6 ratios increased greatly in week 2 compared to that in week 1 (P=0.004 and P=0.0005, respectively), indicating that the imbalance of Th1/Th2 ratios recovered to some degree in week 2 in patients without diabetes, while there was no difference in patients with diabetes between week 1 and week 2. Thus, patients with diabetes showed longer imbalance of Th1/Th2 than in patients without diabetes.

Greatly Increased Levels of Cytokines in Non-Survival Diabetic COVID-19 Cases

To assess the association between the mortality of COVID-19 and the levels of cytokines, we analyzed the longitudinal expression profiles of cytokines from week 1 to week 2 after admission in survivors and non-survivors (**Figure 3**). Compared to that at week 1, the levels of IL-6 and IL-8 were significantly elevated at week 2 in non-survivors of diabetic cases, whereas there were greatly reductions in survivors of diabetes at week 2 than at week 1 (P<0.05, respectively). The ratios of IL-2R/IL-6 in diabetic non-survivors at week 2 were much declined compared to that at week 1, whereas they were lifted greatly in non-diabetic survivors, or there were no significant changes in the diabetic survivors and non-diabetic non-survivors from week 1 to week 2.

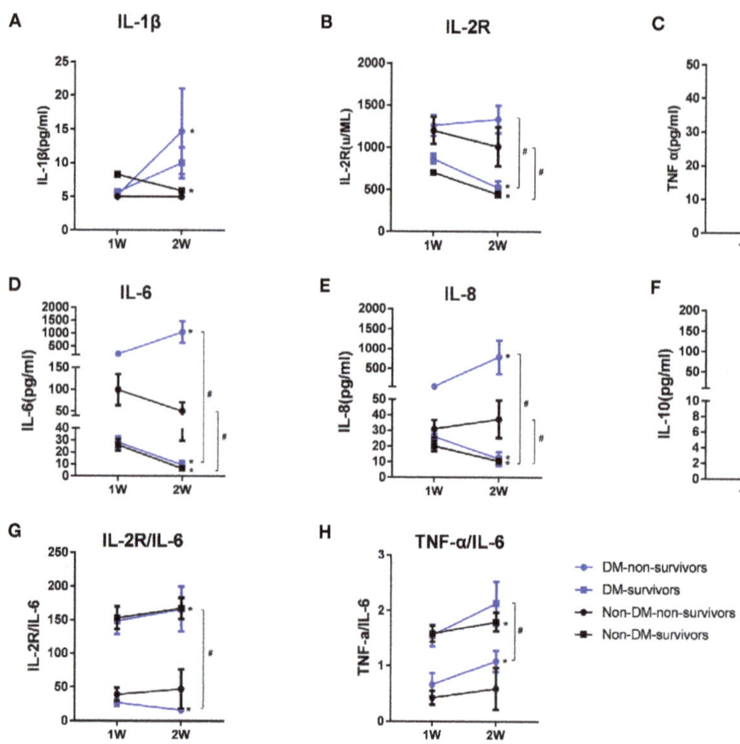

FIGURE 3 | Dynamic changes of serum cytokine levels and Th1/Th2 ratios in groups of diabetic non-survivors, diabetic survivors, non-diabetic non-survivors and non-diabetic survivors from week 1 to week 2. Dynamic changes in Th1 cytokines including IL-1β **(A)**, IL-2R **(B)**, and TNF-α **(C)**; Th2 cytokines, including IL-6 **(D)**, IL-8 **(E)**, and IL-10 **(F)**, and ratios of IL-2R/IL-6 **(G)** and TNF-α/IL-6 **(H)** representing the Th1/Th2 ratios from week 1 to week 2 after admission in survivors and non-survivors with COVID-19 infection. Data shown are median (IQR). *represents $P < 0.05$, week 2 vs. week 1. # represents $P < 0.05$, non-survivors vs. survivors at week 2 in diabetic or non-diabetic patients. DM, diabetes mellitus.

Compared with diabetic survival patients, diabetic non-survival cases showed distinct higher serum concentrations of IL-6, IL-8 and TNF-α and lower Th1/Th2 cytokines ratios (IL-2R/IL-6 and TNF-α/IL-6) at week 2 (P<0.05, respectively), suggesting that these higher levels of cytokines and much greater imbalance of Th1/Th2 cytokines ratios might be involved in the pathogenic mechanisms of mortality for diabetic COVID-19 patients. The median values of cytokines and P values of comparing the levels of cytokines among different groups including diabetic non-survivors, diabetic survivors, non-diabetic non-survivors and non- diabetic survivors patients were displayed in **Supplementary Table 1**.

Greatly Decreased Numbers of $CD4^+$ T Cells, $CD8^+$ T Cells, and NK Cells in Diabetic Cases

Then, we examined the proportion and counts of immune cells in the peripheral blood from nine patients with diabetes and 11 patients without diabetes among the patients with COVID-19 (**Table 2** and **Figure 4**). It was found that absolute numbers of total T lymphocytes were more seriously reduced in the patients with diabetes compared to those in patients without diabetes (448.0 vs. 962.0 × 10^6/L, P=0.002), while the absolute numbers of total B lymphocytes did not differ between the two groups. Furthermore, the numbers of $CD4^+$ T cells and $CD8^+$ T cells were reduced below the lower limit of normal (LLN) in the vast majority of patients with diabetes with COVID-19, and the medians of the diabetic group were reduced more profoundly than in the non-diabetic group (204.0 vs. 583.0 ×10^6/L, P=0.007 and 115.0 vs. 352 ×10^6/L, P=0.002, respectively). As for the NK cell count, it could be known that a lower NK cell count was observed in patients with diabetes compared to that in patients without diabetes (35.0 vs 252.0×10^{6}/L, P=0.004) (**Figure 4E**). Moreover, we found a greater reduction in the total absolute numbers of T, B, and NK cells in the diabetic group than in the non-diabetic group (P=0.002). In addition, all diabetic cases showed a significant decrease in total T lymphocyte counts < 955 × 10^{6}/L (LLN), $CD8^+$ T cell counts < 320 × 10^6/L (LLN), and NK cell counts < 150 × 10^6/L (LLN). Of 9 patients with diabetes, 7 (77.8%) showed obvious broad decrease in all lymphocyte subsets, including total B cell count < 90 × 10 ^{6}/L, $CD4^+$ T cell count < 550 × 10^{6}/L, and the abovementioned total T lymphocyte, $CD8^+$ T cell, and NK cell counts. Of these nine diabetic patients, 3 (33.3%) eventually died, and an image of the flow cytometry of one dead patient is shown in **Figures 4A–D**. The proportion of NK cells (3.58%) obviously decreased.

Among these 20 COVID-19 patients, there were six non-survivors including three diabetic and three non-diabetic

TABLE 2 | Comparing the counts and frequencies of immune cells on admission between T2DM and non-T2DM cases.

	Total n = 20	T2DM n = 9	Non-T2DM n = 11	p value
Total T lymphocytes (%)	70.4(56.6–76.2)	69.0(53.7–75.7)	71.4(60.1–76.9)	0.569
Total T lymphocytes count (10^6/L)	640.5(396.3–1219.3)	448.0(193.0–587.0)	962.0(652.0–1,399.0)	0.002
Decreased, <955, n/N (%)	14(70.0%)	9(100.0%)	5(45.5%)	0.014
<400, n/N (%)	5(25.0%)	4(44.4%)	1(9.1%)	0.127
Total B lymphocytes (%)	17.2(8.9–19.7)	19.9(13.4–36.4)	13.3(7.9–17.5)	0.025
increased, n/N (%)	8(40.0%)	6(66.7%)	2(18.2%)	0.065
Total B lymphocytes count (10*6/L)	135.5(65.5–258.3)	72.0(27.0–261.0)	141.0(103.0–269.0)	0.239
decreased, n/N (%)	7(35.0%)	5(55.6%)	2(18.2%)	0.160
CD4+T cells (%)	39.0(27.7–50.3)	29.5(25.7–58.3)	39.5(28.6–48.9)	0.970
CD4+T cells count (10^6/L)	368.5(201.0–661.8)	204.0(95.0–395.5)	583.0(345.0–872.0)	0.007
decreased, n/N (%)	13(65.0%)	8(88.9%)	5(45.5%)	0.070
CD8+T cells (%)	22.2(17.3–36.5)	23.6(13.2–36.4)	21.7(20.1–37.8)	0.569
CD8+T cells count (10^6/L)	248.0(125.8–379.0)	115.0(38.0–238.0)	352.0(248.0–522.0)	0.002
decreased, n/N (%)	12(60.0%)	8(88.9%)	4(36.4%)	0.028
NK cells (%)	11.4(4.6–23.67)	10.3(3.5–12.3)	14.4(10.2–28.9)	0.074
NK cells count (10^6/L)	148.0(34.3–258.8)	35.0(7.5–99.5)	252.0(182.0–326.0)	0.004
Decreased, <150, n/N (%)	10(50.0%)	8(88.9%)	2(18.2%)	0.005
<77, n/N (%)	8(40.0%)	6(66.7%)	2(18.2%)	0.065
T+B+NK(%)	99.3(98.9–99.5)	99.3(98.9–99.4)	99.4(98.7–99.6)	0.761
T+B+NK(#)	984.5(695.3–1,693.5)	685.0(241.0–899.0)	1584.0(1016.0–1795.0)	0.002
Th/Ts	1.6(0.9–2.4)	1.8(0.7–4.8)	1.4(1.0–2.4)	0.970

patients and 14 survivors including six diabetic and eight non-diabetic patients. When compared with the survivors, non-survivors displayed the greater reductions in the absolute numbers of total T lymphocytes, $CD8^+$ T cells and NK cells (P<0.05) (**Figure 4F**). The proportion and counts of immune cells in the peripheral blood from six non-survivors and 11 survivors with COVID-19 were showed in **Supplementary Table 2**.

DISCUSSION

Patients with COVID-19 with T2DM are likely to develop a severe form of the disease (22). In this retrospective cohort with 306 severe patients with SARS-CoV-2 infection, including 129 patients with diabetes and 177 patients without diabetes, we found that the patients with diabetes had much higher mortality rates (42.6%) than patients without diabetes (10.7%) and first proved that patients with FPG level > 7.0 mmol/L or RPG level > 11.1 mmol/L on admission have a significantly decreased chance of survival, which profoundly indicates that diabetes or hyperglycaemia might be a potential risk factor of fatality in COVID-19. To further investigate the reason for this high mortality, we reviewed the immune status of patients and found that T2DM showed markedly reduced numbers of immune cells, such as $CD4^+$, $CD8^+$ T, NK cells, and obvious imbalance of Th1/Th2 cytokine signalling over-activated Th2 cell function, thus aggravating the severity of COVID-19.

This study reports that patients with T2DM have higher SOFA and CURB-65 scores than patients without diabetes, suggesting that higher rates of multiple organ failure and fatal pneumonia lead to higher mortality in patients with T2DM. Diabetes, with its high morbidity and mortality, has grown to a global health problem in recent decades, owing to increasing risks of infection, cardiovascular disease, and other diseases (17). Recently, a retrospective, multicentered study of COVID-19 found that patients with T2DM required more medical interventions and had a significantly higher mortality rate (7.8% vs. 2.7%) (33). The relationship between diabetes and infection has long been recognised (34). Infections, particularly influenza and pneumonia, are often common and more serious in elderly patients with T2DM (35). T2DM has been recognised as a risk factor for disease progression and mortality in SARS-CoV, MERS-CoV, and novel SARS-CoV-2 infections (22, 36–41).

Patients with T2DM with higher plasma glucose level (FPG level > 7 mmol/L or RPG level > 11.1 mmol/L) in our study were demonstrated to have a greatly decreased survival compared to patients with FPG level < 7.0 mmol/L or RPG level < 11.1 mmol/L, separately. Similar to this conclusion, a recent study indicated that a well-controlled blood glucose level (3.9 to 10.0 mmol/L) was associated with markedly lower mortality rate compared to poorly controlled blood glucose level (> 10.0 mmol/L) during hospitalisation. A meta-analysis showed that diabetes was associated with poor outcomes, including mortality, severity status, acute respiratory distress syndrome, need for intensive care, and disease progression (42). Recently, a large national investigation in England show that type 1 and type 2 diabetes were both independently associated with a significant increased odds of in-hospital death with COVID-19, which supported our conclusions furtherly (43) and BMI was identified to be independently associated with the severity of COVID-19 in French CORONADO study (44).

So far, there has been scarce data regarding the relationship between glucose metabolism and immune response in patients with COVID-19. In this study, we first presented markedly elevated Th1 cytokine IL-2R and TNF-α levels and increased levels of Th2 cytokines, including IL-6, IL-8, and IL-10, in

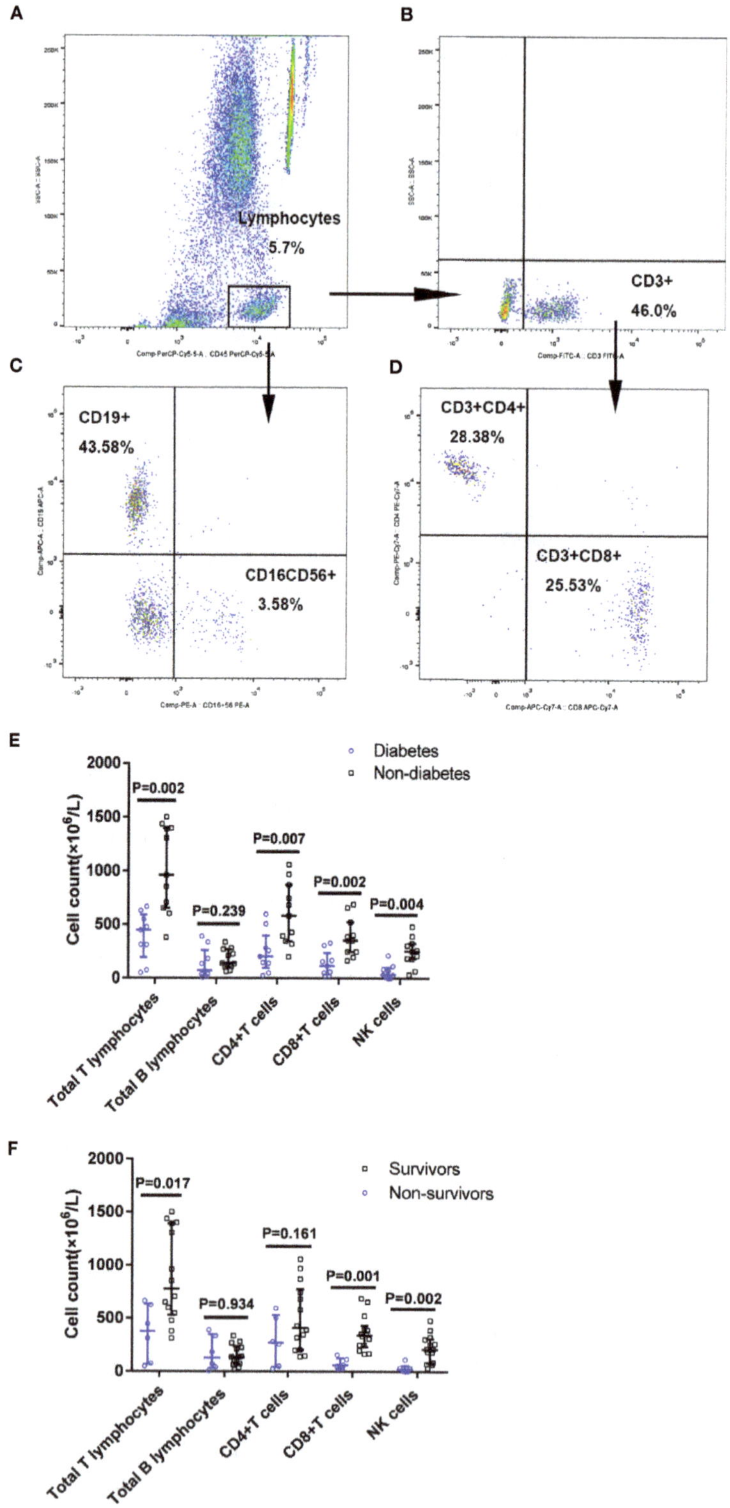

FIGURE 4 | Proportion of immune cells subsets in patients with diabetes with COVID-19. Flow cytometric analysis of B cells, NK cells, CD4+ T cells, and CD8+ T cells from a representative patient **(A–D)**. A series of comparisons of absolute counts of total T and B lymphocytes, $CD4^+$ T cells, $CD8^+$ T cells, and NK cells between patients with diabetes (n=9) and patients without diabetes (n=11) **(E)**, as well as between survivors (n=14) and non-survivors (n=6) **(F)**. All data represent median (IQR). Differences were tested using nonparametric test.

patients with diabetes compared with patients without diabetes among patients with COVID-19 pneumonia. Our results provide novel evidence that the imbalance of Th1/Th2 cytokines, a significant decrease in the Th1/Th2 cytokine ratio in patients with diabetes, suggested the over-activation of Th2 cells, which may account for the disturbance of the immune system, causing poor prognosis. We furtherly found that the lifted expression levels of cytokines were associated with the mortality of COVID-19 patients with T2DM. Non-survivors of diabetic cases showed the significant increases of IL-6 and IL-8 at week 2 compared to that at week 1, whereas there were greatly reductions in survivors of diabetes cases. The ratios of IL-2R/IL-6 in diabetic non-survivors at week 2 were much declined compared to that at week 1, whereas they were raised greatly in non-diabetic survivors, and there were no significant changes in the survivors with or without T2DM from week 1 to week 2. The data indicated that elevated cytokines and greater imbalance of Th1/Th2 ratios might be involved the immune pathogenic mechanisms of COVID-19 patients with T2DM and lead to higher mortality compared with non-diabetic patients.

To the best of our knowledge, Th2 cells typically produce IL-4, IL-6, Il-8, IL-10, and IL-13, whereas cytokines, such as IL-1β, IL-2R, and TNF-α, belong to the Th1 cell response. As two extremes on a scale, Th1 and Th2 responses play different roles and may contribute to immunopathology. Distinct from Th1 cell pro-inflammatory function and antiviral response by stimulating macrophages and cell-mediated immunity, Th2 cells tend to oppose the inflammatory reaction and promote antibody response and inhibit Th1 cell-induced antiviral function (45). Under normal conditions, IFN-γ can induce the differentiation of Th0 cells into Th1 cells, whereas, during SARS-CoV-2 infection, the lower level of IFN-γ production would reduce the production of Th1, resulting in further weakening of the antiviral immune response of $CD4^+$ T cells. In addition, T2DM is a chronic inflammatory condition characterised by multiple metabolic and vascular abnormalities that can affect the immune response to pathogens (46). Both cytokine disturbances and T-cell exhaustion in patients with diabetes indicated poor clinical outcomes (10, 12, 16, 47–49). Hyperglycaemia and insulin resistance promote increased synthesis of glycosylation end products and pro-inflammatory cytokines, oxidative stress, and adhesion molecules, which may be the underlying mechanism that leads to a higher propensity to infections, with worse outcomes in patients with diabetes (50). Targeting the overexpression of IL-6 effects with a monoclonal antibody against IL-6 receptor or using Janus Kinase inhibitors may be particularly helpful for treatment of COVID-19 pneumonia in diabetes in the future (51). A previous study found Th1 cytokines including IFN-γ, TNF-α, and CRP but not Th2 cytokines appeared significantly higher in the T2DM group than in the non-T2DM group. Unlike the above study, we found both Th1 and Th2 cytokines were greatly elevated in T2DM compared with non-T2DM when infected with SARS-CoV-2 (52).

Our study reported that patients with diabetes present a greatly reduced number of lymphocytes, especially the decreased counts of peripheral $CD4^+$ T cells, $CD8^+$ T cells, and NK cells compared to patients without diabetes in SARS-CoV-2 infections. Guo et al.'s study on viral pneumonia, such as influenza A, adenovirus, bocavirus, human rhinovirus, and coronavirus, but not SARS-CoV-2, revealed a higher mortality rate in patients with lower absolute counts of $CD8^+$ T and $CD4^+$ T cells (53). As for COVID-19 pneumonia, T cell counts are reduced significantly in patients with COVID-19, and the surviving T cells appear functional exhausted (54, 55).

SARS-CoV infection can significantly reduce peripheral $CD4^+$ and $CD8^+$ T lymphocyte subsets, which is related to the onset of the disease (56). Similarly, MERS-CoV could effectively induce apoptosis of T cells in the peripheral blood and human lymphoid organs, involving activation pathways of extrinsic and intrinsic apoptosis (57). Presumably, infection of epithelial cells in the airways and subsequent replication of the virus in these tissues might cause high levels of virus-linked apoptosis or pyroptosis, triggering inflammatory responses marked by the activation of pro-inflammatory cytokines or chemokines. Based on recent clinical data obtained from COVID-19 patients, cytokine storm, pulmonary, and endothelial dysfunction, and hypercoagulation condition may contributes to pathogenic mechanisms of COVID-19 patients with T2DM (58). Hyperglycaemia can damage the hypothalamic–pituitary–adrenal axis, resulting in high cortisol secretion. The over-secreted cortisol might not only elevate the serum glucose level but also suppress the immune system and immune cells, leading to a vicious circle (59).

Our study provides distinct evidence that T2DM or hyperglycaemia patients showed an obvious decrease in immune cells and imbalance of TH1/Th2 cytokines, which were associated with the high mortality of COVID-19 patients with T2DM.

CONCLUSIONS

In COVID-19, T2DM or hyperglycaemia affected the numbers of immune cells, including $CD4^+$, $CD8^+$ T cells, and NK cells, and reduced Th1/Th2 cytokine ratios, which might aggravate the severity of COVID-19. This study may shed light on the complex immunological mechanisms and relationship between T2DM and COVID-19.

AUTHOR CONTRIBUTIONS

All authors have been fully involved in the preparation of the manuscript at all stages and approved it for publication. All authors contributed to the article and approved the submitted version.

ACKNOWLEDGMENTS

We thank the subjects and their families, as well as all doctors and nurses of the Department of Infectious Diseases, Tongji Hospital, HUST. We would like to thank Editage (www.editage.cn) for English language editing.

REFERENCES

1. Chen N, Zhou M, Dong X, Qu J, Gong F, Han Y, et al. Epidemiological and clinical characteristics of 99 cases of 2019 novel coronavirus pneumonia in Wuhan, China: a descriptive study. *Lancet* (2020) 395:507–13. doi: 10.1016/S0140-6736(20)30211-7
2. Zhu N, Zhang D, Wang W, Li X, Yang B, Song J, et al. A Novel Coronavirus from Patients with Pneumonia in China, 2019. *N Engl J Med* (2020) 382:727–33. doi: 10.1056/NEJMoa2001017
3. Holshue ML, DeBolt C, Lindquist S, Lofy KH, Wiesman J, Bruce H, et al. First Case of 2019 Novel Coronavirus in the United States. *N Engl J Med* (2020) 382:929–36. doi: 10.1056/NEJMoa2001191
4. Silverstein WK, Stroud L, Cleghorn GE, Leis JA. First imported case of 2019 novel coronavirus in Canada, presenting as mild pneumonia. *Lancet* (2020) 395:734. doi: 10.1016/S0140-6736(20)30370-6
5. Huang C, Wang Y, Li X, Ren L, Zhao J, Hu Y, et al. Clinical features of patients infected with 2019 novel coronavirus in Wuhan, China. *Lancet* (2020) 395:497–506. doi: 10.1016/S0140-6736(20)30183-5
6. Tan W, Zhao X, Ma X, Wang W, Nui P, Xu W, et al. A novel coronavirus genome identified in a cluster of pneumonia cases - Wuhan, China 2019-2020. *China CDC Weekly* (2020) 2:61–2. doi: 10.46234/ccdcw2020.017
7. Lu R, Zhao X, Li J, Niu P, Yang B, Wu H, et al. Genomic characterisation and epidemiology of 2019 novel coronavirus: implications for virus origins and receptor binding. *Lancet* (2020) 395:565–74. doi: 10.1016/S0140-6736(20)30251-8
8. Chen G, Wu D, Guo W, Cao Y, Huang D, Wang H, et al. Clinical and immunological features of severe and moderate coronavirus disease 2019. *J Clin Invest* (2020) 130:2620–9. doi: 10.1172/JCI137244
9. Chen T, Wu D, Chen H, Yan W, Yang D, Chen G, et al. Clinical characteristics of 113 deceased patients with coronavirus disease 2019: retrospective study. *Bmj* (2020), 368:m1091. doi: 10.1136/bmj.m1091
10. Diao B, Wang C, Tan Y, Chen X, Liu Y, Ning L, et al. Reduction and Functional Exhaustion of T Cells in Patients With Coronavirus Disease 2019 (COVID-19). *Front Immunol* (2020) 11:827–7. doi: 10.3389/fimmu.2020.00827
11. Channappanavar R, Perlman S. Pathogenic human coronavirus infections: causes and consequences of cytokine storm and immunopathology. *Semin Immunopathol* (2017) 39:529–39. doi: 10.1007/s00281-017-0629-x
12. Mehta P, McAuley DF, Brown M, Sanchez E, Tattersall RS, Manson JJ, et al. COVID-19: consider cytokine storm syndromes and immunosuppression. *Lancet* (2020) 395:1033–4. doi: 10.1016/S0140-6736(20)30628-0
13. Vaninov N. In the eye of the COVID-19 cytokine storm. *Nat Rev Immunol* (2020) 20:277–7. doi: 10.1038/s41577-020-0305-6
14. Zeng Z, Yu H, Chen H, Qi W, Chen L, Chen G, et al. Longitudinal changes of inflammatory parameters and their correlation with disease severity and outcomes in patients with COVID-19 from Wuhan, China. *Crit Care (London England)* (2020) 24:525. doi: 10.1186/s13054-020-03255-0
15. Lagunas-Rangel FA, Chávez-Valencia V. High IL-6/IFN-γ ratio could be associated with severe disease in COVID-19 patients. *J Med Virol* (2020) 92:1789–90. doi: 10.1002/jmv.25900
16. Hou H, Zhang B, Huang H, Luo Y, Wu S, Tang G, et al. Using IL-2R/lymphocytes for predicting the clinical progression of patients with COVID-19. *Clin Exp Immunol* (2020) 201:76–84. doi: 10.1111/cei.13450
17. WHO: GLOBAL REPORT ON DIABETES. (2016). https://www.who.int/publications-detail/global-report-on-diabetes.
18. Xu B, Fan C-Y, Wang A-L, Zou Y-L, Yu Y-H, He C, et al. Suppressed T cell-mediated immunity in patients with COVID-19: A clinical retrospective study in Wuhan, China. *J Infect* (2020). 81(1):e51–e60 doi: 10.1016/j.jinf.2020.04.012
19. Zhou F, Yu T, Du R, Fan G, Liu Y, Liu Z, et al. Clinical course and risk factors for mortality of adult inpatients with COVID-19 in Wuhan, China: a retrospective cohort study. *Lancet* (2020). 395(10229):1054–62 doi: 10.1016/S0140-6736(20)30566-3
20. Bloomgarden ZT. Diabetes and COVID-19. *J Diabetes* (2020) 12:347–8. doi: 10.1111/1753-0407.13027
21. Hussain A, Bhowmik B, do Vale Moreira NC. COVID-19 and diabetes: Knowledge in progress. *Diabetes Res Clin Pract* (2020) 162:108142. doi: 10.1016/j.diabres.2020.108142
22. Guo W, Li M, Dong Y, Zhou H, Zhang Z, Tian C, et al. Diabetes is a risk factor for the progression and prognosis of COVID-19. *Diabetes Metab Res Rev* (2020), e3319. doi: 10.1002/dmrr.3319
23. Guan WJ, Ni ZY, Hu Y, Liang WH, Ou CQ, He JX, et al. China Medical Treatment Expert Group for C: Clinical Characteristics of Coronavirus Disease 2019 in China. *N Engl J Med* (2020). 382:1708–20. doi: 10.1056/NEJMoa2002032
24. Wu Z, McGoogan JM. Characteristics of and Important Lessons From the Coronavirus Disease 2019 (COVID-19) Outbreak in China: Summary of a Report of 72314 Cases From the Chinese Center for Disease Control and Prevention. *JAMA* (2020). 323(13):1239–42. doi: 10.1001/jama.2020.2648
25. Onder G, Rezza G, Brusaferro S. Case-Fatality Rate and Characteristics of Patients Dying in Relation to COVID-19 in Italy. *JAMA* (2020). 323(18):1775–6 doi: 10.1001/jama.2020.4683
26. China. NHCotPsRo. *Chinese management guideline for COVID-19 (version 6.0). March 7th.* National Health Commission (2020). Available at: http://wwwnhcgovcn/jkj/s3577/202003/4856d5b0458141fa9f376853224d41d7shtml.
27. American Diabetes A. Standards of Medical Care in Diabetes-2020. *Diabetes Care* (2020) 43:S14–31. doi: 10.2337/dc20-S002
28. Ferreira FL, Bota DP, Bross A, Mélot C, Vincent JL. Serial evaluation of the SOFA score to predict outcome in critically ill patients. *JAMA* (2001) 286:1754–8. doi: 10.1001/jama.286.14.1754
29. Guo Q, Li HY, Zhou YP, Li M, Chen XK, Liu H, et al. CURB-65 score predicted mortality in community-acquired pneumonia better than IDSA/ATS minor criteria in a low-mortality-rate setting. *Eur J Clin Microbiol Infect Dis* (2012) 31:3281–6. doi: 10.1007/s10096-012-1693-8
30. Orioli L, Servais T, Belkhir L, Laterre P-F, Thissen J-P, Vandeleene B, et al. Clinical characteristics of seventy fatal patients with Coronavirus Disease 2019. *BMJ* (2020) 15(1):149–57. doi: 10.1016/j.dsx.2020.12.020
31. Ruan Q, Yang K. Clinical predictors of mortality due to COVID-19 based on an analysis of data of 150 patients from Wuhan, China. *Intensive Care Med* (2020) 46:846–8. doi: 10.1007/s00134-020-05991-x
32. Pan F, Ye T, Sun P, Gui S, Liang B, Li L, et al. Time Course of Lung Changes On Chest CT During Recovery From 2019 Novel Coronavirus (COVID-19) Pneumonia. *Radiology* (2020), 295.(3):715–21. 200370–0. doi: 10.1148/radiol.2020200370
33. Zhu L, She ZG, Cheng X, Qin JJ, Zhang XJ, Cai J, et al. Association of Blood Glucose Control and Outcomes in Patients with COVID-19 and Pre-existing Type 2 Diabetes. *Cell Metab* (2020) 31:1068–1077.e1063. doi: 10.1016/j.cmet.2020.04.021
34. Pearson-Stuttard J, Blundell S, Harris T, Cook DG, Critchley J. Diabetes and infection: assessing the association with glycaemic control in population-based studies. *Lancet Diabetes Endocrinol* (2016) 4:148–58. doi: 10.1016/S2213-8587(15)00379-4
35. McDonald HI, Nitsch D, Millett ER, Sinclair A, Thomas SL. New estimates of the burden of acute community-acquired infections among older people with diabetes mellitus: a retrospective cohort study using linked electronic health records. *Diabetes Med* (2014) 31:606–14. doi: 10.1111/dme.12384
36. Chan-Yeung M, Xu RH. SARS: Epidemiology. *Respirology* (2003) 8:S9–S14. doi: 10.1046/j.1440-1843.2003.00518.x
37. Gupta R, Ghosh A, Singh AK, Misra A. Clinical considerations for patients with diabetes in times of COVID-19 epidemic. *Diabetes Metab Syndrome* (2020) 14:211–2. doi: 10.1016/j.dsx.2020.03.002
38. Marhl M, Grubelnik V, Magdic M, Markovic R. Diabetes and metabolic syndrome as risk factors for COVID-19. *Diabetes Metab Syndrome* (2020) 14:671–7. doi: 10.1016/j.dsx.2020.05.013
39. Yang JK, Feng Y, Yuan MY, Yuan SY, Fu HJ, Wu BY, et al. Plasma glucose levels and diabetes are independent predictors for mortality and morbidity in patients with SARS. *Diabetes Med* (2006) 23:623–8. doi: 10.1111/j.1464-5491.2006.01861.x
40. Banik GR, Alqahtani AS, Booy R, Rashid H. Risk factors for severity and mortality in patients with MERS-CoV: Analysis of publicly available data from Saudi Arabia. *Virol Sin* (2016) 31:81–4. doi: 10.1007/s12250-015-3679-z
41. The Lancet Diabetes E. COVID-19 and diabetes: a co-conspiracy? *Lancet Diabetes Endocrinol* (2020) 8:801. doi: 10.1016/S2213-8587(20)30315-6
42. Huang I, Lim MA, Pranata R. Diabetes mellitus is associated with increased mortality and severity of disease in COVID-19 pneumonia - A systematic review, meta-analysis, and meta-regression. *Diabetes Metab Syndrome* (2020) 14:395–403. doi: 10.1016/j.dsx.2020.04.018

43. Barron E, Bakhai C, Kar P, Weaver A, Bradley D, Ismail H, et al. Associations of type 1 and type 2 diabetes with COVID-19-related mortality in England: a whole-population study. *Lancet Diabetes Endocrinol* (2020) 8:813–22. doi: 10.1016/S2213-8587(20)30272-2
44. Cariou B, Hadjadj S. Phenotypic characteristics and prognosis of inpatients with COVID-19 and diabetes: the CORONADO study. (2020) 63:1500–15. doi: 10.1007/s00125-020-05180-x
45. Mahlangu T, Dludla PV, Nyambuya TM, Mxinwa V, Mazibuko-Mbeje SE, Cirilli I, et al. A systematic review on the functional role of Th1/Th2 cytokines in type 2 Diabetologia and related metabolic complications. *Cytokine* (2020) 126:154892. doi: 10.1016/j.cyto.2019.154892
46. Knapp S. Diabetes and infection: is there a link?–A mini-review. *Gerontology* (2013) 59:99–104. doi: 10.1159/000345107
47. Ruscitti P, Berardicurti O, Iagnocco A, Giacomelli R. Cytokine storm syndrome in severe COVID-19. *Autoimmun Rev* (2020), 19(7):102562–2. doi: 10.1016/j.autrev.2020.102562
48. Lagunas-Rangel FA, Chavez-Valencia V. High IL-6/IFN-gamma ratio could be associated with severe disease in COVID-19 patients. *J Med Virol* (2020). 92(10):1789–90. doi: 10.1002/jmv.25900
49. Liu R, Wang Y, Li J, Han H, Xia Z, Liu F, et al. Decreased T cell populations contribute to the increased severity of COVID-19. *Clin Chim Acta; Int J Clin Chem* (2020) 508:110–4. doi: 10.1016/j.cca.2020.05.019
50. Petrie JR, Guzik TJ, Touyz RM. Diabetes, Hypertension, and Cardiovascular Disease: Clinical Insights and Vascular Mechanisms. *Can J Cardiol* (2018) 34:575–84. doi: 10.1016/j.cjca.2017.12.005
51. Maddaloni E, Buzzetti R. Covid-19 and diabetes mellitus: unveiling the interaction of two pandemics. *Diabetes Metab Res Rev* (2020), e33213321. doi: 10.1002/dmrr.3321
52. Zhao R, Sun Y, Zhang Y, Wang W, Wang S, Wang C, et al. Distinguishable Immunologic Characteristics of COVID-19 Patients with Comorbid Type 2 Diabetes Compared with Nondiabetic Individuals. *Mediators Inflamm* (2020) 2020:6914878. doi: 10.1155/2020/6914878
53. Guo L, Wei D, Zhang X, Wu Y, Li Q, Zhou M, et al. Clinical Features Predicting Mortality Risk in Patients With Viral Pneumonia: The MuLBSTA Score. *Front Microbiol* (2019) 10:2752. doi: 10.3389/fmicb.2019.02752
54. Xu Z, Shi L, Wang Y, Zhang J, Huang L, Zhang C, et al. Pathological findings of COVID-19 associated with acute respiratory distress syndrome. *Lancet Respir Med* (2020). 8(4):420–2. doi: 10.1016/S2213-2600(20)30076-X
55. Song JW, Zhang C, Fan X. Immunological and inflammatory profiles in mild and severe cases of COVID-19. *Nat Commun* (2020) 11:3410. doi: 10.1038/s41467-020-17240-2
56. He ZP, Zhao CH, Dong QM, Zhuang H, Song SJ, Peng G, et al. Effects of severe acute respiratory syndrome (SARS) coronavirus infection on peripheral blood lymphocytes and their subsets. *Int J Infect Dis* (2005) 9:323–30. doi: 10.1016/j.ijid.2004.07.014
57. Chu H, Zhou J, Wong BH, Li C, Chan JF, Cheng ZS, et al. Middle East Respiratory Syndrome Coronavirus Efficiently Infects Human Primary T Lymphocytes and Activates the Extrinsic and Intrinsic Apoptosis Pathways. *J Infect Dis* (2016) 213:904–14. doi: 10.1093/infdis/jiv380
58. Erener S. Diabetes, infection risk and COVID-19. *Mol Metab* (2020) 39:101044. doi: 10.1016/j.molmet.2020.101044
59. Joseph JJ, Golden SH. Cortisol dysregulation: the bidirectional link between stress, depression, and type 2 diabetes mellitus. *Ann New Y Acad Sci* (2017) 1391:20–34. doi: 10.1111/nyas.13217

9

The Impact of COVID-19 on Blood Glucose

Juan Chen [1†], *Chunhua Wu* [2†], *Xiaohang Wang* [3], *Jiangyi Yu* [1*] and *Zilin Sun* [3*]

[1] Department of Endocrinology, Jiangsu Province Hospital of Chinese Medicine, Affiliated Hospital of Nanjing University of Chinese Medicine, Nanjing, China, [2] Department of General Practice, Zhongda Hospital, Medical School, Southeast University, Nanjing, China, [3] Department of Endocrinology, Zhongda Hospital, Institute of Diabetes, Medical School, Southeast University, Nanjing, China

***Correspondence:**
Jiangyi Yu
YuJY1961@outlook.com
Zilin Sun
Sunzilin1963@126.com

†These authors have contributed equally to this work

Background: Diabetes mellitus is considered a common comorbidity of COVID-19, which has a wide spectrum of clinical manifestations ranging from asymptomatic infection to severe respiratory symptoms and even death. However, the impact of COVID-19 on blood glucose has not been fully understood. This meta-analysis aimed to summarize available data on the association between glycemic parameters and severity of COVID-19.

Methods: PubMed, EMBASE, and Cochrane Library were searched from December 1, 2019 to May 15, 2020. Observational studies investigating blood glucose or glycated hemoglobin A1c (HbA1c) according to the severity of COVID-19 were considered for inclusion. Two independent researchers extracted data from eligible studies using a standardized data extraction sheet and then proceeded to cross check the results. Data were pooled using a fixed- or random-effects model to calculate the weighted mean differences (WMDs) and 95% confidence intervals (CIs).

Results: Three studies reported blood glucose and HbA1c according to the severity of COVID-19 and were included in this meta-analysis. The combined results showed that severe COVID-19 was associated with higher blood glucose (WMD 2.21, 95% CI: 1.30–3.13, $P < 0.001$). In addition, HbA1c was slightly higher in patients with severe COVID-19 than those with mild COVID-19, yet this difference did not reach significance (WMD 0.29, 95% CI: −0.59 to 1.16, $P = 0.52$).

Conclusions: This meta-analysis provides evidence that severe COVID-19 is associated with increased blood glucose. This highlights the need to effectively monitor blood glucose to improve prognosis in patients infected with COVID-19.

Keywords: COVID-19, glucose, glycated hemoglobin A1c, systematic review, meta-analysis

INTRODUCTION

Coronavirus disease 2019 (COVID-19), caused by severe acute respiratory syndrome coronavirus 2 (SARS-CoV-2), has a wide spectrum of clinical manifestations ranging from asymptomatic infection to severe respiratory symptoms, and even death (1). According to recent researches, the overall mortality of COVID-19 ranged from 1.4 to 15% (2–4). Furthermore, an epidemiological study from Italy reported that the mortality of patients requiring intensive care unit admission was 26% (5). Of note, once the disease progresses to acute respiratory distress syndrome, the mortality would be ~40% (6). Because of efficient person-to-person transmission, it has become an emerging worldwide threat for human health.

Currently, several studies have been designed to focus on details of the clinical and virological course of SARS-CoV-2 infection. Subsequently, studies suggest that individuals with older age and comorbidities, such as diabetes and hypertension, are more likely to have COVID-19, as well as a higher risk of mortality (2, 3, 7). As we all know, diabetes mellitus is considered a public health concern worldwide due to its increasing prevalence and involvement in the development of several diseases, including stroke, kidney failure, and heart disease (8). Since diabetes has been reported to be associated with poor prognosis of COVID-19, glycemic management for patients with both diabetes and COVID-19 has gained much more attention (9, 10). There are evidences that better glycemic control is closely associated with improvement in clinical outcomes in COVID-19 patients (4, 11). Nevertheless, at the same time, it is confused that whether COVID-19 contributes to hyperglycemia. A previous study suggested that pancreas could be the target of coronavirus attack since SARS-CoV was detected in pancreas (12). Furthermore, another research found SARS-CoV damaged the endocrine part of pancreas, indicating that SARS-CoV may cause acute insulin dependent diabetes mellitus (13). In addition, it is worth noting that infection leads to profound alterations in whole-body metabolism, including glucose, fat, and protein (14). Although many studies suggest that diabetes is an important risk factor for COVID-19. It remains unclear regarding the effect of severity of COVID-19 infection on glycemic parameters, including blood glucose and glycated haemoglobinA1c (HbA1c).

At present, the rapid worldwide spread of COVID-19 requires continual improvement of knowledge about glycemic management during COVID-19 infection. Therefore, we conducted this meta-analysis by incorporating the latest evidence with focus on association between glycemic parameters and severity of COVID-19, which may be instructive for clinical practice.

METHODS

Search Strategy

An extensive search strategy was designed on PubMed, Embase and the Cochrane Library to retrieve all articles published from December 1, 2019 to May 15, 2020, following the MOOSE group guidelines of observational meta-analyses (15). No language restrictions were applied. The details of the search strategy are available in the **Supplementary Table 1**. The primary outcome measure was blood glucose or glycated haemoglobinA1c (HbA1c). Two authors (JC and CHW) independently reviewed the titles and abstracts to identify potentially relevant articles. After being identified as relevant articles, the full texts were individually analyzed by both authors, independently, to determine whether the article was qualified for eligibility criteria. During the study selection process, disagreements were resolved through consultation with a third investigator (JYY). In addition, the reference lists of included studies, relevant review articles and meta-analyses were screened for other suitable studies to maximize the search for articles on the same topic.

Study Selection and Quality Assessment

Studies were considered eligible if they fulfilled the following criteria: (1) participants were diagnosed with COVID-19; (2) separate data for patients with mild and severe COVID-19 infection (those who required mechanical ventilation, intensive care unit admission or those who died) were provided; (3) information on any of the prespecified primary outcomes were provided. If suitable data were not available or unclear in the published papers, the corresponding authors were contacted to request this information. Studies were excluded if they were conference abstracts, editorials, commentary, case reports, reviews, nonhuman studies, or did not expressly report the values of glycemic parameters in COVID-19 patients according to the severity. The quality of studies was assessed using the Newcastle-Ottawa Scale (16). We rated cohort studies a maximum of four stars for selection, two stars for comparability, and three stars for outcome assessment. Disagreements were resolved by discussion between two authors or consulting a third investigator (JYY) if necessary.

Data Extraction

Two independent reviewers (JC and CHW) extracted data from eligible studies using a standardized data extraction sheet and then proceeded to cross check the results. Disagreements between two reviewers regarding extracted data were resolved by discussion or consulting a third investigator (JYY) if necessary. The following information was extracted: first author name, publication year, country, sample size, study design, age, gender, primary outcomes including blood glucose and HbA1c.

Data Synthesis and Statistical Analysis

For studies reporting interquartile range, the standard deviations were obtained using the methods described in Cochrane Handbook for Systematic Reviews. The weighted mean differences (WMDs) with 95% confidence intervals (CIs) were calculated. The heterogeneity was evaluated using the Q test and I^2 statistic. $I^2 > 50\%$ or $P < 0.1$ was considered to have a significant heterogeneity. A fixed-effects model was used when the result showed no significant heterogeneity, otherwise a random-effects model was applied. All the analyses were conducted using STATA software (Version 12.0, StataCorp LP, College Station, Texas). A 2-sided $P < 0.05$ was set for statistical significance.

RESULTS

Study Selection and Characteristics

The literature search result and study selection process are presented in **Figure 1**. Overall, 107 citations of interest were found in the initial electronic searches of PubMed, Embase, and the Cochrane Library. After excluding 28 duplicates, 79 potentially eligible articles were selected.

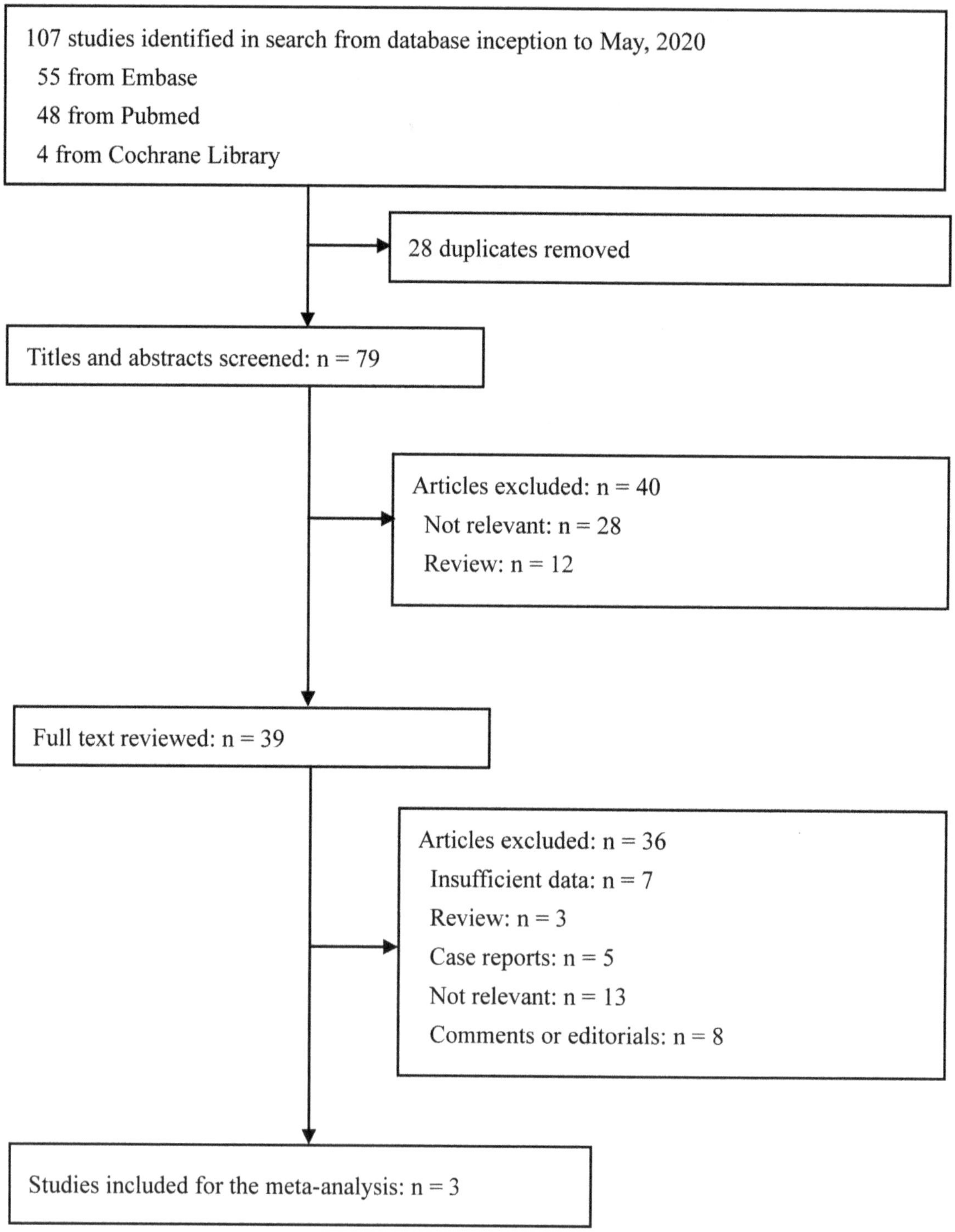

FIGURE 1 | Flow diagram of study selection.

Of these, 39 full text papers were potentially relevant and assessed for eligibility. Finally, three papers were included in the meta-analysis that evaluated blood glucose and/or HbA1c levels according to the severity of COVID-19 (17–19).

Of the three included studies, two articles reported data on both blood glucose and HbA1c, one article only reported data on blood glucose, and all studies used retrospective design. Study sample sizes ranged from 28 to 151, with a total of 222 COVID-19 patients, including 131 patients in mild group and 91 in severe group. Compared with women, men were more likely to have COVID-19 infection. Moreover, patients with severe COVID-19 were older than those with mild COVID-19. The detailed characteristics of the studies included in the meta-analysis are presented in **Table 1**.

Study Quality and Publication Bias

Supplementary Table 2 shows the assessment of quality using Newcastle-Ottawa Scale for three studies included in this meta-analysis. Higher scores indicate better quality. Based on the Newcastle-Ottawa Scale, a maximum of eight points can be awarded to each article. Since only three studies were included in this meta-analysis, a linear regression test of funnel plot asymmetry (Egger's test) could not be carried out.

Association Between Severity of COVID-19 Infection and Blood Glucose

Three trials with 222 patients compared blood glucose between severe group and mild group. Forest plot for the overall effect of severity on blood glucose is presented in **Figure 2**. The pooled WMD was 2.21 (95% CI: 1.30–3.13). Since the evidence collected in our meta-analysis showed no heterogeneity ($I^2 = 0\%$), a fix-effects model was performed. The z-test result for overall effects was statistically significant ($P < 0.001$), indicating a significantly greater elevation in blood glucose in patients with severe COVID-19 infection than those in the mild group.

Association of Severity With HbA1c

Two trials reported data on HbA1c both in severe group and mild group. Forest plot for the overall effect of severity on HbA1c is presented in **Figure 3**. In the overall pooled estimate of two studies with 179 COVID-19 infected patients, the pooled WMD was 0.29 (95% CI: −0.59 to 1.16). Since the evidence collected in our meta-analysis showed heterogeneity ($I^2 = 68.3\%$), a random-effects model was conducted. The z-test result for overall effects showed no statistical significance ($P = 0.52$), which suggested that severity of COVID-19 did not significantly impact HbA1c.

DISCUSSION

Until now, there are accumulating evidences that diabetes is closely correlated with increased risk of COVID-19, as well as poor outcomes (9, 20). However, it remains unclear regarding the effect of severity of COVID-19 on glycemic parameters. Our analyses found that severe COVID-19 infection was significantly associated with increased blood glucose. Meanwhile, we investigated the correlation between severity and HbA1c. However, we did not provide adequate evidence that patients with severe COVID-19 were more likely to have higher HbA1c than those with mild COVID-19. Since viral infection and hyperglycemia adversely affect each other, this study highlights the need to effectively monitor blood glucose to improve prognosis in patients infected with COVID-19.

Due to defects in innate immunity affecting phagocytosis, neutrophil chemotaxis, and cell-mediated immunity, individuals with diabetes are more likely to have infection (21). A population-based study pointed out that nearly half of patients with diabetes had at least one hospitalization or physician claim because of an infectious disease in each cohort year (22). Additionally, study has demonstrated that people with diabetes are at increased risk for lower respiratory tract infection, urinary tract infection, and skin and mucous membrane infection (23). Furthermore, Kornum et al. suggested that subjects with type 1 diabetes had a 4.4-fold increased risk of a pneumonia-related hospitalization, and subjects with type 2 diabetes displayed a 1.2-fold increased risk of a pneumonia-related hospitalization compared with those without diabetes (24). Recently, COVID-19, caused by SARS-CoV-2, has become a global catastrophe. Numerous studies have been performed to focus on the association between diabetes and COVID-19. Based on the available data, patients with diabetes are more susceptible to COVID-19 than those without diabetes.

However, it is worth noting that infection leads to profound alterations in whole-body metabolism (14). Sustained inflammation affects systemic glucose homeostasis and contributes to hyperglycemia (25). Besides, Šestan et al. reported that the activated immune system drove systemic insulin resistance in response to viral infection (26). Another study found that long-term innate immune activation could impair insulin secretion and action, and play an important role in the pathology of diabetes (27). Therefore, we speculated that there may be a strong relationship between the severity of COVID-19 and glycemic parameters, even in those without diabetes. In the present meta-analysis, we found that blood glucose was significantly higher in patients with severe COVID-19 than those with mild COVID-19 (WMD 2.21, 95% CI: 1.30–3.13, $P < 0.001$, $I^2 = 0\%$). A recent study by Zhang et al. reported that COVID-19 infection induced an increase in blood glucose, even those not diagnosed with diabetes before admission (4). However, this study did not compare blood glucose between severe and mild COVID-19 patients. Guan et al. indicated that the prevalence of diabetes was significantly higher in patients with severe COVID-19 (28). Notably, other studies have demonstrated that hyperglycemia is associated with poor prognoses, while better glycemic control is closely associated with improvement in clinical outcomes in COVID-19 patients (4, 11). Therefore, clinicians should pay more attention to the blood glucose status in patients with COVID-19.

Additionally, our study found that HbA1c was slightly higher in individuals with severe COVID-19 than those with mild COVID-19, yet this difference did not reach significance ($P = 0.52$). However, it is noteworthy that there were only two studies with small sample size that explored the influence of severity of COVID-19 on HbA1c, which might affect the outcomes of interest. Moreover, HbA1c reflects the average blood glucose concentration over the past 2–3 months. Therefore, the effect of short-term viral infection on HbA1c levels may not be prominent. Nevertheless, additional researches with large sample size are needed to verify our results.

The COVID-19 outbreak highlights the importance of understanding the shared diseases pathophysiology with diabetes

TABLE 1 | Characteristics of studies included in this meta-analysis.

Study	Period	Study type	Country	No.	Age (year)	Male (%)	BG (mmol/L)	HbA1c (%)	Diabetes (%)
Ren et al. (17)	January 12, 2020 to February 13, 2020	Retrospective cohort study	China	151	Mild case: 53.9 ± 16.2 Severe case: 67.6 ± 11.6	78 (52%)	Mild case: 6.2 ± 1.7 Severe case: 8.4 ± 4.3	Mild case: 6.0 ± 1.5 Severe case: 6.7 ± 2.1	Mild case: 16 (18.0%) Severe case: 23 (37%)
Wang et al. (18)	January 29, 2020 to February 10, 2020	Retrospective cohort study	China	28	Mild case: 65.8 ± 9.4 Severe case: 71.4 ± 7.9	21 (75%)	Mild case: 9.8 ± 3.4 Severe case: 13.7 ± 5.1	Mild case: 7.5 ± 1.2 Severe case: 7.3 ± 0.90	100%
Gao et al. (19)	January 23, 2020 to February 2, 2020	Retrospective cohort study	China	43	Mild case: 43.0 ± 14.0 Severe case: 45.2 ± 7.7	26 (60%)	Mild case: 6.0 ± 1.2 Severe case: 7.7 ± 3.4	NR	Mild case: 1 (4%) Severe case: 6 (40%)

BG, blood glucose; HbA1c, glycated hemoglobin A1c; NR, not reported.

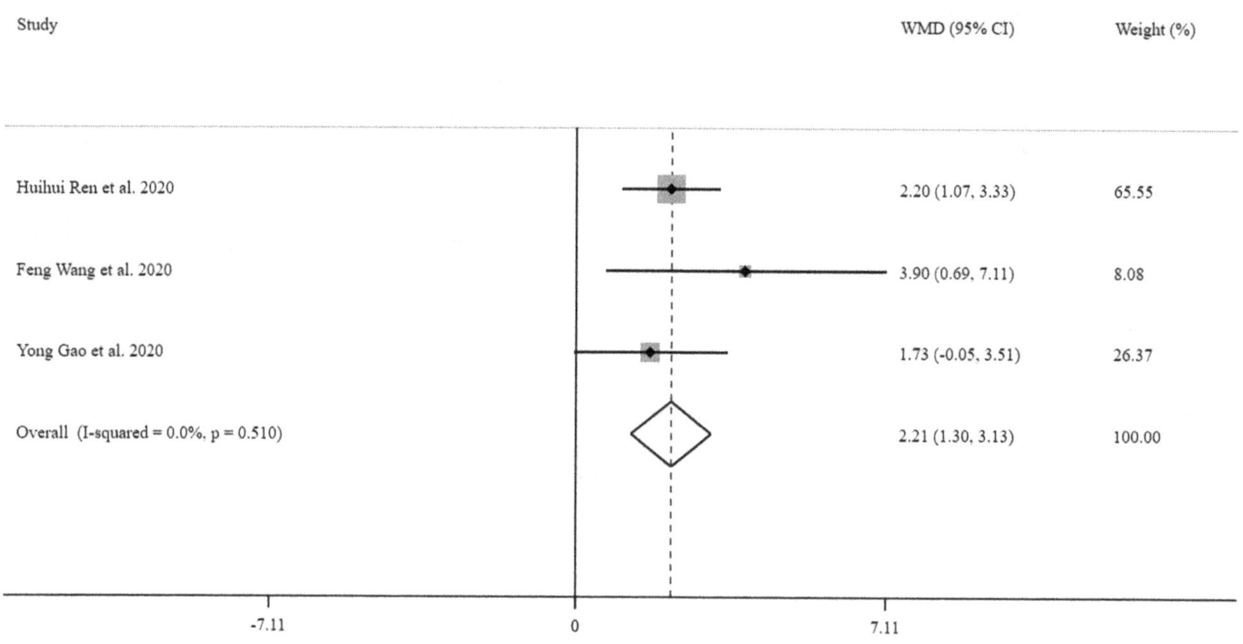

FIGURE 2 | Forest plot of meta-analysis of the effect of severity of COVID-19 on blood glucose. Data are pooled WMDs with 95% CIs. WMD, weighted mean difference; CIs, confidence intervals.

(29). Over a decade ago, SARS-CoV was detected in pancreas, in addition to lung, suggesting pancreas is the target of coronavirus attack (12). Furtherly, another research found SARS-CoV damaged the endocrine part of pancreas, indicating that SARS-CoV may cause acute insulin dependent diabetes mellitus (13). Noteworthy, pathological changes in pancreas, mainly focal enlargement of the pancreas or dilatation of the pancreatic duct, were observed in patients with severe COVID-19, indicating SARS-CoV-2 may cause pancreatic injury (30). This may be one of the reasons that increased blood glucose was observed in COVID-19 patients without a prior history of diabetes (4).

Furtherly, it was hypothesized that angiotensin converting enzyme 2 (ACE2) may be the key regulator that involved in the association between COVID-19 and hyperglycemia. The main role of ACE2 is to incise angiotensin II to generate angiotensin 1–7 and thereby mediates the protective effects of vasodilation, anti-inflammatory and anti-proliferation. In addition, ACE2 is identified as a receptor that facilitates coronavirus entry into cells (31). A recent research noted that ACE2 expression was substantially increased in patients with diabetes mellitus than those without diabetes (32). Consequently, enhanced susceptibility to COVID-19 infection in patients with diabetes may be attributed to overexpression of ACE2. However, ACE2 expression is not limited to the lung. It has been found in pancreas islets (33), which highlights the need for vigilance in consideration of whether SARS-CoV-2 infection may contribute to the exacerbation or development of diabetes. Individuals with diabetes are more susceptible to COVID-19 than

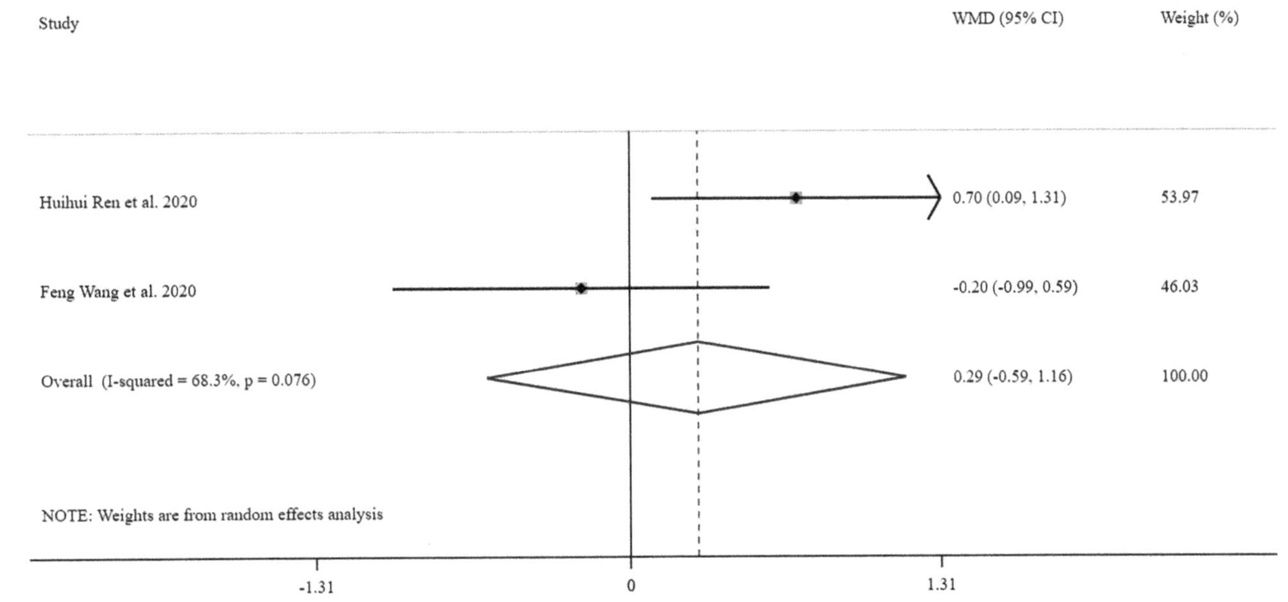

FIGURE 3 | Forest plot of meta-analysis of the effect of severity of COVID-19 on HbA1c. Data are pooled WMDs with 95% CIs. HbA1c, glycated hemoglobin A1c; WMD, weighted mean difference; CIs, confidence intervals.

those without diabetes. Meanwhile, SARS-CoV-2 infection could induce hyperglycemia. The pathogenic mechanism of the two may overlap partially, which may be related to ACE2. However, at present, no data are available on ACE2 expression in islets according to the severity of COVID-19. In addition, the study by Ren et al. revealed that triglyceride and glucose index, a marker of insulin resistance, was closely associated with the severity of COVID-19 (17). Insulin resistance may be another explanation for hyperglycemia in patients with COVID-19 infection.

Researches of COVID-19 outbreaks offer important insights that the management of blood glucose is an urgent need. Our study confirmed a strong relationship between the severity of COVID-19 and blood glucose. Future research is required into the effectiveness of improving blood glucose on the prognosis of COVID-19. In addition, this meta-analysis has some limitations. First, we aimed to investigate the association of severity with glycemic parameters in the overall population, including other countries and races. Yet all patients in our meta-analysis were Chinese. Thus, our findings may not be applicable to other regions of the world. Second, although numerous studies have been conducted to focus on the association between diabetes and COVID-19 and we searched all the relevant articles and tried to include as many researches as possible. Studies that provided detailed glycemic parameters according to the severity of COVID-19 were quite limited. It is necessary to update the meta-analysis in the future when more researches were performed to focus on this topic. Third, interpretation of our findings might be limited by the sample size. Therefore, additional researches with large sample size are necessary to confirm our findings. In addition, the presence of diabetes may have an important impact on this association. Besides, it is unclear whether there are differences in the effect of severity of COVID-19 on glycemic parameters between subjects with diabetes and those without diabetes. However, studies included in this meta-analysis were carried out in a mixed population with and without diabetes and no separated data were provided based on diabetes status. Future studies are required to confirm the association of COVID-19 with glycemic parameters in patients with and without diabetes. Finally, details on medications used during COVID-19 infection is not clear. Yet it may have an impact on the results. Future studies should take this into consideration.

CONCLUSIONS

In conclusion, this meta-analysis suggests that sever COVID-19 is associated with increased blood glucose. Attention should be paid to monitor blood glucose status in patients with COVID-19 and better glycemic control may be an important supportive treatment.

AUTHOR CONTRIBUTIONS

JY had full access to all of the data in the study and take responsibility for the integrity of the data and the accuracy of the data analysis. JC and CW contributed to the study concept and design, drafted the manuscript, and performed the statistical analyses. JC, CW, and XW contributed to the acquisition and analysis and interpretation of the data. JC, CW, XW, ZS, and JY critically revised the manuscript. All authors contributed to the article and approved the submitted version.

REFERENCES

1. Zhou F, Yu T, Du R, Fan G, Liu Y, Liu Z, et al. Clinical course and risk factors for mortality of adult inpatients with COVID-19 in Wuhan, China: a retrospective cohort study. *Lancet.* (2020) 395:1054–62. doi: 10.1016/S0140-6736(20)30566-3
2. Wang D, Hu B, Hu C, Zhu F, Liu X, Zhang J, et al. Clinical characteristics of 138 hospitalized patients with 2019 novel coronavirus-infected pneumonia in Wuhan, China. *JAMA.* (2020) 323:1061–9. doi: 10.1001/jama.2020.1585
3. Chen N, Zhou M, Dong X, Qu J, Gong F, Han Y, et al. Epidemiological and clinical characteristics of 99 cases of 2019 novel coronavirus pneumonia in Wuhan, China: a descriptive study. *Lancet.* (2020) 395:507–13. doi: 10.1016/S0140-6736(20)30211-7
4. Zhang Y, Li H, Zhang J, Cao Y, Zhao X, Yu N, et al. The clinical characteristics and outcomes of diabetes mellitus and secondary hyperglycaemia patients with coronavirus disease 2019: a single-center, retrospective, observational study in Wuhan. *Diabetes Obes Metab.* (2020) 22:1443–54. doi: 10.1111/dom.14086
5. Grasselli G, Zangrillo A, Zanella A, Antonelli M, Cabrini L, Castelli A, et al. Baseline characteristics and outcomes of 1591 patients infected with SARS-CoV-2 admitted to ICUs of the Lombardy Region, Italy. *JAMA.* (2020) 323:1574–81. doi: 10.1001/jama.2020.5394
6. Bellani G, Laffey JG, Pham T, Fan E, Brochard L, Esteban A, et al. Epidemiology, patterns of care, and mortality for patients with acute respiratory distress syndrome in intensive care units in 50 countries. *JAMA.* (2016) 315:788–800. doi: 10.1001/jama.2016.0291
7. Zheng Z, Peng F, Xu B, Zhao J, Liu H, Peng J, et al. Risk factors of critical & mortal COVID-19 cases: a systematic literature review and meta-analysis. *J Infect.* (2020) 8:e16–25. doi: 10.1016/j.jinf.2020.04.021
8. Laiteerapong N, Cifu AS. Screening for prediabetes and type 2 diabetes mellitus. *JAMA.* (2016) 315:697–8. doi: 10.1001/jama.2015.17545
9. Katulanda P, Dissanayake HA, Ranathunga I, Ratnasamy V, Wijewickrama P, Yogendranathan N, et al. Prevention and management of COVID-19 among patients with diabetes: an appraisal of the literature. *Diabetologia.* (2020) 63:1440–52. doi: 10.1007/s00125-020-05164-x
10. Shehav-Zaltzman G, Segal G, Konvalina N, Tirosh A. Remote glucose monitoring of hospitalized, quarantined patients with diabetes and COVID-19. *Diabetes Care.* (2020) 43:e75–6. doi: 10.2337/dc20-0696
11. Zhu L, She ZG, Cheng X, Qin JJ, Zhang XJ, Cai J, et al. Association of blood glucose control and outcomes in patients with COVID-19 and pre-existing type 2 diabetes. *Cell Metab.* (2020) 31:1068–77.e3. doi: 10.1016/j.cmet.2020.04.021
12. Ding Y, He L, Zhang Q, Huang Z, Che X, Hou J, et al. Organ distribution of severe acute respiratory syndrome (SARS) associated coronavirus (SARS-CoV) in SARS patients: implications for pathogenesis and virus transmission pathways. *J Pathol.* (2004) 203:622–30. doi: 10.1002/path.1560
13. Yang JK, Lin SS, Ji XJ, Guo LM. Binding of SARS coronavirus to its receptor damages islets and causes acute diabetes. *Acta Diabetol.* (2010) 47:193–9. doi: 10.1007/s00592-009-0109-4
14. McGuinness OP. Defective glucose homeostasis during infection. *Annu Rev Nutr.* (2005) 25:9–35. doi: 10.1146/annurev.nutr.24.012003.132159
15. Stroup DF, Berlin JA, Morton SC, Olkin I, Williamson GD, Rennie D, et al. Meta-analysis of observational studies in epidemiology: a proposal for reporting. Meta-analysis Of Observational Studies in Epidemiology (MOOSE) group. *JAMA.* (2000) 283:2008–12. doi: 10.1001/jama.283.15.2008
16. Stang A. Critical evaluation of the Newcastle-Ottawa scale for the assessment of the quality of nonrandomized studies in meta-analyses. *Eur J Epidemiol.* (2010) 25:603–5. doi: 10.1007/s10654-010-9491-z
17. Ren H, Yang Y, Wang F, Yan Y, Shi X, Dong K, et al. Association of the insulin resistance marker TyG index with the severity and mortality of COVID-19. *Cardiovasc Diabetol.* (2020) 19:58. doi: 10.1186/s12933-020-01035-2
18. Wang F, Yang Y, Dong K, Yan Y, Zhang S, Ren H, et al. Clinical characteristics of 28 patients with diabetes and COVID-19 in Wuhan, China. *Endocr Pract.* (2020) 26:668–74. doi: 10.4158/EP-2020-0108
19. Gao Y, Li T, Han M, Li X, Wu D, Xu Y, et al. Diagnostic utility of clinical laboratory data determinations for patients with the severe COVID-19. *J Med Virol.* (2020) 92:791–6. doi: 10.1002/jmv.25770
20. Argenziano MG, Bruce SL, Slater CL, Tiao JR, Baldwin MR, Barr RG, et al. Characterization and clinical course of 1000 patients with coronavirus disease 2019 in New York: retrospective case series. *BMJ.* (2020) 369:m1996. doi: 10.1136/bmj.m1996
21. Bornstein SR, Rubino F, Khunti K, Mingrone G, Hopkins D, Birkenfeld AL, et al. Practical recommendations for the management of diabetes in patients with COVID-19. *Lancet Diabetes Endocrinol.* (2020) 8:546–50. doi: 10.1016/S2213-8587(20)30152-2
22. Shah BR, Hux JE. Quantifying the risk of infectious diseases for people with diabetes. *Diabetes Care.* (2003) 26:510–3. doi: 10.2337/diacare.26.2.510
23. Pearson-Stuttard J, Blundell S, Harris T, Cook DG, Critchley J. Diabetes and infection: assessing the association with glycaemic control in population-based studies. *Lancet Diabetes Endocrinol.* (2016) 4:148–58. doi: 10.1016/S2213-8587(15)00379-4
24. Kornum JB, Thomsen RW, Riis A, Lervang HH, Schønheyder HC, Sørensen HT. Diabetes, glycemic control, and risk of hospitalization with pneumonia: a population-based case-control study. *Diabetes Care.* (2008) 31:1541–5. doi: 10.2337/dc08-0138
25. Okin D, Medzhitov R. The effect of sustained inflammation on hepatic mevalonate pathway results in hyperglycemia. *Cell.* (2016) 165:343–56. doi: 10.1016/j.cell.2016.02.023
26. Šestan M, Marinović S, Kavazović I, Cekinović ðD, Wueest S, Turk Wensveen T, et al. Virus-induced interferon-γ causes insulin resistance in skeletal muscle and derails glycemic control in obesity. *Immunity.* (2018) 49:164–77.e6. doi: 10.1016/j.immuni.2018.05.005
27. Donath MY, Dinarello CA, Mandrup-Poulsen T. Targeting innate immune mediators in type 1 and type 2 diabetes. *Nat Rev Immunol.* (2019) 19:734–46. doi: 10.1038/s41577-019-0213-9
28. Guan WJ, Ni ZY, Hu Y, Liang WH, Ou CQ, He JX, et al. Clinical characteristics of coronavirus disease 2019 in China. *N Engl J Med.* (2020) 382:1708–20. doi: 10.1056/NEJMoa2002032
29. Drucker DJ. Coronavirus infections and type 2 diabetes-shared pathways with therapeutic implications. *Endocr Rev.* (2020) 41:bnaa011. doi: 10.1210/endrev/bnaa011
30. Liu F, Long X, Zhang B, Zhang W, Chen X, Zhang Z. ACE2 expression in pancreas may cause pancreatic damage After SARS-CoV-2 infection. *Clin Gastroenterol Hepatol.* (2020) 18:2128–30.e2. doi: 10.1101/2020.02.28.20029181
31. Hoffmann M, Kleine-Weber H, Schroeder S, Krüger N, Herrler T, Erichsen S, et al. SARS-CoV-2 cell entry depends on ACE2 and TMPRSS2 and is blocked by a clinically proven protease inhibitor. *Cell.* (2020) 181:271–80.e8. doi: 10.1016/j.cell.2020.02.052
32. Peters MC, Sajuthi S, Deford P, Christenson S, Rios CL, Montgomery MT, et al. COVID-19 related genes in sputum cells in asthma: relationship to demographic features and corticosteroids. *Am J Respir Crit Care Med.* (2020) 202:83–90. doi: 10.1164/rccm.202003-0821OC
33. Xuan X, Gao F, Ma X, Huang C, Wang Y, Deng H, et al. Activation of ACE2/angiotensin (1-7) attenuates pancreatic β cell dedifferentiation in a high-fat-diet mouse model. *Metabolism.* (2018) 81:83–96. doi: 10.1016/j.metabol.2017.12.003

10

Association Between the Concentration and Rangeability of Cystatin C and Mortality of COVID-19 Patients with or without Type 2 Diabetes Mellitus

Lei Yang[1†], Dou Xu[2†], Yiqing Tan[3†], Bolin Li[1], Dan Zhu[4], Jingbo Wang[4], Hui Sun[5], Xinglong Liu[5], Xiaopu Zheng[1], Ling Zhu[4] and Zhongyu Li[2*]*

[1] Department of Cardiology, The First Affiliated Hospital of Xi'an Jiaotong University, Xi'an, China, [2] School of Software Engineering, Xi'an Jiaotong University, Xi'an, China, [3] Department of Radiology, Wuhan Third Hospital, Tongren Hospital of Wuhan University, Wuhan, China, [4] Department of Radiology, Shanghai Ninth People's Hospital Affiliated to JiaoTong University School of Medicine, Shanghai, China, [5] SenseTime Research, Beijing, China

***Correspondence:**
Zhongyu Li
zhongyuli@xjtu.edu.cn
Ling Zhu
puxuke12@126.com*

[†]These authors have contributed equally to this work and share first authorship

Background: We investigated if the concentration and "rangeability" of cystatin C (CysC) influenced the prognosis of coronavirus disease 2019 (COVID-19) in patients suffering from, or not suffering from, type 2 diabetes mellitus (T2DM).

Methods: A total of 675 T2DM patients and 572 non-T2DM patients were divided into "low" and "high" CysC groups and low and high CysC-rangeability groups according to serum CysC level and range of change of CysC level, respectively. Demographic characteristics, clinical data, and laboratory results of the four groups were analyzed.

Results: COVID-19 patients with a high level and rangeability of CysC had more organ damage and a higher risk of death compared with those with a low level or low rangeability of CysC. Patients with a higher level and rangeability of CysC had more blood lymphocytes and higher levels of C-reactive protein, alanine aminotransferase, and aspartate aminotransferase. After adjustment for possible confounders, multivariate analysis revealed that CysC >0.93 mg/dL was significantly associated with the risk of heart failure (OR = 2.231, 95% CI: 1.125–5.312) and all-cause death (2.694, 1.161–6.252). CysC rangeability >0 was significantly associated with all-cause death (OR = 4.217, 95% CI: 1.953–9.106). These associations were stronger in patients suffering from T2DM than in those not suffering from T2DM.

Conclusions: The level and rangeability of CysC may influence the prognosis of COVID-19. Special care and appropriate intervention should be undertaken in COVID-19 patients with an increased CysC level during hospitalization and follow-up, especially for those with T2DM.

Keywords: COVID-19, cystatin C, renal function, all-cause death, type 2 diabetes mellitus

INTRODUCTION

In late December 2019 in Wuhan City (China), many patients with undefined pneumonia were reported to be infected with a novel coronavirus. The latter was named "severe acute respiratory syndrome coronavirus 2" (SARS-CoV-2) (1–3). The disease that SARS-CoV-2 causes was named "coronavirus disease 2019" (COVID-19). The pandemic of COVID-19 has now infected over 170 million people worldwide until June of 2021 (4).

Kidney involvement is frequent in COVID-19; >40% of cases have abnormal proteinuria at hospital admission (5). Acute kidney injury (AKI) has been observed in 3%–15% of COVID-19 patients (6) and ≤25% in critically-ill COVID-19 patients (7). Greater possibility can be presented for AKI among patients with severe acute respiratory distress syndrome (ARDS), which necessitates invasive mechanical ventilation, especially for older patients or those with comorbidities such as hypertension or type 2 diabetes mellitus (T2DM) (8). Recent studies have suggested that acute renal damage can occur in the early stages of COVID-19, which is associated with death (5, 9, 10).

Xu G and colleagues stated that preexisting renal disease can be associated with an increased risk of adverse outcomes (adjusted hazard ratio of 2.0 (95% confidence interval (CI), 1.32–3.15)) for hospitalized patients (5). That study emphasized that AKI and severe kidney disease are independent risk factors for a poor prognosis of COVID-19, but included indices representing deterioration of renal function - rapid development of urea nitrogen and creatinine in this study. However accumulating evidence has shown that these biomarkers are suboptimal to detect kidney disease in early stages (11).

In the past decade, various studies have been proposed in measuring the serum level of certain biomarkers for early diagnosis of AKI (12), among which major attention has been drawn to cystatin C (CysC) (13). CysC is an early diagnostic biomarkers of AKI in different settings. Evidence points out that it is present approximately 2 days before the clinical syndrome of AKI develops (14), which has been shown to be useful in diagnosing AKI and predicting its outcomes (15).

Whereas the contribution of CysC and changes in the level of CysC with respect to outcomes in COVID-19 patients are poorly understood.

Like many countries, China has an aging population, and an increasing population of T2DM patients. The latter are more likely to develop COVID-19 and have worse clinical outcomes in comparison with COVID-19 patients not suffering from T2DM (16). We hypothesized that CysC and changes in the levels of CysC are associated with worse organ function and a higher risk of death in COVID-19 patients.

We focused on COVID-19 patients with T2DM and investigated the association between CysC and changes in CysC levels with regard to clinical outcomes. Moreover, we investigated whether the relationship between CysC and changes in CysC levels and COVID-19 prognosis differed between T2DM and non-T2DM patients.

METHODS

Ethical Approval of the Study Protocol

This was a retrospective study conducted in Wuhan Third Hospital (Wuhan, China). The study protocol was approved by the Ethics Committees of Wuhan Third Hospital.

Study Population and Data Collection

We considered all consecutive patients with severe COVID-19 admitted to Wuhan Third Hospital between January 11 to March 1, 2020. All patients were diagnosed based on the recommendations (fifth edition) set by the National Institute for Viral Disease Control and Prevention in China. Patients were included in this study if they met the following requirements: (1) 18 years of age or older; (2) had a contact history with patients diagnosed with COVID-19 and presented with the typical features of COVID-19 on computed tomography (CT); (3) a positive result for the nucleic acids of SARS-CoV-2 on the polymerase chain reaction test.

Exclusive criteria of this study: (1) missing data on renal chemistries (creatinine, urea nitrogen, CysC), important clinical covariates such as inflammation indicator, liver function, and hospital treatment; (2) had end-stage kidney disease (ESKD), (3) had prior kidney transplant; (4) had <2 serum CysC levels during admission; (5) with elevated glucose (fasting blood glucose ≥6.1 mmol/L or random glucose ≥11.1 mmol/L) from the nondiabetic group; and (6) type 1 diabetes. A total of COVID-19 patients were included in the current study.

Demographic characteristics, clinical information, laboratory test results, and clinical-outcome data were obtained using data collection forms from electronic medical records. The duration of disease onset to hospital admission and hospital discharge or death was recorded. Information recorded included demographic data, medical history, underlying comorbidities, laboratory findings (e.g., random blood glucose on admission, CysC level duration of hospital stay), and drugs (e.g., insulin and antihyperglycemic agents). Fasting plasma glucose (FPG) was measured for all patients during hospitalization. Comorbidities, including diabetes, cerebral diseases, cardiovascular diseases, and chronic renal diseases were defined as documented history in the admission notes. Cerebral diseases refer to cerebral infarction, epilepsy, Alzheimer's disease, and Parkinson's disease. Cardiovascular diseases refer to hypertension, coronary heart disease, arrhythmia, cardiomyopathy, and heart failure. Chronic renal diseases refer to chronic renal insufficiency, chronic renal failure, chronic nephritis, and nephrotic syndrome.

Definitions

We encountered many difficulties in justifying requests for some tests during the outbreak of COVID-19. Oral glucose tolerance tests to diagnose T2DM and glycosylated hemoglobin were not routinely requested since they were considered low priorities for COVID-19 patients, making the diagnosis of new onset T2DM impossible. We therefore included patients with known T2DM history in the diabetes group and excluded patients with elevated glucose (fasting blood glucose ≥6.1 mmol/L or random glucose

≥11.1 mmol/L) from the nondiabetic group to make the analysis more coherent. The severity of kidney injury was denoted by the CysC level, which was measured upon hospital admission. Changes in renal function were defined as "CysC rangeability", which was calculated as the difference in the CysC level between the time of hospital admission and the highest CysC level recorded during hospitalization. "Severe inflammation" was defined as the highest neutrophil:lymphocyte ratio >6.11 during hospitalization (17). "Liver injury" was defined as degree of alanine transaminase (ALT) ≥the upper limit of normal. ALT was selected to represent liver injury rather than aspartate transaminase (AST) due to the more predominant extra-hepatic sources of AST rendering it less liver-specific (18). "Heart failure" was defined as clinical symptoms (e.g., breathlessness, ankle swelling, and fatigue) are present with the level of N terminal pro B type natriuretic peptide (NT-proBNP) >300 pg/mL during hospitalization (19).

Statistical Analyses

Continuous variables are presented as the mean ± SD if they have a normal distribution or median (lower quartile, upper quartile) value if they do not have a normal distribution. The Shapiro–Wilk test was used to test for normality. Categorical variables are presented as numbers and percentages. Differences in parameters among groups were analyzed using the Student's *t*-test for variables with a normal distribution. The Mann–Whitney *U*-test was employed for continuous variables with a non-normal distribution, and the Chi-square test was used for categorical variables. Logistic regression models were used in univariate analyses and multivariate analyses to determine the prognostic value of the CysC level. Multivariate analyses were adjusted for significant baseline variables and the factors closely related to the outcome of patients with cardiovascular disease (e.g., age, sex, severe pneumonia, serum level of albumin, blood glucose, and log-BNP).

RESULTS

Characteristics of Hospitalized Patients With COVID-19

A total of 1247 COVID-19-associated hospitalized adults from Wuhan City formed the study cohort. The median age was 63 (interquartile range, 51–70) years. Also, 9.4% of the COVID-19 patients were diagnosed with severe pneumonia and 48% were men. There were 675 patients with T2DM and 572 patients did not have T2DM. Severe pneumonia was diagnosed in 8.6% of non-T2DM patients and 10.2% of T2DM patients (**Table 1**).

The entire cohort was divided into two groups according to T2DM or the absence of T2DM. Laboratory testing comprised routine hematology, organ function (heart, liver, kidney), coagulation function, and infection indicators (**Table S1**). Compared with the non-T2DM patients, patients with diabetes were older and were more likely to have cerebral diseases and cardiovascular disease, and the prevalence of severe inflammation and liver injury in hospital was higher in T2DM patients. Neither severe pneumonia, heart failure in hospital, nor other comorbidities were significantly different between patients with T2DM and those without. Patients with T2DM also had a shorter duration of hospital stay (DoHS). T2DM contributed to the prevalence of all-cause death (**Table 1**).

Characteristics of T2DM Patients and Non-T2DM Patients According to the CysC Level

T2DM and non-T2DM patients were divided into two groups according to the CysC level at a cut-off of 0.93 mg/dL.

Among T2DM patients with CysC >0.93 mg/dL, we noted a higher prevalence of severe pneumonia, heart failure, all-cause death, and older age than those in T2DM patients with CysC ≤0.93 mg/dL. The difference in the number of men, comorbidities (cerebral diseases, cardiovascular diseases, chronic renal diseases, and pulmonary diseases), severe inflammation, diabetes duration, medicine control for diabetes, glucocorticoid use, and DoHS between these two groups was not significant (**Table 2**).

Among non-T2DM patients with CysC >0.93 mg/dL, we noted a higher prevalence of men, heart failure, and older age than those in T2DM patients with CysC ≤0.93 mg/dL. The difference in the prevalence of comorbidities (cerebral diseases, cardiovascular diseases, chronic renal diseases, and pulmonary diseases), severe pneumonia, glucocorticoid use, DoHS, liver injury, and severe inflammation between these two groups was not significant (**Table 2**).

The difference in routine hematology, indicators of organ function (heart, liver, kidney), coagulation function, and infection indicators between these two groups with T2DM or without T2DM are shown in **Table S2**.

Characteristics of T2DM Patients and Non-T2DM Patients Grouped by CysC Rangeability

T2DM patients and non-T2DM patients were divided into two groups according to CysC rangeability.

Among T2DM patients with CysC rangeability >0, we noted a higher prevalence of severe pneumonia, severe inflammation, liver injury, and older age than T2DM patients with CysC rangeability ≤0. The difference in the number of men, DoHS, diabetes duration, medicine control for diabetes, glucocorticoid use, comorbidities (cerebral diseases, cardiovascular diseases, chronic renal diseases, and pulmonary diseases), heart failure, and death between these two groups was not significant (**Table 3**).

Among non-T2DM patients with CysC rangeability >0, we documented a higher prevalence of severe pneumonia, DoHS, and older age than those with CysC rangeability ≤0. The difference in the prevalence of glucocorticoid use, comorbidities (cerebral diseases, cardiovascular diseases, chronic renal diseases, and pulmonary diseases), liver injury, severe inflammation, and heart failure between these two groups was not significant (**Table 3**).

TABLE 1 | Characteristics of hospitalized patients with COVID-19.

Variables	Total (n = 1247)	Non-T2DM (n = 572)	T2DM (n = 675)	p
Age	63 (51, 70)	66 (55, 72)	61 (47.5, 68)	<0.001
Men	598 (48)	270 (47)	328 (49)	0.53
Severe pneumonia, n (%)	118 (9.4)	49 (8.6)	69 (10.2)	0.285
CysC baseline, mg/L	0.93 (0.77, 1.14)	0.96 (0.79, 1.19)	0.9 (0.74, 1.12)	<0.001
Hospital stays (days)	15 (11, 17)	16 (14, 17)	14 (11, 17)	0.003
Glucocorticoid use				0.362
0 (no)	1123 (90%)	520 (91.0)	603 (89.3)	
1 (yes)	124 (10.0)	52 (9.0)	72 (10.7)	
Comorbidities				
Cerebral diseases, n (%)				0.003
0 (no)	1193 (95.7)	561 (98)	632 (93.6)	
1(yes)	54 (4.3)	11 (2.0)	43 (6.4)	
Cardiovascular diseases, n (%)				0.045
0 (no)	761 (61.0)	373 (65.2)	388 (57.5)	
1 (yes)	486 (39.0)	199 (34.8)	287 (42.5)	
Chronic renal diseases, n (%)				0.576
0 (no)	1221 (97.9)	565 (98.8)	656 (97.2)	
1 (yes)	26 (2.1)	7 (1.2)	19 (2.8)	
Complications during hospitalization				
Liver injury, n (%)				0.02
0 (no)	989 (79)	486 (85)	503 (75)	
1 (yes)	258 (21)	86 (15)	172 (25)	
Heart failure, n (%)				0.318
0 (no)	1203 (96)	548 (96)	655 (97)	
1 (yes)	44 (4)	24 (4)	20 (3)	
Severe inflammatory, n (%)				<0.001
0 (no)	1057 (85)	516 (90)	541 (80)	
1 (yes)	190 (15)	56 (10)	134 (20)	
All-cause death, n (%)				<0.001
0 (no)	1191 (96)	572 (100)	619 (92)	
1(yes)	56 (4)	0 (0)	56 (8)	

Data are reported as mean ± SD, median (IQR) or number and percentage. T2DM, type 2 diabetes mellitus; NT-proBNP, N terminal pro B type natriuretic peptide; CysC, cystatin C; BNP, brain natriuretic peptide. Severe inflammation was defined as the highest neutrophil:lymphocyte ratio >6.11 during hospitalization; liver injury was defined as a level of alanine transaminase >40 U/L at any time during hospitalization; and heart failure was defined as clinical symptoms present with the level of NT-proBNP >300 pg/mL during hospitalization.

The difference in routine hematology, heart, organ function (liver, kidney), coagulation function, and infection indicators between these two groups of T2DM and non-T2DM patients is shown in **Table S3**.

Association Between the CysC Level and Organ Dysfunction and All-Cause Death as Classified by T2DM

Multivariate logistic analysis for organ dysfunction and all-cause death showed that if CysC ≤0.93 mg/dL was employed as a cut-off, then CysC >0.93 mg/dL was associated significantly with a risk of heart failure (odds ratio (OR) = 2.231, 95% CI: 1.125–5.321) and all-cause death (2.694, 1.161–6.252), but not with severe inflammation (1.142, 0.769–1.695) or liver injury (1.072, 0.871–1.672) (**Figure 1**).

Using CysC ≤0.93 mg/dL as a cut-off, then CysC >0.93 mg/dL was associated with an increased risk of heart failure (OR = 2.962, 95% CI: 1.006–8.724) and all-cause death (5.585, 2.328–13.397), but not with severe inflammation (0.997, 0.980–1.701) or liver injury (0.854, 0.711–1.514) for T2DM patients. The relationship between CysC >0.93 mg/dL and severe inflammation or liver injury was not significant in the non-T2DM group. CysC >0.93 mg/dL is associated with heart failure (4.357, 1.132-10.874), but adjusted by age, prevalence of severe pneumonia, as well as serum levels of albumin, glucose, and log NT-proBNP, the association between CysC >0.93 mg/dL and heart failure was not significant in the non-T2DM group (**Figure 1**).

In T2DM patients adjusted by age, prevalence of severe pneumonia, as well as serum levels of albumin, glucose, and log NT-proBNP, there was a significantly increased contribution of CysC >0.93 mg/dL to all-cause death (OR = 4.059, 95% CI: 1.045–14.340) in women but not in men. Using a cut-off of CysC ≤0.93 mg/dL, then CysC >0.93 mg/dL did not show an obvious link to severe inflammation, liver injury, or heart failure in men or women (**Figure 2**).

Association Between CysC Rangeability and All-Cause Death Classified by T2DM

Compared with patients with CysC rangeability ≤0, those with CysC rangeability >0 had a high correlation with all-cause death (OR = 4.217, 95% CI: 1.953–9.106). For T2DM patients, there was a significantly increased contribution of CysC rangeability >0 to all-cause death (OR = 5.585, 95% CI: 2.328–13.397) (**Figure 3**).

TABLE 2 | Characteristics of T2DM patients and non-T2DM patients according to the CysC level.

Variables **T2DM**	Total N = 675	CysC ≤ 0.93 mg/dl N = 344	CysC > 0.93 mg/dl N = 331	p
Age, y	61 (47.5, 68)	56 (41, 65)	63 (55, 71)	<0.001
Men, n (%)	328 (49)	165 (48)	163 (49)	0.798
Severe pneumonia, n (%)	69 (10.2)	14 (4.1)	55 (16.6)	<0.001
Hospital stays (days)	14 (11, 17)	14 (11, 17)	14 (10.5, 18)	0.842
Diabetes duration, y	4 (1, 7)	4 (0.5, 6)	4 (1, 7)	0.305
Medicine control for diabetes				0.310
No medication, n (%)	405 (60)	219 (63.7)	186 (56.2)	
Oral medication, n (%)	205 (30.5)	96 (28.0)	109 (33.0)	
Insulin, n (%)	83 (12.3)	39 (11.4)	41 (13.2)	
Glucocorticoid use				0.271
0 (no)	603 (89.3)	306 (89.0)	297 (89.7)	
1 (yes)	72 (10.7)	38 (11.0)	34 (10.3)	
Comorbidities				
Cerebral diseases, n (%)				0.376
0 (no)	632 (93.6)	324 (94.1)	308 (93.1)	
1 (yes)	43 (6.4)	20 (5.9)	23 (6.9)	
Cardiovascular diseases, n (%)				0.051
0 (no)	388 (57.5)	206 (59.9)	182 (55.0)	
1 (yes)	287 (42.5)	138 (40.1)	149 (45.0)	
Chronic renal diseases, n (%)				0.056
0 (no)	656 (97.2)	565 (98.8)	656 (97.2)	
1 (yes)	19 (2.8)	9 (2.6)	10 (3.0)	
Complications during hospitalization				
Liver injury, n (%)				0.332
0 (no)	503 (75)	260 (76)	243 (73)	
1 (yes)	172 (25)	84 (24)	88 (27)	
Heart failure, n (%)				0.033
0 (no)	655 (97)	339 (99)	316 (95)	
1 (yes)	20 (3)	5 (1)	15 (5)	
Severe inflammatory, n (%)				0.952
0 (no)	541 (80)	275 (80)	266 (81)	
1 (yes)	134 (20)	69 (20)	65 (19)	
All-cause death, n (%)				<0.001
0 (no)	619 (92)	334 (97)	285 (86.1)	
1 (yes)	56 (8.0)	10 (3.0)	46 (13.9)	
Non-T2DM	**N = 572**	**N = 290**	**N = 282**	
Age	66 (55, 72)	60 (48, 67)	70 (62, 77)	<0.001
Men, n (%)	270 (47)	120 (41)	150 (53)	
Severe pneumonia, n (%)	49 (8.6)	18 (6.2)	31 (11.0)	0.034
Hospital stays (days)	16 (14, 17)	16 (14, 17)	16 (13, 18)	0.317
Glucocorticoid use				0.298
0 (no)	520 (91.0)	261 (90.0)	259 (91.8)	
1 (yes)	52 (9.0)	29 (10.0)	23 (8.2)	
Comorbidities				
Cerebral diseases, n (%)				0.062
0 (no)	561 (98)	284 (97.9)	277 (93.6)	
1 (yes)	11 (2.0)	6 (2.1)	5 (1.7)	
Cardiovascular diseases, n (%)				0.058
0 (no)	373 (65.2)	195 (67.0)	178 (63.1)	
1 (yes)	199 (34.8)	95 (33.0)	104 (36.9)	
Chronic renal diseases, n (%)				0.268
0 (no)	565 (98.8)	286 (98.6)	279 (98.9)	
1 (yes)	7 (1.2)	4 (1.4)	3 (1.1)	
Complications during hospitalization				
Liver injury, n (%)				0.896
0	486 (85)	246 (85)	240 (86)	
1	86 (15)	44 (15)	42 (14)	
Heart failure, n (%)				0.003
0	548 (96)	285 (98)	263 (93)	
1	24 (4)	5 (2)	19 (7)	
Severe inflammatory, n (%)				0.937
0	516 (90)	258 (89)	248 (88)	

(Continued)

TABLE 2 | Continued

Variables T2DM	Total N = 675	CysC ≤ 0.93 mg/dl N = 344	CysC > 0.93 mg/dl N = 331	p
1	56 (10)	32 (11)	34 (12)	
All-cause death, n (%)				1
0	602 (100)	301 (100)	301 (100)	

Data are reported as mean ± SD, median (IQR) or number and percentage. T2DM, type 2 diabetes mellitus; NT-proBNP, N terminal pro B type natriuretic peptide; CysC, cystatin C; BNP, brain natriuretic peptide. Severe inflammation was defined as the highest neutrophil:lymphocyte ratio >6.11 during hospitalization; liver injury was defined as a level of alanine transaminase >40 U/L at any time during hospitalization; and heart failure was defined as clinical symptoms present with the level of NT-proBNP >300 pg/mL during hospitalization.

TABLE 3 | Characteristics of T2DM patients and non-T2DM patients grouped by CysC rangeability.

Variables T2DM	Total N = 675	CysC rangeability ≤ 0 N = 407	CysC rangeability > 0 N = 268	p
Age, years	61 (47.5, 68)	56 (41, 65)	63 (55, 71)	<0.001
Men, n (%)	328 (49)	193 (47.4)	135 (50.4)	
Severe pneumonia, n (%)	69 (10.2)	12 (2.9)	57 (21.3)	<0.001
Hospital stays (days)	14 (11, 17)	14 (10, 17)	14 (11, 18)	0.071
Diabetes duration, y	4 (1, 7)	4 (1,6)	5(2, 7)	0.293
Medicine control for diabetes				0.237
No medication, n (%)	405 (60.0)	248 (61.0)	157 (58.6)	
Oral medication, n (%)	205 (30.5)	130 (32.0)	75 (28.0)	
Insulin, n (%)	83 (12.3)	56 (13.7)	27 (10.0)	
Glucocorticoid use				0.112
0 (no)	603 (89.3)	361 (88.6)	242 (90.3)	
1 (yes)	72 (10.7)	46 (11.4)	26 (9.7)	
Comorbidities				
Cerebral diseases, n (%)				0.237
0 (no)	632 (93.6)	380 (93.3)	252 (94.0)	
1 (yes)	43 (6.4)	27 (6.7)	16 (6.0)	
Cardiovascular diseases, n (%)				0.549
0 (no)	388 (57.5)	232 (57.0)	156 (58.3)	
1 (yes)	287 (42.5)	175 (43.0)	112 (41.7)	
Chronic renal diseases, n (%)				0.576
0 (no)	656 (97.2)	395 (97.0)	261 (97.4)	
1 (yes)	19 (2.8)	12 (3.0)	7 (2.6)	
Complications during hospitalization				
Liver injury, n (%)				0.033
0 (no)	503 (75.0)	365 (89.7)	224 (83.6)	
1 (yes)	172 (25.0)	42 (10.3)	44 (16.4)	
Heart failure, n (%)				0.685
0 (no)	655 (97)	396 (97.3)	259 (96.6)	
1 (yes)	20 (3)	11 (2.7)	9 (3.4)	
Severe inflammation, n (%)				0.035
0 (no)	541 (85)	392 (96.3)	249 (92.9)	
1 (yes)	134 (20)	15 (3.7)	19 (7.1)	
All-cause Death, n (%)				<0.001
0 (no)	619 (92)	395 (97.1)	224 (83.6)	
1 (yes)	56 (8)	12 (2.9)	44 (16.4)	
Non-T2DM	**N = 572**	**N = 372**	**N = 200**	
Age	66 (55, 72)	60 (48, 67)	70 (62, 77)	<0.001
Men, n (%)	270 (47)	176 (45.6)	105 (48.6)	0.477
Severe pneumonia, n (%)	49 (8.6)	15 (3.9)	34 (17)	<0.001
Hospital stays (days)	16 (14, 17)	16 (9, 17)	16 (14, 18)	0.004
Glucocorticoid use				0.380
0 (no)	520 (91.0)	337 (90.5)	183 (91.5)	
1 (yes)	52 (9.0)	35 (9.5)	17 (8.5)	
Comorbidities				
Cerebral diseases, n (%)				0.479
0 (no)	561 (98)	365 (98.1)	196 (98.0)	
1 (yes)	11 (2.0)	7 (1.9)	4 (2.0)	
Cardiovascular diseases, n (%)				0.067

(Continued)

TABLE 3 | Continued

Variables T2DM	Total N = 675	CysC rangeability ≤ 0 N = 407	CysC rangeability > 0 N = 268	p
0 (no)	373 (65.2)	234 (62.8)	133 (66.5)	
1 (yes)	199 (34.8)	138 (37.2)	67 (33.5)	
Chronic renal diseases, n (%)				0.078
0 (no)	565 (98.8)	368 (98.9)	197 (98.5)	
1 (yes)	7 (1.2)	4 (1.1)	3 (1.5)	
Complications during hospitalization				
Liver injury, n (%)				0.387
0 (no)	486 (95)	318 (85.5)	168 (84.0)	
1 (yes)	86 (15)	54 (14.5)	32 (16.0)	
Heart failure, n (%)				0.754
0 (no)	548 (96)	358 (96.3)	190 (95.0)	
1 (yes)	24 (4)	14 (3.7)	10 (5.0)	
Severe inflammation, n (%)				0.325
0 (no)	516 (90)	341 (90.9)	180 (89.0)	
1 (yes)	56 (10)	34 (9.1)	22 (11.0)	
All-cause death, n (%)				1
0 (no)	602 (100)	301 (100)	301 (100)	

Data are reported as mean ± SD, median (IQR) or number and percentage. T2DM, type 2 diabetes mellitus; NT-proBNP, N terminal pro B type natriuretic peptide; CysC, cystatin C; BNP, brain natriuretic peptide. Severe inflammation was defined as the highest neutrophil:lymphocyte ratio >6.11 during hospitalization; liver injury was defined as a level of alanine transaminase >40 U/L at any time during hospitalization; and heart failure was defined as clinical symptoms present with the level of NT-proBNP >300 pg/mL during hospitalization.

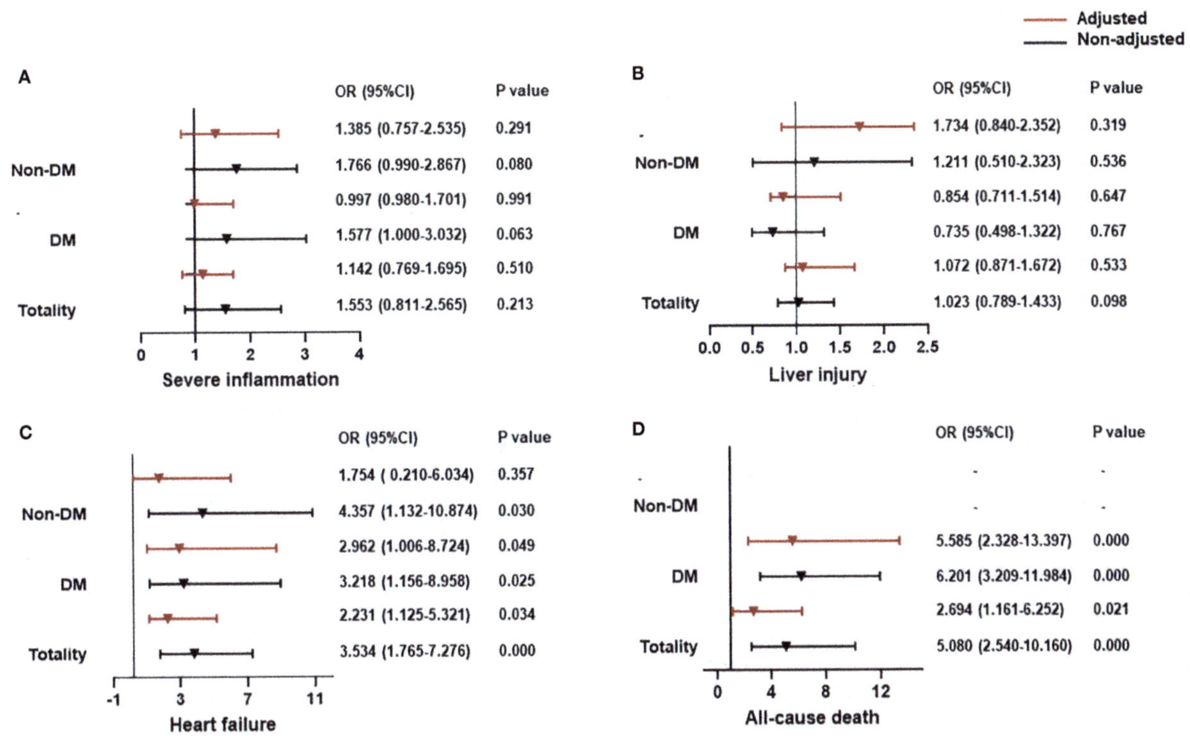

FIGURE 1 | The association between CysC and organ dysfunction and all-cause death classified by T2DM. **(A)** The association between CysC and severe inflammation classified by T2DM. **(B)** The association between CysC and liver injury classified by T2DM. **(C)** The association between CysC and heart failure classified by T2DM. **(D)** The association between CysC and all-cause death classified by T2DM. Severe inflammation was defined as the highest NLR >6.11 during hospitalization; liver injury was defined as a level of ALT >40 U/L at any time during hospitalization; and heart failure was defined as the highest level of NT-proBNP>300 pg/mL during hospitalization. Adjusted by age, severe pneumonia, serum albumin, blood glucose, log NT-proBNP baseline. T2DM, type 2 diabetes mellitus; CysC, cystatin C; NLR, neutrophil-to-lymphocyte ratio; ALT, alanine aminotransferase; NT-proBNP: N terminal pro B type natriuretic peptide.

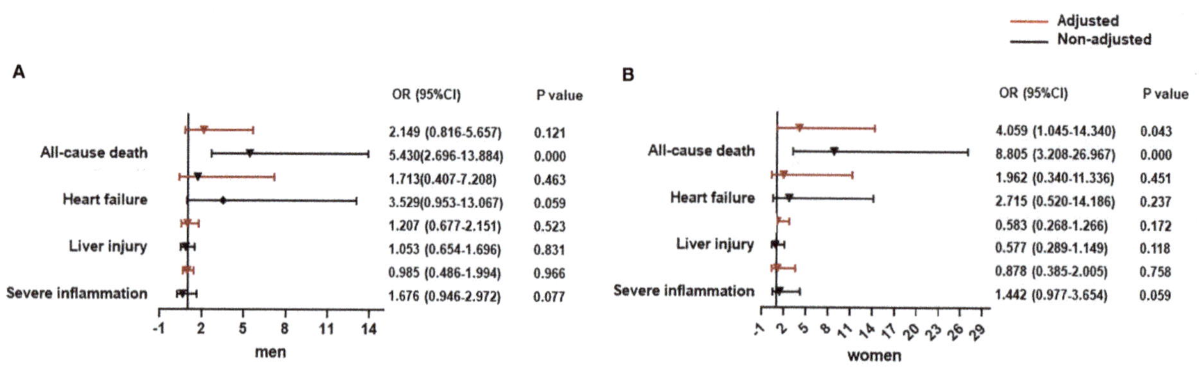

FIGURE 2 | The association between CysC and organ dysfunction and all-cause death in diabetes population classified by sex. **(A)** The association between CysC and organ dysfunction and all-cause death in the male diabetes population. **(B)** The association between CysC and in the female diabetes population. Severe inflammation was defined as the highest NLR >6.11 during hospitalization; liver injury was defined as a level of ALT >40 U/L at any time during hospitalization; and heart failure was defined as the highest level of NT-proBNP>300 pg/mL during hospitalization. Adjusted by age, severe pneumonia, serum albumin, blood glucose, log NT-proBNP baseline. T2DM, type 2 diabetes mellitus; CysC, cystatin C; NLR, neutrophil-to-lymphocyte ratio; ALT, alanine aminotransferase; AST, aspartate aminotransferase; NT-proBNP, N terminal pro B type natriuretic peptide.

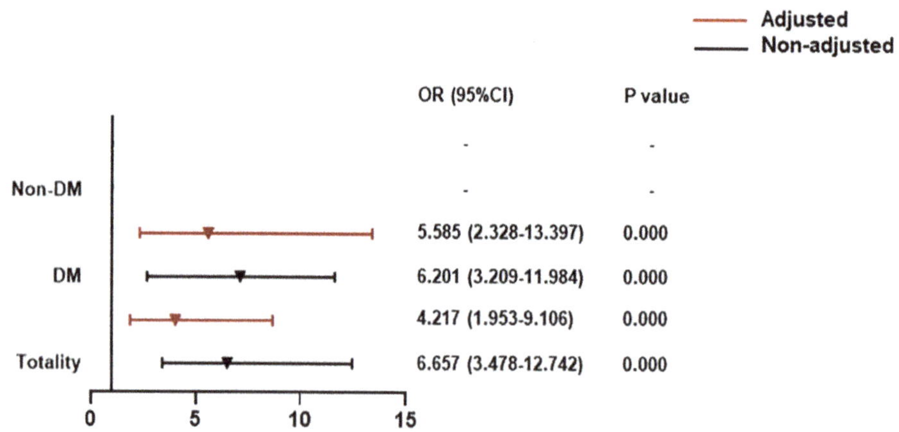

FIGURE 3 | The association between CysC rangeability and all-cause death classified by T2DM. CysC rangeability (changes in renal function) calculated as the difference in the CysC level between the time of hospital admission and the highest CysC level recorded during hospitalization. Adjusted by age, severe pneumonia, serum albumin, blood glucose, log NT-proBNP baseline. T2DM, type 2 diabetes mellitus; NT-proBNP, N terminal pro B type natriuretic peptide.

For T2DM patients adjusted by age, prevalence of severe pneumonia, as well as serum levels of albumin, glucose, and log NT-proBNP, there was a significant contribution of CysC rangeability >0 to all-cause death for men (OR = 4.699, 95% CI: 1.604–13.767). Notably, this association was increased significantly for women (OR = 13.514, 95% CI: 1.398–30.675) (**Figure 4**).

DISCUSSION

We found that CysC >0.93 mg/dL and CysC rangeability >0 were independently associated with mortality among COVID-19-associated hospitalized adults with T2DM, and that CysC rangeability contributed a greater risk for in-hospital death than a single concentration of CysC. More importantly, when classified by sex, this association was stronger in women. Notably, we also observed these associations in patients with mild pneumonia, and all causes of death were contributed by T2DM.

No studies have looked at the association between CysC level and all-cause death in COVID-19-associated hospitalized adults, or the effect of a combination of T2DM and sex.

CysC is an endogenous biomarker of renal function. It can be used to indirectly assess the glomerular filtration rate (20), which has been shown to be useful in diagnosing AKI and predicting its outcomes (15). But there remain a few controversial issues, a study by Hamed HM et al. in 2013 included 32 critically ill

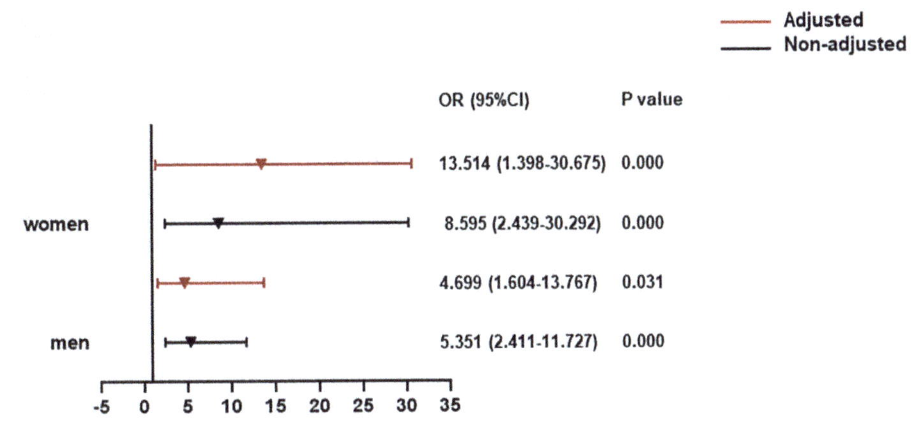

FIGURE 4 | The association between CysC rangeability and all-cause death in T2DM patients. CysC rangeability (changes in renal function) calculated as the difference in the CysC level between the time of hospital admission and the highest CysC level recorded during hospitalization. Adjusted by age, severe pneumonia, serum albumin, blood glucose, log NT-proBNP baseline. T2DM, type 2 diabetes mellitus; NT-proBNP, N terminal pro B type natriuretic peptide.

children who were at risk for developing AKI with a high rate of multi-organ system failure (34.4%) and mortality (62.5%) (21). The study concluded an opposite perspective that CysC is a poor biomarker for diagnosing acute kidney injury. Why the conclusion of this study is different from other studies which included adult patients is uncertain (13, 15, 22), but one reason may be that these children were all critically ill patients with a high incidence of multiple organ dysfunction and death, but the use of glucocorticoids as treatment was not mentioned, however glucocorticoid use can affect serum CysC levels (11). And Hamed HM's study included neonatal patients whose minimum age is 1 month. Whereas in a review study, Jason H and colleagues concluded that the pathophysiology of neonatal AKI is unique and can be affected by high plasma renin activity, high renal vascular resistance, low baseline GFR, ongoing tubular development, and nephrogenesis (23). Furthermore, compared with older adults with diminishing nephron mass, children's ongoing growth, greater renal reserve, and superior renal regenerative potential make AKI in children and adults very different (24). Finally, children have unique comorbidities, of which there are no adult equivalents. Comorbidities may affect the course and management of their AKI, such as bronchopulmonary dysplasia, patent ductus arteriosus, and necrotizing enterocolitis (25). Our study included adults with a median age of 63 (interquartile range [51, 70]), and we also analyzed the data of glucocorticoid use and found that glucocorticoid use showed no difference between the T2DM group and non-T2DM group. The difference of glucocorticoid use between low and high CysC groups and low and high CysC-rangeability groups was also no statistically significant. Thus, considering CysC as a superior biomarker of renal function is reasonable in our study.

CysC is produced in nucleated cells, and is influenced less by reduced muscle mass, acute/chronic illness, and nutritional status than creatinine (26). CysC has been found to be a sensitive serum marker of the glomerular filtration rate and a stronger predictor than creatinine as a risk factor of cardiovascular events and all-cause death in older patients (26). Some studies have suggested that a high serum level of CysC is associated with the severity and poor prognosis of cardiovascular disease (27), neurodegeneration (28), chronic kidney disease (29), AKI (30), and chronic liver disease (31) in critically ill ICU patients (32) as well as the general population (33). Thus, CysC could be a molecular marker in serum for predicting a poor prognosis of various acute and chronic diseases.

Since the COVID-19 pandemic, increasing numbers of studies have been devoted to discovering its clinical features and the organ damage it causes. Some studies have shown that organ (heart, liver, kidney) function is impaired in SARS-CoV-2-infected patients (7, 34–36). Moreover, the outcome of COVID-19 patients is associated with organ damage. An observational study from South Korea by Kim YL and colleagues showed that COVID-19 patients with severe AKI had fatal outcomes (37). Kim YL and colleagues used the rapid development of urea nitrogen and creatinine to evaluate the deterioration of renal function, but not the more stable biomarker CysC. Our study is the first to focus on CysC and CysC rangeability to observe the impact on organ function and mortality in COVID-19 patients.

Researchers have observed that SARS-CoV-2 can directly infect the kidney and cause renal impairment. In an autopsy study, Victor and colleagues quantified the SARS-CoV-2 load in the organs and tissues of 22 patients who had died from COVID-19. They found that the highest number of SARS-CoV-2 copies/cells was detected in the respiratory tract, with lower levels in the kidney, heart, liver, brain, and blood. Those findings indicate that the kidneys are among the most common targets of SARS-CoV-2 (35).

RNA enrichment for transmembrane serine protease 2, angiotensin-converting enzyme 2, and cathepsin L are considered to facilitate SARS-CoV-2 infection. The RNA of genes is enriched in multiple kidney cell types from fetal development through to adulthood. Such enrichment may promote SARS-CoV-2-associated kidney injury (38, 39).

CysC is one of the most reliable parameters of renal function in the general population. Thus, upon SARS-CoV-2 infection, kidney injury can be reflected in the CysC level. Chen X and coworkers studied CTs of the chest in the first week of COVID-19 and CysC levels. They showed that COVID-19 patients with a high CysC level showed more progressive lung lesions on CT. A predictive value of the CysC level upon hospital admission to disease progression was observed rather than dynamic changes (40). Also, COVID-19 severity was closely related to death. We not only found that the CysC level was associated with in-hospital death from COVID-19, we also observed that the change in CysC level during hospitalization was important for predicting death.

Feldman EL and collaborators discovered that T2DM worsened COVID-19 but was also an independent risk factor for severe pneumonia and a poor prognosis (41), data that are in accordance with our results. T2DM can be defined as the phenotype of hyperglycemia that manifests a group of common metabolic disorders. The metabolic disorders related to T2DM cause secondary pathophysiological changes in multiple organs and tissues, and result in various complications that contribute to the morbidity and mortality associated with T2DM (41).

The pathophysiology of SARS-CoV-2 infection is not completely understood. However, studies have demonstrated that SARS-CoV-2 can trigger severe inflammation in certain organs and cause tissue tropism, and shares the same features of chronic inflammation and multi-organ damage observed in T2DM (41). SARS-CoV-2 infection causes intense acute responses to hyperglycemia, inflammation, and tissue damage that are also observed in T2DM. T2DM is characterized by impaired glycemic regulation, chronic low-grade inflammation, slowly progressive multi-organ damage, as well as microvascular (neuropathy, chronic kidney disease) and macrovascular (cerebrovascular disease) complications. Acute COVID-19-associated adverse responses may overlap with glucose instability, preexisting inflammation, and multi-organ damage in T2DM patients and, eventually, worsen outcomes (41). Increased CysC level in COVID-19 patients complicated with AKI is also an indicator for the early detection of diabetic nephropathy in T2DM. Thus, monitoring change in the CysC level may be important for assessing COVID-19 progression.

The CysC level upon hospital admission was strongly associated with death in women, but not in men, in our study. Although the relationship between CysC rangeability and death was not sex-specific, a greater contribution was observed in women than in men. This result may have been because the CysC level is significantly higher in men than that in age-matched women (42), and because if men and women have the same level of CysC, women tend to have worse kidney function. Wang Y and coworkers showed that SARS-CoV-2 infection can aggravate kidney injury in patients with chronic kidney disease (43). Therefore, renal injury in patients with chronic renal disease should be monitored.

Our study had four main limitations. First, it was a single-center observational study, so the generalizability of our results is limited. Second, this study was retrospective. Third, multiple tests for renal function were carried out at different times for each patient. Fourth, biases may have occurred due to the increased number of tests in patients with renal injury. Finally, serum CysC levels are affected by thyroid disease, glucocorticoid use, and obesity (11). However, due to the emergency situation, thyroid diseases were not included in our disease data, and thyroid function of patients in our study were not assessed. Our complication status of T2DM was also deficient.

CONCLUSIONS

CysC may influence the progression and prognosis of COVID-19, and an increased risk of severe complications and death may be seen with COVID-19 patients suffering from T2DM. Attention should be paid to COVID-19 patients with a high level of CysC and CysC rangeability, especially those with T2DM. The exact mechanism underlying CysC-related changes in the course of COVID-19 merit further investigation.

AUTHOR CONTRIBUTIONS

LY, DX, and YT contributed equally to the study and manuscript. LY, DX, and YT contributed to the conception and design of the study, analysis and interpretation of the data, wrote the manuscript, and approved submission. BL contributed to the data acquisition and analysis. DZ, JW, and HS collected the data. XL and XZ contributed to analysis of the data and provided critical revision of the paper. LZ and ZL provided critical revision of the paper for important intellectual content. All authors contributed to the article and approved the submitted version.

REFERENCES

1. Acter T, Uddin N, Das J, Akhter A, Choudhury TR, Kim S. Evolution of Severe Acute Respiratory Syndrome Coronavirus 2 (SARS-Cov-2) as Coronavirus Disease 2019 (COVID-19) Pandemic: A Global Health Emergency. *Sci Total Environ* (2020) 15:730:138996. doi: 10.1016/j.scitotenv.2020.138996
2. Li Q, Guan X, Wu P, Wang X, Zhou L, Tong Y, et al. Early Transmission Dynamics in Wuhan, China, of Novel Coronavirus-Infected Pneumonia. *N Engl J Med* (2020) 382(13):1199–207. doi: 10.1056/NEJMoa2001316
3. Wu JT, Leung K, Leung GM. Nowcasting and Forecasting the Potential Domestic and International Spread of the 2019-Ncov Outbreak Originating in Wuhan, China: A Modelling Study. *Lancet* (2020) 29;395(10225):689–97. doi: 10.1016/S0140-6736(20)30260-9
4. World Health Organization. *Coronavirus Disease 2019 (COVID-19) Situation Report.* Available at: https://www.who.int/emergencies/diseases/novel-coronavirus-2019/situation-reports (Accessed June, 2021).
5. Cheng Y, Luo R, Wang K, Zhang M, Wang Z, Dong L, et al. Kidney Disease is Associated With In-Hospital Death of Patients With COVID-19. *Kidney Int* (2020) 97(5):829–38. doi: 10.1016/j.kint.2020.03.005
6. Zaim S, Chong JH, Sankaranarayanan V, Harky A. COVID-19 and Multiorgan Response. *Curr Probl Cardiol* (2020) 45(8):100618. doi: 10.1016/j.cpcardiol.2020.100618
7. Gabarre P, Dumas G, Dupont T, Darmon M, Azoulay E, Zafrani L. Acute Kidney Injury in Critically Ill Patients With COVID-19. *Intensive Care Med* (2020) 46(7):1339–48. doi: 10.1007/s00134-020-06153-9
8. Fu L, Fei J, Xu S, Xiang HX, Xiang Y, Hu B, et al. Liver Dysfunction and Its Association With the Risk of Death in COVID-19 Patients: A Prospective

Cohort Study. *J Clin Transl Hepatol* (2020) 28;8(3):246–54. doi: 10.14218/JCTH.2020.00043

9. Hong XW, Chi ZP, Liu GY, Huang H, Guo SQ, Fan JR, et al. Characteristics of Renal Function in Patients Diagnosed With COVID-19: An Observational Study. *Front Med (Lausanne)* (2020) 7:409. doi: 10.3389/fmed.2020.00409
10. Uribarri A, Núñez-Gil IJ, Aparisi A, Becerra-Muñoz VM, Feltes G, Trabattoni D, et al. Impact of Renal Function on Admission in COVID-19 Patients: An Analysis of the International HOPE COVID-19 (Health Outcome Predictive Evaluation for COVID 19) Registry. *J Nephrol* (2020) 33(4):737–45. doi: 10.1007/s40620-020-00790-5
11. Wasung ME, Chawla LS, Madero M. Biomarkers of Renal Function, Which and When? *Clin Chim Acta* (2015) 1;438:350–7. doi: 10.1016/j.cca.2014.08.039
12. Parikh CR, Mansour SG. Perspective on Clinical Application of Biomarkers in AKI. *J Am Soc Nephrol* (2017) 28(6):1677–85. doi: 10.1681/ASN.2016101127
13. Dharnidharka VR, Kwon C, Stevens G. Serum Cystatin C is Superior to Serum Creatinine as a Marker of Kidney Function: A Meta-Analysis. *Am J Kidney Dis* (2002) 40(2):221–6. doi: 10.1053/ajkd.2002.34487
14. Soni SS, Ronco C, Katz N, Cruz DN. Early Diagnosis of Acute Kidney Injury: The Promise of Novel Biomarkers. *Blood Purif* (2009) 28(3):165–74. doi: 10.1159/000227785
15. Roos JF, Doust J, Tett SE, Kirkpatrick CM. Diagnostic Accuracy of Cystatin C Compared to Serum Creatinine for the Estimation of Renal Dysfunction in Adults and Children–A Meta-Analysis. *Clin Biochem* (2007) 40(5-6):383–91. doi: 10.1016/j.clinbiochem.2006.10.026
16. Wang X, Wang S, Sun L, Qin G. Prevalence of Diabetes Mellitus in 2019 Novel Coronavirus: A Meta-Analysis. *Diabetes Res Clin Pract* (2020) 164:108200. doi: 10.1016/j.diabres.2020.108200
17. Cai J, Li H, Zhang C, Chen Z, Liu H, Lei F, et al. the Neutrophil-to-Lymphocyte Ratio Determines Clinical Efficacy of Corticosteroid Therapy in Patients With COVID-19. *Cell Metab* (2021) 33(2):258–69.e3. doi: 10.1016/j.cmet.2021.01.002
18. Newsome PN, Cramb R, Davison SM, Dillon JF, Foulerton M, Godfrey EM, et al. Guidelines on the Management of Abnormal Liver Blood Tests. *Gut* (2018) 67(1):6–19. doi: 10.1136/gutjnl-2017-314924
19. Ponikowski P, Voors AA, Anker SD, Bueno H, Cleland JGF, Coats AJS, et al. ESC Scientific Document Group. 2016 ESC Guidelines for the Diagnosis and Treatment of Acute and Chronic Heart Failure: The Task Force for the Diagnosis and Treatment of Acute and Chronic Heart Failure of the European Society of Cardiology (ESC) Developed With the Special Contribution of the Heart Failure Association (HFA) of the ESC. *Eur Heart J* (2016) 37(27):2129–200. doi: 10.1093/eurheartj/ehw12822
20. Carlier M, Dumoulin A, Janssen A, Picavet S, Vanthuyne S, Van Eynde R, et al. Comparison of Different Equations to Assess Glomerular Filtration in Critically Ill Patients. *Intensive Care Med* (2015) 41(3):427–35. doi: 10.1007/s00134-014-3641-9
21. Hamed HM, El-Sherbini SA, Barakat NA, Farid TM, Rasheed EA. Serum Cystatin C Is a Poor Biomarker for Diagnosing Acute Kidney Injury in Critically-Ill Children. *Indian J Crit Care Med* (2013) 17(2):92–8. doi: 10.4103/0972-5229.114829
22. Zhang Z, Lu B, Sheng X, Jin N. Cystatin C in Prediction of Acute Kidney Injury: A Systemic Review and Meta-Analysis. *Am J Kidney Dis* (2011) 58 (3):356–65. doi: 10.1053/j.ajkd.2011.02.389
23. Greenberg JH, Parikh CR. Biomarkers for Diagnosis and Prognosis of AKI in Children: One Size Does Not Fit All. *Clin J Am Soc Nephrol* (2017) 12 (9):1551–7. doi: 10.2215/CJN.12851216
24. Goldstein SL. Renal Recovery at Different Ages. *Nephron Clin Pract* (2014) 127(1-4):21–4. doi: 10.1159/000363679
25. Goldman J, Becker ML, Jones B, Clements M, Leeder JS. Development of Biomarkers to Optimize Pediatric Patient Management: What Makes Children Different? *Biomark Med* (2011) 5(6):781–94. doi: 10.2217/bmm.11.96
26. Kashani KB, Frazee EN, Kukrálová L, Sarvottam K, Herasevich V, Young PM, et al. Evaluating Muscle Mass by Using Markers of Kidney Function: Development of the Sarcopenia Index. *Crit Care Med* (2017) 45(1):e23–9. doi: 10.1097/CCM.0000000000002013
27. Luo J, Wang LP, Hu HF, Zhang L, Li YL, Ai LM, et al. Cystatin C and Cardiovascular or All-Cause Mortality Risk in the General Population: A Meta-Analysis. *Clin Chim Acta* (2015) 23;450:39–45. doi: 10.1016/j.cca.2015.07.016
28. Gauthier S, Kaur G, Mi W, Tizon B, Levy E. Protective Mechanisms by Cystatin C in Neurodegenerative Diseases. *Front Biosci (Schol Ed)* (2011) 3:541–54. doi: 10.2741/s170
29. Bevc S, Hojs N, Knehtl M, Ekart R, Hojs R. Cystatin C as a Predictor of Mortality in Elderly Patients With Chronic Kidney Disease. *Aging Male* (2019) 22(1):62–7. doi: 10.1080/13685538.2018.1479386
30. Maiwall R, Kumar A, Bhardwaj A, Kumar G, Bhadoria AS, Sarin SK. Cystatin C Predicts Acute Kidney Injury and Mortality in Cirrhotics: A Prospective Cohort Study. *Liver Int* (2018) 38(4):654–64. doi: 10.1111/liv.13600
31. Uguen T, Jezequel C, Ropert M, Houssel-Debry P, Latournerie M, Lainé F, et al. Pretransplant Renal Function According to CKD-EPI Cystatin C Equation Is a Prognostic Factor of Death After Liver Transplantation. *Liver Int* (2016) 36(4):547–54. doi: 10.1111/liv.12989
32. Ravn B, Prowle JR, Mårtensson J, Martling CR, Bell M. Superiority of Serum Cystatin C Over Creatinine in Prediction of Long-Term Prognosis at Discharge From ICU. *Crit Care Med* (2017) 45(9):e932–40. doi: 10.1097/CCM.0000000000002537
33. Helmersson-Karlqvist J, Ärnlöv J, Larsson A. Cystatin C-Based Glomerular Filtration Rate Associates More Closely With Mortality Than Creatinine-Based or Combined Glomerular Filtration Rate Equations in Unselected Patients. *Eur J Prev Cardiol* (2016) 23(15):1649–57. doi: 10.1177/2047487316642086
34. Phipps MM, Barraza LH, LaSota ED, Sobieszczyk ME, Pereira MR, Zheng EX, et al. Acute Liver Injury in COVID-19: Prevalence and Association With Clinical Outcomes in a Large U.S. Cohort. *Hepatology* (2020) 72(3):807–17. doi: 10.1002/hep.31404
35. Puelles VG, Lütgehetmann M, Lindenmeyer MT, Sperhake JP, Wong MN, Allweiss L, et al. Multiorgan and Renal Tropism of SARS-Cov-2. *N Engl J Med* (2020) 383(6):590–2. doi: 10.1056/NEJMc2011400
36. Shi S, Qin M, Cai Y, Liu T, Shen B, Yang F, et al. Characteristics and Clinical Significance of Myocardial Injury in Patients With Severe Coronavirus Disease 2019. *Eur Heart J* (2020) 41(22):2070–9. doi: 10.1093/eurheartj/ehaa408
37. Lim JH, Park SH, Jeon Y, Cho JH, Jung HY, Choi JY, et al. Fatal Outcomes of COVID-19 in Patients With Severe Acute Kidney Injury. *J Clin Med* (2020) 9 (6):1718. doi: 10.3390/jcm9061718
38. Sungnak W, Huang N, Bécavin C, Berg M, Queen R, Litvinukova M, et al. SARS-Cov-2 Entry Factors are Highly Expressed in Nasal Epithelial Cells Together With Innate Immune Genes. *Nat Med* (2020) 26(5):681–7. doi: 10.1038/s41591-020-0868-6
39. Zhang YM, Zhang H. Genetic Roadmap for Kidney Involvement of Severe Acute Respiratory Syndrome Coronavirus 2 (SARS-Cov-2) Infection. *Clin J Am Soc Nephrol* (2020) 15(7):1044–6. doi: 10.2215/CJN.04370420
40. Yang Z, Shi J, He Z, Lü Y, Xu Q, Ye C, et al. Predictors for Imaging Progression on Chest CT From Coronavirus Disease 2019 (COVID-19) Patients. *Aging (Albany NY)* (2020) 12(7):6037–48. doi: 10.18632/aging.102999
41. Feldman EL, Savelieff MG, Hayek SS, Pennathur S, Kretzler M, Pop-Busui R. COVID-19 and Diabetes: A Collision and Collusion of Two Diseases. *Diabetes* (2020) 69(12):2549–65. doi: 10.2337/dbi20-0032
42. Marmarinos A, Garoufi A, Panagoulia A, Dimou S, Drakatos A, Paraskakis I, et al. Cystatin-C Levels in Healthy Children and Adolescents: Influence of Age, Gender, Body Mass Index and Blood Pressure. *Clin Biochem* (2016) 49(1-2):150–3. doi: 10.1016/j.clinbiochem.2015.10.012
43. Wang Y, Lv Y, Liu Q. SARS-Cov-2 Infection Associated Acute Kidney Injury in Patients With Pre-Existing Chronic Renal Disease: A Report of Two Cases. *Immun Inflammation Dis* (2020) 8(4):506–11. doi: 10.1002/iid3.333

11

Covid-19 and Diabetes: A Complex Bidirectional Relationship

Hermine Muniangi-Muhitu[1]*, Elina Akalestou*[1]*, Victoria Salem*[2]*, Shivani Misra*[3]*, Nicholas S. Oliver*[3] *and Guy A. Rutter*[1,4*]

[1] Section of Cell Biology and Functional Genomics, Division of Diabetes, Endocrinology and Metabolism, Department of Metabolism, Digestion and Reproduction, Imperial College London, London, United Kingdom, *[2] Section of Endocrinology, Division of Diabetes, Endocrinology and Metabolism, Department of Metabolism, Digestion and Reproduction, Imperial College London, London, United Kingdom,* *[3] Section of Metabolic Medicine, Division of Diabetes, Endocrinology and Metabolism, Department of Metabolism, Digestion and Reproduction, Imperial College London, London, United Kingdom,* *[4] Lee Kong Chian School of Medicine, Nan Yang Technological University, Singapore, Singapore*

Correspondence:
Guy A. Rutter
g.rutter@imperial.ac.uk

Covid-19 is a recently-emerged infectious disease caused by the novel severe acute respiratory syndrome coronavirus SARS-CoV2. SARS-CoV2 differs from previous coronavirus infections (SARS and MERS) due to its high infectivity (reproduction value, R_0, typically 2–4) and pre- or asymptomatic transmission, properties that have contributed to the current global Covid-19 pandemic. Identified risk factors for disease severity and death from SARS-Cov2 infection include older age, male sex, diabetes, obesity and hypertension. The reasons for these associations are still largely obscure. Evidence is also emerging that SARS-CoV2 infection exacerbates the underlying pathophysiology of hyperglycemia in people with diabetes. Here, we discuss potential mechanisms through which diabetes may affect the risk of more severe outcomes in Covid-19 and, additionally, how diabetic emergencies and longer term pathology may be aggravated by infection with the virus. We consider roles for the immune system, the observed phenomenon of microangiopathy in severe Covid-19 infection and the potential for direct viral toxicity on metabolically-relevant tissues including pancreatic beta cells and targets of insulin action.

Keywords: diabetes, Covid-19, ketoacidosis, management, microangiopathy

COVID-19 PANDEMIC

Since its emergence in December 2019 in Wuhan, China, severe acute respiratory syndrome caused by coronavirus 2 (SARS-CoV-2), subsequently called coronavirus disease 19 (Covid-19), has ravaged the world (1) and was declared a pandemic by the World Health Organization (WHO) in March 2020 (2). As of June 15, 2020, 8,014,146 people with Covid-19 have been reported in more than 213 countries and territories, causing more than 436,005 deaths (3, 4). SARS-CoV-2 is a beta coronavirus with sequence homologies with SARS-CoV (79%) and distant similarities (50%) with Middle East respiratory syndrome coronavirus (MERS-CoV) (5, 6). It is highly contagious and transmitted between individuals through aerosolized droplets and contact with infected surfaces (7).

Abbreviations: ACE2, angiotensin-converting enzyme 2; DKA, diabetic ketoacidosis; SARS-CoV2, severe acute respiratory syndrome coronavirus-2; T2D, type 2 diabetes.

Data published at the beginning of the pandemic showed that Covid-19 can cause significant respiratory morbidity and mortality (8). At ~1% the mortality rate, or case fatality rate, of Covid-19 is ten times that of seasonal influenza (9–11). Age, male sex, ethnicity and existing health problems are all additional risk factors for in-hospital death from Covid-19, with age being the greatest of these: those over 80 years of age have a >500-fold higher probability of death than those under 40 (4, 12). Individuals with comorbidities are more likely to suffer a more severe disease course or die (10). The most common comorbidities with Covid-19 infection are metabolic diseases including diabetes, hypertension, obesity and cardiovascular disease (9, 10, 13). The mechanisms behind these increased risks remain unclear, and will be discussed in the present review, with a focus on the possibility that direct actions of the virus on disease-relevant tissues outside of the respiratory tract are involved.

Whereas diabetes rates in the U.K are ~4.7%, 32% of those who have died from Covid-19 had type 1 or type 2 diabetes (4). Estimates of diabetes prevalence in those who have died as a result of Covid-19 in other populations range from 20-50% (14). While obesity is associated with increased risk of a requirement for intensive care or death (15), a recent study from NHS England (16) indicates that below a body mass index (BMI) of 35 (at which point challenges are associated with adequate mechanical ventilation), increased risk is largely ascribed to altered predominance of diabetes and its complications. Similar findings were reported by Goldacre et al. (12).

In a recent study from France on ~1,300 patients (17) multivariate analysis indicated that BMI, micro- and macrovascular complications were associated with the risk of tracheal intubation or death, whereas no association was apparent for diabetes type or glycated hemoglobin (HbA1c). These apparent differences with the NHS England study may, however, reflect the fact that data on diabetes duration and HbA1c were available for ~60% of subjects in the smaller French cohort, which was also limited to patients admitted to hospital, potentially limiting the power to detect an HbA1c signal.

INTERACTION BETWEEN COVID-19 AND DIABETES, HYPERTENSION, AND OBESITY: EPIDEMIOLOGICAL EVIDENCE

Since the beginning of the Covid-19 outbreak much energy has been devoted to identifying risk factors for infection and severe outcomes, and understanding their underlying molecular mechanisms. Diabetes (22%) and cerebrovascular (22%) disease were identified in numerous studies as the most common distinctive comorbidities (2, 18, 19). Other retrospective studies (9–11), have revealed that the most frequent comorbidities in people infected with Covid-19 virus were hypertension (24.7%), followed by diabetes (21.2%) and coronary heart disease (8%) when these variables are assessed individually. In England, 19% of people admitted to intensive care with Covid-19 suffered from diabetes, 1/3 of whom died in hospital (4). The risk of serious complications and death from coronavirus disease in diabetic patients with diabetes in the UK population is 50% higher than that of non-diabetic people (14).

An independent association between HbA_{1C} and Covid-19 death rates was revealed in a recent cohort study based on the British population with type 1 (T1D) or type 2 (T2D) diabetes (4). This rate increased in patients with an HbA_{1C} > 58 mmol/mol, suggesting an association with hyperglycemia. Similar findings were reported by Guo and colleagues (9, 20).

Obesity is another comorbidity associated with poor outcomes after Covid-19 infection (21), and is associated with poor ventilation of the base of the lungs decreasing oxygen saturation of the blood (13). Indeed, a recent report from the National Research Center (ICNARC) (22) in the UK demonstrated that out of 196 obese patients (the majority of whom were men over 60 years old) with a BMI >35kg/m^2 admitted to intensive care, most (3/4) needed mechanical respiration 2 h after admission. According to another study published recently in the newspaper "Le Monde", in France, 15% of overweight or obese adults and 41% of British obese patients admitted to intensive care, were more likely to contract a SARS-CoV-2 infection and to develop severe forms (13). The main factors determining the severity of viral infection in obese patients are hormonal environment, the defective response of the innate and adaptive immune system as well as the sedentary lifestyle (4, 23). Luzi et al. (23) suggest that obesity not only increases the risk of infection and complications but also the risk of developing a more virulent viral layer, prolonging the transmission of the virus across the whole population and increasing the overall mortality rate as was the case during the H1N1 pandemic in 2009 (23). In summary, obesity and diabetes increase the duration of the disease, the requirement for intensive organ support, and increased risk of mortality.

Finally, hypertension is further, independent risk factor (though less predictive than those above) (12, 16, 24) and comorbidity in patients with Covid-19 (25).

ANGIOTENSIN-CONVERTING ENZYME, ACE2: ROLES AND ACTION

Multiple receptors are involved in SARS-CoV2 binding and uptake into cells, as discussed further below. The role of Angiotensin converting enzyme 2, encoded by the *ACE2* gene (26), in infection by coronaviruses including SARS (27) and SARS-Cov2 (28) is now well-established. Indeed, changes in *ACE2* expression with age and differences between sexes may contribute to the altered risks of Covid-19 infection (29). Both hypertension and diabetes are often treated with ACE inhibitors (11, 14, 30) and it has been suggested that altered ACE2 levels resulting from treatment may a contributor to disease severity in Covid-19. In results from Fang et al. (18), patients with diabetes and hypertension who had been treated with ACE inhibitors or angiotensin receptor blockers (ARB) had a high number of ACE2 receptors in the lung, and could therefore be at higher risk of developing severe symptoms, if infected with Covid-19. This hypothesis was further examined by Sardu et al. (31) in hospitalized hypertensive patients with Covid-19. Nonetheless, no firm link was established between ACEi/ARB and the prognosis of Covid-19 infection.

In normal physiology, ACE2 plays an essential role in the renin-angiotensin-aldosterone system (RAAS) (26, 32). Activation of the RAAS system takes place during a loss of blood volume, a decrease in blood pressure or when the serum concentration of Na^+ falls, promoting in juxtaglomerular cells in the kidney to release renin. The latter cleaves angiotensinogen to release angiotensin I (1–10), which is further converted by ACE1 into angiotensin II a potent vasoconstrictor. Angiotensin II is degraded by ACE2, which cleaves angiotensin II to generate Ang (1–7).

Ang (1–7) is specific for AT1Ra (AGTRAP) and Mas receptors, which are associated with vasodilation (26, 32, 33). Therefore, viral depletion of ACE2 in SARS-CoV2 may reduce vasodilatory tone, contributing to the microangiopathy. Of note, AT1R are present on both pancreatic beta and alpha cells in mice (34) and humans (35). Hence lowered ACE2 levels, and consequently of Ang (1–7), may impact hormone secretion from islets.

Could ACE2 present on beta cells represent a direct target for virus entry, potentially leading to the dysregulation or destruction of these cells, promoting a (potentially irreversible) loss of insulin production? Low but detectable (1–4 reads per kilobase of transcript per million reads, RPKM) levels of *ACE2* mRNA are reported in purified human beta cells (35), and ACE2 immunoreactivity has also been described on these cells (36). However, the selectivity of the antibodies used in the latter study was not tested directly, and ACE2-mediated SARS-CoV2 entry into beta cells entry remains unproven.

Might elevated levels of ACE2, facilitating viral entry, contribute to increased disease risk and mortality in metabolic disease? *In vitro* and *in vivo* studies in disease settings have indicated that *ACE2* expression is increased in heart failure, systemic and pulmonary hypertension and diabetes mellitus (33). ACE2 is expressed in several tissues and organs (**Table 1**). These include endothelial cells as well as vascular smooth muscle cells (26). In the kidney, ACE2 is expressed on the apical surface on the proximal tubules and glomerulus. Its expression has also been observed in the gastrointestinal tract (42). ACE2 has also been reported in the central nervous system and in glial cells (37, 38), and SARS-CoV2 infection *via* the receptor may contribute to the loss of smell (anosmia) observed in many patients (https://covid.joinzoe.com/post/uk-anosmia-covid). Whether ACE2 is expressed by olfactory neurons remains to be demonstrated. ACE2 levels throughout the rest of the human brain appear to be low (42). Finally, thyroid tissue has been shown to express high levels of ACE2 (43). To date, there is limited information regarding the risk of SARS-CoV2 infection in patients with thyroid disease. However, some knowledge regarding an impact of SARS-CoV2 on thyroid function can be inferred from the severe acute respiratory syndrome (SARS) epidemic, when a decrease in serum levels of hormones triiodothyronine (T3) and thyroxines (T4) had been observed in infected patients (44).

SARS-COV-2 AND THE IMMUNE SYSTEM IN DIABETES

As discussed below, infection with SARS-CoV2 appears to have actions on both immune cells and on endothelial cells pertinent to its interactions with metabolic disease (23, 45).

Infection of individual cells with the virus begins with the cleavage of the Spike protein (S), a surface glycoprotein carried by the spicules, in 2 subunits S1 and S2. The S1 subunit of the Spike protein binds to the N-terminal region of ACE2 (33). The second subunit, S2, then interacts with the transmarine protease assisted with serine 2 (TMPRSS2) which cleaves Protein S to allow viral entry (46). RNA from the viral genome is then released into the cytoplasm, allowing viral replication (47) (**Figure 1**). Thereafter, the virus' genomic RNA, together with the envelope glycoprotein and nucleocapsid protein, form vesicles containing virions *via* the cell's secretory pathway, which go on to fuse with the plasma membrane and release the virus from the host cell (5, 6).

Cytokine production is a key element of the inflammatory and immune response to viral infection. After release from the host, the virus is first recognized by the innate immune system *via* molecular pattern recognition receptors (PRR), such as type C lectin receptors, and the Toll Like Receptor (TLR) NOD receptor. Exposure to virus causes the expression of inflammatory factors by

TABLE 1 | Summary of the various organs/tissues expressing ACE2.

Organs	Type of cells expressing ACE2	Impacts in term of risk	Type of Receptors	References
Heart	Myocytes	Cardiac failure	ACE2	Burrell et al. (26)
Brain	Glial cells and neurons	Loss of smell, CV stroke, epilepsy	ACE2 receptors present in the central nervous system (CNS)	Gupta et al. (37), Bittman et al. (38)
Liver	Biliary epithelial cells	Proteinuria	ACE2	Sun et al. (39)
Intestine	Enterocytes	/	ACE2	Ziegler et al. (40)
Lungs	Pneumocytes	Respiratory failure	ACE2	Mourad et al. (33)
Pancreas	Beta cells	Decreased insulin production	ACE2	Luzi et al. (23), Yang et al. (36)
Kidney	Nephron proximal bypass tube cell	Renal failure	ACE2	Burrell et al. (26)
Adipose tissue	Adipocytes	Severe obesity	ACE2	Shoemaker et al. (41)

The third column highlights the failures that the various organs will undergo when the virus binds to the ACE2 receptors present in the different types of cells expressing the angiotensin 2 converting enzyme.

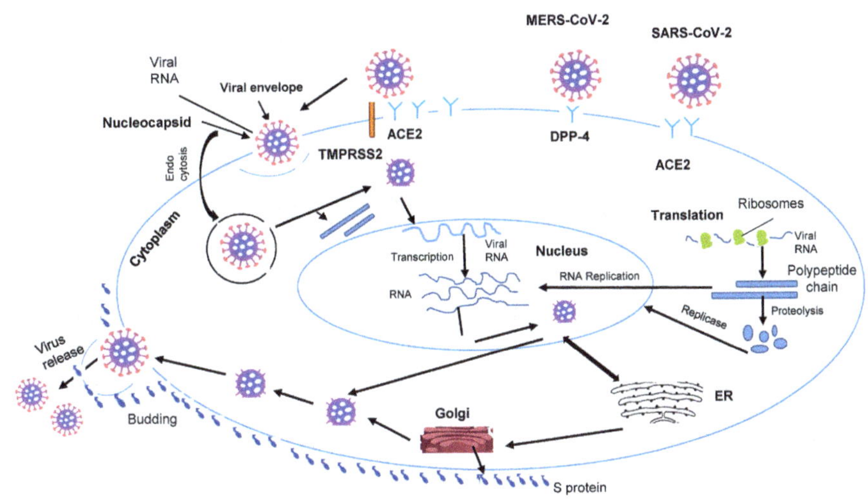

FIGURE 1 | Cellular pathogenesis of coronavirus infection. The lipid envelope (viral) includes spike glycoprotein binding to receptors (ACE2) on the surface of the host. The, entry of cell by endocytosis followed by membrane fusion and release of the virion into the cytosol. Entry of viral RNA into the nucleus and production of new strands of viral RNA and viral proteins. Viral RNA output from the nucleus. Assembly, budding and release of new viruses, impact on organs.

various pathways, in particular the maturation of dendritic cells, and the synthesis of interferons whose role is to limit the spread of the virus and accelerate the phagocytosis of viral antigens (5).

An important feature of Covid-19 infection is a lowered level of lymphocytes in the blood. Implying a similar process after infection with SARS-Cov2, monocytes and T cells are infected with MERS-CoV *via* dipeptidyl peptidase 4 (DPP-4), while SARS-CoV infects primary human monocytes as well as dendritic cells (48). This could be due to destruction of these key cells, which might be a contributor to a weakened immune response, facilitating virus proliferation in Covid-19. However, it is important to bear in mind that a failure to observe lymphocytes in the blood might reflect their homing or recruitment to other infected organs such as the lung (49).

The binding of the virus to immune cells also leads to the synthesis of interleukin 6 (IL-6) which, in turn, leads to signaling both in *cis* and in *trans*. In *cis* signaling, IL-6 binds to lymphocytes *via* cognate receptors. The overproduction of these cytokines (in a "cytokine storm") leads to the risk of multiorganic lesions (35) this might be the main cause of morbidity in subjects with Covid-19. On the other hand, in *trans* signaling, IL-6 binds to receptors on endothelial cells and may lead to hyper-coagulation, an important risk factor for pulmonary embolism and death (50). The fact that patients with severe forms of SARS-CoV-2 infection express higher than normal plasma concentrations of IL-6 (7) which prompted Mehta and colleagues (51) to propose that secondary hemaphagocytic lymphoistiocytosis (sHLH), characterized by an overproduction of cytokines and expansion of macrophages, is found in severe cases of Covid-19 since the main target cells of SARS-CoV-2 are alveolar macrophages expressing ACE2. A recent clinical trial (52) with Kevzara (Sarilumab), an IL-6 receptor antibody, has, however given mixed results, with positive effects observed in "critical" cases but negative in "severe" cases.

COVID-19 AND THROMBOTIC MICROANGIOPATHY

Microangiopathy involves damage to smallest blood vessels and can be the result of the formation of small blood clots, termed thrombotic microangiopathy (TMA) that contribute to renal and neuronal pathology (53). A preexisting microangiopathic disease burden (and markers thereof, e.g. poor glycaemic control and duration of diabetes) are strong risk factors for disease severity (54). TMA is reported as a frequent event in Covid-19 and is likely to involve endothelium-mediated complement activation (55). Given high levels of expression of ACE2 in endothelial cells and podocytes, activation of this process may present a unifying mechanism for viral action in a range of susceptible tissues, including kidney and heart. Clinical observations (56) suggest that SARS-CoV-2 infection facilitates the induction of endotheliitis in several organs as a direct consequence of viral infection. This could contribute markedly to life-threatening complications, such as venous thromboembolic disease and multiple organ failure. Complement inhibition (57) may thus represent an important therapeutic target. Moreover, the inflammatory effects of cytokines may also result in vascular endothelial cell injury which could result in thrombosis (58). Therefore, it is possible that the so-called Covid-19 Associated Coagulopathy (CAC) may be a result of the increased inflammatory response (59).

COVID-19 AND DIABETES: A VICIOUS CIRCLE?

Emerging data indicate a bidirectional relationship between T2D and Covid-19 (**Figure 2**). Firstly, and as described above, preexisting diabetes is a risk factor for poor outcomes and death after Covid-19. Several explanations for this association are possible. Of these the impairment, at different levels, of the innate and adaptive immune response is likely to be involved in the poorer ability to fight infection in patients with diabetes, and particularly in those who are obese (19, 23, 30). People with all forms of diabetes are at increased risk due to defective innate immunity as well as adaptive immunity (14) Severe Covid-19 infection significantly reduces the numbers of natural killer cells, notably $CD4^+$ and $CD8^+$ cells, as well as $CD4^+$ as $CD8^+$ lymphocytes (7). The mechanisms behind these very recent findings are unclear: whether they involve interactions of the virus with beta cells or target tissues for insulin action, or are the result of an indirect effect of an immune response ("cytokine storm"), is unclear (**Figure 2**).

The association between Covid-19 and hyperglycemia in elderly patients with T2D (60) seems likely to reflect metabolic inflammation and exaggerated cytokine release. Strikingly, recent data suggest that SARS-CoV2 infection can lead to a deterioration in glycemic control, involving both profound insulin resistance (requiring as much as 50–100 U insulin/h) and impaired insulin secretion, together leading to diabetic ketoacidosis, DKA (61, 62). Thus, frequent cases of severe DKA have been observed on admission to hospital of patients with Covid-19 (14) and contribute to mortality and morbidity (9).

With respect to the glycemic deterioration seen in patients with preexisting T2D during Covid-19, a very recent report (63) provides the intriguing observation that *ACE2* expression at both the mRNA and protein is increased substantially in human beta cells in response to response to inflammatory cytokines, presumably rendering these cells more susceptible to infection.

TYPE 2 DIABETES MANAGEMENT IN COVID-19

The appropriate management of Covid-19 in people with T2D has been debated actively during the present pandemic, especially with regards to the range of drugs best suited for glycemic control that may also reduce the risk of infection and attenuate the severity of complications. This discussion is of great importance since early glycaemic control may be an important therapeutic option to reduce the poor outcomes in hyperglycaemic Covid-19 patients (64). As an example, it has been shown recently that Covid-19 infection management with the drug tocilizumab was not optimally achieved during hyperglycaemia in both diabetic and non-diabetic patients. Moreover, preclinical models found an indirect link between ACE2 upregulation and several anti-diabetic drugs (65–68). We discuss here presently used treatments both in the context of diabetic emergencies (such as DKA; see above) and for less acute management of hyperglycemia, where different regimens may be required. Given that a number of treatments are now re-purposed as potential therapeutics for Covid-19 (69), the anti-

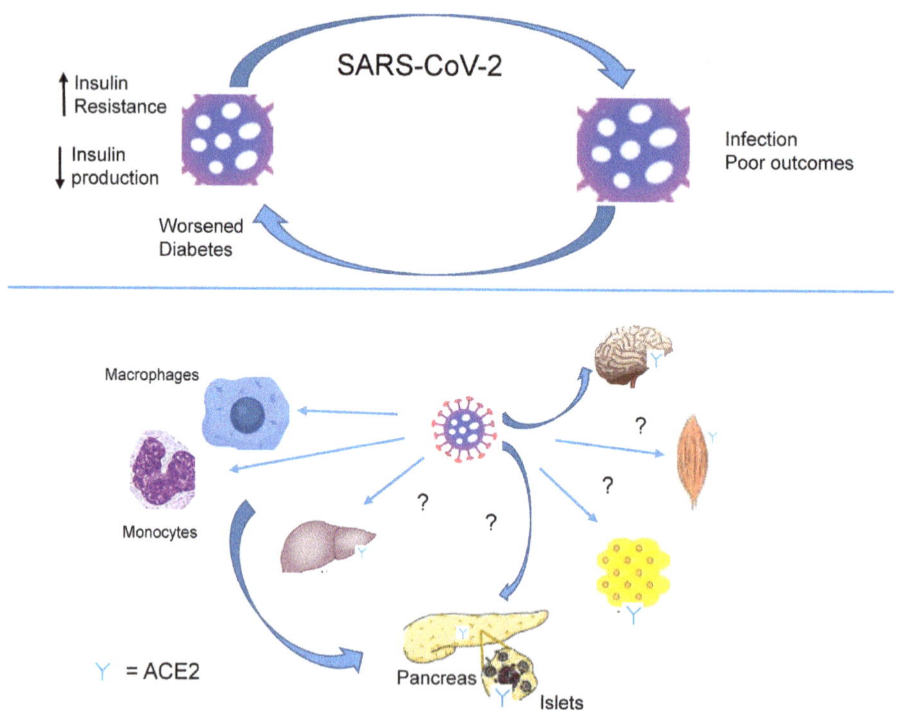

FIGURE 2 | SARS-CoV-2 infection worsens diabetes. Recognition by SAR-CoV-2 of receptors present on immune cells (macrophages, monocytes.) and ACE2 receptors, expressed in several tissues (brain, muscle, adipose tissue, liver, pancreas). Infection causes lowered insulin production and insulin resistance by presently undefined mechanisms.

inflammatory action of several anti-diabetic drugs may also be explored in this light.

Insulin remains a safe choice under all circumstances and is considered the first-line treatment in hyperglycemic critically-ill patients, and may require very high doses (see above). In patients infected with Covid-19, insulin infusion has been shown to be an effective method for achieving glycemic targets as well as reducing the risk of severe symptoms, when compared to patients that did not receive an infusion (70). It has been shown to modulate inflammatory mediators, suppress toll-like receptors (TLRs) implicated in innate immune responses, and suppress pro-inflammatory transcription factors in mononuclear cells (71). Importantly, insulin reduces activation of the pro-inflammatory nuclear transcription factor κB (NF-κB), both in obese non-diabetic and critically ill patients (72, 73). Even though there is no direct link between insulin and ACE2, it has been demonstrated that, in diabetic mice, insulin treatment can attenuate a disintegrin and metalloproteinase-17 (ADAM-17) expression in the kidney.

Glucagon-Like Peptide 1 Receptor Agonists (GLP-1RAs) are an important line of pharmaceutical agents that are especially effective in obese people with T2D to address post-prandial hyperglycaemia. Like insulin, they are also exerting anti-inflammatory activity, as a growing amount of evidence suggests that they may have beneficial effects on lipid profiles and blood pressure, as well as reduced markers of systemic inflammation and improved endothelial dysfunction (74, 75). Specifically in respiratory diseases, GLP-1RAs reduced cytokine concentration and attenuated pulmonary inflammation in preclinical models of lung infection and injury (76–78). Moreover, the GLP-1RA liraglutide has been shown to downregulate immune cell infiltration and protein expression of cytokines, and markedly attenuate NF-κB activation in a chronic asthma preclinical model (79, 80).

Dipeptidyl peptidase 4 (DPP4) inhibitors are often prescribed in combination with other agents for the treatment of T2D. Unlike the majority of anti-diabetic treatments, DPP4 inhibitors do not appear to alter the immune system response in patients with or without T2D (81). However, DPP4 inhibitors have recently been associated with a better clinical outcome in patients with COVID-19 (82) potentially due to the fact that DPP4 is a predicted coronavirus receptor (83). Further details on DPP4 molecular mechanisms and clinical importance have recently been reviewed (20).

Metformin is an oral hypoglycemic agent which is widely used as first-line therapy for T2D as it suppresses hepatic glucose production and increases muscle glucose uptake (84). Similarly to insulin and GLP-1RA, metformin has been suggested to improve chronic inflammation indirectly, *via* insulin resistance and hyperglycemia improvement, but also directly by inhibiting NF-κB *via* AMP-activated protein kinase (AMPK)-dependent and independent pathways (85–88). Another suggested mechanism of the anti-inflammatory action of metformin is inhibition of advanced glycation end products (AGEs) formation, which promote inflammation and glycoxidation (89). However, metformin is not indicated for use in critically-ill hospitalized patients, especially if their hepatic function is impaired, and in cases of dehydration: lactic acidosis is a risk in these circumstances (14). Although concerns have been raised over the use of the anti-rheumatic drug chloroquine or hydroxychloroquine as a potential Covid-19 therapeutic based on studies in animals (90), these were, until recently, used safely together with metformin in humans: however, the licensing of chloroquine use in Covid-19 has recently been withdrawn by the FDA.

Thiazolidinediones are a class of T2D drugs which includes the oral agent pioglitazone. Pioglitazone improves insulin sensitivity through its action at peroxisome proliferator-activated receptor γ1 (PPARγ1) and PPARγ2, and affects lipid metabolism through action at PPARα (91). Although potentially indirect, pioglitazone has been proven to reduce monocyte gene and protein expression of cytokines in patients with impaired glucose tolerance (92). Of note, pioglitazone was found to reduce lung injury by controlling adipose inflammation in a cecal ligation puncture model in mice (93) as well as exert a direct effect on lung inflammation and fibrosis (94). As a result, it has been hypothesized that it should be considered among the drugs currently used against COVID-19 (95). However, use of this drug class in Covid-19 patients is presently very limited.

An additional class of anti-diabetic medications associated with lowering inflammation are the glifozins, or SGLT2 (sodium-glucose cotransporter-2/SLC5A2) inhibitors, which attenuate reabsorption of glucose in the kidney to lower blood sugar. So far, this reported anti-inflammatory effect focuses on the kidney, cardiovascular system and pancreas, rather than lungs (96, 97), though it has been shown to indirectly reduce pulmonary infection in diabetic mice (98). Although SGLT2 inhibitors are associated with dehydration and anorexia and therefore may pose a risk for critically ill patients, a new study focusing on hospitalized adult patients with Covid-19 commenced in April 2020, with the aim of understanding the substantial cardio- and nephroprotective effects of SLGT2 inhibitors in reducing disease progression, complications, and all-cause mortality (99). Recent U.K. guidelines (100) have, nonetheless, advised suspending the use of SGLT2 inhibitors in people with Covid-19 due to the risk of euglycaemic ketoacidosis.

It is important to note that many of the therapeutics mentioned, such as GLP-1RA and SGLT2 inhibitors, have also been strongly associated with improved cardiovascular outcomes (9, 31, 34). This may be of great importance, as growing evidence links Covid-19 with cardiovascular complications (35), in addition to respiratory disease, especially since SARS-CoV-2 can directly infect engineered human blood vessel organoids (36).

Overall, most anti-diabetic therapeutics demonstrate anti-inflammatory effects (**Figure 3**), either indirectly by improving insulin resistance or directly by down-regulating proinflammatory pathways such as those involving nuclear factor κB (NF-κB). Moreover, several drugs have been shown to act directly on the lungs and have a pulmonary effect in respiratory infection and injury. However, most of the studies reporting this utilized preclinical models. It will therefore be

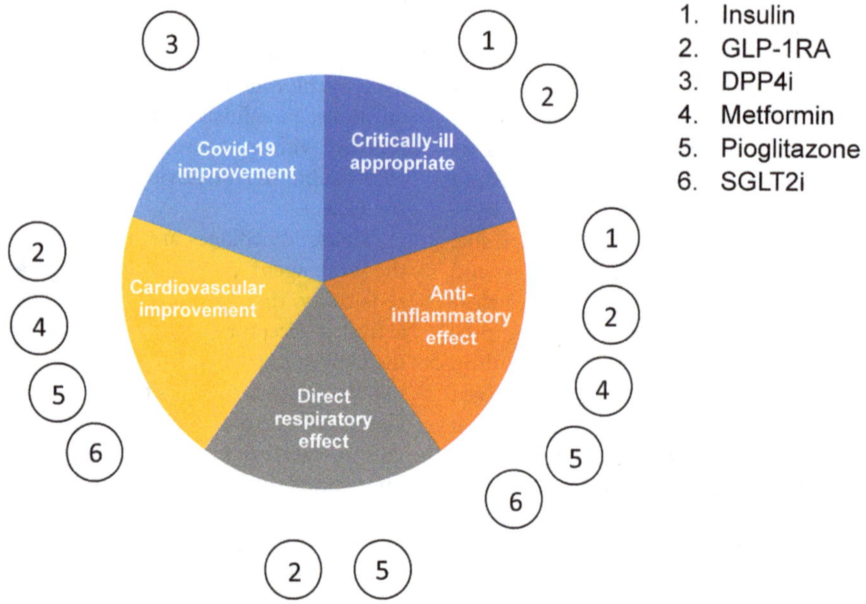

FIGURE 3 | Type 2 diabetes management therapeutics in Covid-19. The six main classes of glucose-lowering drugs summarized according to their reported effect on inflammation, cardiovascular disease, respiratory disease and critically ill patient safety.

important to validate these findings clinically in the context of experimental coronavirus infection in order to determine which anti-diabetic treatments are optimal for a combined management of T2D and Covid-19.

CONCLUSIONS AND PERSPECTIVES

There is now considerable evidence that diabetes is both a risk factor for, and a condition worsened by, SARS-CoV-2 infection. Whereas weakened immunity, alongside impaired kidney function – both features of both aging and diabetes – likely drive the former, exaggerated immune responses probably underlie the latter. Further research will be needed to answer these closely interlinked questions, and we provide suggestions for prioritization below.

With respect to heightened susceptibility to poor Covid-19 outcomes in people with diabetes, key questions include the role of the endothelium and blood hyper-coagulation. Could this affect islet or kidney function? Most evidence suggests that levels of the relevant SARS-Cov2 receptors (ACE2 and DPP4) are low, but not zero, in these tissues - DPP4 is detectable in islets, liver and kidney - suggesting that immune cell-mediated effects are the more likely. More detailed and robust assessment of the expression at the protein level, and sub-cellular localization, of these receptors in the above tissues, and their susceptibility to SARS-Cov2 infection *in vitro* and *in vivo*, are needed.

Regarding the effects of viral infection on glucose control: there is as yet little evidence to suggest that deteriorating glycemia and metabolic control in patients with diabetes outlasts infection, suggesting that immune-mediated destruction of pancreatic beta cells akin to Type 1 diabetes is unlikely to be involved. Nevertheless, formal analysis of this question, i.e. epidemiological assessment of the reversion of glycemic symptoms post Covid-19, as well as histological quantitation *post mortem* of beta cell numbers, and islet infiltration with immune cells, are now called for. The most question remains: are the effects of the virus on glycemic control purely the result of an over-active immune system, with immune cells and inflammatory cytokines acting on multiple tissues (which)?, or are there *direct* actions of the virus on tissues and organs relevant to metabolic homoeostasis (beta cells, other islet hormone-secreting cells, liver, fat, muscle, brain, kidney etc.)? Studies in animal models overexpressing or inactivated for ACE2 (101) or other SARS-CoV2 receptors may be informative here. Where feasible, more in-depth physiological studies (e.g. glucose tolerance tests, hyperinsulimic or hyperglycemic clamps) are required in patients to assess insulin sensitivity (102) and beta cell glucose responsiveness (103) with greater precision. Follow-up studies will then be required at the cellular level to understand the molecular mechanisms behind altered beta (or other) cell function or insulin action, and to understand whether, and through what membrane trafficking pathways, viral replication and shedding occurs in these cell types. Finally, clinical trials in man, informed by the results of the above, will be needed to determine which of the existing, and potentially new, treatments, are likely to be efficacious in reducing glycemia-related medical emergencies as well as the more severe manifestations of Covid-19.

AUTHOR CONTRIBUTIONS

GR, HM-M, and EA prepared the figures. All authors contributed to the article and approved the submitted version.

MR/J0003042/1, MR/L020149/1) and by Diabetes UK (BDA/11/0004210, BDA/15/0005275, BDA 16/0005485) project grants. VS is the recipient of a Diabetes UK Harry Keen Clinician Scientist Fellowship. This project has received funding from the European Union's Horizon 2020 research and innovation programme *via* the Innovative Medicines Initiative 2 Joint Undertaking under grant agreement No 115881 (RHAPSODY). This Joint Undertaking receives support from the European Union's Horizon 2020 research and innovation programme and EFPIA.

REFERENCES

1. Andersen KG, Rambaut A, Lipkin WI, Holmes EC, Garry RF. The proximal origin of SARS-CoV-2. *Nat Med* (2020) 26:450–2. doi: 10.1038/s41591-020-0820-9
2. Pal R, Bhansali A. COVID-19, diabetes mellitus and ACE2: The conundrum. *Diabetes Res Clin Pract* (2020) 162:108132. doi: 10.1016/j.diabres.2020.108132
3. Worldometer. - *real time world statistics.* Worldometer. Available at: http://www.worldometers.info/ (Accessed June 7, 2020).
4. Barron E, Bakhai C, Kar P, Weaver A, Bradley D, Ismail H, et al. Associations of type 1 and type 2 diabetes with COVID-19-related mortality in England: a whole-population study. *Lancet Diabetes Endocrinol* 8(10):813–22. doi: 10.1016/S2213-8587(20)30272-2.
5. Yi Y, Lagniton PNP, Ye S, Li E, Xu R-H. COVID-19: what has been learned and to be learned about the novel coronavirus disease. *Int J Biol Sci* (2020) 16:1753–66. doi: 10.7150/ijbs.45134
6. Neurath MF. COVID-19 and immunomodulation in IBD. *Gut* (2020) 69:1335–42. doi: 10.1136/gutjnl-2020-321269
7. Zhong J, Tang J, Ye C, Dong L. The immunology of COVID-19: is immune modulation an option for treatment? *Lancet Rheumatol* (2020). doi: 10.1016/S2665-9913(20)30120-X
8. Zhu N, Zhang D, Wang W, Li X, Yang B, Song J, et al. A Novel Coronavirus from Patients with Pneumonia in China, 2019. *N Engl J Med* (2020) 382:727–33. doi: 10.1056/NEJMoa2001017
9. Guo W, Li M, Dong Y, Zhou H, Zhang Z, Tian C, et al. Diabetes is a risk factor for the progression and prognosis of COVID-19. *Diabetes Metab Res Rev* (2020). doi: 10.1002/dmrr.3319
10. Guan W, Liang W, Zhao Y, Liang H, Chen Z, Li Y, et al. Comorbidity and its impact on 1590 patients with Covid-19 in China: A Nationwide Analysis. *Eur Respir J* (2020) 55(5):2000547. doi: 10.1183/13993003.00547-2020
11. Zhou F, Yu T, Du R, Fan G, Liu Y, Liu Z, et al. Clinical course and risk factors for mortality of adult inpatients with COVID-19 in Wuhan, China: a retrospective cohort study. *Lancet* (2020) 395:1054–62. doi: 10.1016/S0140-6736(20)30566-3
12. Williamson EJ, Walker AJ, Bhaskaran K, Bacon S, Bates C, Morton CE, et al. Factors associated with COVID-19-related death using OpenSAFELY. *Nature* (2020) 584:430–6. doi: 10.1038/s41586-020-2521-4
13. Simonnet A, Chetboun M, Poissy J, Raverdy V, Noulette J, Duhamel A, et al. High prevalence of obesity in severe acute respiratory syndrome coronavirus-2 (SARS-CoV-2) requiring invasive mechanical ventilation. *Obesity* (2020) 1195–9. doi: 10.1002/oby.22831
14. Bornstein SR, Rubino F, Khunti K, Mingrone G, Hopkins D, Birkenfeld AL, et al. Practical recommendations for the management of diabetes in patients with COVID-19. *Lancet Diabetes Endocrinol* (2020) 546–50. doi: 10.1016/S2213-8587(20)30152-2
15. Caussy C, Pattou F, Wallet F, Simon C, Chalopin S, Telliam C, et al. Prevalence of obesity among adult inpatients with COVID-19 in France. *Lancet Diabetes Endocrinol* (2020) 30160–1. doi: 10.1016/S2213-8587(20)30160-1
16. NHS England. *Type 1 and Type 2 diabetes and COVID-19 related mortality in England.* Available at: https://www.england.nhs.uk/publication/type-1-and-type-2-diabetes-and-covid-19-related-mortality-in-england/ (Accessed June 7, 2020).
17. Cariou B, Hadjadj S, Wargny M, Pichelin M, Al-Salameh A, Allix I, et al. Phenotypic characteristics and prognosis of inpatients with COVID-19 and diabetes: the CORONADO study. *Diabetologia* (2020) 63(8):1500–15. doi: 10.1007/s00125-020-05180-x
18. Fang L, Karakiulakis G, Roth M. Are patients with hypertension and diabetes mellitus at increased risk for COVID-19 infection? *Lancet Respir Med* (2020) 8:e21. doi: 10.1016/S2213-2600(20)30116-8
19. *COVID-19 Infection in People with Diabetes.* touchENDOCRINOLOGY. Available at: https://www.touchendocrinology.com/insight/covid-19-infection-in-people-with-diabetes/ (Accessed April 29, 2020).
20. Drucker DJ. Coronavirus Infections and Type 2 Diabetes—Shared Pathways with Therapeutic Implications. *Endocr Rev* (2020) 41:457–70. doi: 10.1210/endrev/bnaa011
21. *Obesity Link to Severe COVID-19, Especially in the Under 60s.* Medscape. Available at: http://www.medscape.com/viewarticle/928836 (Accessed May 4, 2020).
22. *Early study into UK Covid-19 critical care points to risk factors.* Pulse Today. Available at: http://www.pulsetoday.co.uk/clinical/clinical-specialties/respiratory-/early-study-into-uk-covid-19-critical-care-points-to-risk-factors/20040459.article (Accessed May 14, 2020).
23. Luzi L, Radaelli MG. Influenza and obesity: its odd relationship and the lessons for COVID-19 pandemic. *Acta Diabetol* (2020) 57(6):759–64. doi: 10.1007/s00592-020-01522-8
24. Huang C, Wang Y, Li X, Ren L, Zhao J, Hu Y, et al. Clinical features of patients infected with 2019 novel coronavirus in Wuhan, China. *Lancet Lond Engl* (2020) 395:497–506. doi: 10.1016/S0140-6736(20)30183-5
25. Schiffrin EL, Flack JM, Ito S, Muntner P, Webb RC. Hypertension and COVID-19. *Am J Hypertens* (2020) 33:373–4. doi: 10.1093/ajh/hpaa057
26. Burrell LM, Johnston CI, Tikellis C, Cooper ME. ACE2, a new regulator of the renin–angiotensin system. *Trends Endocrinol Metab* (2004) 15:166–9. doi: 10.1016/j.tem.2004.03.001
27. Li W, Moore MJ, Vasilieva N, Sui J, Wong SK, Berne MA, et al. Angiotensin-converting enzyme 2 is a functional receptor for the SARS coronavirus. *Nature* (2003) 426:450–4. doi: 10.1038/nature02145
28. Zhou P, Yang X-L, Wang X-G, Hu B, Zhang L, Zhang W, et al. A pneumonia outbreak associated with a new coronavirus of probable bat origin. *Nature* (2020) 579:270–3. doi: 10.1038/s41586-020-2012-7
29. Li Y, Zhou W, Yang L, You R. Physiological and pathological regulation of ACE2, the SARS-CoV-2 receptor. *Pharmacol Res* (2020) 157:104833. doi: 10.1016/j.phrs.2020.104833
30. Stefan N, Birkenfeld AL, Schulze MB, Ludwig DS. Obesity and impaired metabolic health in patients with COVID-19. *Nat Rev Endocrinol* (2020) 16:341–2. doi: 10.1038/s41574-020-0364-6
31. Sardu C, Maggi P, Messina V, Iuliano P, Sardu A, Iovinella V, et al. Could anti-hypertensive drug therapy affect the clinical prognosis of hypertensive patients with COVID-19 infection? Data from centers of southern Italy. *J Am Heart Assoc* (2020) 0:e016948. doi: 10.1161/JAHA.120.016948
32. Batlle D, Soler MJ, Ye M. ACE2 and Diabetes: ACE of ACEs? *Diabetes* (2010) 59:2994–6. doi: 10.2337/db10-1205
33. Mourad J-J, Levy BI. Interaction between RAAS inhibitors and ACE2 in the context of COVID-19. *Nat Rev Cardiol* (2020) 17:313–3. doi: 10.1038/s41569-020-0368-x
34. Benner C, van der Meulen T, Caceres E, Tigyi K, Donaldson CJ, Huising MO. The transcriptional landscape of mouse beta cells compared to human beta cells reveals notable species differences in long non-coding RNA and

protein-coding gene expression. *BMC Genomics* (2014) 15:620. doi: 10.1186/1471-2164-15-620
35. Blodgett DM, Nowosielska A, Afik S, Pechhold S, Cura AJ, Kennedy NJ, et al. Novel Observations From Next-Generation RNA Sequencing of Highly Purified Human Adult and Fetal Islet Cell Subsets. *Diabetes* (2015) 64:3172–81. doi: 10.2337/db15-0039
36. Yang J-K, Lin S-S, Ji X-J, Guo L-M. Binding of SARS coronavirus to its receptor damages islets and causes acute diabetes. *Acta Diabetol* (2010) 47:193–9. doi: 10.1007/s00592-009-0109-4
37. *How COVID-19 Affects the Brain*. Medscape. Available at: http://www.medscape.com/viewarticle/928903 (Accessed May 14, 2020).
38. *COVID 19 Expression Of ACE2 Receptors In The Brain Suggest Neurotropic Damage*. MaplesPub. Available at: https://www.maplespub.com/article/COVID-19-Expression-of-ACE2-receptors-in-the-Brain-Suggest-Neurotropic-Damage#article_tab (Accessed May 14, 2020).
39. Sun J, Aghemo A, Forner A, Valenti L. COVID-19 and liver disease. *Liver Int* (2020) 40(6):1278–81. doi: 10.1111/liv.14470 n/a.
40. Ziegler CGK, Allon SJ, Nyquist SK, Mbano IM, Miao VN, Tzouanas CN, et al. SARS-CoV-2 receptor ACE2 is an interferon-stimulated gene in human airway epithelial cells and is detected in specific cell subsets across tissues. *Cell* (2020) 181(5):1016–35.e19. doi: 10.1016/j.cell.2020.04.035
41. Shoemaker R, Tannock LR, Su W, Gong M, Gurley SB, Thatcher SE, et al. Adipocyte deficiency of ACE2 increases systolic blood pressures of obese female C57BL/6 mice. *Biol Sex Differ* (2019) 10:45. doi: 10.1186/s13293-019-0260-8
42. BioGPS. - *your Gene Portal System*. Available at: http://biogps.org/#goto=welcome (Accessed June 8, 2020).
43. Li M-Y, Li L, Zhang Y, Wang X-S. Expression of the SARS-CoV-2 cell receptor gene ACE2 in a wide variety of human tissues. *Infect Dis Poverty* (2020) 9:45. doi: 10.1186/s40249-020-00662-x
44. Guo Y, Korteweg C, McNutt MA, Gu J. Pathogenetic mechanisms of severe acute respiratory syndrome. *Virus Res* (2007) 133:4–12. doi: 10.1016/j.virusres.2007.01.022
45. Gheblawi M, Wang K, Viveiros A, Nguyen Q, Zhong J-C, Turner AJ, et al. Angiotensin-Converting Enzyme 2: SARS-CoV-2 Receptor and Regulator of the Renin-Angiotensin System. *Circ Res* (2020) 126:1456–74. doi: 10.1161/CIRCRESAHA.120.317015
46. Hoffmann M, Kleine-Weber H, Schroeder S, Krüger N, Herrler T, Erichsen S, et al. SARS-CoV-2 Cell Entry Depends on ACE2 and TMPRSS2 and Is Blocked by a Clinically Proven Protease Inhibitor. *Cell* (2020) 181:271–80. doi: 10.1016/j.cell.2020.02.052
47. Wadman M, Couzin-Frankel J, Kaiser J, Matacic C. *How does coronavirus kill? Clinicians trace a ferocious rampage through the body, from brain to toes* (2020). Sci AAAS. Available at: https://www.sciencemag.org/news/2020/04/how-does-coronavirus-kill-clinicians-trace-ferocious-rampage-through-body-brain-toes (Accessed April 29, 2020).
48. Moore JB, June CH. Cytokine release syndrome in severe COVID-19. *Science* (2020) 368:473–4. doi: 10.1126/science.abb8925
49. Xu Z, Shi L, Wang Y, Zhang J, Huang L, Zhang C, et al. Pathological findings of COVID-19 associated with acute respiratory distress syndrome. *Lancet Respir Med* (2020) 8:420–2. doi: 10.1016/S2213-2600(20)30076-X
50. Jose RJ, Manuel A. COVID-19 cytokine storm: the interplay between inflammation and coagulation. *Lancet Respir Med* (2020) 30216–2. doi: 10.1016/S2213-2600(20)30216-2
51. Mehta P, McAuley DF, Brown M, Sanchez E, Tattersall RS, Manson JJ. COVID-19: consider cytokine storm syndromes and immunosuppression. *Lancet* (2020) 395:1033–4. doi: 10.1016/S0140-6736(20)30628-0
52. Sanofi. *Press Releases, Monday, April 27, 2020. Httpswwwsanoficomenmedia-Roompress-Releases20202020-04-27-12-58-00*. Available at: https://www.sanofi.com/media-room/press-releases/2020/2020-04-27 (Accessed June 15, 2020). 12-58-00 2022288.
53. Benz K, Amann K. Thrombotic microangiopathy: new insights. *Curr Opin Nephrol Hypertens* (2010) 19:242–7. doi: 10.1097/MNH.0b013e3283378f25
54. Sharma S, Schaper D, Rayman G. Microangiopathy: Is it relevant to wound healing in diabetic foot disease? *Diabetes Metab Res Rev* (2020) 36 Suppl 1: e3244. doi: 10.1002/dmrr.3244
55. Gavriilaki E, Brodsky RA. Severe COVID-19 infection and thrombotic microangiopathy: success does not come easily. *Br J Haematol* (2020) e227–30. doi: 10.1111/bjh.16783
56. Varga Z, Flammer AJ, Steiger P, Haberecker M, Andermatt R, Zinkernagel AS, et al. Endothelial cell infection and endotheliitis in COVID-19. *Lancet* (2020) 395:1417–8. doi: 10.1016/S0140-6736(20)30937-5
57. Campbell Courtney M. Kahwash Rami. Will Complement Inhibition Be the New Target in Treating COVID-19–Related Systemic Thrombosis? *Circulation* (2020) 141:1739–41. doi: 10.1161/CIRCULATIONAHA.120.047419
58. Leisman DE, Deutschman CS, Legrand M. Facing COVID-19 in the ICU: vascular dysfunction, thrombosis, and dysregulated inflammation. *Intensive Care Med* (2020) 46:1105–8. doi: 10.1007/s00134-020-06059-6
59. Becker RC. COVID-19 update: Covid-19-associated coagulopathy. *J Thromb Thrombolysis* (2020) 50:54–67. doi: 10.1007/s11239-020-02134-3
60. Xue T, Li Q, Zhang Q, Lin W, Wen J, Li L, et al. Blood glucose levels in elderly subjects with type 2 diabetes during COVID-19 outbreak: a retrospective study in a single center. *medRxiv* (2020). doi: 10.1101/2020.03.31.20048579
61. Rayman G, Lumb A, Kennon B, Cottrell C, Nagi D, Page E, et al. Guidance on the management of Diabetic Ketoacidosis in the exceptional circumstances of the COVID-19 pandemic. *Diabetes Med* (2020) 37(7):1214–16. doi: 10.1111/dme.14328 n/a.
62. ADA. *How COVID-19 Impacts People with Diabetes*. Available at: https://www.diabetes.org/coronavirus-covid-19/how-coronavirus-impacts-people-with-diabetes (Accessed April 29, 2020).
63. Fignani D, Licata G, Brusco N, Nigi L, Grieco GE, Marselli L, et al. SARS-CoV-2 receptor Angiotensin I-Converting Enzyme type 2 is expressed in human pancreatic islet β-cells and is upregulated by inflammatory stress. *bioRxiv* (2020). doi: 10.1101/2020.07.23.208041 2020.07.23.208041.
64. Sardu C, D'Onofrio N, Balestrieri ML, Barbieri M, Rizzo MR, Messina V, et al. Hyperglycaemia on admission to hospital and COVID-19. *Diabetologia* (2020). doi: 10.1007/s00125-020-05216-2
65. Tripathy D, Daniele G, Fiorentino TV, Perez-Cadena Z, Chavez-Velasquez A, Kamath S, et al. Pioglitazone improves glucose metabolism and modulates skeletal muscle TIMP-3-TACE dyad in type 2 diabetes mellitus: a randomised, double-blind, placebo-controlled, mechanistic study. *Diabetologia* (2013) 56:2153–63. doi: 10.1007/s00125-013-2976-z
66. Salem ESB, Grobe N, Elased K. Insulin treatment attenuates renal ADAM17 and ACE2 shedding in diabetic Akita mice. *Am J Physiol Renal Physiol* (2014) 306:F629–39. doi: 10.1152/ajprenal.00516.2013
67. Romaní-Pérez M, Outeiriño-Iglesias V, Moya CM, Santisteban P, González-Matías LC, Vigo E, et al. Activation of the GLP-1 Receptor by Liraglutide Increases ACE2 Expression, Reversing Right Ventricle Hypertrophy, and Improving the Production of SP-A and SP-B in the Lungs of Type 1 Diabetes Rats. *Endocrinology* (2015) 156:3559–69. doi: 10.1210/en.2014-1685
68. Dambha-Miller H, Albasri A, Hodgson S, Wilcox CR, Khan S, Islam NN, et al. Currently prescribed drugs in the UK that could up or downregulate ACE2 in COVID-19 disease: A systematic review. *medRxiv* (2020). doi: 10.1101/2020.05.19.20106856
69. Johnson RM, Vinetz JM. Dexamethasone in the management of covid -19. *BMJ* (2020) 370:2648. doi: 10.1136/bmj.m2648
70. Sardu C, D'Onofrio N, Balestrieri ML, Barbieri M, Rizzo MR, Messina V, et al. Outcomes in Patients With Hyperglycemia Affected by COVID-19: Can We Do More on Glycemic Control? *Diabetes Care* (2020) 43:1408–15. doi: 10.2337/dc20-0723
71. Sun Q, Li J, Gao F. New insights into insulin: The anti-inflammatory effect and its clinical relevance. *World J Diabetes* (2014) 5:89–96. doi: 10.4239/wjd.v5.i2.89
72. Dandona P, Aljada A, Mohanty P, Ghanim H, Hamouda W, Assian E, et al. Insulin inhibits intranuclear nuclear factor kappaB and stimulates IkappaB in mononuclear cells in obese subjects: evidence for an anti-inflammatory effect? *J Clin Endocrinol Metab* (2001) 86:3257–65. doi: 10.1210/jcem.86.7.7623
73. Ma C, Liu W, Cui Q, Gu C, Dou Y, Zhao R, et al. [Effects of intensive insulin therapy on plasma nitric oxide and endothelin-1 levels in patients undergoing cardiac surgery under cardiopulmonary bypass]. *Zhonghua Wai Ke Za Zhi* (2008) 46:443–5. doi: 10.4330/wjc.v6.i11.1209
74. Lee Y-S, Jun H-S. Anti-Inflammatory Effects of GLP-1-Based Therapies beyond Glucose Control. *Mediators Inflammation* (2016) 2016:3094642. doi: 10.1155/2016/3094642
75. Rizzo M, Nikolic D, Banach M, Patti AM, Montalto G, Rizvi AA. Incretin-based therapies, glucometabolic health and endovascular inflammation. *Curr Pharm Des* (2014) 20:4953–60. doi: 10.2174/1381612819666131206102255

76. Viby N-E, Isidor MS, Buggeskov KB, Poulsen SS, Hansen JB, Kissow H. Glucagon-like peptide-1 (GLP-1) reduces mortality and improves lung function in a model of experimental obstructive lung disease in female mice. *Endocrinology* (2013) 154:4503–11. doi: 10.1210/en.2013-1666
77. Zhou F, Zhang Y, Chen J, Hu X, Xu Y. Liraglutide attenuates lipopolysaccharide-induced acute lung injury in mice. *Eur J Pharmacol* (2016) 791:735–40. doi: 10.1016/j.ejphar.2016.10.016
78. Bloodworth MH, Rusznak M, Pfister CC, Zhang J, Bastarache L, Calvillo SA, et al. Glucagon-like peptide 1 receptor signaling attenuates respiratory syncytial virus-induced type 2 responses and immunopathology. *J Allergy Clin Immunol* (2018) 142:683–7. doi: 10.1016/j.jaci.2018.01.053
79. Gou S, Zhu T, Wang W, Xiao M, Wang X, Chen Z. Glucagon like peptide-1 attenuates bleomycin-induced pulmonary fibrosis, involving the inactivation of NF-κB in mice. *Int Immunopharmacol* (2014) 22:498–504. doi: 10.1016/j.intimp.2014.07.010
80. Zhu T, Wu X-L, Zhang W, Xiao M. Glucagon Like Peptide-1 (GLP-1) Modulates OVA-Induced Airway Inflammation and Mucus Secretion Involving a Protein Kinase A (PKA)-Dependent Nuclear Factor-κB (NF-κB) Signaling Pathway in Mice. *Int J Mol Sci* (2015) 16:20195–211. doi: 10.3390/ijms160920195
81. Poppel PCM, van, Gresnigt MS, Smits P, Netea MG, Tack CJ. The dipeptidyl peptidase-4 inhibitor vildagliptin does not affect ex vivo cytokine response and lymphocyte function in patients with type 2 diabetes mellitus. *Diabetes Res Clin Pract* (2014) 103:395–401. doi: 10.1016/j.diabres.2013.12.039
82. Rhee SY, Lee J, Nam H, Kyoung D-S, Kim DJ. Effects of a DPP-4 inhibitor and RAS blockade on clinical outcomes of patients with diabetes and COVID-19. *medRxiv* (2020). doi: 10.1101/2020.05.20.20108555 2020.05.20.20108555.
83. Li Y, Zhang Z, Yang L, Lian X, Xie Y, Li S, et al. The MERS-CoV Receptor DPP4 as a Candidate Binding Target of the SARS-CoV-2 Spike. *iScience* (2020) 23(8):101400. doi: 10.1016/j.isci.2020.101400
84. Stumvoll M, Nurjhan N, Perriello G, Dailey G, Gerich JE. Metabolic effects of metformin in non-insulin-dependent diabetes mellitus. *N Engl J Med* (1995) 333:550–4. doi: 10.1056/NEJM199508313330903
85. Li S-N, Wang X, Zeng Q-T, Feng Y-B, Cheng X, Mao X-B, et al. Metformin inhibits nuclear factor kappaB activation and decreases serum high-sensitivity C-reactive protein level in experimental atherogenesis of rabbits. *Heart Vessels* (2009) 24:446–53. doi: 10.1007/s00380-008-1137-7
86. Hattori Y, Suzuki K, Hattori S, Kasai K. Metformin inhibits cytokine-induced nuclear factor kappaB activation via AMP-activated protein kinase activation in vascular endothelial cells. *Hypertens. Dallas Tex 1979* (2006) 47:1183–8. doi: 10.1161/01.HYP.0000221429.94591.72
87. Saisho Y. Metformin and Inflammation: Its Potential Beyond Glucose-lowering Effect. *Endocr Metab Immune Disord - Drug Targets* (2015) 15:196–205. doi: 10.2174/1871530315666150316124019
88. Cameron AR, Morrison VL, Levin D, Mohan M, Forteath C, Beall C, et al. Anti-Inflammatory Effects of Metformin Irrespective of Diabetes Status. *Circ Res* (2016) 119:652–65. doi: 10.1161/CIRCRESAHA.116.308445
89. Beisswenger P, Ruggiero-Lopez D. Metformin inhibition of glycation processes. *Diabetes Metab* (2003) 29:6S95–103. doi: 10.1016/s1262-3636(03)72793-1
90. Zhou L, Xu Z, Castiglione GM, Soiberman US, Eberhart CG, Duh EJ. ACE2 and TMPRSS2 are expressed on the human ocular surface, suggesting susceptibility to SARS-CoV-2 infection. *bioRxiv* (2020). doi: 10.1101/2020.05.09.086165 2020.05.09.086165.
91. Smith U. Pioglitazone: mechanism of action. *Int J Clin Pract Suppl* (2001) 121:13–8. doi: 10.1049/PBPC003E_ch2
92. Zhang W-Y, Schwartz EA, Permana PA, Reaven PD. Pioglitazone inhibits the expression of inflammatory cytokines from both monocytes and lymphocytes in patients with impaired glucose tolerance. *Arterioscler. Thromb Vasc Biol* (2008) 28:2312–8. doi: 10.1161/ATVBAHA.108.175687
93. Kutsukake M, Matsutani T, Tamura K, Matsuda A, Kobayashi M, Tachikawa E, et al. Pioglitazone attenuates lung injury by modulating adipose inflammation. *J Surg Res* (2014) 189:295–303. doi: 10.1016/j.jss.2014.03.007
94. Aoki Y, Maeno T, Aoyagi K, Ueno M, Aoki F, Aoki N, et al. Pioglitazone, a Peroxisome Proliferator-Activated Receptor Gamma Ligand, Suppresses Bleomycin-Induced Acute Lung Injury and Fibrosis. *Respiration* (2009) 77:311–9. doi: 10.1159/000168676
95. Carboni E, Carta AR, Carboni E. Can pioglitazone be potentially useful therapeutically in treating patients with COVID-19? *Med Hypotheses* (2020) 140:109776. doi: 10.1016/j.mehy.2020.109776
96. Heerspink HJL, Perco P, Mulder S, Leierer J, Hansen MK, Heinzel A, et al. Canagliflozin reduces inflammation and fibrosis biomarkers: a potential mechanism of action for beneficial effects of SGLT2 inhibitors in diabetic kidney disease. *Diabetologia* (2019) 62:1154–66. doi: 10.1007/s00125-019-4859-4
97. Bonnet F, Scheen AJ. Effects of SGLT2 inhibitors on systemic and tissue low-grade inflammation: The potential contribution to diabetes complications and cardiovascular disease. *Diabetes Metab* (2018) 44:457–64. doi: 10.1016/j.diabet.2018.09.005
98. Åstrand A, Wingren C, Benjamin A, Tregoning JS, Garnett JP, Groves H, et al. Dapagliflozin-lowered blood glucose reduces respiratory Pseudomonas aeruginosa infection in diabetic mice. *Br J Pharmacol* (2017) 174:836–47. doi: 10.1111/bph.13741
99. *Dapagliflozin in Respiratory Failure in Patients With COVID-19 - Full Text View - ClinicalTrials.gov*. Available at: https://clinicaltrials.gov/ct2/show/NCT04350593 (Accessed June 8, 2020).
100. *Summary of COVID-19 medicines guidance: Diabetes*. SPS - Spec Pharm Serv. Available at: https://www.sps.nhs.uk/articles/summary-of-covid-19-medicines-guidance-diabetes/ (Accessed June 15, 2020).
101. Jiang RD, Liu M-Q, Chen Y, Shan C, Zhou Y-W, Shen X-R. Pathogenesis of SARS-CoV-2 in Transgenic Mice Expressing Human Angiotensin-Converting Enzyme 2. *Cell* (2020) 182(1):50–8.e8. doi: 10.1016/j.cell.2020.05.027
102. Swan JW, Walton C, Godsland IF. Assessment of insulin sensitivity in man: a comparison of minimal model- and euglycaemic clamp-derived measures in health and heart failure. *Clin Sci* (Lond) (1994) 86(3):317–22. doi: 10.1042/cs0860317
103. Ferrannini E, Mari A. β-Cell function in type 2 diabetes. *Metabolism* (2014) 63(10):1217–27. doi: 10.1016/j.metabol.2014.05.012

12

The Efficacy and Potential Mechanisms of Metformin in the Treatment of COVID-19 in the Diabetics

Moein Zangiabadian[1], *Seyed Aria Nejadghaderi*[1], *Mohammad Mahdi Zahmatkesh*[1], *Bahareh Hajikhani*[2], *Mehdi Mirsaeidi*[3*] *and Mohammad Javad Nasiri*[2*]

[1] *Student Research Committee, School of Medicine, Shahid Beheshti University of Medical Sciences, Tehran, Iran,*
[2] *Department of Microbiology, School of Medicine, Shahid Beheshti University of Medical Sciences, Tehran, Iran,*
[3] *Department of Medicine, Division of Pulmonary, Critical Care, Sleep and Allergy, University of Miami, Coral Gables, FL, United States*

Correspondence:
Mohammad Javad Nasiri
mj.nasiri@hotmail.com
Mehdi Mirsaeidi
Msm249@med.miami.edu

Introduction: Diabetes mellitus (DM) is one of the most common comorbidities among patients with coronavirus disease 2019 (COVID-19) which may exacerbate complications of this new viral infection. Metformin is an anti-hyperglycemic agent with host-directed immune-modulatory effects, which relieve exaggerated inflammation and reduce lung tissue damage. The current systematic review aimed to summarize the available evidence on the potential mechanism of action and the efficacy of metformin in COVID-19 patients with DM.

Methods: A systematic search was carried out in PubMed/Medline, EMBASE, the Cochrane Controlled Register of Trials (CENTRAL), and Web of Science up to July 30, 2020. The following keywords were used: "COVID-19", "SARS-CoV-2", "2019-nCoV", "metformin", and "antidiabetic drug".

Results: Fourteen studies were included in our systematic review. Three of them were observational with 6,659 participants. Decreasing insulin resistance, reduction of some inflammatory cytokines like IL-6 and TNF-α, modulation of angiotensin-converting enzyme 2 (ACE2) receptor, and improving neutrophil to lymphocyte ratio are some of the potential mechanisms of metformin in COVID-19 patients with DM. Nine out of fourteen articles revealed the positive effect of metformin on the prognosis of COVID-19 in diabetic or even non-diabetic patients. Moreover, different studies have shown that metformin is more effective in women than men.

Conclusions: The use of metformin may lead to improve the clinical outcomes of patients with mild to moderate SARS-CoV-2, especially in diabetic women. Further observational studies should be conducted to clarify the effects of metformin as a part of the treatment strategy of COVID-19.

Keywords: metformin, diabetes mellitus, SARS-CoV-2, COVID-19, 2019-nCoV, systematic review

INTRODUCTION

In late December 2019, a cluster of patients with pneumonia was referred to hospitals in Wuhan city, Hubei province, China (1). Further clinical investigations showed that a novel coronavirus called Severe Acute Respiratory Syndrome Coronavirus-2 (SARS-CoV-2) caused the disease, COVID-19 (2). Rapidly, COVID-19 affected almost all countries and territories worldwide, so that the World Health Organization (WHO) declared it as a pandemic on March 11, 2020 (3). As of late February 2021, more than 112 million prevalent numbers and above 2.5 million deaths were due to affecting by SARS-CoV-2 (4). Some pharmacologic therapeutic approaches like chloroquine, lopinavir/ritonavir, favipiravir, and tocilizumab have been used in clinical practice without any proven effect (5), while some drugs such as remdesivir have shown some effects on reducing time to recovery (6). Seniors, patients with preexisting diseases including hypertension, diabetes, coronary heart disease, and chronic obstructive pulmonary disease are at a higher risk of morbidity and mortality of COVID-19 (7).

Based on findings of a study on diabetic patients compared to controls, inflammatory responses and levels of inflammation-related biomarkers are higher among patients with diabetes mellitus (DM), which suggests considering DM as a major risk factor in the progression and prognosis of SARS-CoV-2 (8). DM is one of the most common comorbidities among COVID-19 patients, which leads to the intensive care unit (ICU) admission in 14%-32% of cases (9). Different potential mechanisms were mentioned for severity and increased risk of COVID-19 in patients with DM, including upregulation of angiotensin-converting-enzyme-2 (ACE2) expression (10), increased interleukin-6 (IL-6) expression (11), and decreasing CD4-positive T-cells in diabetic patients with Mediterranean Eastern respiratory syndrome coronavirus (MERS-CoV) (12) that may have the similar mechanism with COVID-19.

Metformin is a well-known antidiabetic drug, which showed immunomodulatory effects by phosphorylation of adenosine monophosphate (AMP)-activated protein kinase in animal models (13). A large-scale observational study showed that metformin reduced the mortality of chronic lower respiratory diseases significantly compared to the overall population (14).

This systematic review aimed to determine the potential efficacy of metformin in COVID-19 and the underlying mechanism of action in patients with preexisting DM.

METHODS

This systematic review was according to the "Preferred Reporting Items for Systematic Reviews and Meta-analyses" (PRISMA) statement (15).

Search Strategy

A systematic search was carried out in the literature from the following bibliographical databases: PubMed/Medline, EMBASE, the Cochrane Controlled Register of Trials (CENTRAL), and Web of Science up to July 30, 2020. The following search terms were used: "COVID-19", "SARS-CoV-2", "2019-nCoV", "metformin", and "antidiabetic drug". Lists of references of selected articles and relevant review articles were hand-searched to identify further studies. There were no restrictions on publication date and type of article but only studies written in English were selected.

Study Selection

All potentially English relevant articles were screened in two stages for eligibility. In the first stage, two reviewers independently reviewed titles and abstracts and chose those fitting selection criteria for full-text evaluation. Discrepancies were discussed with a third reviewer. In the second stage of assessment with full-text evaluation, all types of studies except reviews that discussed the effect of metformin in different stages of the COVID-19 and represented its mechanism were considered by the same authors. Disagreements and technical uncertainties were discussed and resolved between review authors.

Data Extraction

The following variables were extracted from all included studies: first author, year of publication, type of study, country/ies where the study was conducted, viral entrance pathway of SARS-CoV-2, mechanism of action of metformin against COVID-19, other effective drugs with the role of them, Possibility of using metformin in COVID-19 treatment and target society. In three analytic studies the extracted data included: study population (number of cases with metformin and number of controls without metformin), mean age (both in metformin and no-metformin group), COVID-19 diagnosis technique (clinical and confirmed diagnosis), and the effect of metformin on outcomes (effect on the duration of hospitalization, the effect on in-hospital death, and effect on poor prognosis). Two authors independently extracted the data from the selected studies. The data was jointly reconciled, and disagreements were discussed and resolved between review authors.

RESULTS

The selection process of articles is shown in **Figure 1**. Fourteen articles were included and classified into the followings: three commentaries (16–18), six letters to the editor (19–24), three observational studies (25–27), one personal view (28), and one research prospective study (29) (**Table 1**). Two of the three observational studies were conducted in China and one in the USA. The total population of the observational articles was 6,659. History of exposure, clinical symptoms, imaging findings, and laboratory assessments was included in clinical diagnosis. Also, PCR or immunoglobulin (Ig)-M and IgG tests were used to confirm the diagnosis (**Tables 1** and **2**).

Possibility of Using Metformin in COVID-19 Treatment

Nine out of fourteen articles showed the efficacy of metformin on COVID-19 that not only can be continued in diabetic patients as an anti-hyperglycemic drug but also may be offered in non-diabetics as

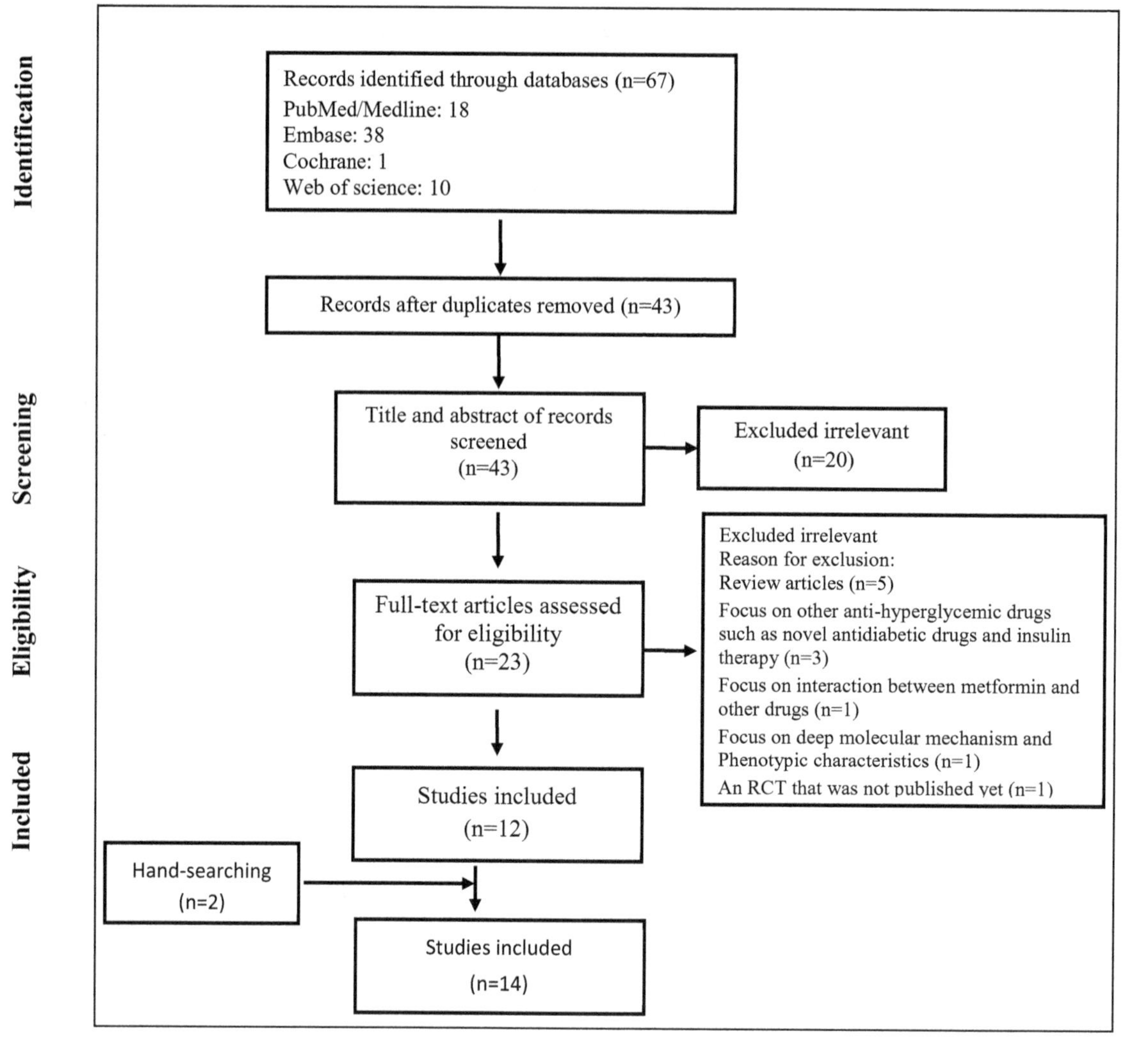

FIGURE 1 | Flow chart of study selection for inclusion in the systematic review.

a part of treatment protocol (17–19, 21, 23, 25–27, 29). Three articles did not provide a definitive opinion on the use of metformin for therapeutic purposes (16, 22, 24), and two articles reported that metformin should not be used in patients with SARS-CoV-2 infection (20, 28) (**Table 3**). Among these articles, Bramante et al. (25) by designing a retrospective cohort analysis study noticed that metformin has sex-specific effects and is useful for diabetic or obese women. Chen et al. (26) reported the positive effect of metformin in the course of the disease, whereas this effect was not statistically significant. On the contrary, Bornstein et al. (28) reported that metformin should not be used in patients with severe symptoms of COVID-19, but it is not contraindicated in patients with mild or moderate symptoms.

Effect of Metformin on Clinical Outcomes

Duration of hospitalization, in-hospital death, and poor prognosis (progression to severe or critical illness) was discussed as major outcomes in three retrospective analytical studies. Luo et al. (27) and Chen et al. (26) did not report any significant effect of metformin on the duration of hospitalization. Furthermore, according to Luo et al. study (27), there was no significant relationship between metformin and poor prognosis. For in-hospital death, Luo et al. (27) represented a significant decrease in the metformin group and Bramante et al. (25) reported this significant effect only in women. On the other hand, the article by Chen et al. (26) did not represent any significant relationship between the administration of metformin and in-hospital mortality reduction. More details on the three mentioned studies are available in **Table 2**.

Potential Mechanisms of Metformin and Other Drugs Against SARS-CoV-2

The suggested mechanisms of action for metformin within the fourteen included papers can be classified into some major

TABLE 1 | Characteristics of all included studies.

Title of article	Author	Year	Country	Type of study
Metformin, neutrophils and COVID-19 infection	Dalan et al. (16)	2020	Singapore	Commentary
Metformin in COVID-19: A possible role beyond diabetes	Sharma et al. (17)	2020	India	Commentary
Is metformin ahead in the race as a repurposed host-directed therapy for atients with diabetes and COVID-19?	Singh et al. (9)	2020	India	Commentary
COVID-19 and Diabetes Mellitus: May Old Antidiabetic Agents Become the New Philosopher's Stone?	Penlioglu et al. (23)	2020	Greece	Letter to the editor
COVID-19 and diabetes: Is metformin a friend or foe?	Ursini et al. (24)	2020	Italy	Letter to the editor
Metformin use amid coronavirus disease 2019 pandemic	Kow et al. (22)	2020	Malaysia and UK	Letter to the editor
Metformin and COVID-19: A novel deal of an old drug	El-arabey et al. (19)	2020	Egypt and China	Letter to the editor
A proposed mechanism for the possible therapeutic potential of Metformin in COVID-19	Esam et al. (21)	2020	Iran	Letter to the editor
Comment on "Should anti-diabetic medications be reconsidered amid COVID-19 pandemic?"	Cure et al. (20)	2020	Turkey	Letter to the editor
Metformin Treatment Was Associated with Decreased Mortality in COVID-19 Patients with Diabetes in a Retrospective Analysis	Luo et al. (27)	2020	China	Retrospective analysis
Observational Study of Metformin and Risk of Mortality in Persons Hospitalized with COVID-19	Bramante et al. (25)	2020	USA	Retrospective cohort analysis
Clinical Characteristics and Outcomes of Patients With Diabetes and COVID-19 in Association With Glucose-Lowering Medication	Chen et al. (26)	2020	China	Retrospective analysis
Practical recommendations for the management of diabetes in patients with COVID-19	Bornstein et al. (28)	2020	Switzerland, Germany, UK, Italy, Singapore, USA, Netherlands, France, Australia, Brazil, Spain, China	Personal view
Metformin and SARS-CoV-2: mechanistic lessons on air pollution to weather the cytokine/thrombotic storm in COVID-19	Menendez et al. (29)	2020	Spain	Research perspective

UK, United Kingdom; USA, United States of America; COVID-19: Coronavirus disease 2019; SARS-CoV-2, Severe acute respiratory syndrome coronavirus 2.

TABLE 2 | Detailed characteristics and statistical information of three retrospective analytical studies.

Authors	Study population			Age (mean)[4]		COVID-19 diagnosis technique		Outcome		
	Used metformin	Did not use metformin	total	Metformin group	No metformin group	Clinical diagnosis	Confirmed diagnosis	Effect on duration of hospitalization	Effect on in-hospital death	Effect on poor prognosis
Luo et al.	104	179	283	63	65	History and clinical symptoms. Imaging (CT scan) Laboratory assessment	Nuclear acid test or IgM-IgG test	No significant effect[1]	Significantly decreased OR:0.21 (0.06-0.73) P-value:0.02	–
Bramante et al.	2333	3923	6256	73	76	–	PCR	–	Significantly decreased in women[2] OR:0.792 (0.640-0.979) P-value:0.031	–
Chen et al.	43	77	120	62	67	Clinical symptoms, exposure, imaging findings	NGS, fluorescent RT-PCR	No significant effect[3]	No significant effect OR:0.62 (0.17-2.20) P-value:0.456	No significant effect OR:2.49 (0.92-6.76) P-value:0.074

COVID-19, Coronavirus disease 2019; Ig, immunoglobulin; CT, computed tomography; OR, odds ratio; RT-PCR, real-time polymerase chain reaction; NGS, next generation sequencing.

1) Duration of hospitalization was 21 days in metformin group while it was 19.5 days in no-metformin group.

2) In overall population metformin was not significantly effective. OR: 0.904 (0.782-1.045); P-value: 0.173

3) Duration of hospitalization was 24 days in metformin group while it was 23 days in no-metformin group.

4) The total mean age in studies were 64.2, 74.8 and 65.2 respectively.

TABLE 3 | Possibility of using metformin in COVID-19 treatment.

Author	Possibility of using metformin in COVID-19 treatment	suggested for/not suggested for
Dalan et al.	May	Uncertain
Sharma et al.	Yes	Not mentioned
Singh et al.	Yes	Suggested: Patients with diabetes and COVID-19
Penlioglu et al.	Yes	Suggested: Patients with or without diabetes
Ursini et al.	May	Uncertain
Kow et al.	May	Uncertain
El-arabey et al.	Yes	Suggested: Elderly, obese and diabetics
Esam et al.	Yes	Suggested: patients in acute, chronic and recovery phases of COVID-19
Cure et al.	No	Not suggested in diabetics
Luo et al.	Yes	Both diabetics and non-diabetics
Bramante et al.	Yes in women	Diabetic or obese women
Chen et al.	Yes but not strongly recommended	Not mentioned
Bornstein et al.	No (in patients with severe symptoms of COVID-19)	Not Suggested: patients with severe COVID-19 symptoms
Mendez et al.	Yes	Suggested: patients with severe COVID-19

COVID-19, Coronavirus disease 2019.

categories. First, El-Arabey et al. (19) and Kow et al. (22) mentioned that weight reduction might have moderate protective effects against SARS-CoV-2, especially in the elderly. Second, adenosine monophosphate-activated protein kinase (AMPK) pathways that can affect the expression of ACE2, the receptor for SARS-CoV-2, is another pathway that can be modulated by metformin (17, 23–25). The articles by Penlioglou et al. (23), Sharma et al. (17), and Bramante et al. (25) mentioned protective roles of metformin by different mechanisms such as a reduction in insulin resistance (23), improving ACE2 stability (17), balancing renin-angiotensin-aldosterone system (17), modulation of ACE2 receptor (25), and controlling blood glucose levels (25). However, Ursini et al. (24) suggested that overexpression of ACE2 as a result of the AMPK pathway can put diabetic patients at higher risk of affecting by SARS-CoV-2. Third, high production of lactate and lactic acidosis due to metformin might be another potential mechanism for the high rate of infection in patients using metformin (20, 22, 28). Fourth, anti-inflammatory effects of metformin can protect patients administrating metformin from SARS-CoV-2 in different ways like inhibition of cytokine storms (18, 27, 29), inhibition of IL-6 crisis (18), and modulation of gut microbiota composition (18). Fifth, reduction of neutrophil count and improving neutrophil to lymphocyte ratio is another mechanism of metformin against COVID-19 in patients with preexisting diabetes mellitus (16, 25). In addition to these main mechanisms, metformin can play roles in protecting from or predisposing diabetic patients to SARS-CoV-2 infection in other various pathways, including reduction of vitamin B12 and immunosuppression (22), inhibition of PI3K/AKT/mTOR pathway (17), reducing thrombosis formation (25), prevention of lung damage and fibrosis (21, 27), interruption of the endocytic cycle due to decreasing acidity of endosomes and lysosomes (21), and reduction of some inflammatory cytokines like IL-6 (18, 25, 26) and TNF-α (25). **Table 4** shows the mechanisms of metformin and other drugs on SARS-CoV-2 infection in diabetic patients.

DISCUSSION

In the present work, most of the evaluated studies have shown that the use of metformin in the treatment regimen of diabetic and non-diabetic patients with COVID-19 is beneficial. Only two studies found that metformin should not be used in severe forms of the COVID-19, however, they did not prohibit its use in moderate to mild cases of infection.

COVID-19 is associated with poor prognosis and increased mortality rate in patients with DM. Also, diabetes management in patients suffering from COVID-19 is a great clinical challenge. Most of the studies evaluated in the current systematic review point to the beneficial effect of metformin in the treatment of COVID-19 patients with diabetes. Metformin as an agent of host-directed therapy can modulate immune mechanisms and therefore might prevent progression to acute respiratory distress syndrome (ARDS). Since there are some metabolic similarities between COVID-19 and DM such as hyperglycemia, oxidative stress, and pro-inflammatory cytokines, it is not unreasonable to expect that metformin with effects such as decreasing the levels of inflammatory cytokines IL-6 and TNF-alpha as well as increasing IL-10, an anti-inflammatory cytokine can play a beneficial role in reducing the complications of COVID-19 in patients with DM (30). Metformin induces the formation of M2 macrophages and T-regulatory as well as CD8 memory T cells which in turn minimize the inflammatory reactions (31). However, some studies have suggested not using this medication in the COVID-19 treatment protocol. In fact, in patients suffering from heart failure, respiratory distress, sepsis or renal impairment use of metformin should be stopped due to the risk of lactic acidosis (28). Of course, it should be noted that the risk of acidosis following the use of metformin is not very high, however, it should be considered, especially in hospitalized patients. Another issue to be considered is that metformin reduces intestinal absorption of vitamin B12 and lowers serum vitamin B12 concentrations in some metformin-treated patients. Due to the role of vitamin B12 in regulating the immune system its deficiency may negatively affect the cellular immune

TABLE 4 | Suggested potential mechanisms of action of metformin and other drugs on Severe Acute Respiratory Syndrome-Coronavirus-2 (SARS-CoV-2).

Author	Suggested viral entrance pathway of SARS-CoV-2	Suggested mechanism of action of metformin on COVID-19.	Other effective drugs	Role of other dugs
El-arabey et al.	Not mentioned	Reduction of weight and pneumonia in elderly, obese and diabetic patients.	Not mentioned	Not mentioned
Mendez et al.	Not mentioned	Preventing ROS/CRAC mediated IL-6 release, preventing cytokine and thrombotic-like storms, ameliorate immunometabolism- related inflammation thus alleviating ARDS.	CM4620 might be useful.	CM4620 is a direct inhibitor of CRAC channel.
Singh et al.	Not mentioned	Anti-inflammatory properties: induction of AMPK, anti-oxidant role by altering activity of catalase and superoxide dismutase, altering composition of gut microbiota to reduce inflammation. Collectively combating cytokine storm and preventing excessive rise in IL-6.	Not mentioned	Not mentioned
Penlioglou et al.	Not mentioned	Reduction in insulin resistance in infected subjects by AMPK, reduction in liver fibrosis and also protective role on liver.	Pioglitazone	Anti-inflammatory, improving liver injury
Ursini et al.	ACE2 acts as docking site for SARS-CoV-2	AMPK Increases ACE2 expression and stability thus promoting SARS-CoV-2 infection. Optimal management of glucose levels and the immune-modulation properties of metformin may result on a beneficial effect on patients' outcome.	Not mentioned	Not mentioned
Kow et al.	Not mentioned	Only modest weight reduction (may not be the main mechanism to protect against, if any, toward mortality from COVID-19), metformin-induced vitamin B12 deficiency may weaken immune system (patients should undergo routine B12 monitoring). Metformin may cause lactic acidosis.	Not mentioned	Not mentioned
Sharma et al.	ACE2 acts as docking site for SARS-CoV-2	AMPK Increases ACE2 expression. AMPK increases ACE2 stability by phosphorylation. This could lead to decreased binding with SARS-CoV-2 due to steric hindrance. Metformin prevents the detrimental sequelae of imbalance RAS by causing activation of ACE2 through AMPK signaling. Inhibition of P13k/AKT/mTOR pathway. Prevention of viral replication and pathogenesis through inhibition of mTOR pathway. Activated AMPK potentiates expression of certain genes with known antiviral properties such as IFNs, OAS2, ISG15, and MX1 while inhibiting inflammatory mediators like TNF-alpha and CCL5. Role of metformin in optimal control of T2DM, for both chronic and transient cases, might help in the treatment of COVID-19.	2-DG	Inhibition of glycosis
Esam et al.	Endocytosis	Metformin increases endosomal and lysosomal pH through acting directly on V-ATPase as proton pumping or acidifier compartment, and eNHEs as proton leaking or alkalizing compartment on the endosomal membrane and subsequently interferes with the endocytic cycle. Metformin is a strong base drug (pKa= 12.4) which might enhance the pH of the acidic vesicles containing viruses. Metformin can reverse established lung fibrosis.	Not mentioned	Not mentioned
Dalan et al.	Not mentioned	Metformin can reduce neutrophil count and neutrophil to lymphocyte ratio in patients with diabetes. Metformin can reduce NETs formation in diabetics and prediabetes patients. Metformin can reduce neutrophil and macrophage infiltration in hyperoxia induced lung injury (described in neonatal rats).	Not mentioned	Not mentioned
Bornstein et al.	ACE2 acts as docking site for SARS-CoV-2	Metformin can cause lactic acidosis.	1. ACEi and ARB 2. statins	1) Could protect against severe lung injury following infection 2) administration is not recommended but statins should not be discontinued because of the long-term benefits and the potential for tipping the balance toward a cytokine storm by rebound rises in IL-6 and IL-1β if they were to be discontinued.
Luo et al.	Not mentioned	Metformin can modulate immune mechanisms that relieve cytokine storms and exaggerated inflammation to reduce lung tissue damage.	Chinese traditional medicine such as Lianhua Qingwen capsules	Not mentioned
Bramante et al.	ACE2 acts as docking site for	Metformin decreases levels of TNF-α and IL-6, and boosts levels of IL-10, significantly more in females than males. ACE2 receptor modulation (via AMPK) improved neutrophil to lymphocyte	Beta 2 agonists (used in asthmatics)	IL-10 boosting and TNF-α decreasing in asthmatics

(Continued)

TABLE 4 | Continued

Author	Suggested viral entrance pathway of SARS-CoV-2	Suggested mechanism of action of metformin on COVID-19.	Other effective drugs	Role of other dugs
	SARS-CoV-2	ratio, decreased glycemia (via AMPK), mast cell stabilization, decreased thrombosis, and improved endothelial function.		
Chen et al.	ACE2 acts as docking site for SARS-CoV-2	Metformin can reduce IL-6.	Not mentioned	Not mentioned
Cure et al.	Penetration to ACE2 at low pH	Metformin increases lactate production.	1. Insulin 2. Dapagliflozin	1) Lowers ADAM-17 activation and thus reduces ACE2 level. Increases NHE activation. Both reducing possibility of virus adhering cell. 2) Lowers lactate levels.

ROS, reactive oxygen species; CRAC, calcium release-activated channel; ARDS, acute respiratory distress syndrome; ACE2, angiotensin-converting enzyme 2; 2-DG, 2-deoxy-D-glucose; RAS, renin-angiotensin-aldosterone system; mTOR, mammalian target of rapamycin; IL, interleukin; IFN, interferon; TNF, tumor necrosis factor; CCL5, chemokine ligand 5; T2DM, type 2 diabetes mellitus; V-ATPase, Vacuolar ATPase; eNHE, endosomal Na+/H+ exchanger; NET, neutrophil extracellular traps; ACEi, angiotensin-converting enzyme inhibitor; ARB, angiotensin receptor blocker; NHE, Na+/H+ exchanger.

responses and thereafter facilitates infection from COVID-19 (32, 33). So, routine monitoring of vitamin B12 is suggested in metformin-treated patients.

Ursini et al. speculated that metformin synergistically with ACEi or ARBs may theoretically result in increasing ACE2 availability in the respiratory tract thus promoting Coivid-19 (24).

Nevertheless, it has been shown that poorly controlled blood glucose levels make patients prone to experience more complications or in-hospital death due to COVID-19. In other words, hospitalized patients with COVID-19 and diabetes had a longer length of stay in the hospital than patients without diabetes (34). Metformin by enhancing the activity of existing insulin and reducing hepatic glucose production exerts its glucose-lowering effect. That's why it does not generally cause hypoglycemia in patients with or without diabetes (27). However, since the effects of host-directed therapy agents such as metformin on the virus itself are limited, we do not expect a reduction in the hospitalization period and the time it takes for the patient to be free of the virus (27). Luo et al. (27) and Chen et al. (26) findings are consistent with this theory. However, it has been proposed that metformin may have an inhibitory effect on the virus, by increasing insulin sensitivity (35).

The next issue is the more effective effects of metformin in women compared to men (25, 36). Also, metformin causes a greater reduction in TNF-α and IL-6 in women (36–38). The article by Mackey et al. suggests that this might be due to a higher secretion of TNF-α from mast cells in response to inflammation in women (39). Moreover, Klein et al. claim that sex hormones and epigenetic changes of the Y chromosome may be responsible for the sex-specific effects of metformin (40). Also, Li et al. proposed that although metformin increases the expression of ACE2 in both sexes equally, the subsequent inflammatory response can be different between men and women, which can also have a relation to the sex-specific benefits of metformin (41). Last, of all, metformin can increase the levels of IL-10, an anti-inflammatory cytokine, in women more than men (42, 43). According to the above, it is proven that Metformin is more beneficial in women with DM and COVID-19 compared to similar men.

The beneficial effects of metformin to reduce the duration of hospitalization, in-hospital death and poor prognosis are controversial. Since the studies performed in these cases are limited, evidence may not be sufficient to confirm or deny the adequacy of metformin in reducing these complications in patients with diabetes suffering from COVID-19.

The current study has been limited with a lack of clinical trials and the number of cohort studies. So we couldn't design a meta-analysis study. Furthermore, only the efficacy of metformin is discussed in our study, and the effects, mechanisms, complications, and interactions of other diabetic and non-diabetic drugs that may use in combination therapy in diabetic patients have not been studied.

CONCLUSIONS

According to the current knowledge, it can be concluded that the use of metformin can have beneficial effects on COVID-19, especially in diabetic patients, while more studies such as retrospective analysis of COVID-19 diabetic cohorts are suggested to be conducted. These beneficial effects of metformin should be considered, especially among female patients. On the other side, in the case of hospitalized patients with severe symptoms of COVID-19 and underlying diseases, the possibility of adverse effects of metformin like lactate acidosis should be taken into account.

AUTHOR CONTRIBUTIONS

MZ, MJN, MM: designed the study. MZ, SAN, MMZ: performed the search, study selection, and data synthesis. MJN, MZ, BH, SAN, MMZ: wrote the first draft of the manuscript. MJN, MM: revised the article. All authors contributed to the article and approved the submitted version.

ACKNOWLEDGMENTS

This study is related to the project NO 1399/62228 From Student Research Committee, Shahid Beheshti University of Medical Sciences, Tehran, Iran. We also appreciate the "Student Research Committee" and "Research & Technology Chancellor" in Shahid Beheshti University of Medical Sciences for their financial support of this study.

REFERENCES

1. Li Q, Guan X, Wu P, Wang X, Zhou L, Tong Y, et al. Early Transmission Dynamics in Wuhan, China, of Novel Coronavirus-Infected Pneumonia. *N Engl J Med* (2020) 382(13):1199–207. doi: 10.1056/NEJMoa2001316
2. Park SE. Epidemiology, virology, and clinical features of severe acute respiratory syndrome -coronavirus-2 (SARS-CoV-2; Coronavirus Disease-19). *Clin Exp Pediatr* (2020) 63(4):119–24. doi: 10.3345/cep.2020.00493
3. (WHO) WHO. *WHO Director-General"s opening remarks at the media briefing on COVID-19 - 11 March 2020.* (2020). Available at: https://www.who.int/dg/speeches/detail/who-director-general-s-opening-remarks-at-the-media-briefing-on-covid-19—11-march-2020.
4. (WHO) WHO. *Coronavirus disease (COVID-2019) situation reports.* (2020). Available at: https://www.who.int/emergencies/diseases/novel-coronavirus-2019/situation-reports/.
5. Sanders JM, Monogue ML, Jodlowski TZ, Cutrell JB. Pharmacologic Treatments for Coronavirus Disease 2019 (COVID-19): A Review. *JAMA* (2020) 323(18):1824–36. doi: 10.1001/jama.2020.6019
6. Beigel JH, Tomashek KM, Dodd LE, Mehta AK, Zingman BS, Kalil AC, et al. Remdesivir for the Treatment of Covid-19 - Final Report. *N Engl J Med* (2020) 383(19):1813–26. doi: 10.1056/NEJMoa2007764
7. Zhou F, Yu T, Du R, Fan G, Liu Y, Liu Z, et al. Clinical course and risk factors for mortality of adult inpatients with COVID-19 in Wuhan, China: a retrospective cohort study. *Lancet* (2020) 395(10229):1054–62. doi: 10.1016/S0140-6736(20)30566-3
8. Guo W, Li M, Dong Y, Zhou H, Zhang Z, Tian C, et al. Diabetes is a risk factor for the progression and prognosis of COVID-19. *Diabetes/Metabol Res Rev* (2020), e3319. doi: 10.1002/dmrr.3319
9. Singh AK, Gupta R, Ghosh A, Misra A. Diabetes in COVID-19: Prevalence, pathophysiology, prognosis and practical considerations. *Diabetes Metab Syndr* (2020) 14(4):303–10. doi: 10.1016/j.dsx.2020.04.004
10. Rao S, Lau A, So HC. Exploring Diseases/Traits and Blood Proteins Causally Related to Expression of ACE2, the Putative Receptor of SARS-CoV-2: A Mendelian Randomization Analysis Highlights Tentative Relevance of Diabetes-Related Traits. *Diabetes Care* (2020) 43(7):1416–26. doi: 10.2337/dc20-0643
11. Maddaloni E, Buzzetti R. Covid-19 and diabetes mellitus: unveiling the interaction of two pandemics. *Diabetes/Metabol Res Rev* (2020), e33213321–e33213321. doi: 10.1002/dmrr.3321
12. Kulcsar KA, Coleman CM, Beck SE, Frieman MB. Comorbid diabetes results in immune dysregulation and enhanced disease severity following MERS-CoV infection. *JCI Insight* (2019) 4:(20). doi: 10.1172/jci.insight.131774
13. Kajiwara C, Kusaka Y, Kimura S, Yamaguchi T, Nanjo Y, Ishii Y, et al. Metformin Mediates Protection against Legionella Pneumonia through Activation of AMPK and Mitochondrial Reactive Oxygen Species. *J Immunol (Baltimore Md 1950)* (2018) 200(2):623–31. doi: 10.4049/jimmunol.1700474
14. Mendy A, Gopal R, Alcorn JF, Forno E. Reduced mortality from lower respiratory tract disease in adult diabetic patients treated with metformin. *Respirology* (2019) 24(7):646–51. doi: 10.1111/resp.13486
15. Moher D, Liberati A, Tetzlaff J, Altman DG, Group P. Preferred reporting items for systematic reviews and meta-analyses: the PRISMA statement. *PloS Med* (2009) 6(7):e1000097. doi: 10.1371/journal.pmed.1000097
16. Dalan R. Metformin, neutrophils and COVID-19 infection. *Diabetes Res Clin Pract* (2020) 164:108230. doi: 10.1016/j.diabres.2020.108230
17. Sharma S, Ray A, Sadasivam B. Metformin in COVID-19: A possible role beyond diabetes. *Diabetes Res Clin Pract* (2020) 164:108183. doi: 10.1016/j.diabres.2020.108183
18. Singh AK, Singh R. Is metformin ahead in the race as a repurposed host-directed therapy for patients with diabetes and COVID-19? *Diabetes Res Clin Pract* (2020) 165:108268. doi: 10.1016/j.diabres.2020.108268
19. EL-Arabey AA, Abdalla M. Metformin and COVID-19: A novel deal of an Old Drug. *J Med Virol* (2020) 92:2293–4. doi: 10.1002/jmv.25958
20. Cure E, Cumhur Cure M. Comment on "Should anti-diabetic medications be reconsidered amid COVID-19 pandemic?" *Diabetes Res Clin Pract* (2020) 164:108184. doi: 10.1016/j.diabres.2020.108184
21. Esam Z. A proposed mechanism for the possible therapeutic potential of Metformin in COVID-19. *Diabetes Res Clin Pract* (2020) 167:108282. doi: 10.1016/j.diabres.2020.108282
22. Kow CS, Hasan SS. Metformin use amid coronavirus disease 2019 pandemic. *J Med Virol* (2020) 92:2401–2. doi: 10.1002/jmv.26090
23. Penlioglou T, Papachristou S, Papanas N. COVID-19 and Diabetes Mellitus: May Old Anti-diabetic Agents Become the New Philosopher's Stone? *Diabetes Ther Res Treat Educ Diabetes Related Disord* (2020) 11(6):1–3. doi: 10.1007/s13300-020-00830-0
24. Ursini F, Ciaffi J, Landini MP, Meliconi R. COVID-19 and diabetes: Is metformin a friend or foe? *Diabetes Res Clin Pract* (2020) 164:108167. doi: 10.1016/j.diabres.2020.108167
25. Bramante C, Ingraham N, Murray T, Marmor S, Hoversten S, Gronski J, et al. Observational Study of Metformin and Risk of Mortality in Patients Hospitalized with Covid-19. *MedRxiv Prepr Server Health Sci* (2020). doi: 10.1101/2020.06.19.20135095
26. Chen Y, Yang D, Cheng B, Chen J, Peng A, Yang C, et al. Clinical Characteristics and Outcomes of Patients With Diabetes and COVID-19 in Association With Glucose-Lowering Medication. *Diabetes Care* (2020) 43 (7):1399. doi: 10.2337/dc20-0660
27. Luo P, Qiu L, Liu Y, Liu XL, Zheng JL, Xue HY, et al. Metformin Treatment Was Associated with Decreased Mortality in COVID-19 Patients with Diabetes in a Retrospective Analysis. *Am J Trop Med Hygiene* (2020) 103 (1):69–72. doi: 10.4269/ajtmh.20-0375
28. Bornstein SR, Rubino F, Khunti K, Mingrone G, Hopkins D, Birkenfeld AL, et al. Practical recommendations for the management of diabetes in patients with COVID-19. *Lancet Diabetes Endocrinol* (2020) 8(6):546–50. doi: 10.1016/S2213-8587(20)30152-2
29. Menendez JA. Metformin and SARS-CoV-2: mechanistic lessons on air pollution to weather the cytokine/thrombotic storm in COVID-19. *Aging* (2020) 12(10):8760–5. doi: 10.18632/aging.103347
30. Zumla A, Hui DS, Azhar EI, Memish ZA, Maeurer M. Reducing mortality from 2019-nCoV: host-directed therapies should be an option. *Lancet* (2020) 395(10224):e35–6. doi: 10.1016/S0140-6736(20)30305-6
31. Schuiveling M, Vazirpanah N, Radstake T, Zimmermann M, Broen JCA. Metformin, A New Era for an Old Drug in the Treatment of Immune Mediated Disease? *Curr Drug Targets* (2018) 19(8):945–59. doi: 10.2174/1389450118666170613081730
32. de Jager J, Kooy A, Lehert P, Wulffele MG, van der Kolk J, Bets D, et al. Long term treatment with metformin in patients with type 2 diabetes and risk of vitamin B-12 deficiency: randomised placebo controlled trial. *BMJ* (2010) 340: c2181. doi: 10.1136/bmj.c2181

33. Tamura J, Kubota K, Murakami H, Sawamura M, Matsushima T, Tamura T, et al. Immunomodulation by vitamin B12: augmentation of CD8+ T lymphocytes and natural killer (NK) cell activity in vitamin B12-deficient patients by methyl-B12 treatment. *Clin Exp Immunol* (1999) 116(1):28–32. doi: 10.1046/j.1365-2249.1999.00870.x
34. Al-Salameh A, Lanoix JP, Bennis Y, Andrejak C, Brochot E, Deschasse G, et al. Characteristics and outcomes of COVID-19 in hospitalized patients with and without diabetes. *Diabetes Metab Res Rev* (2020), e3388. doi: 10.1002/dmrr.3388
35. Chen Y, Gu F, Guan JL. Metformin Might Inhibit Virus through Increasing Insulin Sensitivity. *Chin Med J (Engl)* (2018) 131(3):376–7. doi: 10.4103/0366-6999.223856
36. Park JW, Lee JH, Park YH, Park SJ, Cheon JH, Kim WH, et al. Sex-dependent difference in the effect of metformin on colorectal cancer-specific mortality of diabetic colorectal cancer patients. *World J Gastroenterol* (2017) 23(28):5196–205. doi: 10.3748/wjg.v23.i28.5196
37. Kelly B, Tannahill GM, Murphy MP, O'Neill LAJ. Metformin Inhibits the Production of Reactive Oxygen Species from NADH:Ubiquinone Oxidoreductase to Limit Induction of Interleukin-1β (IL-1β) and Boosts Interleukin-10 (IL-10) in Lipopolysaccharide (LPS)-activated Macrophages. *J Biol Chem* (2015) 290(33):20348–59. doi: 10.1074/jbc.M115.662114
38. Matsiukevich D, Piraino G, Lahni P, Hake PW, Wolfe V, O Connor M, et al. Metformin ameliorates gender-and age-dependent hemodynamic instability and myocardial injury in murine hemorrhagic shock. *Biochim Biophys Acta (BBA) Mol Basis Dis* (2017) 1863(10, Part B):2680–91. doi: 10.1016/j.bbadis.2017.05.027
39. Mackey E, Ayyadurai S, Pohl CS, D' Costa S, Li Y, Moeser AJ. Sexual dimorphism in the mast cell transcriptome and the pathophysiological responses to immunological and psychological stress. *Biol Sex Differ* (2016) 7:60–0. doi: 10.1186/s13293-016-0113-7
40. Klein SL, Flanagan KL. Sex differences in immune responses. *Nat Rev Immunol* (2016) 16(10):626–38. doi: 10.1038/nri.2016.90
41. Li M-Y, Li L, Zhang Y, Wang X-S. Expression of the SARS-CoV-2 cell receptor gene ACE2 in a wide variety of human tissues. *Infect Dis Poverty* (2020) 9(1):45. doi: 10.1186/s40249-020-00662-x
42. Berlin DA, Gulick RM, Martinez FJ. Severe Covid-19. *N Engl J Med* (2020) 383 (25):2451–60. doi: 10.1056/NEJMcp2009575
43. Mehta P, McAuley DF, Brown M, Sanchez E, Tattersall RS, Manson JJ. Hlh Across Speciality Collaboration UK (2020) COVID-19: consider cytokine storm syndromes and immunosuppression. *Lancet* (2020) 395(10229):1033–4. doi: 10.1016/S0140-6736(20)30628-0

13

COVID-19 and Diabetes: The Importance of Controlling RAGE

Ernestina M. De Francesco†, Veronica Vella† and Antonino Belfiore**

Department of Clinical and Experimental Medicine, University of Catania, and ARNAS Garibaldi, P.O. Garibaldi-Nesima, Catania, Italy

Keywords: COVID-19, diabetes, RAGE (receptor for advanced glycation end products), HMGB-1 (high mobility group box 1), pneumonia, coagulation disorders

***Correspondence:**
Ernestina M. De Francesco
ernestina.defrancesco@unict.it
Antonino Belfiore
antonino.belfiore@unict.it

†These authors have contributed equally to this work

INTRODUCTION

The recent looming pandemic of Coronavirus disease 2019 (COVID-19) is caused by the novel severe acute respiratory syndrome coronavirus 2 (SARS-CoV-2), which has 80% homology with SARS-CoV-1 and 50% homology with the Middle East respiratory syndrome (MERS) viruses, both pathogens most likely originating from bats (1). While up to 80% of COVID-19 patients experience mild symptoms or remain asymptomatic, ~20% of them develop pneumonia that in nearly one third of cases presents as acute respiratory distress syndrome (ARDS) leading to severe hypoxia and possibly death (1). The risk of ARDS and mortality are increased in the presence of concomitant comorbidities like diabetes mellitus (DM). Herein, we propose that the Receptor for Advanced Glycation End Products (RAGE) and its ligands may play a pivotal role in COVID-19 pneumonia and ARDS, particularly in DM patients. While this paper was in preparation others have hypothesized a role for RAGE axis in COVID-19 pathogenesis and lung inflammation (2–4). In this opinion article, we extend these studies, and propose that targeting RAGE signaling system may hold potential in the clinical management of COVID-19 DM patients.

PATHOGENESIS OF COVID-19 RELATED MORTALITY

In the majority of patients, a finely tuned, and spatio-temporally coordinated response of both local innate and systemic adaptive immunity effectively clears SARS-CoV-2-infection. However, the cytopathic effect of the virus at the level of alveolar cells and vascular endothelium may induce massive pyroptosis, an inflammatory form of cell death linked to caspase 1 dependent activation of proinflammatory cytokines IL-1β and IL-18 by the NLR family pyrin domain containing 3 (NLRP3) inflammasome (5). In a minority of patients, a dysfunctional immune response occurs, leading to ARDS, multiorgan failure, and death, anticipated by the massive release of interleukin-17 (IL17), IL22, IL6, tumor necrosis factor-α (TNF), and other cytokines/chemokines. This so-called cytokine storm is associated with unbalanced immune responses including lymphocytopenia, impaired T cell function and deregulated Th17 cells differentiation, which leads to enhanced recruitment and activity of neutrophils and macrophages (1). In particular, IL6 tends to progressively increase in patients with severe ARDS; these patients may benefit from the treatment with anti-IL6 antibodies, such as Tocilizumab (6). Notably, an important component of ARDS is a lung-centric intravascular coagulopathy, which may evolve to multiorgan dysfunction with impaired microcirculatory function, thrombotic manifestations, and more rarely to disseminated intravascular coagulation (7, 8). Consistently, anticoagulation therapy with low molecular weight heparins (LMWH) is associated with decreased mortality in these patients. However, LMWHs may not be sufficient to revert pulmonary intravascular coagulopathy (7, 8).

On the basis of these observations, an unopposed inflammatory response mediated by hyperactivated immune effectors may play a key pathogenic role in ARDS of COVID-19 patients.

When it comes to unwarranted host immune response of COVID-19, lessons from studying bats are to be learnt. Bats are unique natural hosts for a number of RNA viruses with high pathogenic potential for humans, including SARS-CoV-1, and MERS related coronavirus. Notably, bats' ability to host these pathogens showing minimal or no signs of disease seems to be associated with a peculiar enhancement of innate immunity provided by constitutive expression of IFN-α and IFN-stimulated genes (9). Moreover, bats' extraordinary lifespan and viral tolerance, which seem to have evolved as protective mechanisms against flight-induced metabolic stress, appear to be related to a better overall execution of anti-inflammatory responses. Indeed, after viral infection, bats dampen excessive inflammation associated with the production of IL1β and IL18 by the NLRP3 inflammasome (10). Therefore, the enriched and highly competent innate immunity of bats halts the spread of pathogens and simultaneously freezes inflammatory pathways, thereby permitting a better control of infectious diseases.

Bringing this relevant piece of information back to the current pandemic might be useful to elaborate a therapeutic strategy in order to cope more efficiently with the severe clinical manifestations of COVID-19.

DIABETES MELLITUS AS RISK FACTOR FOR COVID-19 MORTALITY

In COVID-19 patients, the development of severe ARDS is associated with advanced age, hypertension, severe obesity, and DM (1). In particular, a recent metanalysis indicates that DM significantly increases the risk of Intensive Care Unit (ICU) admission (OR: 2.79) as well as mortality (OR: 3.21) (11). The majority of DM patients suffer from Type 2 DM (T2DM) which is typically associated with obesity, insulin resistance, and multiple alterations of both the innate and adaptive immune responses (12, 13). Corroborating the role of dysregulated innate immunity in the progression of T2DM, peripheral blood mononuclear cells from diabetic patients have increased Th17 cytokine production, owing to dysregulated fatty acid oxidation occurring in these patients (14).

Moreover, T2DM patients are affected by chronic low-grade inflammation and endothelial dysfunction characterized by increased vessel permeability, and enhanced thrombotic propensity (15), these inflammatory-driven conditions are persistently supported by chronic hyperglycemia.

In this intricate scenario, RAGE, and its ligands have been involved in weight gain, insulin resistance, poor glycemic control, and inflammation, contributing to T2DM progression. Moreover, this complex signaling system does play a pivotal role in innate immunity, thereby representing one the first barriers against pathogens. However, unrestrained RAGE signaling supports and propagates inflammation thereby triggering tissue damage.

RAGE AND ITS LIGANDS AS KEY REGULATORS OF THE INNATE IMMUNITY AND INFLAMMATION AND THEIR ROLE IN DM

RAGE has been named for its ability to bind advanced glycation end products (AGEs) that are found at increased levels in patients with hyperglycemia and contribute to chronic vascular complications of DM patients (16). In fact, AGEs-mediated RAGE activation is a major trigger of chronic endothelial dysfunction characterized by vascular hyper-permeability, increased of leucocytes adhesion, extravasation, and consequent acquisition of procoagulant status (17).

Moreover, RAGE is a transmembrane pattern recognition receptor (PPR) and a critical component of the innate immune system with the remarkable ability to bind numerous ligands including exogenous pathogen-associated molecular patterns (PAMPs), and danger-associated molecular patterns (DAMPs) released by cells undergoing damage or death (18).

Notably, RAGE is constitutively expressed at high levels only in the lung, at the basal membrane of type 1 alveolar epithelial cells (19), where it may contribute to cell adhesion and morphology that are functional to gas exchange. Its expression in type 2 alveolar epithelial cells is more controversial. In other cells, including endothelial cells, airway smooth muscle cells, vascular smooth muscle cells, neurons, and immune cells, RAGE expression is induced by inflammation and by local expression of RAGE ligands in a feed-forward loop that perpetuates inflammation. In the absence of ligands, RAGE may preassemble in multimeric complexes that are a prerequisite for activation and that are stabilized by ligand binding (20, 21). In DM patients RAGE is upregulated and chronically activated by AGEs (16).

Besides AGEs, RAGE binds also several other ligands (**Figure 1**), among which protein HMGB1 (high mobility group box 1) and S100/calgranulin proteins have been extensively characterized. HMGB1 and S100 share the ability to be passively released from damaged cells and to be actively secreted by immune cells, such as macrophages, natural killer cells, and dendritic cells. Both classes of proteins contribute to the inflammatory response by binding to RAGE and members of the Toll-like Receptors (TLRs) family.

In particular, RAGE activation triggers the NF-κβ-mediated transcription of inflammatory genes, together with the activation of the NRP3 inflammasome. These events may ultimately lead to pyroptosis, which determines the release of further mediators from dying cells and the propagation of the initial damage (10, 22).

RAGE AND LIGANDS IN PNEUMONIA AND ARDS

Direct evidence that RAGE may play a detrimental role in pathogen-induced pneumonia in the context of DM come by recent studies assessing that diabetic mice challenged with Gram-negative bacteria (GNB) show excess mortality from pneumonia (23) that was associated with RAGE mediated

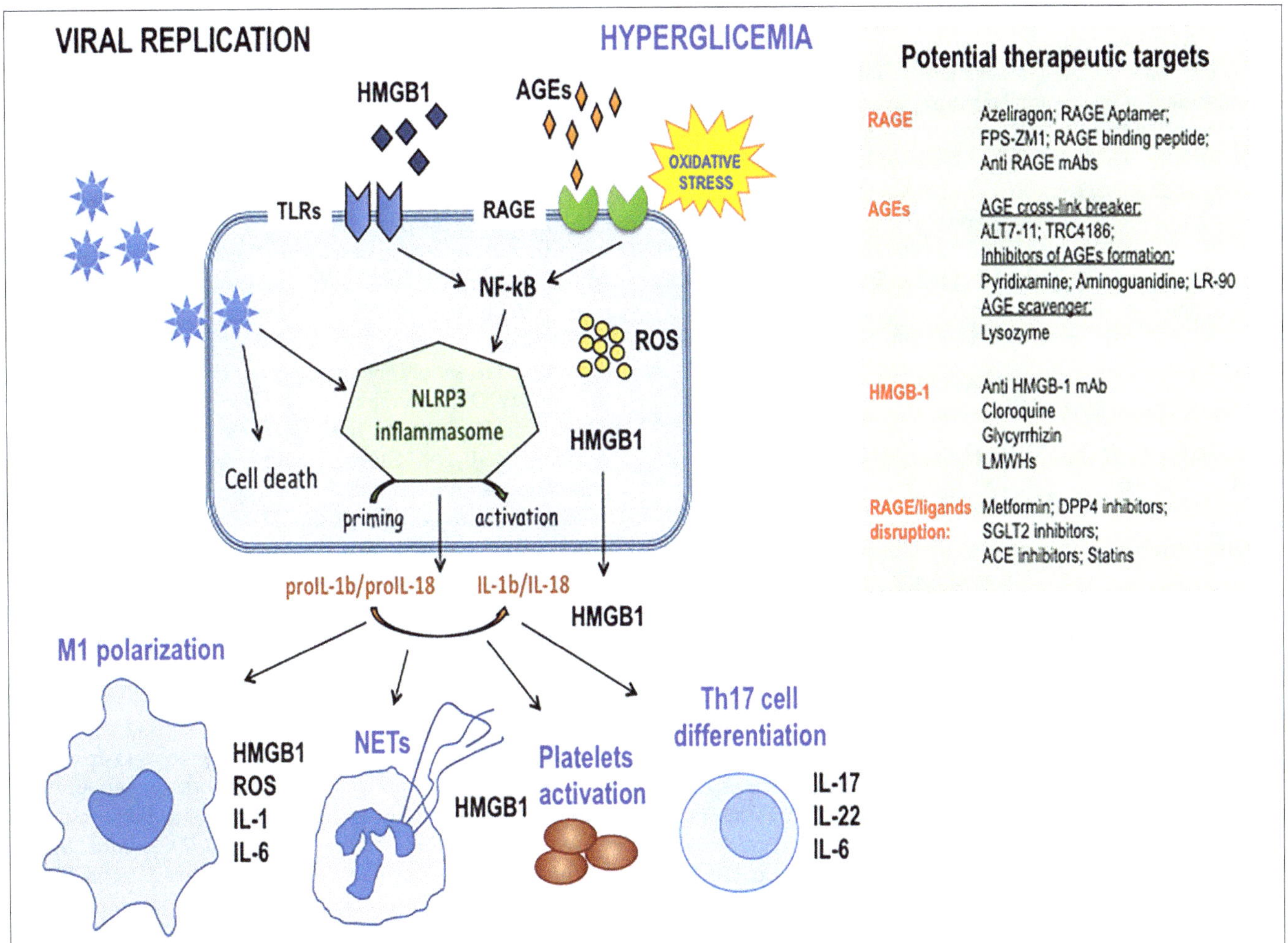

FIGURE 1 | Schematic representation of the activation of RAGE axis in Sars-Cov-2 infected cells in DM patients. Hyperglycemia enhances the production of RAGE ligands that prompt viral replication and increase RAGE signaling activation thus contributing to NRLP3 inflammasome priming and activation. Cytokine production and HMGB1 passive secretion contribute to dysregulated immune cell responses like M1 macrophages polarization, NETs formation, altered Th17 lymphocytes differentiation, thus paving the way for the cytokine storm. The preexisting endothelial dysfunction of DM patients and the ability of HMGB1 to activate platelets contribute to the pathogenesis of lung-centric and eventually multiorgan intravascular coagulopathy. Side panel shows druggable targets of molecular and clinical intervention. Targeting the RAGE pathway may represent a useful and feasible strategy for controlling severe ARDS and coagulopathy, particularly in DM patients. DPP4, Dipeptidyl-peptidase 4; SGLT2, Sodium-Glucose Cotransporter 2; LMWH, Low Molecular Weights Heparins.

hyperinflammation. Accordingly, RAGE blockade improved survival of only diabetic mice during GNB infection (23). Moreover, accumulating evidence suggest that RAGE and its ligands play a significant role also in viral pneumonia and in ARDS.

HMGB1 is also upregulated by hyperglycemia and appears to play a major role in lung inflammation especially in the context of DM. In a mouse model of DM, HMGB1 was found to maintain lung inflammation through the RAGE/AKT1/β-catenin pathway (24). Moreover, HMGB1 is implicated in deregulated differentiation of Th17 cells and, by binding to RAGE, increases the expression of NLRP3 inflammasome components, and of IL1β (25).

In pneumonia and ARDS, HMGB1 is emerging as a biomarker of mortality risk, whereas in child pneumonia HMGB1 permits to discriminate between coinfection (bacterial and viral) vs. single infection. Adding pieces to this puzzle, circulating levels of soluble RAGE (sRAGE, a decoy receptor) positively correlate with ARDS severity and mortality risk, whilst sRAGE drop is associated with disease resolution (18, 19). Therefore, monitoring the levels of sRAGE and ligands may represent an appropriate tool for predictive/prognostic purposes.

Notably, RAGE, HMGB1, and S100 proteins have all been involved in coagulation disorders. In particular, HMGB1 directly stimulates platelets through TLR4, and RAGE, while S100 proteins released from neutrophils and platelets facilitate thrombus formation through RAGE activation (26). In turn, vascular damage induces huge release of HMGB1 from platelets (27). Moreover, HMGB1 and hyperglycemia prime neutrophils for the formation of NETs (Neutrophil Extracellular Traps), complex webs of chromatin and antimicrobial proteins released by neutrophils in an attempt to contain infections (28).

However, unrestrained NETs release, which may especially occur in COVID-19 patients receiving mechanical ventilation (29), may contribute to the propagation of inflammation and the establishment of microvascular thrombosis (30). Reinforcing this self-perpetuating loop, NETs themselves may act as a source of HMGB1 (31), which enhances also vascular permeability (32). Of note, endothelial cells (EC) are a direct target of SARS-CoV-2 infection that induces a widespread endotheliitis characterized by acute ECs dysfunction/death and vascular leakage (33). Together, these observations suggest that chronic EC dysfunction of DM patients predispose to further EC damage by SARS-CoV-2 infection (34) and that RAGE is an important molecular hub in this context.

POSSIBLE ROLE OF RAGE IN SARS-COV-2 CELL ENTRY

Finally, there are evidence that, besides binding to the main receptor ACE2 (35), SARS-CoV-2 spike protein may bind also to CD147 glycoprotein (36), a multiligand protein that is upregulated by hyperglycemia and by RAGE activation (37). CD147 is highly expressed in type II pneumocytes and in a wide range of other cells, including immune cells, endothelial cells, and platelets. Interestingly, CD147 is involved in hyaluronan production, which has a key role in COVID-19 pneumonia and elicits pro-inflammatory and pro-thrombotic actions (38). AGEs—induced CD147 glycosylation in endothelial cells may increase the activity of metalloproteinases (MMPs) and loosen tight junctions. These findings raise the intriguing possibility that RAGE activation may play a role also in viral invasion to host cells.

THERAPEUTICAL PERSPECTIVES

These considerations raise important questions concerning the best therapeutic management of COVID-19 DM patients. Recent evidence indicates that a tighter glucose control is associated with a better outcome and reduced mortality (39, 40). Further studies are actually needed to ascertain whether plasma levels of AGEs, sRAGE, HMGB1, and S100 proteins in DM COVID-19 patients are differentially affected by conventional vs. intensive insulin therapy and are predictive of patients' outcome. An encouragement to chase this track more in depth comes from the observation that in non-COVID-19 critically ill hyperglycemic patients admitted at ICU, plasma levels of sRAGE are higher in DM vs. non-DM patients, and reduced by intensive insulin therapy only in DM patients (41). In a similar series of patients, sRAGE levels were associated with circulatory and kidney failure and a higher rate of mortality but were not affected by insulin therapy (42).

Targeting RAGE axis to get a better control of COVID-19-related inflammation has been very recently proposed by independent investigators (2–4). We suggest that COVID-19 DM patients could be the subset most likely to get the highest therapeutic advantage from these strategies.

In this context, several pharmacological approaches are immediately available for controlling aberrant RAGE activation (**Figure 1**), although none of them has been purposely evaluated in patients with COVID-19 pneumonia and ARDS, with or without DM.

The small molecule azeliragon is an orally bioavailable and overall well-tolerated RAGE inhibitor that prevents the interactions with ligands. Additional FDA-approved drugs are known to disrupt RAGE signaling (**Figure 1**), thus suggesting that a drug repositioning effort could provide a fast track for controlling at least some of the negative outcomes associated with severe ARDS.

However, it should be noted that chloroquine, currently used in COVID-19 therapy, inhibits HMGB1 release especially in DM patients (43). In this last clinical setting, interfering with the HMGB-1/RAGE axis could serve as a further tool in combination strategies with IL-6 receptor mAbs, as HMGB-1/RAGE interaction contributes to IL6 expression (44).

Moreover, LMWHs, such as 2-O,3-O-desulfated heparin (ODSH), are able to inhibit interaction of RAGE with HMGB1 and S100 calgranulins (45). Enoxaparin may also elicit similar effects on HMGB1 (46). Accordingly, in experimental models the use of neutralizing anti-HMGB1 monoclonal antibody confers protection against lung injury and pneumonia, including pneumonia from influenza virus (47).

Additionally, thrombomodulin (TM) a protein expressed by the vascular endothelium that interacts with various proteins and inhibits coagulation and inflammation, has been shown to bind and block HMGB1 binding to RAGE (48). Administration of soluble recombinant TM (srTM) has shown some benefit in a mouse model of surgical ARDS via suppression of HMGB1 (49). In humans, administration of srTM significantly reduced 28-day mortality in patients with sepsis-associated coagulopathy (50).

Recently, human recombinant soluble (s)ACE2 has been shown to inhibit the early stages of SARS-CoV-2 infections (51). As ACE2 has a protective role in lung injury (52, 53) and it may downregulate HMGB1 (54), the use of sACE2 might be beneficial also at later stages of COVID-19.

DISCUSSION

Several mechanisms have been implicated for the increased risk of DM patients to develop severe COVID-19 disease (11). For the first time, we suggest that chronically activated RAGE/RAGE ligands axis, may be an additional and important mechanism. The RAGE system is a critical player in innate immunity and coagulation homeostasis, therefore, there is hope that targeting this system could halt the cytokine storm and the thrombotic manifestations associated with dysregulated immune responses to SARS-CoV-2 infection, especially in DM patients.

AUTHOR CONTRIBUTIONS

All authors collected and discussed the literature, with special participation of AB and VV for clinical aspects of Covid-19 and their relation with diabetes mellitus, of ED for the RAGE system and of AB for ARDS and viral pneumonia. VV and ED prepared the figure. AB wrote the manuscript which was substantially integrated, revised, and approved in its final version by all authors. All Authors contributed to the conceptualization and design of the review.

REFERENCES

1. Guo YR, Qing-Dong C, Hong ZS, Tan YY, Chen SD, Jin HJ, et al. The origin, transmission and clinical therapies on coronavirus disease 2019 (COVID-19) outbreak - an update on the status. *Mil Med Res.* (2020) 7:11. doi: 10.1186/s40779-020-00240-0
2. Kerkeni M, Gharbi J. RAGE receptor: may be a potential inflammatory mediator for SARS-COV-2 infection? *Med Hypotheses.* (2020) 144:109950. doi: 10.1016/j.mehy.2020.109950
3. Rojas A, Gonzalez I, Morales MA. SARS-CoV-2-mediated inflammatory response in lungs: should we look at RAGE? *Inflamm Res.* (2020) 69:641–3. doi: 10.1007/s00011-020-01353-x
4. Andersson U, Ottestad, Tracey KJ. Extracellular HMGB1: a therapeutic target in severe pulmonary inflammation including COVID-19? *Mol Med.* (2020) 26:42. doi: 10.1186/s10020-020-00172-4
5. Tay MZ, Poh CM, Rénia L, MacAry PA, Ng LFP. The trinity of COVID-19: immunity, inflammation and intervention. *Nat Rev Immunol.* (2020) 20:363–74. doi: 10.1038/s41577-020-0311-8
6. Zhang C, Wu Z, Li JW, Zhao H, Wang GQ. The cytokine release syndrome (CRS) of severe COVID-19 and Interleukin-6 receptor (IL-6R) antagonist Tocilizumab may be the key to reduce the mortality. *Int J Antimicrob Agents.* (2020) 55:105954. doi: 10.1016/j.ijantimicag.2020.105954
7. Jabaudon M, Blondonnet R, Roszyk L, Bouvier D, Audard J, Clairefond G, et al. Soluble receptor for advanced glycation end-products predicts impaired alveolar fluid clearance in acute respiratory distress syndrome. *Am J Respir Crit Care Med.* (2015) 192:191–9. doi: 10.1164/rccm.201501-0020OC
8. Tang N, Bai H, Chen X, Gong J, Li D, Sun Z. Anticoagulant treatment is associated with decreased mortality in severe coronavirus disease 2019 patients with coagulopathy. *J Thromb Haemost JTH.* (2020) 40:1094–9. doi: 10.1111/jth.14817
9. Zhou P, Tachedjian M, Wynne JW, Boyd V, Cui J, Smith I, et al. Contraction of the type I IFN locus and unusual constitutive expression of IFN-α in bats. *Proc Natl Acad Sci USA.* (2016) 113:2696–701. doi: 10.1073/pnas.1518240113
10. Ahn M, Anderson DE, Zhang Q, Tan CW, Lim BL, Luko K, et al. Dampened NLRP3-mediated inflammation in bats and implications for a special viral reservoir host. *Nat Microbiol.* (2019) 4:789–99. doi: 10.1038/s41564-019-0371-3
11. Roncon L, Zuin M, Rigatelli G, Zuliani G. Diabetic patients with COVID-19 infection are at higher risk of ICU admission and poor short-term outcome. *J Clin Virol.* (2020) 127:104354. doi: 10.1016/j.jcv.2020.104354
12. Geerlings SE, Hoepelman AI. Immune dysfunction in patients with diabetes mellitus (DM). *FEMS Immunol Med Microbiol.* (1999) 26:259–65. doi: 10.1111/j.1574-695X.1999.tb01397.x
13. Donath MY, Dinarello CA, Mandrup-Poulsen T. Targeting innate immune mediators in type 1 and type 2 diabetes. *Nat Rev Immunol.* (2019) 19:734–46. doi: 10.1038/s41577-019-0213-9
14. Nicholas DA, Proctor EA, Agrawal M, Belkina AC, Van Nostrand SC, Panneerseelan-Bharath L, et al. Fatty acid metabolites combine with reduced β oxidation to activate Th17 inflammation in human type 2 diabetes. *Cell Metab.* (2019) 30:447–61.e5. doi: 10.1016/j.cmet.2019.07.004
15. Di Marco E, Gray SP, Jandeleit-Dahm K. Diabetes alters activation and repression of pro- and anti-inflammatory signaling pathways in the vasculature. *Front Endocrinol.* (2013) 4:68. doi: 10.3389/fendo.2013.00068
16. Hudson BI, Lippman ME. Targeting RAGE signaling in inflammatory disease. *Annu Rev Med.* (2018) 69:349–64. doi: 10.1146/annurev-med-041316-085215
17. Suresh R, Mosser DM. Pattern recognition receptors in innate immunity, host defense, and immunopathology. *Adv Physiol Educ.* (2013) 37:284–91. doi: 10.1152/advan.00058.2013
18. Fehrenbach H, Kasper M, Tschernig T, Shearman MS, Schuh D, Müller M. Receptor for advanced glycation endproducts (RAGE) exhibits highly differential cellular and subcellular localisation in rat and human lung. *Cell Mol Biol.* (1998) 44:1147–57.
19. Sirois CM, Jin T, Miller AL, Bertheloot D, Nakamura H, Horvath GL, et al. RAGE is a nucleic acid receptor that promotes inflammatory responses to DNA. *J Exp Med.* (2013) 210:2447–63. doi: 10.1084/jem.20120201
20. Yatime L, Andersen GR. Structural insights into the oligomerization mode of the human receptor for advanced glycation end-products. *FEBS J.* (2013) 280:6556–68. doi: 10.1111/febs.12556
21. Andersson U, Yang H, Harris H. High-mobility group box 1 protein (HMGB1) operates as an alarmin outside as well as inside cells. *Semin Immunol.* (2018) 38:40–8. doi: 10.1016/j.smim.2018.02.011
22. Nielsen TB, Pantapalangkoor P, Yan J, Luna BM, Dekitani K, Bruhn K, et al. Diabetes exacerbates infection via hyperinflammation by signaling through TLR4 and RAGE. *mBio.* (2017) 8:e00818–17. doi: 10.1128/mBio.00818-17
23. Boteanu RM, Uyy E, Suica VI, Antohe F. High-mobility group box 1 enhances the inflammatory process in diabetic lung. *Arch Biochem Biophys.* (2015) 583:55–64. doi: 10.1016/j.abb.2015.07.020
24. Kim EJ, Park SY, Baek SE, Jang MA, Lee WS, Bae SS, et al. HMGB1 increases IL-1β production in vascular smooth muscle cells via NLRP3 inflammasome. *Front Physiol.* (2018) 9:313. doi: 10.3389/fphys.2018.00313
25. Uchida T, Shirasawa M, Ware LB, Kojima K, Hata Y, Makita K, et al. Receptor for advanced glycation end-products is a marker of type I cell injury in acute lung injury. *Am J Respir Crit Care Med.* (2006) 173:1008–15. doi: 10.1164/rccm.200509-1477OC
26. Wu H, Li R, Pei LG, Wei ZH, Kang LN, Wang L, et al. Emerging role of high mobility group box-1 in thrombosis-related diseases. *Cell Physiol Biochem Int J Exp Cell Physiol Biochem Pharmacol.* (2018) 47:1319–37. doi: 10.1159/000490818
27. Vogel S, Bodenstein R, Chen Q, Feil S, Feil R, Rheinlaender J, et al. Platelet-derived HMGB1 is a critical mediator of thrombosis. *J Clin Invest.* (2015) 125:4638–54. doi: 10.1172/JCI81660
28. Hoste E, Maueröder C, van Hove L, Catrysse L, Vikkula HK, Sze M, et al. Epithelial HMGB1 delays skin wound healing and drives tumor initiation by priming neutrophils for NET formation. *Cell Rep.* (2019) 29:2689–701.e4. doi: 10.1016/j.celrep.2019.10.104
29. Zuo Y, Yalavarthi S, Shi H, Gockman K, Zuo M, Madison JA, et al. Neutrophil extracellular traps in COVID-19. *JCI Insight.* (2020) 5:e138999. doi: 10.1172/jci.insight.138999
30. Hashimoto H, Watanabe M, Inoue N, Hirai N, Haga E, Kinoshita R, et al. Association of IFNG gene methylation in peripheral blood cells with the development and prognosis of autoimmune thyroid diseases. *Cytokine.* (2019) 123:154770. doi: 10.1016/j.cyto.2019.154770
31. *Neutrophil Extracellular Traps Are a Source of Extracellular HMGB1 in Lupus Nephritis: Associations With Clinical and Histopathological Features.* Available online at: https://www.ncbi.nlm.nih.gov/pubmed/?term=31619143 (accessed April 28, 2020).
32. Jeong J, Lee J, Lim J, Cho S, An S, Lee M, et al. Soluble RAGE attenuates AngII-induced endothelial hyperpermeability by disrupting HMGB1-mediated crosstalk between AT1R and RAGE. *Exp Mol Med.* (2019) 51:1–15. doi: 10.1038/s12276-019-0312-5
33. Varga Z, Flammer AJ, Steiger P, Haberecker M, Andermatt R, Zinkernagel AS, et al. Endothelial cell infection and endotheliitis in COVID-19. *Lancet.* (2020) 395:1417–8. doi: 10.1016/S0140-6736(20)30937-5
34. Bermejo-Martin JF, Martín-Fernandez M, López-Mestanza C, Duque P, Almansa R. Shared features of endothelial dysfunction between sepsis and its preceding risk factors (aging and chronic disease). *J Clin Med.* (2018) 7:400. doi: 10.3390/jcm7110400
35. Ziegler CGK, Allon SJ, Nyquist SK, Mbano IM, Miao VN, Tzouanas CN, et al. SARS-CoV-2 receptor ACE2 is an interferon-stimulated gene in human airway epithelial cells and is detected in specific cell subsets across tissues. *Cell.* (2020) 181:1016–035.e19. doi: 10.1016/j.cell.2020.04.035
36. Wang K, Chen W, Zhou YS, Lian JQ, Zhang Z, Du P, et al. SARS-CoV-2 invades host cells via a novel route: CD147-spike protein. *bioRxiv.* (2020). doi: 10.1101/2020.03.14.988345

36. Wang K, Chen W, Zhou YS, Lian JQ, Zhang Z, Du P, et al. SARS-CoV-2 invades host cells via a novel route: CD147-spike protein. *bioRxiv.* (2020). doi: 10.1101/2020.03.14.988345
37. Bao W, Min D, Twigg SM, Shackel NA, Warner FJ, Yue DK, et al. Monocyte CD147 is induced by advanced glycation end products and high glucose concentration: possible role in diabetic complications. *Am J Physiol Cell Physiol.* (2010) 299:C1212–9. doi: 10.1152/ajpcell.00228.2010
38. Heinzmann D, Noethel M, Ungern-Sternberg SV, Mitroulis I, Gawaz M, Chavakis T, et al. CD147 is a novel interaction partner of integrin αMβ2 mediating leukocyte and platelet adhesion. *Biomolecules.* (2020) 10:541. doi: 10.3390/biom10040541
39. Sardu C, D'Onofrio N, Balestrieri ML, Barbieri M, Rizzo MR, Messina V, et al. Diabetes care outcomes in patients with hyperglycemia affected by COVID-19: can we do more on glycemic control? *Diabetes Care.* (2020) 43:1408–15. doi: 10.2337/dc20-0723
40. Zhu L, She ZG, Cheng X, Qin JJ, Zhang XJ, Cai J, et al. Association of blood glucose control and outcomes in patients with COVID-19 and pre-existing type 2 diabetes. *Cell Metab.* (2020) 31:1068–77.e3. doi: 10.1016/j.cmet.2020.04.021
41. Arabi YM, Dehbi M, Rishu AH, Baturcam E, Kahoul SH, Brits RJ, et al. sRAGE in diabetic and non-diabetic critically Ill patients: effects of intensive insulin therapy. *Crit Care.* (2011) 15:R203. doi: 10.1186/cc10420
42. Ingels C, Derese I, Wouters PJ, Van den Berghe G, Vanhorebeek I. Soluble RAGE and the RAGE ligands HMGB1 and S100A12 in critical illness: impact of glycemic control with insulin and relation with clinical outcome. *Shock.* (2015) 43:109–16. doi: 10.1097/SHK.0000000000000278
43. Fang H, Liu A, Dahmen U, Dirsch O. Dual role of chloroquine in liver ischemia reperfusion injury: reduction of liver damage in early phase, but aggravation in late phase. *Cell Death Dis.* (2013) 4:e694. doi: 10.1038/cddis.2013.225
44. Mi L, Zhang Y, Xu Y, Zheng X, Zhang X, Wang Z, et al. HMGB1/RAGE pro-inflammatory axis promotes vascular endothelial cell apoptosis in limb ischemia/reperfusion injury. *Biomed Pharmacother.* (2019) 116:109005. doi: 10.1016/j.biopha.2019.109005
45. Rao NV, Argyle B, Xu X, Reynolds PR, Walenga JM, Prechel M, et al. Low anticoagulant heparin targets multiple sites of inflammation suppresses heparin-induced thrombocytopenia, and inhibits interaction of RAGE with its ligands. *Am J Physiol Cell Physiol.* (2010) 299:C97–110. doi: 10.1152/ajpcell.00009.2010
46. Xie Y, Wang Y, Ding H, Guo M, Wang X, Dong Q, et al. Highly glycosylated CD147 promotes hemorrhagic transformation after rt-PA treatment in diabetes: a novel therapeutic target? *J Neuroinflammation.* (2019) 16:72. doi: 10.1186/s12974-019-1460-1
47. Ding J, Cui X, Liu Q. Emerging role of HMGB1 in lung diseases: friend or foe. *J Cell Mol Med.* (2017) 21:1046–57. doi: 10.1111/jcmm.13048
48. Abeyama K, Stern DM, Ito Y, Kawahara K, Yoshimoto Y, Tanaka M, et al. The N-terminal domain of thrombomodulin sequesters high-mobility group-B1 protein, a novel antiinflammatory mechanism. *J Clin Invest.* (2005) 115:1267–74. doi: 10.1172/JCI22782
49. Takahashi Y, Matsutani N, Dejima H, Nakayama T, Okamura R, Uehara H, et al. Therapeutic potential of recombinant thrombomodulin for lung injury after pneumonectomy via inhibition of high-mobility group box 1 in mice. *J Trauma Acute Care Surg.* (2016) 81:868–75. doi: 10.1097/TA.0000000000001208
50. Valeriani E, Squizzato A, Gallo A, Porreca E, Vincent JL, Iba T, et al. Efficacy and safety of recombinant human soluble thrombomodulin in patients with sepsis-associated coagulopathy: a systematic review and meta-analysis. *J Thromb Haemost JTH.* (2020) doi: 10.1111/jth.14812. [Epub ahead of print].
51. Monteil V, Kwon H, Prado P, Hagelkrüys A, Wimmer RA, Stahl M, et al. Inhibition of SARS-CoV-2 infections in engineered human tissues using clinical-grade soluble human ACE2. *Cell.* (2020) 181:905–13.e7. doi: 10.1016/j.cell.2020.04.004
52. Haga S, Yamamoto N, Nakai-Murakami C, Osawa Y, Tokunaga K, Sata T, et al. Modulation of TNF-alpha-converting enzyme by the spike protein of SARS-CoV and ACE2 induces TNF-alpha production and facilitates viral entry. *Proc Natl Acad Sci USA.* (2008) 105:7809–14. doi: 10.1073/pnas.0711241105
53. Imai Y, Kuba K, Rao S, Huan Y, Guo F, Guan B, et al. Angiotensin-converting enzyme 2 protects from severe acute lung failure. *Nature.* (2005) 436:112–6. doi: 10.1038/nature03712
54. Qi YF, Zhang J, Wang L, Shenoy V, Krause E, Oh SP, et al. Angiotensin-converting enzyme 2 inhibits high-mobility group box 1 and attenuates cardiac dysfunction post-myocardial ischemia. *J Mol Med Berl Ger.* (2016) 94:37–49. doi: 10.1007/s00109-015-1356-1

14

The Urgent Need for Recommending Physical Activity for the Management of Diabetes During and Beyond COVID-19 Outbreak

*Isabela Roque Marçal, Bianca Fernandes, Ariane Aparecida Viana and Emmanuel Gomes Ciolac**

Exercise and Chronic Disease Research Laboratory (ECDR), Department of Physical Education, School of Sciences, Campus Bauru (UNESP), São Paulo State University, Bauru, Brazil

***Correspondence:**
Emmanuel Gomes Ciolac
emmanuel.ciolac@unesp.br

Diabetes is the second most prevalent non-communicable chronic diseases (NCDs) in patients with coronavirus disease 2019 (COVID-19) and is highly associated with increased incidence of disease severity and mortality. Individuals with diabetes and poor glycemic control have an even worse prognosis. Despite of the need/effectiveness of social distancing measures (i.e.: home confinement, quarantine and/or lockdown) during COVID-19 outbreak, preliminary findings showed an increase in negative behaviors during COVID-19 home confinement (i.e.: ~33.5% reduction in physical activity, ~28.6% (~3.10h) increase in sedentary behavior (i.e.: daily sitting, reclining and lying down time), and more unhealthy food consumption and meal pattern), which may have important clinical implications. For example, we estimated that this reduction in physical activity can increase the cases of type 2 diabetes (from ~7.2% to ~9.6%; ~11.1 million cases per year) and all-cause mortality (from ~9.4% to ~12.5%; ~1.7 million deaths per year) worldwide. Few weeks of reduction in physical activity levels result in deleterious effects on several cardiometabolic (i.e.: glycemic control, body composition, inflammatory cytokines, blood pressure, vascular function…) and functional parameters (i.e.: cardiorespiratory/muscle fitness, balance, agility…). In contrast, physical activity and exercise are important tools for preventing and treating diabetes and others NCDs. Home-based exercise programs are useful, safe and effective for the management of diabetes, and could be widely used during COVID-19 outbreak. In this context, there is an urgent need for recommending physical activity/exercise, during and beyond COVID-19 outbreak, for improving the management of diabetes, as well as to prevent the increase in global burden of COVID-19, diabetes and others NCDs.

Keywords: burden of disease, disease severity, exercise, noncommunicable chronic diseases, mortality, pandemic (COVID-19)

KEY POINTS

- Diabetes is highly associated with increased disease severity and mortality of coronavirus disease 2019 (COVID-19), and poor glycemic control have an even worse prognosis.
- Physical inactivity during home confinement may increase global cases of type 2 diabetes (more ~11.1 million cases per year) and all-cause mortality (more ~1.7 million deaths per year), and impairs several cardiometabolic (i.e.: glycemic control, body composition, inflammatory cytokines, blood pressure, vascular function…) and functional parameters (i.e.: cardiorespiratory/muscle fitness, balance, agility…).
- Physical activity and exercise are important tools for preventing and treating diabetes and others noncommunicable chronic diseases (NCDs); home-based exercise programs are a useful, safe, and effective strategy that could be widely used during COVID-19 outbreak.
- There is an urgent need for recommending physical activity/exercise, during and beyond COVID-19 outbreak, for improving the management of diabetes, as well as to prevent the increase of global burden of COVID-19, diabetes and others NCDs.

INTRODUCTION

The pandemic of coronavirus disease 2019 (COVID-19) is an unprecedented public health emergency of global concern that resulted in more than 813.406 deaths worldwide in only 8 months (as of August 24, 2020) (1). Individuals with non-communicable chronic diseases (NCDs) are at high-risk of severe cases and mortality for COVID-19 (2, 3). Diabetes is the second most prevalent NCDs in individuals requiring treatment for COVID-19 (prevalence = 10.0%, 95% confidence interval [CI] 8.0% to 12.0%) and is highly correlated with disease severity (odds ratio [OR] 2.61, 95% CI 1.93 to 3.52) (2). In addition, a recent study showed that COVID-19 patients with diabetes required more medical interventions, and had higher mortality (7.8% *versus* 2.7%, adjusted hazard ratio [HR] = 1.49) and multiple organ injury than those without diabetes (3).

The high contamination and rapid spread capacity of COVID-19 represents a high risk of collapse to health systems, because of the exponential increase demand for healthcare professionals, and semi-intensive and intensive care units for the severe cases (4). The absence of specific preventive or therapeutic medical interventions thus lead the governments to adopt urgent measures to contain the spread of the virus, which included recommendations of social distancing, home confinement, quarantine and/or lockdown. However, despite the effectiveness of these measures for reducing incidence and mortality of COVID-19 (5), they result in negative behaviors that have clinical repercussions for both COVID-19 and global burden of diabetes and others NCDs.

Preliminary findings of an international online survey showed substantial reduction in physical activity levels, increase daily sitting time, and more unhealthy food consumption and meal pattern during COVID-19 home confinement (6). A recent meta-analysis suggested that prolonged TV-viewing time (i.e.: sedentary behavior) was associated with increased risk for type 2 diabetes, cardiovascular disease, and all-cause mortality (7). Sedentary behavior (any waking behavior characterized by an energy expenditure ≤1.5 metabolic equivalents, while in a sitting, reclining or lying posture) has also emerged as a potential risk factor for many chronic conditions and mortality during the last decade (7), and has increased concern during home confinement (8). It is important to note that sedentary behavior is distinct from physical activity levels (9). For example, even with high levels of physical activity, the risk of death associated with high TV-viewing time does not attenuate (7). Furthermore, previous studies have showed that the maintenance of these negative behaviors for few weeks result in deleterious metabolic consequences (impairments in glycemic control, total body fat, abdominal fat, and inflammatory cytokine) that impact management of diabetes and others NCDs (10). In addition, physical inactivity-derived metabolic consequences may have more serious consequences for diabetic individuals during the COVID-19 outbreak, because an adequate glycemic control is associated with a markedly lower mortality rate and disease complications in COVID-19 patients with diabetes (3). Moreover, the potential requirement of cocooning (a more severe form of physical distance measures) or prolonging of home confinement of high risk populations (11), will probably exacerbate the deleterious effects of physical inactivity in individuals with or at risk for diabetes.

However, the recommendation for maintaining adequate levels of physical activity and avoiding sedentary behavior is not always addressed in clinical practice. For example, a recent recommendation for clinical management of diabetes during COVID-19 does not mention the key role of physical activity for maintaining adequate glycemic control and others comorbidities that are highly prevalent in individuals with diabetes (12). Therefore, the present manuscript addresses the consequences of physical inactivity and sedentary behavior during COVID-19 pandemic in individuals with or at risk for diabetes, and the urgent need for recommending physical activity and exercise during and beyond the current outbreak.

DIABETES, GLYCEMIC CONTROL, AND COVID-19 OUTCOMES

Diabetes is one of the leading NCDs that affects nearly 1 in 11 adults worldwide (9.3% of prevalence) (13). It is strongly associated with disabling and life-threatening health complications (e.g., cardiovascular disease, neuropathy, nephropathy), and a poor management of the disease can result in innumerous and serious complications (13). In this context, nearly 4.2 million adults died from diabetes or its complications (equivalent to one death every 8 s) in 2019 (13). Not surprisingly, diabetes is the second most prevalent NCDs in individuals requiring treatment for COVID-19 and is highly correlated with disease severity (2). A meta-analyses with 24 studies (10,948 patients with COVID-19) found that diabetes was present in 10.0% (95% CI 8.0% to 12.0%) of patients with COVID-19, and that it was strongly correlated with risk of disease severity (OR 2.61, 95% CI 1.93 to 3.52) (2). In agreement, another recent meta-analysis founded that COVID-19 patients previously diagnosed with diabetes have increased risk of severe COVID-19 infection (OR: 2.60, 95% CI: 1.96 to 3.45) and mortality (OR 2.03, 95%CI: 1.29 to 3.20) (14). A more recent multicenter study from a cohort of 7,337 confirmed COVID-19 cases enrolling among 19 hospitals found that individuals with type 2 diabetes required more medical interventions, and had higher mortality (7.8% *versus* 2.7%, adjusted HR = 1.49) and multiple organ injury than non-diabetic individuals (3).

The current findings are even more alarming when the level of glycemic control is taking into account (**Figure 1**). For example, the above mentioned cohort also compared COVID-19 outcomes between patients with poorly-controlled diabetes (blood glucose >180 mg/dl) and well-controlled diabetes (blood glucose between 70 and 180 mg/dl) and found that patients with poorly-controlled diabetes have significant higher incidence of poor prognostic markers (higher rates of: lymphopenia, 49.6% *vs.* 30.5%; neutrophil count, 19.4% *vs.* 10.7%; leukocyte count, 12.2% *vs.* 6.3%; C-reactive protein, 59.5% *vs.* 47.5%; procalcitonin, 35% *vs.* 24.2%; D-dimer, 55.4% vs. 35.6%; and oxygen saturation of < 95%, 22.7% *vs.* 12.6%), significant increase in severity (Acute Respiratory Distress Syndrome [ARDS], 21.4% *vs.* 7.1%; acute heart injury, 9.9% *vs.* 1.4%; acute kidney injury, 3.8% *vs.* 0.7%; and septic shock, 4.7% *vs.* 0.0%), and higher mortality rate (well-controlled *vs.* poorly-controlled diabetic adjusted HR for all-cause mortality = 0.13, 95% CI 0.04 to 0.44) (3). In addition, the authors also compared outcomes by matching patients 1:1 for other comorbidities (hypertension, cardio- and cerebrovascular disease and chronic kidney disease), and the increase in severity (ARDS, 14.8% *vs.* 7.2%; acute heart injury, 6.8% *vs.* 1.6%; acute kidney injury, 3.2% *vs.* 0.4%), and higher mortality rate (well-controlled *vs.* poorly-controlled diabetic adjusted HR for all-cause mortality = 0.14, 95% CI 0.03 to 0.60) were maintained despite the adjustment (3).

It is important to note that other comorbidities commonly prevalent in individuals with diabetes (i.e.: hypertension, obesity, cardiovascular disease and dyslipidemia) are also associated with high risk of COVID-19 severity and/or mortality (2, 15, 16). For example, the severe acute respiratory syndrome coronavirus 2 (SARS-CoV-2) penetrates human cells through angiotensin-converting enzyme 2 (ACE2), which is more pronounced in adipose tissue and, consequently, in obese population (17). In this context, it is reasonable to suggest that individuals with diabetes should urgently intensify the metabolic control (12), as well as the management of other comorbidities, as a primary prevention of COVID-19.

PHYSICAL INACTIVITY DURING COVID-19 OUTBREAK AND ITS IMPACT ON GLOBAL BURDEN OF DIABETES AND OTHER NCDs

The absence of specific preventive or therapeutic medical interventions for COVID-19 may require the prolonging of preventive measures (i.e.: social distancing, home confinement and quarantine) by high risk populations, which include individuals with diabetes. In addition, it has been suggested that these high-risk populations should adhere to cocooning (a more severe form of physical distance measures) throughout the COVID-19 outbreak (11). However, although these preventive measures are effective for reducing the incidence and mortality of COVID-19 (5), they may result in negative behaviors that have

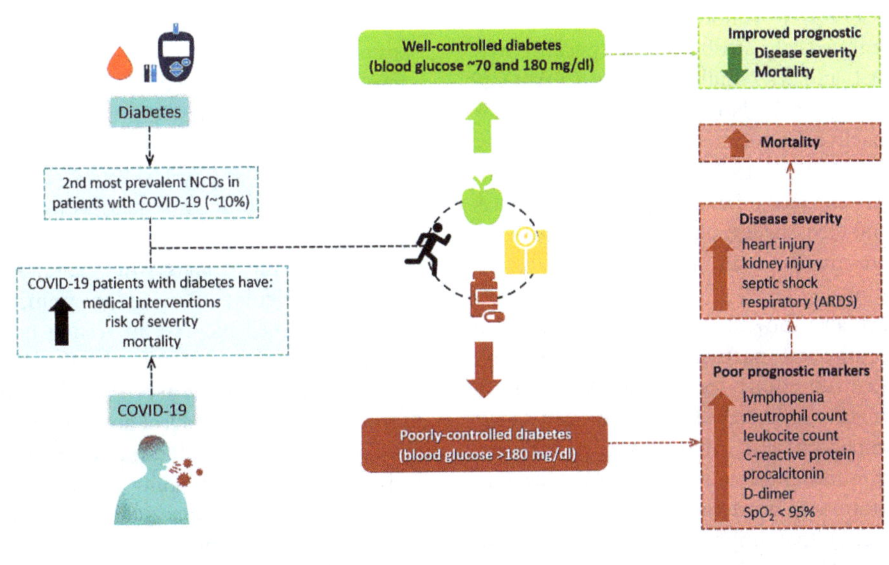

FIGURE 1 | Association between diabetes, glycemic control and COVID-19 severity and mortality.

clinical repercussions for both diabetes and COVID-19 management.

Preliminary results from the ECLB-COVID19 International Online Survey showed substantial reductions in levels of physical activity of all intensities domains (vigorous intensity: ~33.1%, from ~39 to ~26 min/week; moderate intensity: ~33.4%, from ~32 to ~21 min/week; walking: ~34%, from ~37 to ~25 min/week) during COVID-19 home confinement, totaling an average reduction of ~33.5% (from ~108 to ~72 min/week) (6). A ~28.6% (3.10 h) increase in day sitting time (from ~5.31 to ~8.41 h per day), and a more unhealthy food consumption and meal pattern during COVID-19 home confinement (6). Despite of the lack of studies assessing the health impact of these behaviors alterations during the COVID-19 pandemic, it may have important public health implications, which would include an increase of the global burden of diabetes and others NCDs, as well as a poor management of COVID-19 outcomes.

It is estimated that physical inactivity, an activity level insufficient to meet current recommendations (18), is responsible for 7.2% (3.9% to 9.6%) of the cases of type 2 diabetes (~33.3 million cases in 2019) and 9.4% (5.1% to 12.5%) of all-cause mortality (~5.3 million deaths in 2018) worldwide (19). Prior to COVID-19 pandemic, worldwide prevalence of physical inactivity among the population (aged ≥ 40 years) and individuals at risk for type 2 diabetes was estimated to be 42.9% (23.4% to 57.1%) and 43.2% (23.6% to 57.6%), respectively (19). Supposing that the prevalence of physical inactivity during COVID-19 pandemic increased at the same rate as total level of physical activity (~33.5%) (6), the prevalence of physical inactivity is currently 57.3% (31.2% to 76.2%) and 57.7% (31.5% to 76.9%) among the population (aged ≥ 40 years) and individuals at risk for type 2 diabetes, respectively. In this context, by using population attribution factors and the known adjusted relative risk of physical inactivity for type 2 diabetes and all-cause mortality (19), we can estimate that physical inactivity will be responsible for 9.6% (5.3% to 12.8%) of the cases of diabetes and 12.5% (6.8% to 16.7%) of all-cause mortality worldwide during the COVID-19 pandemic. Thus, the cases of type 2 diabetes and all-cause deaths attributed to physical activity would increase by ~11.1 and ~1.7 million during COVID-19 pandemic, respectively (**Figure 2**). Noteworthy, a recent study showed that physical inactive is associated with a greater relative risk for hospitalization for COVID-19, even after adjustment for age, sex, obesity, smoking and alcohol consumption (relative risk 1.32, 95% CI 1.10 to 1.58) (15), suggesting that an increase in the prevalence of physical inactivity may also result in the increase of COVID-19 hospitalizations.

Previous studies have also showed that the maintenance of negative behaviors (i.e.: physical inactivity, sedentary behavior, and unhealthy food consumption) for few weeks result in deleterious effects on metabolic (increases in insulin resistance, total body fat, abdominal fat and inflammatory cytokines), immune function (immunosenescence), and cardiovascular parameters (blood pressure and heart rate increase, endothelial function reduction, etc...) that impact the management of diabetes and others NCDs (10, 20–22). For example, substantial

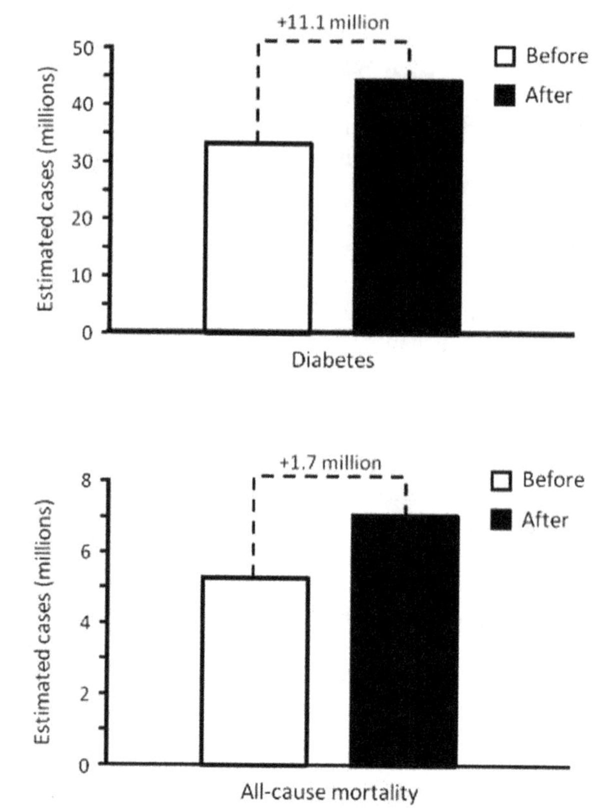

FIGURE 2 | Estimated cases of diabetes and all-cause mortality attributed for physical inactivity, before and after COVID-19 pandemic. Cases were estimated by attribution factors, using the adjusted relative risk of physical inactivity for type 2 diabetes and all-cause mortality (19) and the preliminary findings of physical activity during COVID-19 home confinement (6).

worsening of glycemic control and reduced rate of muscle protein synthesis has occurred in overweight and pre-diabetic older individuals who reduced the daily walking to less than 1,000 steps per day for two weeks (23), which may be easily meet during home confinement. In addition, the impairments in glycemic control and rate of muscle protein synthesis were still present after 2 weeks of resuming to baseline daily walking levels (23).

The reduction of physical activity during home confinement may also have health consequences to individuals with diabetes that are previously active. Studies assessing the effects of exercise detraining in individuals with diabetes that were previously performing regular exercise programs showed innumerous physiological (i.e.: increase in resting heart rate and body fat, dysregulation of insulin and glucose secretion, decrease in the levels of GLUT-4 transporter, loss of training-induced improvements in cholesterol and HbA1C levels) and functional consequences (i.e.: reduction of aerobic, muscle strength, flexibility, balance and agility performance) after short periods of interruption of aerobic and/or resistance exercise programs (24–29). It is important to note that the potential requirement of cocooning (a more severe form of physical distance measures) or prolonging of home confinement of high risk populations (11) will probably exacerbate the above mentioned deleterious effects of physical inactivity, and contribute to negative psychological effects (i.e.: quarantine duration, infection fears, frustration, boredom, inadequate supplies) (30) in individuals with or at risk for diabetes. In this context, the maintenance or increase of physical activity levels, as well as the avoidance of sedentary behavior (**Table 1**), should be emphasized during and beyond COVID-19 pandemic to prevent the severity of COVID-19, as well as to prevent the deleterious effects of physical inactivity on the management of diabetes and others NCDs (**Figure 3**), which may positively impact others syndemics (i.e.: food insecurity, malnutrition and obesity) (31), epidemics (i.e.: obesity) (17) and pandemics (i.e.: sedentary behavior) (32).

PHYSICAL EXERCISE FOR MANAGING DIABETES AND COUNTERACTING DELETERIOUS EFFECTS OF HOME CONFINEMENT DURING COVID-19 OUTBREAK

The benefits of behavioral interventions for promoting metabolic and cardiovascular benefits are well established (33, 34), with the probability that behavioral interventions are 59% more effective than pharmaceutical treatments for reversing of metabolic syndrome components (20, 21). Regarding to prevention and treatment of diabetes, lifestyle interventions are recommended to be based on a well-structured physical activity program (physical

TABLE 1 | Reducing sedentary behavior by WHO guidelines.

	Activity	Description	Action
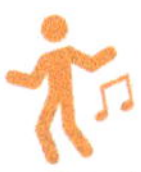	Take short active breaks during the day	Short bouts of physical activity add up to the weekly recommendations;	Dancing, playing with children, and performing domestic chores (i.e.: cleaning and gardening) and other means to stay active at home.
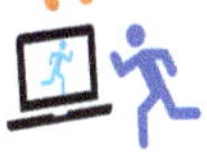	Follow an online exercise class	Take advantage of the wealth of online exercise classes;	Many of these are free and can be found on YouTube. If you have no experience performing these exercises, be cautious and aware of your own limitations.
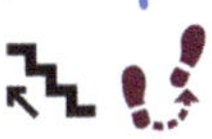	Walk	Walking around or walking on the spot, can help you remain active;	If you have a call, stand, or walk around your home while you speak, instead of sitting down.
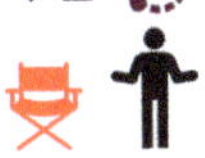	Stand up	Interrupt sitting and reclining time every 30 min;	Reduce your sedentary time by standing up whenever possible. During sedentary leisure time prioritize cognitively stimulating activities (i.e.: reading, board games, and puzzles).
	Relax	Meditation and deep breaths can help you remain calm;	Sit comfortably or legs up the wall. Concentrate on your breath, trying not to focus on any thoughts or concerns. Stay comfortable, relaxing and de-stressing.
	Eat healthily and stay hydrated	Ensure plenty of fruits and vegetables, and limit the intake of salt, sugar and fat. Limit or avoid alcoholic drinks;	Plan your intake. Use fresh ingredients. Be aware of portion sizes. Avoid drinking caffeinated and energy drinks. Drinking water instead of sugar-sweetened beverages.

Available at: https://www.euro.who.int/en/health-topics/health-emergencies/coronavirus-covid-19/technical-guidance/stay-physically-active-during-self-quarantine.

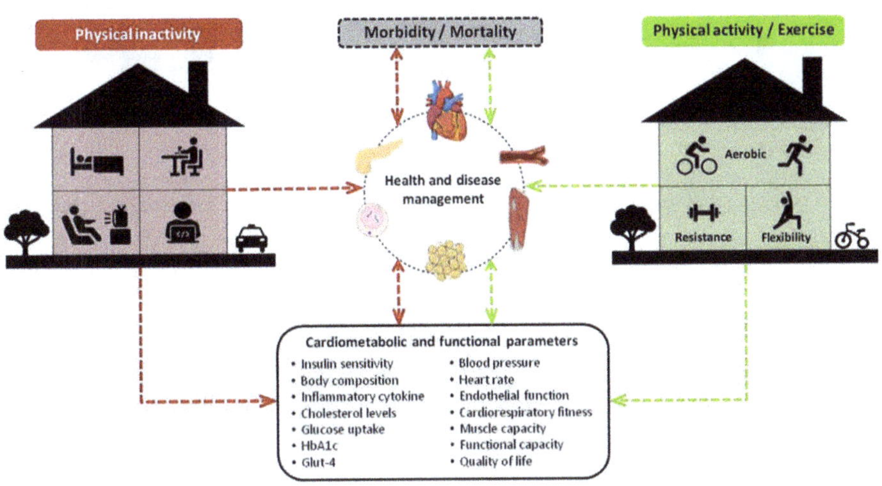

FIGURE 3 | Consequences of physical inactivity (negative effects) and physical active/exercise (positive effects) during home confinement on cardiometabolic and functional parameters, health and disease management, and morbidity/mortality.

exercise) and a healthy nutritional behavior (13), and physical exercise is essential for improving glycemic control, insulin signaling, blood lipids, low-grade inflammation, vascular function, body composition and others health variables (35).

Systematic reviews with meta-analysis have showed that most of above mentioned benefits of physical exercise can be obtained by aerobic and/or resistance exercise programs (25, 36–39). For example, a recent-meta-analysis of 37 studies involving 2208 individuals with diabetes showed that both supervised aerobic or resistance exercise were effective for promoting substantial improvements in HbA1C, total cholesterol and triglycerides; however, only aerobic exercise improved fasting plasma glucose and low-density lipoprotein cholesterol, while only resistance exercise improved systolic blood pressure (37). It is important to note that the benefits of aerobic exercise appears to be associated with its intensity, with high-intensity exercise inducing superior effects in HbA1c, insulin, body weight, body mass index, VO_{2MAX}, lipid profile, C reactive protein, interleukin 6, and systolic blood pressure when compared to low and moderate intensities (25, 36, 38).

In this context, in order to maintain or improve the health condition of individuals with or at risk for diabetes, current guidelines recommends at least 150 min (30 min, 5 d/wk) of moderate-intensity exercise (40-60% VO_{2MAX}) or 75 min (25 min, 3 d/wk) of high-intensity exercise (60-85% of VO_{2MAX}) per week, in association with 2 to 3 sessions per week of resistance exercise (40–43). Flexibility and balance training (i.e.: yoga, tai chi) are also recommended (2-3 d/wk) mainly for older individuals (43). In addition, in order to decrease the daily sedentary behavior, it is also recommended to interrupt prolonged sitting every 30 min (43). Indeed, according with recent findings, the replacement of sedentary behavior with light intensity physical activity (100 to 1951 counts/min) might be beneficial for diabetes risk markers (44). As 10.5 min of light intensity physical activity is equivalent to 1 min of moderate-to-vigorous physical activity, to performing higher volumes of light intensity physical activity is a beneficial alternative to improve cardiometabolic health in individuals who cannot meet the guidelines recommendations due to any reason (45). Finally, these and others recommendations also emphasize the importance of combining aerobic and resistance exercise to optimize improvements on glucose control, HbA1c, blood lipids, body composition, systolic blood pressure and liver and pancreatic function (37, 40, 41, 46, 47).

Despite of the frequency, intensity, time and type (FITT) of exercise recommended for individuals with or at risk for diabetes (40, 41) (**Table 2**), lower frequencies and/or time (duration) of exercise are effective. For example, high-intensity exercise programs with a weekly time commitment 25% to 56% lower than the minimum recommended in current exercise guidelines showed significant improvements in blood glucose, HbA1c, lipid profile (i.e.: total cholesterol, high-density lipoprotein and triglycerides), blood pressure, endurance performance, body composition in individuals type 2 diabetes mellitus (48) or with overweight/obesity and dyslipidemia (49). Only one session of exercise is effective to transiently reduce capillary glycemia, insulin sensitivity, and ambulatory blood pressure in individuals with diabetes (35, 50). In addition, the breaking up of sedentary behavior with very-short bouts of moderate- or high-intensity exercise throughout the day ("exercise snacks") has shown several health-related benefits, including improvements in cardiorespiratory fitness (51), vascular function (52), glycemic control (53) and muscle function (54), being suggested as an effective strategy to prevent some deleterious effects of sedentary behavior and unhealthy food consumption (52). Indeed, the benefits of exercise snacks were reached by simple exercises using body weight (e.g.: stair climbing, sit-to-stand from a

TABLE 2 | Minimal exercise frequency, intensity, time, and type recommendations for individuals at risk or with type 2 diabetes.

Modality	Frequency	Intensity	Time	Type
Aerobic	At least 3 d/wk	Moderate: 40% to 59% of HR reserve, 12 to 13 in the 6-20 RPE, 3 to 4 in the CR-10 or comfortable conversation possible (Talk Test) Vigorous: 60% to 89% of HR reserve, 14 to 17 in the 6-20 RPE, 5 to 7 in the CR-10 or comfortable conversation not likely possible (Talk Test)	25 to 60 min/d (at least 150 min/wk of moderate intensity or 75 min/wk of vigorous intensity) in bouts of 10 min or more	Continuous activities using major muscle groups (e.g.: walking, jogging, running, cycling, dancing, climbing stairs, jumping jacks, skipping rope...)
Resistance	At least 2-3 d/wk	Moderate to vigorous intensity: 60%-80% 1-RM, 14 to 17 in the 6-20 RPE or 5 to 7 in the CR-10	No specific duration. 1 to 4 sets of 8 to 15 reps, with 1 to 2 min of interval between sets, and performed in 6 to 10 exercises (1 exercise for each major muscle groups)	Resistance based-activities (e.g.: weight lifting exercises, body-weighted exercises [squats, push-ups, sit-ups, abdominal crunch]...)
Balance*	2-3 d/wk	No specific intensity	No specific duration	Activities that progressively reduce the base of support, perturb the center of gravity, stress postural muscle groups, and/or reduce sensory input (e.g.: tai chi chuan, two-legged stand, semitandem stand, tandem stand, one-legged stand, tandem walk, circle turns, heel stands, toe stands, standing with eyes closed...)
Flexibility*	2-3 d/wk	Moderate: 13 to 15 in the 6-20 RPE scale or 5 to 6 in the CR-10	No specific duration. All major muscle groups should be stressed	Activities that maintain or increase flexibility (e.g.: yoga, sustained stretches)

*6-20 RPE: 6 to 20 rating of perceived exertion scale; CR-10: category ratio scale. *Balance and flexibility are recommended only for older individuals (age > 65 years).*

TABLE 3 | Overview of studies assessing the effects of home-based exercise programs in individuals with diabetes.

Study/population	Home-based and comparator groups (N/age)/Follow-up	Orientation, monitoring and follow-up	Tools and measurements during home-based intervention	Home-based exercise programs	Home-based exercise improvements
Collins et al. (53) /T2DM+PAD	Home-based: 37/35 (M/F)/66 ± 10 yr Control: 53/20 (M/F)/67 ± 10 yr Follow-up: 6 months	Orientation: 7-min educational video/ orientation on self-management behaviors/ instructional audiotape Monitoring: phone calls (biweekly for 6 months)	Tools: pedometers and questionnaire Measurements: diary (daily glucose, lipid, weekly blood pressures)	Frequency: 4-5 d/wk Intensity: not reported Time: 50 min/session Type: aerobic (walking)	Walking speed; and quality of life
Dadgostar et al. (41) /T2DM	Home-based: 36 (F)/49 ± 6 yr Supervised exercise: 38 (F)/ 50± 5 yr Follow-up: 3 months	Orientation: general information on diabetes, self-care, diet, and exercise (90min) + educational booklet Monitoring: clinical visit (baseline, week 6 and week 12) + phone calls (biweekly for 6 weeks)	Tools: pedometers, elastic bands and activity log Measurements: not reported	Frequency: 3-5 d/wk Intensity: moderate (gradual progress from 2,500-30,00 to 10,000–12,000 steps per day) Time: not reported Type: aerobic (walking) and resistance (elastic bands)	Glycemic control; body composition; lipid profile; and health-related quality of life
Guelfi et al. (50) /Gestational DM	Home-based: 85 (F)/34 ± 4 yr Control: 87 (F)/34 ± 4 yr Follow-up: 3 months	Orientation: not reported Monitoring: supervision by an exercise physiologist at participants' home (3 times-a-week)	Tools: HR monitor and RPE scale Measurements: diary (daily nutritional intake)	Frequency: 3 d/week Intensity: moderate (65-75% HR_{MAX}) with intervals of high (75-85% HR_{MAX}) Time: 20-60 min/session (progressive) Type: aerobic (cycle ergometer)	Cardiorespiratory fitness; exercise automaticity; and general psychological distress
Halse et al. (43) Gestational DM	Home-based: 20 (F)/29 ± 1 yr Control: 20 (F)/29 ± 1 yr Follow-up: 8 months	Orientation: counseling by a diabetes educator and dietician Monitoring: home visit	Tools: exercise diary and RPE scale Measurements: capillary glucose, food diary and questionnaires	Frequency: 5 d/wk Intensity: progressive - moderate- (65-75% HR_{MAX}) to high-intensity interval (75-85% HR_{MAX}) Time: 25 to 45 min/session (progressive) Type: aerobic (cycle ergometer)	Postprandial glycemic control; and post-exercise capillary glucose
Karjalainen et al. (55) /T2DM+CAD	Home-based T2DM+CAD: 32/7 (M/F)/62 ± 5 yr Home-based CAD:???? (32/ 12 (M/F)/62 ± 5 yr Follow-up: 6 months	Orientation: not reported Monitoring: contacted by a sports medicine specialist or physiotherapist (1 and 3 months)	Tools: accelerometer, HR monitor and exercise diary Measurements: daily diary	Frequency: 5 d/wk Intensity: 50-70% $HR_{RESERVE}$ (progressive) Time: 60 min/session Type: aerobic and resistance training	Cardiorespiratory fitness; and daily levels of high-intensity activity
Krousel-Wood et al. (46) /T2DM	Home-based: 37 (not reported)/57 ± 10 yr Control: 39 (not reported)/57 ± 10 yr Follow-up: 3 months	Orientation: education program on diabetes self-management (5 sessions, 2.5h) Monitoring: clinic visit (1 per month up to 3rd month)	Tools: videotape exercise and activity logs Measurements: questionnaires	Frequency: 5 d/w Intensity: low- to moderate-intensity (3-6 METs) Time: 30 min/session Type: aerobic and resistance	Body mass index; and quality of life
Lee et al. (44) /T2DM	Home-based steps group: 19/21 (M/F)/54 ± 10 yr Home-based aerobic group: 21/19 (M/F)/56 ± 8 yr Control: 18/22 (M/F)/56 ± 9 yr Follow-up: 3 months	Orientation: a nurse-oriented session on how to correctly perform the program Monitoring: phone calls (weekly)	Tools: pedometer (steps group) or portable oximeter and RPE scale (aerobic group) Measurements: not reported	Frequency: 5 d/wk Intensity: moderate (13-15 RPE) or not reported (steps group) Time: 10,000 steps/day (steps group) or 30 min/session (aerobic group) Type: aerobic (steps group: walking; aerobic group: brisk walking, jogging and/ or bicycling)	Glucose metabolism; and pancreatic beta cell function (greater improvements in the steps group)
Marios et al. (49)/ T2DM	Tele-monitored home-based: 10/5 (M/F)/60 ± 9 yr Non-monitored home-based (control): 4/9 (M/F)/65 ± 8 yr	Orientation: not reported Monitoring: phone calls (weekly)	Tools: HR monitor Measurements: exercise training diary	Frequency: not reported Intensity: not reported Time: 180 min per week Type: aerobic (walking program)	Cardiorespiratory fitness; and exercise tolerance

(Continued)

TABLE 3 | Continued

Study/population	Home-based and comparator groups (N/age)/Follow-up	Orientation, monitoring and follow-up	Tools and measurements during home-based intervention	Home-based exercise programs	Home-based exercise improvements
	Follow-up: 6 months				
Olse et al. (45)/ T2DM	Home-based T2DM: 9 (M)/60 ± 2 yr Home-based healthy control: 8 (M)/56 ± 1 yr Follow-up: 2 months	Orientation: not reported Orientation: regular phone calls	Tools: HR monitor Measurements: exercise training diary	Frequency: 3-4 d/wk Intensity: 65-70% VO_{2PEAK} Time: 30 min/session Type: aerobic (rowing ergometer)	Submaximal aerobic capacity; and insulin-mediated glucose extraction and clearance
Plotnikoff et al. (42) /T2DM	Home-based: 8/19 (M/F)/55 ± 12 yr Control: 8/13 (M/F)/54 ± 12 yr Follow-up: 4 months	Orientation: one week of learning and practicing of each exercise by supervision of an exercise specialist Monitoring: home visits (18 of 48 sessions) + clinical visits (week 2 and 10)	Tools: multigym apparatus and dumbbells Measurements: exercise training logs	Frequency: 3 d/week Intensity: moderate- (50-60% of 1RM) to high-intensity (70-85% of 1RM) - progressive Time: not reported (2-3 sets of 8-12 reps in 8 exercises) Type: resistance	Muscle strength; fasting insulin; HDL cholesterol; social-cognitive variables; and exercise self-efficacy
Scheede-Bergdahl et al. (52) /T2DM	Home-based T2DM: 12 (M)/ 59 ± 2 yr Home-based healthy control: 9 (M)/55 ± 1 yr Follow-up: 2 months	Orientation: not reported Monitoring: not reported	Tools: HR monitor Measurements: training logs	Frequency: 3-4 d/wk Intensity: 65-70% of VO_{2PEAK} Time: 30 min/session Type: aerobic (rowing ergometer)	Submaximal aerobic capacity; and C-reactive protein
Shinji et al. (51) /T2DM	Home-based high-compliance: 40/24 (M/F) 58 ± 10 yr Home-based low-compliance: 21/17 (M/F)/54 ± 10 yr Follow-up: 3/17 months of intervention/incidence of cardiovascular events	Orientation: diabetes education, health counseling and an exercise prescription Monitoring: phone calls	Tools: not reported Measurements: self-reported adherence	Frequency: 4-6 d/wk Intensity: moderate (adjusted to anaerobic threshold) Time: 20-30 min/session Type: aerobic (walking)	Lower incidence of cardiovascular disease
Wu et al. (47) /at risk for T2DM	Home-based: 22/46 (M/F)/54 ± 5 yr Control: 16/51 (M/F)/54 ± 6 yr Follow-up: 9 months	Orientation: educational orientation with a physiotherapist (1.5h), and guided book on proper diet and diabetes prevention Monitoring: phone calls (weekly–biweekly intervals for 3 months, reducing from 3 to 6 months and ending after 6 months)	Tools: exercise video and stepper Measurements: body weight, exercise training logs and questionnaires (physical activity, self-efficacy)	Frequency: 3-5 d/wk Intensity: moderate to vigorous Time: 30 min/session Type: aerobic	Exercise self-efficacy; body mass index; muscle endurance; flexibility; and physical activity levels
Yang et al. (48) /T2DM	Home-based: 274/309 (M/F)/ 58 ± 1 yr Follow-up: 6 months	Orientation: education on diabetes management and healthy lifestyle behaviors Monitoring: supervised session once-a-week	Tools: not reported Measurements: exercise training diary	Frequency: 5 d/wk Intensity: 60-75% of VO_{2PEAK} or $HR_{RESERVE}$ Time: not reported Type: aerobic (walking) and resistance (free weights/elastic bands)	Cardiorespiratory fitness; and body mass index

CAD, coronary artery disease; DM, diabetes mellitus; F, female; HR, heart rate; M, male; PAD, peripheral arterial disease; RPE, rating of perceived exertion; T2DM, type 2 diabetes mellitus.

chair, marching on the spot…). Other options without specific materials include the use of items with light and moderate weights (e.g.: rice bags, battle of water), walking inside the house, dancing or balance exercise, and stepping over obstacles (30). In this context, low frequencies and/or time (duration) of exercise have several health-related benefits and should be encourage for those individuals unable to meet the minimum FITT recommendation.

As part of the necessary social distancing measures during COVID-19 outbreak, the use of public spaces, athletic clubs, gyms and health centers for practicing exercise is not recommended (or permitted), mainly for high-risk populations. Thus, home-based exercise training emerges as the most important potential approach to control, maintain or increase the exercise practice during the COVID-19 pandemic. Further, home-based training has several potential advantages (i.e.: expanded access, individual programs, flexible scheduling, individuals' privacy and, an integration with regular home routine) (55), and has been safe and effective for individuals with diabetes (**Table 3**). Randomized controlled trials assessing the benefits of home-based exercise programs in individuals with diabetes showed positive effects on glycemic control (56–60), lipid profile (56), body composition (61–63), cardiorespiratory fitness (i.e. exercise capacity, maximal oxygen uptake) (62–65) and psychological variables (62, 65). In addition, the adherence to a home-based exercise program was strongly associated with a reduced incidence of CVD among individuals with type 2 diabetes (a 10-fold higher risk among individuals who dropped out when compared with individuals who completed the home-based exercise program) (66).

Moderate-intensity continuous aerobic exercise (3 to 5 times per week), regulated by $VO_{2PEAK}/HR_{RESERVE}$ (58, 60, 63, 65), METs (61) or steps (59), was the most frequent modality in the studies involving home-based training (**Table 2**); however, programs with combined aerobic and resistance exercise (56, 61) or multicomponent exercise (57) were also used. Some studies provided equipment's to control the exercise performed at home, such as heart rate monitor (60, 64), pedometers (56, 59, 61), potable oximeter (59), cycle and home rowing ergometer (65, 67). However, these tools may be expensive, difficult to administer and not suitable for all participants in unsupervised sessions. In this sense, RPE scale, talking test or questionnaires can be a feasible and cost-effectiveness alternative in controlling the sessions (58, 59, 65). In addition, the use of personal glucometers, food intake diary and body weight variables are also alternatives to control the responses of exercise sessions in physiological variables (58, 62, 65). It is important to emphasize that there were no adverse events reported during the follow-up of all home-based exercise program (57–60, 62–69), which can be explained by the fact that most studies provided a first orientation session involving explanations about exercise program and/or a complex diabetes self-management education (56–59, 61–63, 65, 70). Finally, home-based exercise training appears to be more cost-effective than traditional exercise programs performed in centers (71). In this context, despite the absence of social interaction, as well as the lack of studies assessing the effectiveness in individuals with type 1 diabetes or the safety of high-intensity exercise, home-based exercise programs are useful, safe and effective for the management of diabetes, especially during COVID-19 outbreak.

CONCLUSION

Despite of the lack of studies assessing the health impact of the negative behaviors during the COVID-19 pandemic, physical inactivity may have important public health implications, including an increase in global burden of diabetes and other NCDs, as well as impaired COVID-19 management. These deleterious effects of physical inactivity can be exacerbated by the potential requirement of cocooning or prolonging of home confinement of high-risk populations. In contrast, physical activity and exercise are important tools for preventing and treating diabetes and others NCDs. In addition, home-based exercise programs are useful, safe, and effective for the management of diabetes, and could be widely used during COVID-19 outbreak. In this context, there is an urgent need for recommending physical activity/exercise, during and beyond COVID-19 outbreak, for improving the management of diabetes, as well as to prevent the increase in global burden of COVID-19, diabetes and others NCDs.

AUTHORS' CONTRIBUTIONS

IRM, BF, AAV, and EGC conceived, designed, and drafted the manuscript; IRM and EGC prepared figures and tables. IRM and EGC edited and revised the manuscript. All authors contributed to the article and approved the submitted version.

REFERENCES

1. World Health Organization. *Corona- virus disease (COVID-19) outbreak.* Available at: https://www.who.int/westernpacific/emergencies/covid-19 (Accessed May 2, 2020).
2. Liu H, Chen S, Liu M, Nie H, Lu H. Comorbid Chronic Diseases and Acute Organ Injuries Are Strongly Correlated with Disease Severity and Mortality among COVID-19 Patients: A Systemic Review and Meta-Analysis. *Aging Dis* (2020) 2020:1–17. doi: 10.34133/2020/2402961
3. Zhu L, She Z-G, Cheng X, Guo J, Zhang B-H, Li H. Association of Blood Glucose Control and Outcomes in Patients with COVID-19 and Pre-existing Type 2 Diabetes. *Cell Metab* (2020) 31:1068–77. doi: 10.1016/j.cmet.2020.04.021
4. Lazzeri M, Lanza A, Bellini R, Bellofiore A, Cecchetto S, Colombo A, et al. Respiratory physiotherapy in patients with COVID-19 infection in acute setting: A Position Paper of the Italian Association of Respiratory Physiotherapists (ARIR). *Monaldi Arch Chest Dis* (2020) 90:163–8. doi: 10.4081/monaldi.2020.1285
5. Nussbaumer-Streit B, Mayr V, Mayr V, Dobrescu A, Chapman A, Persad E, et al. Quarantine alone or in combination with other public health measures to control COVID-19: a rapid review. *Cochrane Database Syst Rev* (2020) 4: CD013574. doi: 10.1002/14651858.CD013574
6. Ammar A, Brach M, Trabelsi K, Chtourou H, Boukhris O, Masmoudi L, et al. Effects of COVID-19 home confinement on physical activity and eating behaviour Preliminary results of the ECLB-COVID19 international online-survey. *Nutrients* (2020) 12:1583. doi: 10.3390/nu12061583
7. Ekelund U, Steene-Johannessen J, Brown WJ, Fagerland MW, Owen N, Powell KE, et al. Does physical activity attenuate, or even eliminate, the detrimental association of sitting time with mortality? A harmonised meta-analysis of data from more than 1 million men and women. *Lancet* (2016) 388:1302 10. doi: 10.1016/S0140-6736(16)30370-1

8. Ricci F, Izzicupo P, Moscucci F, Sciomer S, Maffei S, Di Baldassarre A, et al. Recommendations for Physical Inactivity and Sedentary Behavior During the Coronavirus Disease (COVID-19) Pandemic. *Front Public Heal* (2020) 8:199. doi: 10.3389/fpubh.2020.00199
9. Copeland JL, Ashe MC, Biddle SJ, Brown WJ, Buman MP, Chastin S, et al. Sedentary time in older adults: A critical review of measurement, associations with health, and interventions. *Br J Sports Med* (2017) 51:1–8. doi: 10.1136/bjsports-2016-097210
10. Martinez-Ferran M, de la Guía-Galipienso F, Sanchis-Gomar F, Pareja-Galeano H. Metabolic Impacts of Confinement during the COVID-19 Pandemic Due to Modified Diet and Physical Activity Habits. *Nutrients* (2020) 12:1549. doi: 10.3390/nu12061549
11. Wang X, Du Z, Huango G, Pasco RF, Spencer FJ, Galvani AP, et al. Cocooning is essential to relaxing social distancing. *Medrxiv* (2020) 2020.05.03.20089920. doi: 10.1101/2020.05.03.20089920
12. Bornstein RS, Rubino F, Khunti K, Mingrone G, Hopkins D, Birkenfeld LA, et al. Practical recommendations for the management of diabetes in patients with COVID-19. *Lancet Diabetes Endocrinol* (2020) 8:546–50. doi: 10.1016/S2213-8587(20)30152-2
13. International Diabetes Federation. *IDF Diabetes Atlas, 9th edn*. Brussels, Belgium (2019). Available at: http://www.idf.org/about-diabetes/facts-figures.
14. Aggarwal G, Lippi G, Lavie CJ, Henry BM, Sanchis-Gomar F. Diabetes Mellitus Association with Coronavirus Disease 2019 (COVID-19) Severity and Mortality: A Pooled Analysis. *J Diabetes* (2020) 12:851–5. doi: 10.1111/1753-0407.13091
15. Hamer M, Kivimäki M, Gale CR, Batty GD. Lifestyle risk factors, inflammatory mechanisms, and COVID-19 hospitalization: A community-based cohort study of 387,109 adults in UK. *Brain Behav Immun* (2020) 87:184–7. doi: 10.1016/j.bbi.2020.05.05
16. Cao X, Yin R, Albrecht H, Fan D, Tan W. Cholesterol: A new game player accelerating endothelial injuries caused by SARS-CoV-2? *Am J Physiol Endocrinol Metab* (2020) 319:E197–202. doi: 10.1152/ajpendo.00255.2020
17. Sanchis-Gomar F, Lavie J, Mehra M, Henry B, Lippi G. Obesity and Outcomes in COVID-19: When an Epidemic and Pandemic Collide. *Mayo Clin Proc* (2020) 95:1445–53. doi: 10.1017/CBO9781107415324.004
18. World Health Organization. *Global recommendations on physical activity for health, 18-64 years old*. Geneva, Switzerland (2011). doi: 10.1080/11026480410034349
19. Lee I-M, Shiroma EJ, Lobelo F, Puska P, Blair SN, Katzmarzyk PT. Impact of Physical Inactivity on the World's Major Non-Communicable Diseases. *Lancet* (2012) 380:219–29. doi: 10.1016/S0140-6736(12)61031-9
20. Guzmán A, Navarro E, Obando L, Pacheco J, Quirós K, Vásquez L, et al. Efectividad de las intervenciones para revertir el diagnóstico del síndrome metabólico: actualización de un metaanálisis de comparación mixta de tratamientos. *Biomédica* (2019) 39:647–62. doi: 10.7705/biomedica.4684
21. Dunkley AJ, Charles K, Gray LJ, Camosso-Stefinovic J, Davies MJ, Khunti K. Effectiveness of interventions for reducing diabetes and cardiovascular disease risk in people with metabolic syndrome: Systematic review and mixed treatment comparison meta-analysis. *Diabetes Obes Metab* (2012) 14:616–25. doi: 10.1111/j.1463-1326.2012.01571.x
22. Laddu DR, Lavie CJ, Phillips SA, Arena R. Physical activity for immunity protection: Inoculating populations with healthy living medicine in preparation for the next pandemic. *Prog Cardiovasc Dis* (2020) S0033-0620(20)30078-5. doi: 10.1016/j.pcad.2020.04.006
23. McGlory C, Von Allmen MT, Stokes T, Morton RW, Hector AJ, Lago BA, et al. Failed recovery of glycemic control and myofibrillar protein synthesis with 2 wk of physical inactivity in overweight, prediabetic older adults. *J Gerontol - Ser A Biol Sci Med Sci* (2018) 73:1070–7. doi: 10.1093/gerona/glx203
24. Liu JX, Zhu L, Li PJ, Li N, Xu YB. Effectiveness of high-intensity interval training on glycemic control and cardiorespiratory fitness in patients with type 2 diabetes: a systematic review and meta-analysis. *Aging Clin Exp Res* (2019) 31:575–93. doi: 10.1007/s40520-018-1012-z
25. Lora-Pozo I, Lucena-Anton D, Salazar A, Galán-Mercant A, Moral-Munoz JA. Anthropometric, cardiopulmonary and metabolic benefits of the high-intensity interval training versus moderate, low-intensity or control for type 2 diabetes: Systematic review and meta-analysis. *Int J Environ Res Public Health* (2019) 16:4524. doi: 10.3390/ijerph16224524
26. Farias TY, Santos-Lozano A, Urra PS, Cristi-Montero C. Efectos del entrenamiento y el desentrenamiento físico sobre la hemoglobina glucosilada, la glucemia y el perfil lipídico en diabéticos tipo II. *Nutr Hosp* (2015) 32:1729–34. doi: 10.3305/nh.2015.32.4.9341
27. Tokmakidis SP, Touvra AM, Douda HT, Smilios I, Kotsa K, Volaklis KA. Training, detraining, and retraining effects on glycemic control and physical fitness in women with type 2 diabetes. *Horm Metab Res* (2014) 46:974–9. doi: 10.1055/s-0034-1390483
28. Park SY, Lee IH. Effects on training and detraining on physical function, control of diabetes and anthropometrics in type 2 diabetes; A randomized controlled trial. *Physiother Theory Pract* (2015) 31:83–8. doi: 10.3109/09593985.2014.958265
29. Prior SJ, Goldberg AP, Ortmeyer HK, Chin ER, Chen D, Blumenthal JB, et al. Increased skeletal muscle capillarization independently enhances insulin sensitivity in older adults after exercise training and detraining. *Diabetes* (2015) 64:3386–95. doi: 10.2337/db14-1771
30. Jiménez-Pavón D, Carbonell-Baeza A, Lavie CJ. Physical exercise as therapy to fight against the mental and physical consequences of COVID-19 quarantine: Special focus in older people. *Prog Cardiovasc Dis* (2020) 63:386–8. doi: 10.1016/j.pcad.2020.03.009
31. Huizar MI, Arena R, Laddu DR. The global food syndemic: The impact of food insecurity, Malnutrition and obesity on the healthspan amid the COVID-19 pandemic. *Prog Cardiovasc Dis* (2020) S0033-0620(20)30139-0. doi: 10.1016/j.pcad.2020.07.002
32. Hall G, Laddu DR, Phillips SA, Lavie CJ, Arena R. A tale of two pandemics: How will COVID-19 and global trends in physical inactivity and sedentary behavior affect one another? *Prog Cardiovasc Dis* (2020) S0033-0620(20)30077-3. doi: 10.1016/j.pcad.2020.04.005
33. Fletcher GF, Landolfo C, Niebauer J, Ozemek C, Arena R, Lavie CJ. Promoting Physical Activity and Exercise: JACC Health Promotion Series. *J Am Coll Cardiol* (2018) 72:1622–39. doi: 10.1016/j.jacc.2018.08.2141
34. Lavie CJ, Ozemek C, Carbone S, Katzmarzyk PT, Blair SN. Sedentary Behavior, Exercise, and Cardiovascular Health. *Circ Res* (2019) 124:799–815. doi: 10.1161/CIRCRESAHA.118.312669
35. Kirwan JP, Sacks J, Nieuwoudt S. The essential role of exercise in the management of type 2 diabetes. *Cleve Clin J Med* (2017) 84:S15–21. doi: 10.3949/ccjm.84.s1.03
36. Batacan RB, Duncan MJ, Dalbo VJ, Tucker PS, Fenning AS. Effects of high-intensity interval training on cardiometabolic health: A systematic review and meta-analysis of intervention studies. *Br J Sports Med* (2017) 51:494–503. doi: 10.1136/bjsports-2015-095841
37. Pan B, Ge L, Xun Yq, Chen YJ, Gao CY, Han X, et al. Exercise training modalities in patients with type 2 diabetes mellitus: A systematic review and network meta-analysis. *Int J Behav Nutr Phys Act* (2018) 15:1–14. doi: 10.1186/s12966-018-0703-3
38. Liu Y, Ye W, Chen Q, Zhang Y, Kuo CH, Korivi M. Resistance exercise intensity is correlated with attenuation of HbA1c and insulin in patients with type 2 diabetes: A systematic review and meta-analysis. *Int J Environ Res Public Health* (2019) 16:140. doi: 10.3390/ijerph16010140
39. Teo SYM, Kanaley JA, Guelfi KJ, Cook SB, Hebert JJ, Forrest MRL, et al. Exercise timing in type 2 diabetes mellitus: A systematic review. *Med Sci Sports Exerc* (2018) 50:2387–97. doi: 10.1249/MSS.0000000000001732
40. Colberg SR, Sigal RJ, Fernhall B, Regensteiner JG, Blissmer BJ, Rubin RR, et al. Exercise and type 2 diabetes: The American College of Sports Medicine and the American Diabetes Association: Joint position statement. *Diabetes Care* (2010) 33:2692–6. doi: 10.2337/dc10-9990
41. Rydén L, Grant PJ, Anker SD, Berne C, Cosentino F, Danchin N, et al. ESC guidelines on diabetes, pre-diabetes, and cardiovascular diseases developed in collaboration with the EASD. *Eur Heart J* (2013) 34:3035–87. doi: 10.1093/eurheartj/eht108
42. Cosentino F, Grant PJ, Aboyans V, Bailey CJ, Ceriello A, Delgado V, et al. ESC Guidelines on diabetes, pre-diabetes, and cardiovascular diseases developed in collaboration with the EASD. *Eur Heart J* (2020) 41:255–323. doi: 10.1093/eurheartj/ehz486
43. American Diabetes Association. 5. Lifestyle management: Standards of Medical Care in Diabetes - 2019. *Diabetes Care* (2019) 42:S46–60. doi: 10.2337/dc19-S005

44. Chastin SFM, Palarea-Albaladejo J, Dontje ML, Skelton DA. Combined effects of time spent in physical activity, sedentary behaviors and sleep on obesity and cardio-metabolic health markers: A novel compositional data analysis approach. *PloS One* (2015) 10:e0139984. doi: 10.1371/journal.pone.0139984
45. McGregor DE, Palarea-Albaladejo J, Dall PM, Stamatakis E, Chastin SFM. Differences in physical activity time-use composition associated with cardiometabolic risks. *Prev Med Rep* (2019) 13:23–9. doi: 10.1016/j.pmedr.2018.11.006
46. Hansen D, Dendale P, Coninx K, Vanhees L, Piepoli MF, Niebauer J, et al. The European Association of Preventive Cardiology Exercise Prescription in Everyday Practice and Rehabilitative Training (EXPERT) tool: A digital training and decision support system for optimized exercise prescription in cardiovascular disease. Concept. *Eur J Prev Cardiol* (2017) 24:1017–31. doi: 10.1177/2047487317702042
47. Hordern MD, Dunstan DW, Prins JB, Baker MK, Singh MAF, Coombes JS. Exercise prescription for patients with type 2 diabetes and pre-diabetes: A position statement from Exercise and Sport Science Australia. *J Sci Med Sport* (2012) 15:25–31. doi: 10.1016/j.jsams.2011.04.005
48. Alvarez C, Ramirez-Campillo R, Martinez-Salazar C, Mancilla R, Flores-Opazo M, Cano-Montoya J, et al. Low-Volume High-Intensity Interval Training as a Therapy for Type 2 Diabetes. *Int J Sport Med* (2016) 37:723–9. doi: 10.1055/s-0042-104935
49. Alvarez C, Ramirez-campillo R, Martinez-salazar C, Castillo A, Gallardo F, Ciolac EG. High-Intensity Interval Training as a Tool for Counteracting Dyslipidemia in Women. *Int J Sport Med* (2018) 39:397–406. doi: 10.1055/s-0044-100387
50. Viana AA, Fernandes B, Alvarez C, Guimarães GV, Ciolac EG. Prescribing high-intensity interval exercise by RPE in individuals with type 2 diabetes: Metabolic and hemodynamic responses. *Appl Physiol Nutr Metab* (2019) 44:348–56. doi: 10.1139/apnm-2018-0371
51. Jenkins EM, Nairn LN, Skelly LE, Little JP, Gibala MJ. Do stair climbing exercise "snacks" improve cardiorespiratory fitness? *Appl Physiol Nutr Metab* (2019) 44:681–4. doi: 10.1139/apnm-2018-0675
52. Cho MJ, Bunsawat K, Kim HJ, Yoon ES, Jae SY. The acute effects of interrupting prolonged sitting with stair climbing on vascular and metabolic function after a high-fat meal. *Eur J Appl Physiol* (2020) 120:829–39. doi: 10.1007/s00421-020-04321-9
53. Francois ME, Baldi JC, Manning PJ, Lucas SJE, Hawley JA, Williams MJA, et al. "Exercise snacks" before meals: A novel strategy to improve glycaemic control in individuals with insulin resistance. *Diabetologia* (2014) 57:1437–45. doi: 10.1007/s00125-014-3244-6
54. Perkin OJ, McGuigan PM, Stokes KA. Exercise Snacking to Improve Muscle Function in Healthy Older Adults: A Pilot Study. *J Aging Res* (2019) 2019:7516939. doi: 10.1155/2019/7516939
55. Thomas RJ, Beatty AL, Beckie TM, Brewer LPC, Brown TM, Forman DE, et al. Home-Based Cardiac Rehabilitation: A Scientific Statement From the American Association of Cardiovascular and Pulmonary Rehabilitation, the American Heart Association, and the American College of Cardiology. *J Am Coll Cardiol* (2019) 74:133–53. doi: 10.1016/j.jacc.2019.03.008
56. Dadgostar H, Firouzinezhad S, Ansari M, Younespour S, Mahmoudpour A, Khamseh ME. Supervised group-exercise therapy versus home-based exercise therapy: Their effects on Quality of Life and cardiovascular risk factors in women with type 2 diabetes. *Diabetes Metab Syndr Clin Res Rev* (2016) 10:S30–6. doi: 10.1016/j.dsx.2016.01.016
57. Plotnikoff RC, Eves N, Jung M, Sigal RJ, Padwal R, Karunamuni N. Multicomponent, home-based resistance training for obese adults with type 2 diabetes: A randomized controlled trial. *Int J Obes* (2010) 34:1733–41. doi: 10.1038/ijo.2010.109
58. Halse RE, Wallman KE, Newnham JP, Guelfi KJ. Home-based exercise training improves capillary glucose profile in women with gestational diabetes. *Med Sci Sports Exerc* (2014) 46:1702–9. doi: 10.1249/MSS.0000000000000302
59. Lee SF, Pei D, Chi MJ, Jeng C. An investigation and comparison of the effectiveness of different exercise programmes in improving glucose metabolism and pancreatic β cell function of type 2 diabetes patients. *Int J Clin Pract* (2015) 69:1159–70. doi: 10.1111/ijcp.12679
60. Olsen DB, Scheede-Bergdahl C, Reving D, Boushel R, Dela F. The effect of rowing on endothelial function and insulin action in healthy controls and in patients with type 2 diabetes. *Scand J Med Sci Sport* (2011) 21:420–30. doi: 10.1111/j.1600-0838.2009.01012.x
61. Krousel-Wood MA, Berger L, Jiang X, Blonde L, Myers L, Webber L. Does home-based exercise improve body mass index in patients with type 2 diabetes?. Results of a feasibility trial. *Diabetes Res Clin Pract* (2008) 79:230–6. doi: 10.1016/j.diabres.2007.08.028
62. Wu YT, Hwang CL, Chen CN, Chuang LM. Home-based exercise for middle-aged Chinese at diabetic risk: A randomized controlled trial. *Prev Med (Baltim)* (2011) 52:337–43. doi: 10.1016/j.ypmed.2011.02.018
63. Yang P, Oh P. Predicting aerobic fitness improvements after participation in a hybrid supervised and home-based exercise program in people with type 2 diabetes. *Can J Diabetes* (2013) 37:388–93. doi: 10.1016/j.jcjd.2013.09.004
64. Marios T, Dalton S, Smart NA. The effect of tele-monitoring on exercise training adherence, functional capacity, quality of life and glycemic control in patients with type II diabetes. *J Sport Sci Med* (2012) 11:51–6.
65. Guelfi KJ, Ong MJ, Crisp NA, Fournier PA, Wallman KE, Grove JR, et al. Regular Exercise to Prevent the Recurrence of Gestational Diabetes Mellitus: A Randomized Controlled Trial. *Obstet Gynecol* (2016) 128:819–27. doi: 10.1097/AOG.0000000000001632
66. Shinji S, Shigeru M, Ryusei U, Mitsuru M, Shigehiro K. Adherence to a home-based exercise program and incidence of cardiovascular disease in type 2 diabetes patients. *Int J Sports Med* (2007) 28:877–9. doi: 10.1055/s-2007-964967
67. Scheede-Bergdahl C, Olsen DB, Reving D, Boushel R, Dela F. Cardiovascular disease markers in type 2 diabetes: The effects of a moderate home-based exercise training programme. *Diabetes Vasc Dis Res* (2009) 6:291–6. doi: 10.1177/1479164109341689
68. Ellingsen Ø, Halle M, Conraads V, Støylen A, Dalen H, Delagardelle C, et al. High-Intensity Interval Training in Patients with Heart Failure with Reduced Ejection Fraction. *Circulation* (2017) 135:839–49. doi: 10.1161/CIRCULATIONAHA.116.022924
69. Karjalainen JJ, Kiviniemi AM, Hautala AJ, Niva J, Lepojärvi S, Mäkikallio TH, et al. Effects of exercise prescription on daily physical activity and maximal exercise capacity in coronary artery disease patients with and without type 2 diabetes. *Clin Physiol Funct Imaging* (2012) 32:445–54. doi: 10.1111/j.1475-097X.2012.01148.x
70. Collins TC, Lunos S, Carlson T, Henderson K, Lightbourne M, Nelson B, et al. Effects of a home-based walking intervention on mobility and quality of life in people with diabetes and peripheral arterial disease: A randomized controlled trial. *Diabetes Care* (2011) 34:2174–9. doi: 10.2337/dc10-2399
71. Kraal JJ, Elske Van Den Akker-Van Marle M, Abu-Hanna A, Stut W, Peek N, Kemps HMC. Clinical and cost-effectiveness of home-based cardiac rehabilitation compared to conventional, centre-based cardiac rehabilitation: Results of the FIT@Home study. *Eur J Prev Cardiol* (2017) 24:1260–73. doi: 10.1177/2047487317710803

15

Type 2 Diabetes Mellitus and COVID-19

Salvatore Corrao [1,2*], _Karen Pinelli_ [1], _Martina Vacca_ [1], _Massimo Raspanti_ [1] and _Christiano Argano_ [1]

[1] Department of Internal Medicine, National Relevance and High Specialization Hospital Trust ARNAS Civico, Di Cristina, Benfratelli, Palermo, Italy, [2] Dipartimento di Promozione della Salute, Materno Infantile, Medicina Interna e Specialistica di Eccellenza "G. D'Alessandro", PROMISE, University of Palermo, Palermo, Italy

*Correspondence:
Salvatore Corrao
s.corrao@tiscali.it;
salvatore.corrao@unipa.it

The pandemic of coronavirus disease (COVID-19), caused by severe acute respiratory syndrome coronavirus 2 (SARS-CoV-2), has involved more than one hundred million individuals, including more than two million deaths. Diabetes represents one of the most prevalent chronic conditions worldwide and significantly increases the risk of hospitalization and death in COVID-19 patients. In this review, we discuss the prevalence, the pathophysiological mechanisms, and the outcomes of COVID-19 infection in people with diabetes. We propose a rationale for using drugs prescribed in patients with diabetes and some pragmatic clinical recommendations to deal with COVID-19 in this kind of patient.

Keywords: COVID-19, SARS-CoV-2, coronavirus, diabetes, chronic conditions, review

INTRODUCTION

In early December 2019, the first pneumonia cases of unknown origin were identified in Wuhan, the capital city of Hubei province. The novel pathogen was an enveloped RNA-beta-coronavirus-2 named Severe Acute Respiratory Syndrome Coronavirus 2 (SARS-CoV-2), with phylogenetic similarity SARS-CoV (1). Initially, the outbreak was reported starting from a zoonotic transmission in live animal and seafood market. It soon became apparent that efficient person-to-person transmission was also occurring (2). The disease has rapidly spread from Wuhan to other areas. By March 11, 2020, the WHO (World Health Organization) declared the pandemic status (3). Globally, up to February 3, 2021, there have been 103.201.340 confirmed cases of COVID-19, including 2.237.636 deaths, reported to COVID-19 Dashboard by the Center for Systems Science and Engineering (CSSE) at Johns Hopkins University.

Considering the rapid spread and high mortality rate of COVID-19, it is necessary to evaluate the possible risk factors affecting the progression of disease in COVID-19 patients (4).

The pandemic has involved millions of persons, and their related chronic conditions could have prognostic and therapeutic implications. One of the essential chronic conditions is, without any doubt, diabetes for its impact on hospitalization, mortality, and economic burden. To date, about half a billion people have diabetes worldwide, and the number will increase by 25% in 2030 and 51% in 2045 (5). The prevalence is estimated to be 9.3% (463 million people), rising to 10.2% by 2030 and 10.9% by 2045 (5). According to various studies, the prevalence of diabetes in COVID-19 patients ranged from 5% to 36%. Considering that diabetes is one of the most important comorbidities in

SARS patients, it is necessary to clarify all the aspects concerning the links between the two conditions to offer the scientific and clinical community those elements useful to face this pandemic in the best possible way. An extensive search of SCOPUS, PubMed, and CENTRAL was performed using the following string "(SARS-Cov-2 OR COVID-19) AND (diabetes OR hyperglycemia)". The hand-searching of principal generalist and infectious disease Journals was carried out as well. This review aimed to summarize the special aspects of COVID-19 infection in people with diabetes and the relation between diabetes and COVID-19 in epidemiology, pathophysiology, prognosis, and therapeutics to provide practical and clinical recommendations approaching diabetic patients during this pandemic.

PREVALENCE OF DIABETES AND ITS CLINICAL SEVERITY IN PATIENTS WITH COVID-19

Emerging data suggest that COVID-19 is common in patients with diabetes, hypertension, and cardiovascular diseases (CVD), even if the prevalence rate changed in different studies and country-wise data (6). The rates of type 2 diabetes in subjects affected by SARS-CoV-2 vary, depending on the median age, the severity of illness, the location of the study population, and the method of testing.

Table 1 shows a synthesis of various studies from an extensive search on bibliographic citation databases (7–16) that explored the prevalence of diabetes according to the type of study, population, sample size, age, sex, and prevalence of diabetes, hypertension, and obesity.

Data show that the prevalence of diabetes and sex differences (with a higher prevalence of men than women), increases according to the increase of median age. A similar trend regarded hypertension. Current evidence indicates that fatality rates are higher in men than in women. A report on April 23, 2020, from the Italian National Institute of Health, shows that of 23.188 deaths from COVID-19 infection in Italy, approximately 70% were in men (17). Besides, our previously published data in elderly inpatients (18, 19) have shown a higher prevalence of diabetes in men than women. This evidence might explain the higher prevalence of diabetes in elderly patients affected by COVID-19. It could justify an exclusively epidemiological association between diabetes and COVID-19 and not the virus's ability to affect diabetic patients specifically.

There are two other aspects to consider: how much does diabetes affect clinical severity? Since its relationship to, how does obesity? Some data might clarify these issues.

Firstly, U.S.A. Centers for Disease Control and Prevention reported data for laboratory-confirmed SARS-CoV-2 infections in the United States from February 12 to March 28, 2020. Data regards 7,162 subjects with completed case information and revealed a prevalence rate for diabetes of 6%, 24%, and 32%, for non-hospitalized, hospitalized but not requiring intensive care unit (I.C.U.) admission vs hospitalized in the I.C.U., respectively (20). In Italy, a diabetes prevalence of 17% was reported in patients admitted to intensive care units for severe COVID-19 (16). Recent data confirmed the findings mentioned above, outlining a diabetes prevalence of 18.3% in English people with severe COVID- 19 requiring critical care treatment (high dependency unit or intensive care unit) (21). Other study showed a significant prevalence of diabetes (30.05% vs 19.57%) in dead patients compared to survivors in ICU wards in Spain (22). Moreover, Du and colleagues reported a prevalence of 35.3% of diabetes in Wuhan's ICU patients (23). In summary, diabetes resulted associated with a dramatic increase in mortality (OR 3.62; 95% CI 2.11–6.2; p<0.0001) and emerged as an independent risk factor even after correcting for age, race, sex, obesity, and hypertension (24).

Secondly, prevalence rates of diabetes (31.8% vs 5.4%) and obesity (39.8% vs 14.5%) were more significant in the hospitalized vs non-hospitalized subgroups, respectively (12). Additionally, a Body Mass Index (B.M.I.) >40 was among the risk factors most predictive of the need for hospitalization (OR 6.2, 95% CI, 4.2-9.3) (12). In addition, obesity represented by B.M.I. has still increased the mortality (obesity class I HR 1.23; obesity

TABLE 1 | Prevalence of type 2 diabetes, hypertension and cardiovascular disease in various studies on COVID-19 patients.

Authors	Type of study	Population	N of patients	Age (median)	Female (%)	Diabetes (%)	H.T.N. (%)	Obesity (%)
Liang W. et al. (7)	Retrospective study	Chinese	1590	NR	42.7	8.2	16.9	NR
Singh et al. (8)	Systematic Review	Chinese	2209	40-57	41.7	11.0	21.0	NR
Yang et al. (9)	Meta-analysis	Chinese	46.248	49.6	43.5	8.0	17.0	NR
Wu Z. et al. (10)	Retrospective study	Chinese	72314	NR	NR	7.3	6.0	NR
Richardson S. et al. (11)	Case Series	North American	5700	63.0	39.7	33.8	56.6	41.7
Petrilli et al. (12)	Cross-sectional analysis	North American	4103	52.0	49.5	15.0	24.0	30.1
Mandeep et al. (13)	Observational multicentric database	North American, European, Asian	8910	49.0	40.0	14.3	26.3	NR
Onder et al. (14)	Retrospective study	Italian	355	79.5	30.0	35.5	NR	NR
COVID-19 Surveillance group (15)	Registry	Italian	481	80.0	29.4	33.9	7.3	NR
Grasselli et al. (16)	Retrospective case-series	Italian	1043	63.0	28.0	17.0	49.0	NR

NR, not reported.

class II HR 1.81) (25). Severe obesity (BMI ≥ 35 kg/m2), increasing age, and male sex are independently associated with mortality and need for intubation and increasing oxygen requirements during hospitalization (26). An analysis of 124 consecutive I.C.U. admissions in a single center in Lille, France from February 27 to April 5, 2020, revealed higher obesity rates and severe obesity among SARS-CoV-2 patients, relative to historical no SARS-CoV-2 controls. In this observational study, the frequency of obesity was 47.5% compared to 25.8% in a control group of I.C.U. individuals with the non-SARS-CoV-2 illness. In subjects affected by obesity, the requirement for intubation and mechanical ventilation was higher (27).

Moreover, obesity increases the risk of hypoventilation syndrome in I.C.U. patients and it can lead to respiratory failure when ARDS is present (28–33). The likely mechanisms that explain these effects are poorly understood, but mechanical and inflammatory factors might contribute. At the same time, we have shown that obesity (especially the visceral type) is associated with low levels of adiponectin, which could be the link to explain the increased cardiovascular risk in patients who present the association between obesity and COVID-19 (34–36). Finally, according to Crouse et al., 74% of diabetic patients were obese, which may have contributed further to the increased risk observed in this population (24). Given the known epidemiological relationship above mentioned, both conditions' coexistence can be considerate a "cumulative" risk factor for disease severity.

DIABETES AS A RISK FACTOR OF WORST OUTCOMES

In general, people with diabetes are at higher risk of developing complications because of infection, particularly viral one. The differences in response are likely the result of the degree of viral load, host immune response, age of the patient, and presence of comorbidities. The higher risk of mortality and complications among people with diabetes was similar in the two other recent coronavirus outbreaks, the SARS and the Middle East respiratory syndrome (MERS) (37). Type 2 diabetes is associated with low-grade chronic inflammation induced by the excessive visceral adipose tissue. This inflammatory condition affects the homeostatic glucose regulation and peripheral insulin sensitivity. Chronic hyperglycemia and inflammation can determine an abnormal and ineffective immune response (37).

Diabetic patients with COVID-19 are at higher risk of being in an excessively hypercoagulable state and uncontrolled inflammation responses, which may contribute to a poorer outcome (38).

In particular, a known history of diabetes and a fasting plasma glucose ≥ 7.0 mmol/l before steroid treatment were independent predictors of death with an increased risk (odds ratio) of 3.0 and 3.3, respectively (39).

In a recent study on 132 patients with type 2 diabetes, a negative linear correlation between SaO2 and HbA1c was found. At the same time, there was a positive linear correlation between serum ferritin, C-Reactive Protein, Fibrinogen, and Erythro-Sedimentation Rate levels and HbA1c, especially with HbA1c ≥ 7.5% (40).

Developing data also suggest that COVID-19 patients with diabetes are more often associated with severe or critical disease with a percentage ranges from 14-32% in different studies (41–45).

Wu et al. (46) reported a hazard ratio (H.R.) of 2.34 (95% CI, 1.35 to 4.05; p=0.002) for the acute respiratory syndrome (ARDS) in a sample of 201 diabetic patients with COVID-19.

However, in their meta-analysis (n=46,248), Yang et al. reported that the odds ratio (OR) of severe COVID-19 was not significantly higher in people with diabetes (OR, 2.07; 95% CI, 0.89 to 4.82), unlike hypertension (OR, 2.36; 95% CI, 1.46 to 3.83) (9).

The lower prevalence of diabetes might explain this finding, and the lower age of the populations studied. Another meta-analysis of 9 studies from China (n=1936) by Chen et al. found a significant association between COVID-19 severity and diabetes (OR, 2.67, 95% CI; 1.91 to 3.74; p<0.01) (47). Curiously, the prevalence of non-survivors was also higher in diabetic subjects with COVID-19 (42, 48, 49). Also, a summary report of 44,672 patients of COVID-19 from the Chinese Center for Disease Control and Prevention reported a case fatality rate (C.F.R.) of 2.3% (1023 deaths among 44,672 confirmed cases). In any case, the C.F.R. was as high as 7.3% in patients with diabetes and 6.0% in hypertension (50).

However, conflicting data exist. Indeed, in univariate analysis of 191 patients with COVID-19, Zhou et al. (48) found that diabetes had an OR of 2.85 (95% CI, 1.35 to 6.05; p<0.001) for in-hospital mortality. Nevertheless, the association of diabetes and mortality was no longer significant after a multivariate regression analysis showing an independent and positive relationship with age, SOFA score, and D-Dimer levels.

In 174 consecutive patients confirmed with COVID-19, data between diabetics and non-diabetics were compared according to signs and symptoms, laboratory findings, and chest computed tomography. Patients with diabetes had no significant differences in gender and age, less fever (59.5% vs 83.2%), more nausea and vomiting (16.7% vs 0%), and higher mortality (16.7% vs 0%) in comparison with patients without diabetes.

The absolute counts of neutrophils and some inflammation-related biomarkers' serum levels are much higher than those without diabetes, such as IL-6, serum ferritin, E.S.R., C.R.P, and D-dimer. Beyond that, the absolute count of lymphocytes, red blood cells, and haemoglobin level was significantly lower in the diabetes group than in the non-diabetes group. It is crucial to outline that the levels of enzymes such as L.D.H., α-hydroxybutyrate-dehydrogenase, A.L.T., and G-GT, indicating the injury of myocardium, kidney, and liver were even higher in patients with diabetes than patients without diabetes. These data provide a clue that the injure of organs was much more severe in the diabetics group than those without diabetes (38).

Finally, even when chest computed tomography (C.T.) imaging of COVID-19 patients with or without diabetes was compared, the latter showed more severe pathological changes than the former. To confirm this, the diabetes group presented higher C.T. imaging scores in comparison with the non-diabetes group (38).

Proposal of Pathogenetic Mechanisms

There are several specific factors and mechanisms by which diabetes predisposes to infections in general and may increase susceptibility or risk and severity of SARS-CoV-2 disease. Potential mechanisms that may enhance the susceptibility for COVID-19 diabetics include the role of hyperglycemia, higher affinity cellular binding, and efficient virus entry, decreased viral clearance, diminished T cell function, increased susceptibility to hyper-inflammation, cytokine storm syndrome, and presence of CVD (51).

THE ROLE OF HYPERGLYCEMIA

The susceptibility to SARS appears to be primarily dependent on the spike's affinity to bind host ACE2 receptors (ACE2r) in target tissues in the initial viral attachment step (52).

ACE2r has been confirmed recently as the SARS-CoV-2 internalization receptor causing COVID- 19, in concert with the host's TMPRSS2 membrane protease that primes the spike S protein of the virus to facilitate its cell entry (53).

A possible explanation for a link between hyperglycemia and ACE2r levels in the severity of COVID- 19 disease could be the potential changes in glycosylation of the ACE2r and glycosylation of the viral spike protein.

Both possibly resulting from uncontrolled hyperglycemia may alter the viral spike protein binding to ACE2r and the degree of the immune response to the virus (54). Elevated glycemia levels can directly increase glucose concentrations in airway secretion (55). According to Brufsky, potentially, in uncontrolled hyperglycemia, high and aberrantly glycosylated ACE2r in the lung, nasal airways, tongue, and oropharynx could also serve as increased SARS-CoV-2 viral binding sites, thus leading to a higher trend to COVID-19 infection and a more severe form of the disease (54). This indicates the presence of stress hyperglycemia (i.e., a temporary increase in blood sugar in patients with A1C <6.5% after acute illness or surgery) (56), which may have a worse outcome in acute illness, compared to a previously diagnosed diabetes. Given that stress hyperglycemia patients have observed similar worse results in the previous meta-analysis, this finding is not unexpected (57, 58). Stress hyperglycemia was one of the poor prognostic factors and had been associated with a significant increase in respiratory failure and death in subjects with SARS (59).

Glycemic control could reduce levels of glycosylated ACE2r target in the lung. In this way, the number of glycosylated viral binding sites decreases, possibly ameliorate inflammation and symptoms of COVID-19 disease (54). ACE2r is expressed not only in type I and II alveolar epithelial cells in the lungs and upper respiratory tract, but also in several other locations like the heart, endothelium, renal tubular epithelium, intestinal epithelium, and pancreas (54).

Within the pancreas, ACE2 expression has been described in acinar cells and within subsets of islet cells. In preclinical studies, gain and loss of ACE2 function reveal physiological and pharmacological roles for ACE2, both dependent and independent of Angiotensin (1-7), which may antagonize the actions of angiotensin II in glucose control and cell function, renal physiology, blood pressure, atherosclerosis and amelioration of experimental diabetes (60, 61).

An acute viral respiratory infection has been linked to the rapid development of transient insulin resistance, both in otherwise healthy euglycemic normal weight or overweight individuals (62).

This link suggested a mechanism of transient hyperglycemia induced by a temporary inflammation of the pancreas' islet cells by SARS-CoV through SARS-CoV binding to the ACE2r present on islet cells, resulting in a transient insulin-dependent diabetes mellitus, which resolved with the resolution of disease (63).

Hyperglycemia may also affect pulmonary function, such that it is exacerbated by influenza virus-induced respiratory dysfunction in patients with diabetes. In animal models of disease, diabetes is associated with numerous structural changes to the lung such as augmented permeability of the vasculature and a collapsed alveolar epithelium (64).

Until a short time ago, whether D.M. was causally linked to ACE2r expression levels in the lung in humans was unknown. Rao et al., by a phenome-wide Mendelian randomization study, explored diseases that may be causally linked to increased ACE2 expression in the lung, showing that diabetes was causally associated with increased lung ACE2 expression (65).

Despite a possible role of TMPRSS2 in the viral pathogenicity, little information is available about the regulation or dysregulation of TMPRSS2 expression or activity by glucose in the context of experimental or clinical diabetes. In patients with diabetes, higher circulating glucose levels will result in a higher percentage of glycated haemoglobin. SARS-CoV-2 surface proteins seem to bind to and potentially impair the heme molecule within red blood cells. In this way, a separation of iron from the molecule to form a porphyrin occurs, determining in red blood cells less oxygen and carbon dioxide carriage, thereby generating cell death and intense inflammation in the lung.

Because patients with diabetes and older people have more glycated haemoglobin, they may be preferentially affected by SARS-CoV-2 binding and dissociation of iron from heme to form porphyrins, and another receptor (CD147 or basigin) might be involved (66).

IMPAIRED T-CELL FUNCTION AND INCREASED SUSCEPTIBILITY TO HYPERINFLAMMATION

The activation of proinflammatory cytokines or chemokines causes infected cells apoptosis or necrosis and triggers inflammatory responses, which leads to the recruitment of inflammatory cells. Through interferon-gamma (I.F.N) production, CD4 T helper (Th1) cells are involved in regulating antigen presentation against intracellular pathogens such as CoV. The recruitment of neutrophils and macrophages is induced by Th17 cells by producing interleukin-17 (IL-17), IL-21, and IL-22 (67).

SARS-CoV-2 increases apoptosis of lymphocytes (CD3, CD4, and CD8 T cells) and infects circulating immune cells leading to lymphocytopenia.

Lower T cell function diminishes the inhibition of innate immune system resulting in the secretion of high amounts of inflammatory cytokines. This phenomenon is called "cytokine storm" (68). Neutrophil chemotaxis, the intracellular killing of microbes, and phagocytosis were inhibited by diabetes. In the beginning, a delay in the activation of Th1 cell-mediated immunity and a late hyper-inflammatory response is often observed in diabetics (69).

In line with this evidence, in patients with COVID-19, the number of CD4+ and CD8+ T cells are low. However, a higher proportion of highly pro-inflammatory Th17 CD4+ T cells, along with elevated cytokine levels was present. It is possible to speculate that patients with D.M. may have weakened anti-viral I.F.N. responses, and the delayed activation of Th1/Th17 may accentuate inflammatory responses (51).

Several cytokines are increased in COVID-19 infection. At baseline, cytokines such as TNF, IL-1, and IL-6 are more active in diabetics and subjects affected by obesity. Therefore, it is believed that SARS-CoV-2 infection may enhance the cytokine response of such patients, thereby exacerbating the cytokine storm that seems to cause multiple organ failure in COVID-19 (33, 70).

The baseline proinflammatory state found in diabetes and obesity may serve to exacerbate this. Diabetes occurs in part because the increase of activated innate immune cells in metabolic tissues leads to the overproduction of inflammatory mediators, especially IL-1β and TNFα, which can promote systemic insulin resistance and β cell damage (9).

THERAPEUTICAL CONSIDERATIONS

Metformin

In preclinical studies, metformin exerts anti-inflammatory action and reduces circulating biomarkers of inflammation in people with T2D (71). However, there is scant information about the immunomodulatory actions of metformin in the context of coronavirus infection. Recent data showed that the use of metformin significantly reduced the odds of dying. People tested positive who were taking metformin had an 11% risk of dying, which was the same as the general COVID-19 population and dramatically lower than 24% mortality of subjects with diabetes not taking metformin. Interestingly, even after correcting for insulin use, age, race, sex, obese status, and hypertension status, the likelihood of death in subjects with T2D taking metformin was significantly lower than those who did not take metformin (OR 0.33; 95% CI 0.13–0.84; p=0.0210) (24).

Anyway, metformin should be used with caution in unstable hospitalized patients and should be discontinued in people with concomitant sepsis or severe impairment of hepatic and renal function (72). If vomiting or poor oral intake occurs, metformin may also be stopped. Due to the level of blood sugar, the dosage of sulfonylureas and insulin may have to be changed (6).

GLP-1R AGONISTS

GLP-1R agonists exert broad anti-inflammatory actions in animals with experimental inflammation and reduce biomarkers of systemic inflammation in human subjects with T2D and people with obesity (73). It is well known that the most severe form of COVID-19 is the Acute Respiratory Distress Syndrome characterized by the highest levels of inflammatory cytokines known as "Cytokine Storm" which hurts alveolar epithelial cells in the lung, inactivates pulmonary surfactant resulting in the formation of the hyaline membrane and lung parenchyma breakdown.

Different preclinical studies showed that GLP-1R agonists attenuate pulmonary inflammation, reduce cytokine production and preserve lung function in mice and rats with experimental lung injury (74, 75) through the stimulation of pulmonary vasodilator like atrial natriuretic peptide and facilitation of surfactant protein A. GLP-1R agonists exert the repression of the proinflammatory cytokine, the stimulation of eNOS/sGC/PKG signaling and cause the inactivation of the NF-κB signaling. In addition, in the LPS-induced acute lung inflammatory injury mouse model, liraglutide attenuates the expression of key inflammasome components, such as thioredoxin-interacting protein (TxNIP) significantly increased after the administration of lipopolysaccharide (L.P.S.) along with cytokines and chemokine genes (73).

These beneficial effects could identify GLP-1-based drugs as fundamental tools for treating COVID-19 patients with or without diabetes. Although GLP-1 safely lowers blood glucose of ventilated patients with critical illness in short term studies, there is still insufficient safety and experience in using GLP-1R agonists in critically ill patients, and it is impossible to make treatment recommendations for the use of these drugs in new coronavirus infection (76).

In our opinion, GLP-1R agonists must not be suspended if previously prescribed. Moreover, further studies need to evaluate the beneficial effect as the first prescription in diabetes patients with COVID- 19.

DIPEPTIDYL PEPTIDASE-4 (DPP4)

Recently, coronavirus's relationship to cellular type-II transmembrane protein DPP4, also known as adenosine deaminase complexing protein 2 or cluster of differentiation 26 (CD26), has generated a great interest. Just as ACE-2 is the receptor for SARS CoV and SARS CoV2, DPP4 acts as the receptor for MERS-CoV. Whether the use of DPP4 inhibitors (DPP4i) can reduce MERS-CoV's viral entry has aroused great interest. In vitro study, sitagliptin, vildagliptin, and saxagliptin did not prevent the coronavirus from entering the cell (74).

Briefly, DPP4i seem to increase inflammation in type 2 diabetes *via* catalytic and noncatalytic mechanisms. It is crucial to outline that the enzymatic activity of DPP4 causes the cleavage and may affect the function of several chemokines, cytokines, and growth factors (37).

However, in patients with type 2 diabetes, the effects of DPP4 inhibition on the immune response is controversial and not completely understood. A meta-analysis showed that DPP4 inhibitor treatment does not increase significantly upper respiratory tract infections. Compared with placebo or active comparator treatment, risks of respiratory infection for DPP4i were all comparable. The initiation of a DPP4 inhibitor was not associated with an increased risk of respiratory tract infections. On the contrary, anti-inflammatory and anti-adipogenic effects have been related to the use of DPP4 inhibitors and GLP-1 receptor analogues (37). In fact, gliptins can preserve endothelial function by their reported anti-inflammatory, anti-oxidant, and potentially protective effects on the vascular system, which are beneficial aspects in the fight against COVID-19 (77).

INSULIN

Insulin exerts anti-inflammatory actions in humans and reduces biomarkers of inflammations in hospitalized individuals with a critical illness. Among available agents for the treatment of acute disease complicated by diabetes, insulin has been the most extensively used agent in human subjects with bacterial or viral infections and in hospitalized critically ill patients. Most hospitalized patients with COVID-19, especially those with respiratory distress, would require insulin.

However, there is little information surrounding the potential benefits or risks of insulin in the context of acute coronavirus infection (75, 76). On the other hand, one should consider the importance of maintaining a reasonable glycemic control in this patient. This statement may be remarkably faithful to the light of recent evidence that showed, in a sample size of fifty-nine patients, that insulin infusion is beneficial for achieving glycemic targets and improving outcomes in patients with COVID-19 (78).

SGLT2-INHIBITORS

Sodium-glucose cotransporter-2 inhibitors (SGLT2i) are demonstrated to have cardiovascular and renal benefits in addition to its anti-diabetic effects (79). Clinical experiments showed that the combined use of SGLT2i and ACEI/ARB significantly increases intrarenal ACE2 expression, which may be closely related to improving cardiac and renal function (80). However, the increased ACE2 may be detrimental to patients infected with the coronavirus infection 2019 (COVID-19), which is found to invades cells *via* the entry receptor of ACE2. Besides, SGLT2i induced natriuretic effect may also increase the risk of acute kidney injury and affect hemodynamic stability during systemic infection (81). SGLT2i have been reported to prevent the release of various proinflammatory cytokines such as IL 6. Besides, SGLT2i lead to an increase in the ACE-2 levels, which leads to greater production of the angiotensin 17, which is a potent vasodilator, anti-oxidant, and anti-fibrotic, which helps in the prevention of acute respiratory distress syndrome (ARDS) and alleviating cytokine storm (82). This may have a putative role in COVID-19 patients with myocarditis and adverse cardiac remodeling. SGLT2i also downregulates the expression of inflammatory genes and reduces oxidative stress, leading to cardiorenal dysfunction's amelioration (83).

A.C.E. INHIBITORS/A.R.B.S

In the absence of further evidence of risk or benefit, the American Heart Association, the American College of Cardiology, and the American Society of Hypertension have recommended that people continue treatment with their usual antihypertensive therapy ACE-inhibitors or ARBs (84). According to a recent study (13), the use of A.C.E. inhibitors in COVID-19 patients, was associated with lower mortality after hospital discharge (no association was found for the use of A.R.B.s). Whether there is an immunosuppressive state, the presence or absence of hyperlipidemia or diabetes mellitus and the race or ethnic group were not independent predictors of death in the hospital.

STATINS

Besides their lipid-lowering activity, statins exert pleiotropic effects on inflammation and oxidative stress, contributing to their beneficial impact on cardiovascular diseases. Statins modulate the immune response at different levels, including immune cell adhesion and migration, antigen presentation, and cytokine production.

Statins also interfere with ACE2 signaling. After initial entry through ACE2, SARS-CoV-2 down-regulates ACE2 expression, possibly facilitating the initial infiltration by innate immunity cells and causing an unopposed angiotensin II accumulation, leading to organ injury.

Furthermore, in COVID-19 infection, statins' lipid-lowering action could treat the hyperlipidemia associated with the use of protease-inhibitor-based antiretroviral and immunosuppressive drugs. The hepatic isoenzyme CYP3A4 metabolizes simvastatin and, to a lesser extent, atorvastatin. Concomitant administration of CYP3A4 inhibitors such as ritonavir and cobicistat, currently used in COVID-19, could increase the risk of muscle and liver toxicity.

Therefore, starting with a lower dose of statin and monitoring creatine kinase and transaminases would be advisable (85).

Moreover, the same problem occurs with azithromycin. The same study above mentioned (13) pointed out the statins as an independent protective factor for survival to hospital discharge.

CLINICAL CONSIDERATION

Data reported in our review support the notion that diabetes should be considered as a risk factor not only for increased susceptibility to infection but also for a rapid progression and bad prognosis of COVID-19. Therefore, according to pathophysiological consideration, people with diabetes should be paid more intensive attention to the importance of glycosylation of both the viral spike protein and ACE2r.

This consideration argues for better glycemic control in patients with hyperglycemia at hospital admission. Pre-diabetes and diabetes are potential mechanisms to slow the spread of COVID-19 and reduce symptoms and improve outcomes. We know that blood glucose control is essential for patients with COVID-19 and those without the disease. Nevertheless, hyperglycemia is still a powerful predictor of the prognosis of hospitalized Covid-19 patients. Besides, Covid-19 patients with hyperglycemia, compared with subjects normoglycemia, showed a higher cumulative incidence of serious diseases. In addition, optimal blood glucose control mediated by insulin infusion can improve the prognosis of hospitalized Covid-19 and hyperglycemic patients (78). Patients with mild infections, and regular oral doses can continue routine hypoglycemic drugs. However, in today's world, with an unprecedented pandemic, the treatment of diabetes presents challenges. In most places, people are confined to "closed areas", exercise opportunities are limited, and they cannot take regular walks and visit gyms or swimming pools. Due to the unpredictability and social nature of the disease, mental stress is also great. Do not move as well as social immobility. Alterations in the daily routine affect dietary intake as well. Stress could lead to inappropriate eating. All these factors may lead to uncontrolled glycemia or worsening status of comorbid diseases (e.g., hypertension) and predispose the patients to complications like other types of infections, hyperosmolar coma, ketoacidosis, and even acute cardiovascular or cerebrovascular events (6).

In this sense, telemedicine could come to assistance. In a Cochrane review, Flodgren and colleagues analyzing 21 randomized controlled trials of 2768 patients with diabetes showed that a significant reduction of HBA1c by -0.31% ($p < 0.001$) was present in patients on telemedicine in comparison with controls (86). In a recent systematic review and meta-analysis which included patients with type 2 diabetes mellitus and type 1 diabetes mellitus Timpel and colleagues showed that there was a mean reduction in HbA1c levels in type 1 (-0.12 to -0.86%) and type 2 diabetes patients (-0.01% to -1.13%) included in the telemedicine intervention group (87).

According to this view, it is possible to summarize measures for good health in patients with diabetes:

- Diabetics need to maintain a regular diet.
- According to the American Diabetes Association (88), exercises should be continued at home.
- Physical activity improves blood glucose control in type 2 diabetes (aerobic exercise increases muscle glucose uptake up to fivefold through insulin-independent mechanisms), reduces cardiovascular risk factors, contributes to weight loss. Adults affected by type 2 diabetes should ideally perform both aerobic and resistance exercise training for optimal glycemic and health outcomes (89).

Structured lifestyle interventions including at least 150 min/week of physical activity and dietary changes are recommended to promote weight loss of 5%-7% and to prevent or delay the onset of type 2 diabetes in people at high risk and with pre-diabetes.

- Regular intake of ACE2-inhibitors and other antihypertensive and anti-diabetic drugs (including GLP1-R agonists) and, if necessary, insulin is important and should be emphasized for the best blood pressure glucose control.
- Telemedicine can be beneficial in these times. Patients can consult their physicians *via* telemedicine, who can give appropriate advice about treatment (90).

In conclusion, COVID-19, due to its heterogeneity, can be considered a systemic disease as it is more than a single-organ disease (4). The association with diabetes makes the whole condition at a higher risk of poor outcomes. For this reason, from now on, diabetes care has to include a careful, holistic evaluation of all the patients affected by COVID-19.

AUTHOR CONTRIBUTIONS

KP, MV, and MR have collected the various studies. CA and SC were responsible for revising the article critically. All authors contributed to the article and approved the submitted version.

REFERENCES

1. Zhu N, Zhang D, Wang W, Li X, Yang B, Song J, et al. A Novel Coronavirus from Patients with Pneumonia in China, 2019. *N Engl J Med* (2020) 382 (8):727–33. doi: 10.1056/NEJMoa2001017
2. Li Q, Guan X, Wu P, Wang X, Zhou L, Tong Y, et al. Early Transmission Dynamics in Wuhan, China, of Novel Coronavirus- Infected Pneumonia. *N Engl J Med* (2020) 382(13):1199–207. doi: 10.1056/NEJMoa2001316
3. World Health Organization Director-General's Opening Remarks at the Media Briefing on COVID-19–11 (2020).
4. Lenti MV, Corazza GR, Di Sabatino A. Carving out a place for internal medicine during COVID-19 epidemic in Italy. *J Internal Med* (2020) 288(2):263–5. doi: 10.1111/joim.13079
5. Saeedi P, Petersohn I, Salpea P, Malanda B, Karuranga S, Unwin N, et al. Global and regional diabetes prevalence estimates for 2019 and projections for 2030 and 2045: Results from the International Diabetes Federation Diabetes Atlas, 9(th) edition. *Diabetes Res Clin Pract* (2019) 157:107843. doi: 10.1016/j.diabres.2019.107843
6. Singh AK, Gupta R, Ghosh A, Misra A. Diabetes in COVID-19: Prevalence, pathophysiology, prognosis and practical considerations. *Diabetes Metab Syndrome* (2020) 14(4):303–10. doi: 10.1016/j.dsx.2020.04.004
7. Liang W, Liang H, Ou L, Chen B, Chen A, Li C, et al. Development and Validation of a Clinical Risk Score to Predict the Occurrence of Critical Illness in Hospitalized Patients With COVID-19. *JAMA Internal Med* (2020). doi: 10.1001/jamainternmed.2020.2033
8. Singh AK, Gupta R, Misra A. Comorbidities in COVID-19: Outcomes in hypertensive cohort and controversies with renin angiotensin system blockers. *Diabetes Metab Syndrome* (2020) 14(4):283–7. doi: 10.1016/j.dsx.2020.03.016
9. Yang J, Zheng Y, Gou X, Pu K, Chen Z, Guo Q, et al. Prevalence of comorbidities and its effects in coronavirus disease 2019 patients: A systematic review and meta-analysis. *Int J Infect Dis* (2020) 94:91–5. doi: 10.1016/j.ijid.2020.03.017
10. Wu Z, McGoogan JM. Characteristics of and Important Lessons From the Coronavirus Disease 2019 (COVID-19) Outbreak in China: Summary of a

Report of 72314 Cases From the Chinese Center for Disease Control and Prevention. *JAMA* (2020) 323(13):1239–42. doi: 10.1001/jama.2020.2648
11. Richardson S, Hirsch JS, Narasimhan M, Crawford JM, McGinn T, Davidson KW, et al. Presenting Characteristics, Comorbidities, and Outcomes Among 5700 Patients Hospitalized With COVID-19 in the New York City Area. *JAMA* (2020). doi: 10.1001/jama.2020.6775
12. Petrilli CM, Jones SA, Yang J, Rajagopalan H, O'Donnell L, Chernyak Y, et al. Factors associated with hospitalization and critical illness among 4,103 patients with COVID-19 disease in New York City. *medRxiv* (2020) 2020.04.08.20057794.
13. Mandeep R, Mehra MR, Desai SS, Kuy S, Henry TD, Patel AN. Cardiovascular Disease, Drug Therapy, and Mortality in Covid-19. *N Engl J Med* (2020)382 (26):2582. doi: 10.1056/NEJMc2021225
14. Onder G, Rezza G, Brusaferro S. Case-Fatality Rate and Characteristics of Patients Dying in Relation to COVID-19 in Italy. *JAMA* (2020) 323(18): 1775–76. doi: 10.1001/jama.2020.4683
15. https://www.epicentro.iss.it/coronavirus/bollettino/Report-COVID-201920marzoeng.pdf.
16. Grasselli G, Zangrillo A, Zanella A, Antonelli M, Cabrini L, Castelli A, et al. Baseline Characteristics and Outcomes of 1591 Patients Infected With SARS-CoV-2 Admitted to I.C.U.s of the Lombardy Region, Italy. *JAMA* (2020). doi: 10.1001/jama.2020.5394
17. Spagnolo PA, Manson JE, Joffe H. Sex and Gender Differences in Health: What the COVID- 19 Pandemic Can Teach Us. *Ann Internal Med* (2020) 173 (5):385–86. doi: 10.7326/M20-1941
18. Corrao S, Argano C, Natoli G, Nobili A, Corazza GR, Mannucci PM, et al. Sex-Differences in the Pattern of Comorbidities, Functional Independence, and Mortality in Elderly Inpatients: Evidence from the RePoSI Register. *J Clin Med* (2019) 8(1). doi: 10.3390/jcm8010081
19. Corrao S, Santalucia P, Argano C, Djade CD, Barone E, Tettamanti M, et al. Gender-differences in disease distribution and outcome in hospitalized elderly: data from the REPOSI study. *Eur J Internal Med* (2014) 25(7):617–23. doi: 10.1016/j.ejim.2014.06.027
20. Kang MJ. Novel genetic cause of idiopathic short stature. *Ann Pediatr Endocrinol Metab* (2017) 22(3):153–7. doi: 10.6065/apem.2017.22.3.153
21. Dennis JM, Mateen BA, Sonabend R, Thomas NJ, Patel KA, Hattersley AT, et al. Type 2 Diabetes and COVID-19-Related Mortality in the Critical Care Setting: A National Cohort Study in England, March-July 2020. *Diabetes Care* (2021) 44(1):50–7. doi: 10.2337/dc20-1444
22. Ferrando C, Mellado-Artigas R, Gea A, Arruti E, Aldecoa C, Bordell A, et al. de la Red de UCI Española para COVID-19. Patient characteristics, clinical course and factors associated to ICU mortality in critically ill patients infected with SARS-CoV-2 in Spain: A prospective, cohort, multicentre study. *Rev Esp Anestesiol Reanim* (2020) 67(8):425–37. doi: 10.1016/j.redare.2020.07.001
23. Du RH, Liu LM, Yin W, Wang W, Guan LL, Yuan ML, et al. Hospitalization and Critical Care of 109 Decedents with COVID-19 Pneumonia in Wuhan, China. *Ann Am Thorac Soc* (2020) 17(7):839–46. doi: 10.1513/AnnalsATS.202003-225OC
24. Crouse AB, Grimes T, Li P, Might M, Ovalle F, Shalev A, et al. Metformin Use Is Associated With Reduced Mortality in a Diverse Population With COVID-19 and Diabetes. *Front Endocrinol.* doi: 10.3389/fendo.2020.600439
25. Williamson EJ, Walker AJ, Bhaskaran K, Bacon S, Bates C, Morton CE, et al. Factors associated with COVID-19- related death using OpenSAFELY. *Nature* (2020) 584:430–6. doi: 10.1038/s41586-020-2521-4
26. Palaiodimos L, Kokkinidis DG, Li W, Karamanis D, Ognibene J, Arora S, et al. Severe obesity is associated with higher in- hospital mortality in a cohort of patients with COVID-19 in the Bronx, New York. *Metabol: Clin Exp* (2020) 154262. doi: 10.1016/j.metabol.2020.154262
27. Simonnet A, Chetboun M, Poissy J, Raverdy V, Noulette J, Duhamel A, et al. High prevalence of obesity in severe acute respiratory syndrome coronavirus-2 (SARS-CoV-2) requiring invasive mechanical ventilation. *Obesity* (2020). doi: 10.1002/oby.22831
28. Huang JF, Wang XB, Zheng KI, Liu WY, Chen JJ, George J, et al. Obesity hypoventilation syndrome and severe COVID-19. *Metabol: Clin Exp* (2020) 108:154249. doi: 10.1016/j.metabol.2020.154249
29. Chen Q, Zheng Z, Zhang C, Zhang X, Wu H, Wang J, et al. Clinical characteristics of 145 patients with corona virus disease 2019 (COVID-19) in Taizhou, Zhejiang, China. *Infection* (2020). doi: 10.1007/s15010-020-01432-5
30. Kalligeros M, Shehadeh F, Mylona EK, Benitez G, Beckwith CG, Chan PA, et al. Association of Obesity with Disease Severity among Patients with COVID-19. *Obesity* (2020). doi: 10.1002/oby.22859
31. Gupta R, Misra A. Contentious issues and evolving concepts in the clinical presentation and management of patients with COVID-19 infectionwith reference to use of therapeutic and other drugs used in Comorbid diseases (Hypertension, diabetes etc). *Diabetes Metab Syndrome* (2020) 14(3):251–4. doi: 10.1016/j.dsx.2020.03.012
32. Malavazos AE, Corsi Romanelli MM, Bandera F, Iacobellis G. Targeting the Adipose Tissue in COVID-19. *Obesity* (2020) 28(7):1178–79. doi: 10.1002/oby.22844
33. Ryan PM, Caplice NM. Is Adipose Tissue a Reservoir for Viral Spread, Immune Activation and Cytokine Amplification in COVID-19. *Obesity* (2020) 28(7):1191–94. doi: 10.1002/oby.22843
34. Di Chiara T, Licata A, Argano C, Duro G, Corrao S, Scaglione R. Plasma adiponectin: a contributing factor for cardiac changes in visceral obesity-associated hypertension. *Blood Pressure* (2014) 23(3):147–53. doi: 10.3109/08037051.2013.823767
35. Di Chiara T, Argano C, Scaglione A, Duro G, Corrao S, Scaglione R, et al. Hypoadiponectinemia, cardiometabolic comorbidities and left ventricular hypertrophy. *Internal Emergency Med* (2015) 10(1):33–40. doi: 10.1007/s11739-014-1104-5
36. Chiara TD, Argano C, Scaglione A, Corrao S, Pinto A, Scaglione R. Circulating adiponectin: a cardiometabolic marker associated with global cardiovascular risk. *Acta Cardiol* (2015) 70(1):33–40. doi: 10.1080/AC.70.1.3064591
37. Iacobellis G. COVID-19 and diabetes: Can DPP4 inhibition play a role? *Diabetes Res Clin Pract* (2020) 162:108125. doi: 10.1016/j.diabres.2020.108125
38. Guo W, Li M, Dong Y, Zhou H, Zhang Z, Tian C, et al. diabetes is a risk factor for the progression and prognosis of COVID-19. *Diabetes/metabolism Res Rev* (2020) e3319. doi: 10.1002/dmrr.3319
39. Yang JK, Feng Y, Yuan MY, Yuan SY, Fu HJ, Wu BY, et al. Plasma glucose levels and diabetes are independent predictors for mortality and morbidity in patients with SARS. *Diabetic Med* (2006) 23(6):623–8. doi: 10.1111/j.1464-5491.2006.01861.x
40. Wang Z, Du Z, Zhu F. Glycosylated hemoglobin is associated with systemic inflammation, hypercoagulability, and prognosis of COVID-19 patients. *Diabetes Res Clin Pract* (2020) 164:108214. doi: 10.1016/j.diabres.2020.108214
41. Preliminary Estimates of the Prevalence of Selected Underlying Health Conditions Among Patients with Coronavirus Disease 2019 — United States, February 12–March 28, 2020. (2020). doi: 10.15585/mmwr.mm6913e2
42. Guan WJ, Ni ZY, Hu Y, Chen X, Ao Y, Fitzpatrick T, et al. Clinical Characteristics of Coronavirus Disease 2019 in China. *New Engl J Med* (2020) 382(18):1708–20. doi: 10.1016/j.jinf.2020.03.041
43. Huang C, Wang Y, Li X, Ren L, Zhao J, Hu Y, et al. Clinical features of patients infected with 2019 novel coronavirus in Wuhan, China. *Lancet* (2020) 395 (10223):497–506. doi: 10.1016/S0140-6736(20)30183-5
44. Zhang JJ, Dong X, Cao YY, Yuan YD, Yang YB, Yan YQ, et al. Clinical characteristics of 140 patients infected with SARS- CoV-2 in Wuhan, China. *Allergy* (2020). doi: 10.1111/all.14238
45. Wang D, Hu B, Hu C, Zhu F, Liu X, Zhang J, et al. Clinical Characteristics of 138 Hospitalized Patients With 2019 Novel Coronavirus-Infected Pneumonia in Wuhan, China. *Jama* (2020). doi: 10.1001/jama.2020.1585
46. Wu C, Chen X, Cai Y, Xia J, Zhou X, Xu S, et al. Risk Factors Associated With Acute Respiratory Distress Syndrome and Death in Patients With Coronavirus Disease 2019 Pneumonia in Wuhan, China. *JAMA Internal Med* (2020). doi: 10.1001/jamainternmed.2020.0994
47. Chen Y, Gong X, Wang L, Guo J. Effects of hypertension, diabetes and coronary heart disease on COVID-19 diseases severity: a systematic review and meta-analysis. *medRxiv* (2020) 14(4):303–10. 2020.03.25.20043133.
48. Zhou F, Yu T, Du R, Fan G, Liu Y, Liu Z, et al. Clinical course and risk factors for mortality of adult inpatients with COVID-19 in Wuhan, China: a retrospective cohort study. *Lancet* (2020) 395(10229):1054–62. doi: 10.1016/S0140-6736(20)30566-3

49. Chen T, Wu D, Chen H, Yan W, Yang D, Chen G, et al. Clinical characteristics of 113 deceased patients with coronavirus disease 2019: retrospective study. *Bmj* (2020) 368:m1091. doi: 10.1136/bmj.m1295
50. Wu Z, McGoogan JM. Characteristics of and Important Lessons From the Coronavirus Disease 2019 (COVID-19) Outbreak in China: Summary of a Report of 72 314 Cases From the Chinese Center for Disease Control and Prevention. *JAMA* (2020) 323(13):1239–42. doi: 10.1001/jama.2020.2648
51. Muniyappa R, Gubbi S. COVID-19 pandemic, coronaviruses, and diabetes mellitus. *Am J Physiol Endocrinol Metab* (2020) 318(5):E736–E41. doi: 10.1152/ajpendo.00124.2020
52. Li F. Receptor recognition mechanisms of coronaviruses: a decade of structural studies. *J Virol* (2015) 89(4):1954–64. doi: 10.1128/JVI.02615-14
53. Hoffmann M, Kleine-Weber H, Schroeder S, Krüger N, Herrler T, Erichsen S, et al. SARS-CoV-2 Cell Entry Depends on ACE2 and TMPRSS2 and Is Blocked by a Clinically Proven Protease Inhibitor. *Cell* (2020) 181(2):271–80.e8. doi: 10.1016/j.cell.2020.02.052
54. Brufsky A. Hyperglycemia, hydroxychloroquine, and the COVID-19 pandemic. *J Med Virol* (2020) 92(7):770–75. doi: 10.1002/jmv.25887
55. Morra ME, Van Thanh L, Kamel MG, Ghazy A, Altibi AMA, Dat LM, et al. Clinical outcomes of current medical approaches for Middle East respiratory syndrome: A systematic review and meta-analysis. *Rev Med Virol* (2018) 28 (3):e1977. doi: 10.1002/rmv.1977
56. Classification and diagnosis of diabetes American diabetes association. *Diabetes Care* (2017).
57. Olariu E, Pooley N, Danel A, Miret M, Preiser J-C. A systematic scoping review on theconsequences of stress-related hyperglycaemia. *PLoS One* (2018) 13(4):e0194952. doi: 10.1371/journal.pone.0194952
58. Umpierrez GE, Isaacs SD, Bazargan N, You X, Thaler LM, Kitabchi AE. Hyperglycemia: an independent marker of in-hospital mortality in patients with undiagnosed diabetes. *J Clin Endocrinol Metab* (2002) 87(3):978e82. doi: 10.1210/jcem.87.3.8341
59. Yang JK, Feng Y, Yuan MY, Yuan SY, Fu HJ, Wu BY, et al. Plasma glucose levels and diabetes are independent predictors for mortality and morbidity in patients with SARS. *Diabetes Med* (2006) 23:623e8. doi: 10.1111/j.1464-5491.2006.01861.x
60. Jiang F, Yang J, Zhang Y, Dong M, Wang S, Zhang Q, et al. Angiotensin-converting enzyme 2 and angiotensin 1-7: novel therapeutic targets. *Nat Rev Cardiol* (2014) 11(7):413–26. doi: 10.1038/nrcardio.2014.59
61. Liu F, Long X, Zou W, Zhang W, Chen X, Zhang Z, et al. Highly ACE2 Expression in Pancreas May Cause Pancreas Damage After SARS-CoV-2 Infection. *medRxiv* (2020), 2020.02.28.20029181.
62. Sestan M, Marinovic S, Kavazovic I, Cekinović Đ, Wueest S, Turk Wensveen T, et al. Virus-Induced Interferon-gamma Causes Insulin Resistance in Skeletal Muscle and Derails Glycemic Control in Obesity. *Immunity* (2018) 49(1):164–77.e6. doi: 10.1016/j.immuni.2018.05.005
63. Yang JK, Lin SS, Ji XJ, Guo LM. Binding of SARS coronavirus to its receptor damages islets and causes acute diabetes. *Acta Diabetol* (2010) 47(3):193–9. doi: 10.1007/s00592-009-0109-4
64. Philips BJ, Meguer JX, Redman J, Baker EH. Factors determining the appearance of glucose in upper and lower respiratory tract secretions. *Intensive Care Med* (2003) 29(12):2204–10. doi: 10.1007/s00134-003-1961-2
65. Rao S, Lau A, So H-C. Exploring diseases/traits and blood proteins causally related to expression of ACE2, the putative receptor of SARS-CoV-2: A Mendelian Randomization analysis highlights tentative relevance of diabetes-related traits. *medRxiv* (2020) 43(7):1416–26. doi: 10.2337/dc20-0643
66. Wenzhong L, Hualan L. COVID-19: Attacks the 1-Beta Chain of Hemoglobin and captures the porphyrin to inhibit human heme metabolism. (2020). doi: 10.26434/chemrxiv.11938173.v5
67. de Wit E, van Doremalen N, Falzarano D, Munster VJ. SARS and MERS: recent insights into emerging coronaviruses. *Nat Rev Microbiol* (2016) 14 (8):523–34. doi: 10.1038/nrmicro.2016.81
68. Palm NW, Medzhitov R. Not so fast: adaptive suppression of innate immunity. *Nat Med* (2007) 13(10):1142–4. doi: 10.1038/nm1007-1142b
69. Hodgson K, Morris J, Bridson T, Govan B, Rush C, Ketheesan N. Immunological mechanisms contributing to the double burden of diabetes and intracellular bacterial infections. *Immunology* (2015) 144(2):171–85. doi: 10.1111/imm.12394
70. Maddaloni E, Buzzetti R. Covid-19 and diabetes mellitus: unveiling the interaction of two pandemics. *Diabetes/metabolism Res Rev* (2020) (31): e33213321. doi: 10.1002/dmrr.3321
71. Cameron AR, Morrison VL, Levin D, Mohan M, Forteath C, Beall C, et al. Anti-Inflammatory Effects of Metformin Irrespective of Diabetes Status. *Circ Res* (2016) 119(5):652–65. doi: 10.1161/CIRCRESAHA.116.308445
72. Drucker DJ. Coronavirus Infections and Type 2 Diabetes-Shared Pathways with Therapeutic Implications. *Endocr Rev* (2020) 41(3):bnaa011. doi: 10.1210/endrev/bnaa011
73. Jin T, Liu M. Letter to the Editor: Comment on GLP-1-based drugs and COVID-19 treatment. *Acta Pharm Sin B* (2020) 10(7):1249–50. doi: 10.1016/j.apsb.2020.05.006. Epub ahead of print.
74. Raj VS, Mou H, Smits SL, Dekkers DH, Müller MA, Dijkman R, et al. Dipeptidyl peptidase 4 is a functional receptor for the emerging human coronavirus-EMC. *Nature* (2013) 495(7440):251–4. doi: 10.1038/nature12005
75. Drucker DJ. Mechanisms of Action and Therapeutic Application of Glucagon-like Peptide-1. *Cell Metab* (2018) 27(4):740–56. doi: 10.1016/j.cmet.2018.03.001
76. Hansen TK, Thiel S, Wouters PJ, Christiansen JS, Van den Berghe G. Intensive insulin therapy exerts antiinflammatory effects in critically ill patients and counteracts the adverse effect of low mannose-binding lectin levels. *J Clin Endocrinol Metab* (2003) 88(3):1082–8. doi: 10.1210/jc.2002-021478
77. Avogaro A, Fadini GP. The pleiotropic cardiovascular effects of dipeptidyl peptidase-4 inhibitors. *B J Clin Pharmacol* (2018) 84:1686–95. doi: 10.1111/bcp.13611
78. Sardu C, D'Onofrio N, Balestrieri ML, Barbieri M, Rizzo MR, Messina V, et al. Outcomes in Patients With Hyperglycemia Affected by Covid-19: Can We Do More on Glycemic Control? *Diabetes Care* (2020). doi: 10.2337/figshare.12275516
79. Wanner C, Inzucchi SE, Lachin JM, Fitchett D, von Eynatten M, Mattheus M, et al. Empagliflozin and Progression of Kidney Disease in Type 2 Diabetes. *N Engl J Med* (2016) 375(4):323–34. doi: 10.1056/NEJMoa1515920
80. Muskiet MH, van Raalte DH, van Bommel EJ, Smits MM, Tonneijck L. Understanding EMPA- REG OUTCOME. *Lancet Diabetes Endocrinol* (2015) 3(12):928–9. doi: 10.1016/S2213-8587(15)00424-6
81. Chen CF, Chen YT, Chen TH, Chen FY, Yang YP, Wang ML, et al. Judicious Use of Sodium-Glucose Cotransporter 2 Inhibitors in Patients with Diabetes on Coronavirus-19 Pandemic. *J Chin Med Assoc JCMA* (2020). doi: 10.1097/JCMA.0000000000000354
82. Cure E, Cumhur Cure M. Angiotensin-converting enzyme inhibitors and angiotensin receptor blockers may be harmful in patients with diabetes during COVID-19 pandemic. *Diabetes Metab Syndr* (2020) 14:349–50. doi: 10.1016/j.dsx.2020.04.019
83. Kashish G, Shekhar K. SGLT-2 inhibitors as cardioprotective agents in COVID-19. *Heart Lung* (2020) 49(6):875–76. doi: 10.1016/j.hrtlng.2020.09.002
84. Danser AHJ, Epstein M, Batlle D. Renin-Angiotensin System Blockers and the COVID-19 Pandemic: At Present There Is No Evidence to Abandon Renin-Angiotensin System Blockers. *Hypertension* (2020) 75(6):1382–5. doi: 10.1161/HYPERTENSIONAHA.120.15082
85. Castiglione V, Chiriaco M, Emdin M, Taddei S, Vergaro G. Statin therapy in COVID-19 infection. *Eur Heart J Cardiovasc Pharmacother* (2020) 6(4):258–59. doi: 10.1093/ehjcvp/pvaa042
86. Timpel P, Oswald S, Schwarz PEH, Harst L. Mapping the Evidence on the Effectiveness of Telemedicine Interventions in Diabetes, Dyslipidemia, and Hypertension: An Umbrella Review of Systematic Reviews and Meta-Analyses. *J Med Internet Res* (2020) 22(3):e16791. doi: 10.2196/16791
87. Timpel P, Oswald S, Schwarz PEH, Harst L. Mapping the Evidence on the Effectiveness of Telemedicine Interventions in Diabetes, Dyslipidemia, and Hypertension: An Umbrella Review of Systematic Reviews and Meta-Analyses. *J Med Internet Res* (2020) 22(3):e16791. doi: 10.2196/16791
88. Colberg SR, Sigal RJ, Yardley JE, Riddell MC, Dunstan DW, Dempsey PC, et al. Physical Activity/Exercise and Diabetes: A Position Statement of the American Diabetes Association. *Diabetes Care* (2016) 39(11):2065–79. doi: 10.2337/dc16-1728

16

Obesity, Diabetes and COVID-19: An Infectious Disease Spreading from the East Collides with the Consequences of an Unhealthy Western Lifestyle

Jeff M. P. Holly, Kalina Biernacka, Nick Maskell and Claire M. Perks*

Faculty of Medicine, School of Translational Health Science, Southmead Hospital, University of Bristol, Bristol, United Kingdom

***Correspondence:**
Jeff M. P. Holly
jeff.holly@bristol.ac.uk

The pandemic of COVID-19, caused by the coronavirus, SARS-CoV-2, has had a global impact not seen for an infectious disease for over a century. This acute pandemic has spread from the East and has been overlaid onto a slow pandemic of metabolic diseases of obesity and diabetes consequent from the increasing adoption of a Western-lifestyle characterized by excess calorie consumption with limited physical activity. It has become clear that these conditions predispose individuals to a more severe COVID-19 with increased morbidity and mortality. There are many features of diabetes and obesity that may accentuate the clinical response to SARS-CoV-2 infection: including an impaired immune response, an atherothrombotic state, accumulation of advanced glycation end products and a chronic inflammatory state. These could prime an exaggerated cytokine response to viral infection, predisposing to the cytokine storm that triggers progression to septic shock, acute respiratory distress syndrome, and multi-organ failure. Infection leads to an inflammatory response and tissue damage resulting in increased metabolic activity and an associated increase in the mechanisms by which cells ingest and degrade tissue debris and foreign materials. It is becoming clear that viruses have acquired an ability to exploit these mechanisms to invade cells and facilitate their own life-cycle. In obesity and diabetes these mechanisms are chronically activated due to the deteriorating metabolic state and this may provide an increased opportunity for a more profound and sustained viral infection.

Keywords: diabetes, obesity, COVID–19, SARS-CoV-2, pandemic (COVID-19)

The current global pandemic is the third epidemic of a major severe acute respiratory syndrome (SARS) caused by a coronavirus this century. The initial SARS epidemic in 2002 affected 29 countries, primarily in the far east, with 8,098 cases and 774 fatalities (1). This was followed 10 years later by the Middle-East Respiratory Syndrome (MERS) in 2012 that affected 27 countries, mainly in the middle-east, with 2,494 cases and 858 deaths (1). Seven years later another coronavirus, SARS-CoV-2, closely resembling SARS-CoV-1, originated in China in late 2019 but has since spread to 213 countries and as of early August 2020 there have been over 20 million cases worldwide with three-quarters of a million deaths (www.worldometers.info/coronavirus/). As such this is the first coronavirus to have a major impact on Western countries. In contrast to many places in

Asia, Africa, and South America, over the last century most infectious diseases have become well-controlled in the West. However, growing epidemics of chronic diseases linked to lifestyle, such as cardiovascular disease, obesity and diabetes, that first became apparent in the West, have now spread to other regions of the world that have adopted a Western lifestyle and have slowly become global pandemics. The obesity and diabetes epidemics are also now prevalent in the Middle East and in the East; a cross-sectional survey of 170,287 participants in China in 2013 estimated that 47% of the adult population had either diabetes or prediabetes (2), The SARS-CoV-2 is the first acute pandemic in which an infectious disease from the East has collided with the slow pandemic of chronic lifestyle-related conditions from the West with severe consequences.

In contrast to the previous coronavirus epidemics, SARS-CoV-2 has spread more widely because its transmission has been facilitated by being highly contagious, in combination with a long latency period and large numbers of asymptomatic carriers (3). The SARS-CoV-2 virus results in a disease, COVID-19, that in some individuals can progress from a mild respiratory infection to a generalized inflammatory state, acute respiratory distress syndrome (ARDS) and ultimately multi-organ failure (MOF) associated with a high mortality rate (4). There are now seven coronaviruses that have spread to humans with HCov-229E, HCoV-OC43, HCoV-NL63, and HCoV-HKU1 thought to be responsible for around 30% of cases of the common cold (5). In around 80% of individuals, infection with SARS-CoV-2 can similarly result in mild or no discernible symptoms, but in around 20% of those infected COVID-19 can progress to severe outcomes with a high risk of mortality. The risk of severe disease is greatly enhanced by co-morbidities; the most common co-morbidities conferring the greatest risk are the chronic conditions associated with a Western-lifestyle; cardiovascular disease, obesity, and diabetes (6). A Western lifestyle is characterized by increased consumption of energy-dense foods and reduced physical activity leading to metabolic dysregulation with the global incidence of diabetes estimated to be some 463 million people in 2019 (7). The enforced stay-at-home/shield-in-place orders, that became almost universal, potentially resulted in reduced physical activity, altered nutritional intake and increased stress levels; all factors that could aggravate these conditions. In addition, reduced sun-light exposure and consequently reduced Vitamin D, reducing its anti-inflammatory actions (8) could also potentiate insulin-resistance (9). Indeed, using a simulation model that was created using glycemic data measured during previous disasters in India, with a similar impact to the current lockdown, it was predicted that after 45 days of lockdown glycemic control would deteriorate in patients with diabetes with a 3.68% increase in HbA1c (10).

OBESITY, DIABETES EFFECTS ON COVID-19 RISK, AND SEVERITY

That the metabolic disorder of diabetes was associated with COVID-19 was reported during the original outbreak in China and as the epidemic spread to Italy and the USA this was confirmed and similar associations were then also observed with obesity (11) A meta-analysis of 6 studies from China, that included 1,527 confirmed cases with SARS-CoV-2 infections, found a prevalence of diabetes among the patients of 9.7% compared to a prevalence within the general Chinese population of 10.9% (12) and an audit of 146 patients hospitalized with COVID-19 in Padova in Italy observed a prevalence of 8.9% (95% CI 5.3–14.6) compared to a prevalence of 11.0% in the same region (13). These preliminary reports would suggest that subjects with diabetes have no increased susceptibility to being infected; however, such conclusions are premature as there are many confounding issues that are yet to be examined including patients with obesity or diabetes being more likely to stay at home during such epidemics, being less mobile, have fewer social contacts and hence may have less exposure to the virus. Furthermore, the question of whether pre-existing diabetes or obesity predispose to acquiring an infection with SARS-CoV-2 is not possible to assess from reports of incident cases that depend considerably on the existing testing regimes which have varied greatly as the pandemic has developed and across different countries. If these conditions increased the severity of symptoms then there could be ascertainment bias in testing and detection of cases. Whether these preconditions predisposed to infection will only be answered when serological studies, monitoring the presence of viral antibodies in populations, have been completed with appropriate consideration for all confounding issues.

In contrast to the uncertainty regarding potential effects on the risk of infection, it is now clear that pre-existing diabetes and/or obesity have profound effects on the subsequent course of disease with many consistent reports of strong associations with morbidity and mortality. In the original outbreak in Wuhan it was observed that diabetes was associated with a higher risk of severe pneumonia, release of tissue injury-related enzymes, excessive uncontrolled inflammatory responses, and a hypercoagulable state (14). A report from the Center for Disease Control and Prevention in China, summarizing findings from 72,314 cases, observed that the overall case fatality rate was 2.3%, but for cases with diabetes the fatality rate was 7.3% (15). A review of hospital records of 1,099 patients in China found that the overall prevalence of diabetes was 7.4%; however, in those who required intensive care or mechanical ventilation or who died the prevalence was 26.9% compared to a prevalence of 6.1% in those without these indications of severe disease (16). A similar review of patient charts in Italy found that of 355 deaths 35.5% had pre-existing diabetes (6). A review of 5,279 confirmed infections at a single Medical Center in New York observed that overall 22.6% had pre-existing diabetes, but in those not requiring hospital admission only 9.7% had diabetes compared to 34.7% of those admitted (17). An initial assessment of co-morbidities among affected cases in the USA by the Center for Disease Control found that of 7,162 cases with full records overall 10.9% had diabetes but the prevalence was only 6% of those not requiring hospital admission compared to 24% of those requiring admission and 32% of those subsequently admitted to Intensive Care Units (ICU) (18). A study of 1,158 patients admitted to hospital in Kuwait, of which 104 needed ICU care, found the prevalence of diabetes to be 23.4% and in a multivariate analysis diabetes increased the risk of need for subsequent ICU with an OR 5.49 (CI 3.13, 9.65) (19).

There have also now been several meta-analyses of the many studies documenting the effects of diabetes and obesity on the severity and outcomes of COVID-19. A meta-analysis including data from 31 studies with a total of 6,104 cases found that cases with pre-existing diabetes had an OR of 2.61 (CI 2.05, 3.33) for developing severe COVID-19 compared to cases without diabetes (20). Another meta-analysis of 14 studies including 4,659 cases from China and USA with a prevalence of diabetes of 23.8% found that pre-existing diabetes increased the risk of death with OR 2.0 (CI 1.7, 2.3) (21). A larger meta-analysis including 33 studies with 16,003 cases found a prevalence of diabetes overall of 11.2%, but sub-group analysis revealed a prevalence of 10.5% of cases in China and 19.3% of cases outside of China (mainly USA): diabetes increased the risk of severe disease with OR 2.75 (CI 2.09, 3.62) and death with OR 1.90 (CI 1.37, 2.64) (22). A further meta-analysis of 30 studies with 6,452 cases found that diabetes increased the risk of severe COVID-19 with OR 2.45 (CI 1.79, 3.35), of ARDS with OR 4.64 (CI 1.68, 11.58) and of death with OR 2.12 (CI 1.44, 3.11) (23). When all of these outcomes were combined in an analysis of composite poor outcome, diabetes increased the risk with OR 2.38 (CI 1.88, 3.03) and a subgroup analysis revealed the risk was stronger in the younger cases with median age <55 years-old (RR 3.48) compared to older cases ≥55 years-old (RR 1.92) (23).

Associations between obesity and severity of COVID-19 or mortality have similarly been consistently reported. An audit of 124 patients admitted to ICU in France observed that among patients with COVID-19, obesity (BMI >30–<35 kg/m^2) and severe obesity (BMI >35 kg/m^2) were more prevalent than in control patients admitted to ICU for other causes: 47.6 vs. 25.2% and 28.2 vs. 10.8%, respectively, and those requiring invasive mechanical ventilation were also more obese (24). In a multivariate analysis of hospitalized patients in Kuwait, the risk of requirement for ICU was increased in the obese OR 2.7 (CI 1.17, 6.20) and those with morbid obesity (BMI >40) OR 3.95 (CI 1.0–15.2) (19). A similar study from New York that included 1,331 hospitalized COVID-19 patients, of whom 431 were admitted to ICU, found that the association with obesity was only evident in younger patients <60 years old with a higher risk of ICU admission for those with obesity (OR 1.8, CI 1.2, 2.7) and severe obesity (OR 3.6, CI 2.5, 5.3) compared to patients with a BMI <30 (25). An observational study of 20,133 patients admitted to 208 hospitals across the UK found that obesity increased the risk of death OR 1.33 (CI 1.19, 1.49) (26).

These observations are consistent with the long-known effects of obesity and diabetes on the severity and prognosis of infections. Influenza is often more severe and more often results in pneumonia in subjects with diabetes (27, 28). Following the influenza pandemic due to the H1N1 virus in 2009 obesity was recognized as a risk factor for hospitalization, the need for mechanical ventilation and death (29, 30). Plasma glucose and pre-existing diabetes were reported to be independent risk factors for morbidity and mortality in the original SARS epidemic in 2002 (31) and diabetes was strongly associated with mortality in the MERS epidemic in 2012 (32).

OBESITY, DIABETES AFFECT THE HOST RESPONSE TO SARS-COV-2

The metabolic derangements associated with obesity and diabetes have multiple effects on how the body responds to viral infections that could impact on the course of the disease. The most fundamental effect, that underpins the generalized increased predisposition to all infections, is the compromised immune system that is secondary to the metabolic derangements in obesity and diabetes. Interestingly, just a few years ago, as the health problems associated with a Western lifestyle spread to tropical regions, it was prophesized that this would pose a large threat for subjects with diabetes who contracted infectious diseases (33). With SARS-CoV-2 this threat is no longer confined geographically but has now become a global reality. Many aspects of the innate and adaptive immune systems are impaired in diabetes and obesity including inappropriate T-cell action, impaired natural killer cell activity, phagocytic cell dysfunction, inhibition of neutrophil chemotaxis, and defects in complement action (34–37). The compromised immune system in subjects with diabetes results in impaired responses to many of the stimuli activated during infections (38). Another potential consequence of the impaired immune cell function is that viral clearance could be reduced. A recent report measuring the interval between hospital admission and two negative tests for SARS-CoV-2 RNA, at least a day apart, found some evidence that there was delayed viral clearance in patients with diabetes (39). In addition, they found evidence that the use of glucocorticoids could also delay viral clearance (39) which is significant as glucocorticoids are frequently used for patients with ARDS (40). Indeed, glucocorticoid use is known to impair glycaemic control (41) and has been reported to reduce angiotensin-(1-7)-Mas receptor expression (42). However, although glucocorticoid use has been advised against in patients with COVID-19 (43) this advice has been questioned with a suggestion that low-to-moderate dose glucocorticoid could still be beneficial in treating critically ill patients with COVID-19 (44). Critical illness is associated with corticosteroid insufficiency (45) and there are cogent arguments for the use of glucocorticoids in critically ill patients (46) especially for treating ARDS (47). Consistent with this glucocorticoid treatment was found to reduce mortality in critically ill patients with SARS (48). A recent report confirmed similar findings in patients with COVID-19: in 2,014 patients randomized to receive dexamethasone, 28-day mortality was unaffected in subjects receiving no respiratory support but was reduced in critically ill patients receiving oxygen without invasive mechanical ventilation and was even more reduced in those receiving invasive mechanical ventilation (mortality rate ratio, 0.64; 95% CI, 0.51–0.81) (49). The compromised immune system in subjects with diabetes also increases susceptibility to potential secondary bacterial infection in the lungs (50).

Both obesity and type 2 diabetes are associated with chronic low-grade inflammation. Excess calorie intake results in a stimulation of pancreatic β-cell insulin secretion with the increase in oxygen consumption resulting in cell stress and mild inflammation. The insulin promotes glucose uptake and enlargement of adipocytes that in turn causes activation and recruitment of resident macrophages in adipose tissue. The adipocytes and macrophages then release more of a variety of proinflammatory cytokines and chemokines (including interleukin-1 (IL-1), IL-6, IL-8, monocyte chemoattractant protein-1 (MCP-1), C-reactive protein (CRP)) and less anti-inflammatory cytokines and adipokines (including IL-4, IL-10, IL-13, and adiponectin) (51, 52). These factors can then aggravate insulin-resistance leading to increased pancreatic insulin release and establish a vicious cycle. In subjects with obesity and diabetes the chronic low-grade inflammatory state could then aggravate the inflammatory response to SARS-CoV-2 infection and precipitate the hypersensitivity state and cytokine storm that can lead to pneumonia, ARDS and ultimately MOF observed in severe COVID-19 cases (16, 53, 54). Consistent with this, higher levels of IL-6, CRP and fibrinogen were observed in COVID-19 patients with diabetes compared to those without (14). The cytokine storm is part of an evolutionary conserved stress response preparing the body for a severe insult (55) with activation of the hypothalamic-pituitary-adrenal (HPA) axis (to produce cortisol), the sympathetic nervous system (to generate catecholamines), a tissue defense response and an acute-phase reaction, to generate pro-coagulant factors, in preparation for tissue damage.

Insulin-resistance, obesity, and diabetes promote an atherothrombotic state due to a disturbance in the balance of factors regulating coagulation and fibrinolysis with an increase in many clotting factors (such as tissue factor and fibrinogen) and adhesion molecules (such as P-selectin), a reduction in anticoagulant proteins (such as antithrombin) and a reduction in fibrinolysis due to an increase in plasminogen activator inhibitor type-1 (PAI-1) (56, 57). These factors could increase the likelihood of the development of endothelial dysfunction and platelet aggregation promoting the formation of occlusive thrombus in the heart and lungs in COVID-19 patients with diabetes. In patients with COVID-19 however there are increased levels of fibrinogen, CRP, and D-dimer (14, 58), with elevated D-dimer levels being a risk factor for mortality (53) these findings indicate that there appears to be an increase not only in coagulation but also in fibrinolysis. An imbalance or an impairment of coordination between coagulation and fibrinolysis appears to be responsible for much of the pathology observed in COVID-19 (59). The dysregulation of the system in subjects with obesity and diabetes could then exacerbate the effects of COVID-19 (60). Indeed, lung, heart, and brain damage appear to be common pathological findings in COVID-19 associated with fibrotic clots and disseminated intravascular coagulation (61, 62).

Severe obesity is associated with restrictive lung function with decreased expiratory reserve volume, functional capacity, and respiratory system compliance. These factors can complicate the clinical management of obese COVID-19 patients and in subjects with excess abdominal adipose tissue the diaphragmatic excursions are compromised and this can make assisted ventilation more problematic (63).

Diabetes and hyperglycaemia are accompanied by an accumulation of advanced glycation end-products (AGEs) that interact with a specific cell surface protein, the receptor for AGEs (RAGE). This has subsequently been found to be a pattern recognition receptor (PRR) that also recognizes pathogen-associated molecular patterns (PAMPs) from microorganisms, as well as danger-associated molecular patterns (DAMPs) released by stressed or damaged cells and play a key role in the inflammatory response (64). Although RAGE is normally expressed at low levels in most tissues and increased during inflammation, it is expressed at high levels in Type I and Type II alveolar epithelial cells (AT1, AT2) in the lung and appears to be a critical mediator of the pulmonary inflammatory response (65). In addition, it has been shown that activation of the Angiotensin II receptor 1 (AT1R) by Angiotensin II (AngII) can transactivate RAGE and that this mediates the subsequent inflammatory response (66). It has been suggested that RAGE may aggravate the inflammation and coagulation observed in COVID-19 (67) and contributes to the lung pathology (68). Infection with SARS-CoV-2 perturbs the renin–angiotensin system favoring AT1R activation (see below) and hence potentially transactivating RAGE, which is also activated by accumulated AGEs in patients with diabetes, aggravating the inflammatory and fibrotic response and promoting lung damage.

In addition to the general effect of inflammatory cytokines aggravating insulin-resistance, it had previously been reported that the SARS-CoV-1 receptor, which is the same receptor used by SARS-CoV-2, was abundantly expressed in the pancreas and that a proportion of patients with SARS developed transient diabetes during the course of the disease (69). This suggests that infection with SARS-CoV-2 could lead to a deterioration in metabolic control via a number of mechanisms and the metabolic derangements could, in turn, promote a more severe disease; this could be a particular problem in patients with obesity and those with type 2 diabetes who have residual pancreatic function in whom metabolic perturbations were already present.

OBESITY, DIABETES, AND THE VIRAL PATHWAY

In addition to the many established mechanisms whereby metabolic disorders could promote a more severe clinical response to SARS-CoV-2; the emerging evidence, uncovering how the virus infects cells, has indicated many further links to endocrine and metabolic controls. This has raised the prospect that obesity and diabetes could promote the course of the viral infection within the body. In order to enter and infect host cells the virus appears to have hijacked mechanisms that have evolved to ingest and degrade foreign material; with SARS-CoV viral entry occurring mainly by endocytosis via the endosomal/lysosomal route (70)(**Figure 1**).

Angiotensin Converting Enzyme 2 (ACE2)

The initial attachment of SARS-CoV-2 virus to cells has been reported to be mediated by ACE2, a transmembrane protein known to be important in the renin-angiotensin system (RAS) (71, 72). There are two immediate implications: the pattern of expression of ACE2 may determine the tissues in the body that are most affected by infection and secondly the virus may perturb

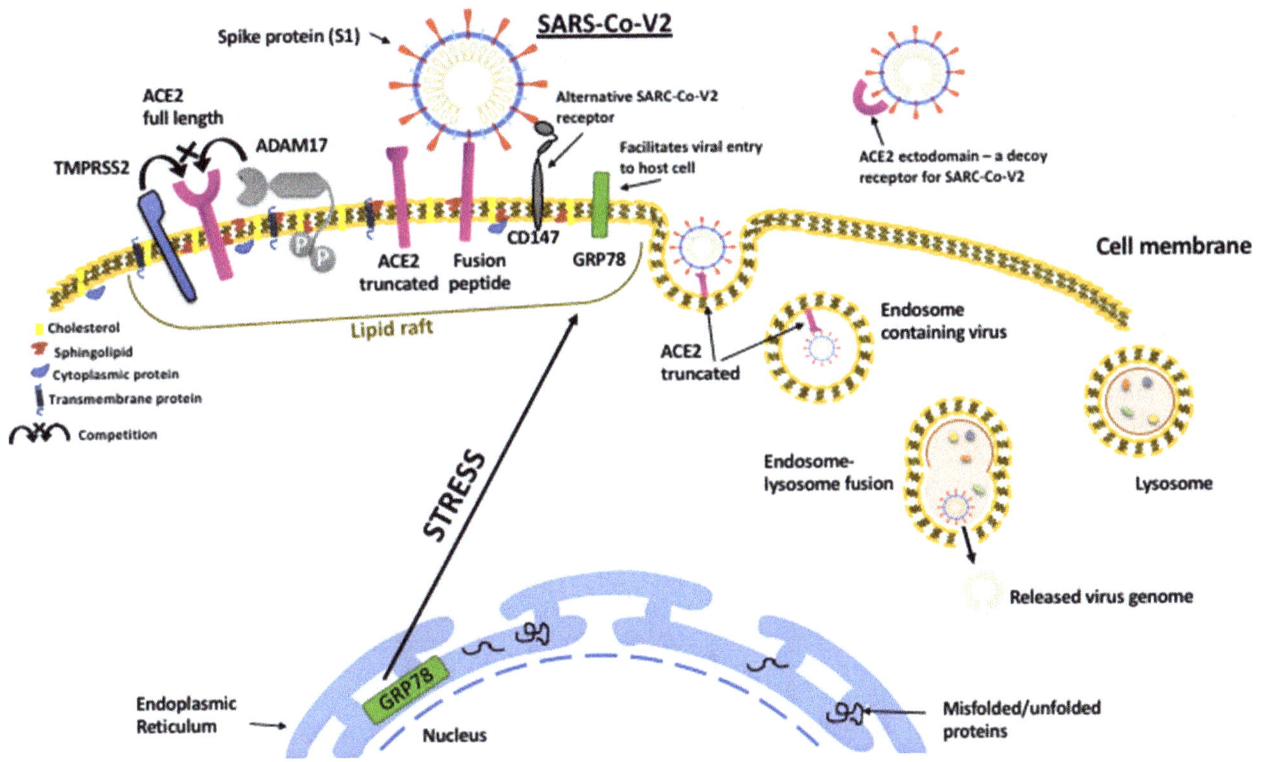

FIGURE 1 | SARS-CoV-2 viral entry to host cell pathway. The SARS-CoV-2 virus attaches to host cell surfaces via specific receptors, ACE2 and CD147, via spike protein (S1) projecting from the viral envelope. The spike protein first has to be "primed" by proteolytic cleavage by TMPRRS2 which can also cleave ACE2 resulting in shedding of the ectodomain. In contrast to TMPRSS2, which facilitates virus binding, ACE2 can also be cleaved by ADAM17, which prevents viral binding and results in shedding of the ACE2 ectodomain that can still bind to SARS-CoV-2 and act as a decoy receptor reducing viral infection. The entry of the virus is facilitated by the protein chaperone, GRP78 that also binds to the spike protein. Metabolic stress in the host cell results in upregulation of GRP78 and its translocation to the cell surface. On the cell surface ACE2, CD147, GRP78, TMPRSS2, and ADAM17 all cluster within organized cholesterol-rich domains called lipid rafts and together can enable viral entry via endocytosis. Viral replication within the cell can also be facilitated by GRP78.

the normal function of RAS which could impact the course of the disease. Two forms of ACE2 are found in the body, the full-length transmembrane form and a soluble form generated by proteolytic shedding of the extracellular domain of ACE2. The normal enzyme function of ACE2 is to degrade AngII to Ang-(1-7) and to a lesser extent AngI to Ang-(1-9); this in effect then opposes the action of ACE which converts Ang I to Ang II (73). The RAS plays an important role in regulating vascular function, blood pressure, and fluid and electrolyte balance. It comprises a dynamic counter-regulatory system with Ang II, the product of ACE, activating the AT1R to promote vasoconstriction, salt and water retention, fibrosis, and inflammation whereas the product of ACE2, Ang-(1-7) activates the G protein-coupled receptor Mas-receptor (MasR) to stimulate vasodilation and anti-inflammatory effects. The expression of ACE2 has been described in a number of tissues including the heart, kidneys, pancreas, and both type I and type II alveolar epithelial cells (ATI, ATII) in the lungs (74, 75). In addition to its well-known role in the cardiovascular system, the RAS also plays a critical role in lung function and disturbances to the ACE/ACE2 balance can lead to pulmonary disease. Knock-out of ACE2 in mice results in severe ARDS (76). In addition, ACE2 was shown to play an important role in lung injury in mice infected with H5N1 (77) and also infected with SARS-CoV-1 (78).

It has also become increasingly clear that ACE2 may play an important role in metabolic regulation. Knock-out of the ACE2 gene in mice resulted in a deficiency of pancreatic insulin secretion that was partially countered by increased glucose utilization in muscle (79, 80). Knock-down of ACE2 also compromises pancreatic function in obese mice (81). In an experimental model in which a high-calorie diet induces insulin resistance in mice, knock-down of ACE2 exaggerates the insulin resistance by reducing glucose uptake into tissues (82). Furthermore, overexpression of ACE2 improved glycaemic control in a model of type II diabetes in mice (83). In addition to SARS-CoV-2 directly infecting the pancreas via ACE2 and causing transient diabetes (69) the interaction of the virus with ACE2 could therefore have other effects to perturb the RAS and further compromise metabolic control.

The levels of ACE2 have been reported to be decreased in some experimental models of diabetes (84) and the loss of the counter-regulatory protective effects of the RAS has been speculated to potentiate lung damage. However, other reports indicate increased levels of ACE2 in the heart, liver, and lungs of mice with diabetes (85) and it has been suggested that this could make these tissues more vulnerable to SARS-CoV-2 infection and contribute to an increased risk of MOF in patients with diabetes. Evidence from humans indicate that levels of ACE2 in urine are increased in patients with type I diabetes (86) and type II diabetes (87) and positively related to blood glucose and HbA1c levels (88). It is not yet clear however, whether increased ACE2 in the urine is due to increased shedding of ACE2 in the kidney or whether it reflects increased circulating or systemic tissue levels. However, increased serum levels of ACE2 have been reported in subjects with diabetes and obesity (89). Expression of ACE2 in sputum cells has also been reported to be increased in subjects with diabetes and to be decreased in subjects using inhaled corticosteroids (90). Furthermore, a Mendelian Randomization study indicated that diabetes was causally related to increased ACE2 expression in lung tissue (91). An increase in ACE2 expression was also recently reported in the kidney of patients with diabetic kidney disease (92) and in the liver of patients with diabetes and also subjects with non-alcoholic fatty liver, which is prevalent in subjects with prediabetes (93). The weight of evidence therefore suggests that ACE2 levels are probably increased in various tissues in humans with diabetes and as evidence from cell biology suggests this may increase viral entry, this implies that infection with SARS-CoV-2 may be increased in tissues such as the lung, liver and kidney.

Following binding of SARS-CoV to ACE2, the complex is endocytosed and proteolyzed resulting in reduced tissue levels of ACE2 (94–96). Consistent with a down-regulation of ACE2, increased levels of AngII have been observed in patients with COVID-19 and these correlated with viral load (97). The increased levels of Ang II, together with potentially reduced levels of Ang-(1-7), would shift the balance of RAS actions to pro-inflammatory, rather than anti-inflammatory, resulting in increased lung damage as has been shown in experimental models of SARS (76, 78). However, it has recently been reported that expression of ACE2 can be upregulated by inflammatory cytokines (98) and this has also been reported to occur in airway epithelium (99). The chronic inflammatory state found in diabetes and obesity could facilitate viral infection via such a mechanism. In addition, insulin decreases expression of ACE2 (85, 100) suggesting that metabolic regulators could play an important role in affecting viral entry and/or in altering the inflammatory response by shifting the balance in the RAS. It has also been reported that the virus itself could upregulate ACE2 expression suggesting a positive feed-forward loop to enhance infection (101).

THE TYPE II TRANSMEMBRANE SERINE PROTEASE (TMPRSS2)

The virus interacts with ACE2 via a specific spike protein (S-protein) projecting from its envelope. The S-proteins of SARS-CoV viruses are typical class I viral fusion proteins that first need to be cleaved by proteases to activate their fusion ability that enables the virus to invade the host cell (70). The S protein is cleaved into two subunits (S1 and S2); the S1 subunit is then further divided into SA and SB domains, with the SB domain predicted to bind to human ACE2. This is often referred to as S-protein priming. The S2 subunit is responsible for fusion of the virus–ACE2 complex with the cell membrane. The enzyme responsible for S-protein priming and SARS-CoV-2 entry has been identified as TMPRSS2 and a clinically approved TMPRSS2 inhibitor, Camostat, markedly reduced viral entry into cultured lung cells (102). Similar results were reported previously for SARS-CoV-1 cell entry (103).

Expression of TMPRSS2 has been described in epithelial cells across a variety of tissues including prostate, colon, small intestine, pancreas, kidney, liver, and lung (104). It has been most studied in the prostate where it is strongly upregulated by androgens via an androgen-responsive promoter enhancer in the TMPRSS2 gene (105). Interestingly, it has also been reported to be upregulated on lung cells by both androgens and glucocorticoids (106). The strong androgen dependence of TMPRSS2 could contribute to the increased risk for men with COVID-19 (107). In addition to cleaving the S-protein, TMPRSS2 also cleaves ACE2 resulting in shedding of its ectodomain creating a soluble form of ACE2. This then competes with the normal shedding of ACE2 due to cleavage by the cell surface protease a disintegrin and metallopeptidase domain 17 (ADAM17) also known as tumor necrosis factor-converting enzyme (TACE) (108). Cleavage and shedding of ACE2 by ADAM17 prevents the action of TMPRSS2 to facilitate viral entry and in addition the soluble shed ACE2 can still bind to the viral S-protein and hence can compete with cell surface binding and protect tissues from infection acting as a decoy receptor (103). Although, as described above, a loss of the counter-regulatory protective effects of the RAS may enhance the damage in already infected lungs.

Whether TMPRSS2 has a role in metabolic regulation has yet to be investigated. The TMPRSS2 inhibitor, Camostat, has been reported to correct some of the metabolic abnormalities present in rats with diabetes and obesity (109), however, it is not clear that these effects were specific to inhibition of TMPRSS2.

LIPID RAFTS

Viral entry depends on an interaction between the virus S-protein and both ACE2 and TMPRSS2 on host cell surfaces and this occurs within organized domains called lipid rafts that are rich in cholesterol and sphingolipids; agents that disrupt lipid rafts prevent SARS-CoV-2 viral entry (110, 111). Lipid rafts were previously shown to play a role in SARS-CoV-1 infection (112), specifically that the interaction of SARS-CoV-1 S-protein with ACE2 occurred within lipid rafts (113). Indeed, lipid rafts have previously been implicated as important cell surface domains for the entry of other viruses (114, 115). An increase in cholesterol increases the availability of SARS-CoV-2 viral entry points (111). As cholesterol levels increase with aging and with metabolic disorders this could contribute to their associations with the severity of COVID-19. In addition, 7-ketocholesterol (7-KC) and 25-hydroxycholesterol (25-HC; a major circulating metabolite of cholesterol), can replace cholesterol in lipid rafts, disrupting their organization and these oxysteroids have been reported to have anti-viral activity (116–119) including against a porcine coronavirus (120). Inflammatory cytokines stimulate the formation of 25-HC, which in turn, promotes adipose tissue inflammation that is found in diabetes and obesity (121). The targeting of cholesterol and lipid metabolism and distribution has been proposed as a novel strategy for treating viral infections (122). The need for clustering of ACE2 and TMPRSS2 within organized domains in lipid rafts for viral entry could help explain some of the seemingly discrepant reports that increased ACE2 could facilitate infection, as described above, or actually protect against infection (123). With ACE2 present as a soluble, shed form that could act as a decoy-receptor and on cell surfaces in raft and non-raft domains, the total abundance may be less important than the localization and distribution of ACE2.

CD147

In addition to the virus gaining entry to host cells via an interaction of the viral S-protein with ACE2, viral entry has also been reported to occur via an interaction between the S-protein and CD147, with viral entry blocked by an antibody to CD147 (124). Again, this route had previously been reported for SARS-CoV-1 (125) and for other viruses including hepatitis B, human cytomegalovirus, Kaposi's sarcoma–associated herpesvirus, measles and HIV-1 (126–128). In turn, viral infection of host cells leads to upregulation of CD147 (129).

CD147, which is also known as Basigin or extracellular matrix metalloproteinase inducer (EMMPRIN), is a transmembrane glycoprotein that belongs to the immunoglobulin superfamily (126). CD147 is expressed in a number of cells in the lungs and its expression is increased in patients with chronic obstructive pulmonary disease (COPD) (130) and at sites of lung fibrosis (131). The expression of CD147 on the cell surface is upregulated by high glucose levels and by AGEs, via activation of RAGE, and has been suggested to play a role in diabetic complications (132). On cell surfaces CD147 is found within lipid rafts associated with caveolin-1 (133). In addition, HMG-CoA reductase inhibitors, statins, inhibit the cholesterol biosynthesis pathway and disrupt lipid raft composition resulting in a reduction of CD147 translocation to the cell surface (134). In addition to playing a role in viral entry, CD147 has a role in the immune response by modulating T-cell activation (135). One of the other prime functions of CD147 appears to be as a chaperone for monocarboxylate transporters (MCTs) that facilitate the transport of monocarboxylates such as lactate across the plasma membrane (136). In addition, CD147 is colocalized and associates with the glucose transporter, GLUT1, on cell surfaces (137) and an increase in CD147 is accompanied by an increase in GLUT1 and a switch to more glycolytic metabolism (138). Therefore, CD147 appears to be an important determinant of cell metabolism and in addition to facilitating SARS-CoV-2 entry and modulating the immune response, the virus interaction with CD147 could affect cell metabolism.

GLUCOSE-REGULATED PROTEIN 78 (GRP78)

A further important component in viral entry appears to be GRP78. Molecular modeling predicts that the SARS-CoV-2 S-protein should bind to GRP78 with high affinity (139). This would be consistent with a previous report that GRP78 bound to the S-protein of other coronavirus and was permissive for their entry to host cells, including MERS-CoV and HKU9 (140). The most well-established role of GRP78 is as a protein chaperone that ensures the correct folding and assembly of proteins in the endoplasmic reticulum (ER) and in the event of accumulation of misfolded proteins aids their degradation or initiates the unfolded protein response (UPR) or the ER stress response (141, 142). The chaperone role of GRP78 acts not only in the ER but also to chaperone proteins entering the cell via endocytosis (143). As viral proteins are foreign to host cells, viruses that acquired an ability to engage with host cell chaperones and disrupt the process designed to degrade unrecognized proteins would have gained a clear advantage. As such GRP78 binding appears to be have been commonly acquired by many viruses to not only ensure safe entry to host cells but also to facilitate viral replication. When a cell starts to make new viral proteins, it is an advantage for the virus if these are not immediately degraded. Infection with Coxsackievirus A9 (CAV-9) causes clustering of GRP78 with integrin receptors within lipid rafts on host cell surfaces which together then facilitate viral entry (144). The endocytosis of Zika virus is also facilitated by cell surface GRP78 (145). Similarly, GRP78 acts as a receptor for Dengue virus and antibodies to GRP78 could inhibit infection (146). Denge virus induces increased expression of GRP78 in host cells which then acts as a chaperone to facilitate viral protein production and viral replication (147). Similarly, Japanese Encephalitis Virus not only employs GRP78 as a receptor for host cell entry but also in facilitating viral replication (148). Although binding to GRP78 appeared not to be required for the entry of Ebola virus into host cells, it did play an essential role in viral protein transcription (149).

While GRP78 belongs to the heat shock protein 70 (HSP70) family, rather than being induced by heat shock it is induced by metabolic stress and was named due to observations of its induction by glycaemic stress (142, 150). The significance of the metabolic regulation of GRP78 is still far from being fully understood. However, it is clear that metabolic disturbances can have profound effects on the expression and functions of GRP78. Cell surface GRP78 can be shed and circulating GRP78 levels were found to be increased in subjects with diabetes and obesity and to correlate with CRP levels, suggesting that the chronic inflammation could be a contributing factor to the observed increase in addition to the metabolic stress (151). Indeed, as well as induction by metabolic stress, inflammatory cytokines also appear to stimulate the translocation of GRP78 to cell surfaces (152). Accumulation of AGEs can also induce GRP78 via activation of RAGE (153, 154). In a cell model of diabetic nephropathy high glucose was shown to upregulate cell surface GRP78 where it associated with integrin receptors and enhanced a fibrotic response (155). Androgens have also been reported to upregulate GRP78 (156, 157) and this could be a further contributing factor to the increased risk of COVID-19 in males. Other relevant functions of cell surface GRP78 are its ability to bind and stabilize ADAM17 (158) and also bind to tissue factor and regulate the initiation of coagulation (159).

The chaperone role of GRP78 acts not only in the ER but also to chaperone proteins entering the cell via endocytosis (143). It seems that viruses have commonly acquired an ability to bind to GRP78 and hijack its chaperone function to both facilitate entry to host cells and to enable the production and assembly of viral proteins. The role of GRP78 in SARS-CoV-2 infections has yet to be defined although in a clinical study serum levels of GRP78 were found to be elevated in patients admitted with COVID-19 compared to patients with pneumonia or healthy controls (160). The available evidence indicates that GRP78 is increased and is translocated to cell surfaces in patients with metabolic disorders and this could play an important role in viral entry to host cells and in viral replication, as well as contributing to the fibrotic and coagulation responses.

CLINICAL IMPLICATIONS

There are a number of implications from these observations. Reducing excess weight gain and improving metabolic health, in addition to all of the obvious well-known health benefits, may help prevent against a severe COVID-19 response to infection. Special protection/shielding should be provided to those with pre-existing obesity and diabetes. However, in contrast to the implication that the androgen dependence of COVID-17 severity may offer a strategy for using counter-measures to protect against COVID-19 (161), the metabolic effect needs more careful consideration. The management of metabolic control in critically ill patients is much more challenging than in those not acutely ill and many of the normal drugs used in diabetes are counter-indicated, with insulin being the most appropriate therapy (162). In addition, there are good reasons why glucocorticoids, which may seem counter-indicated, may actually be very beneficial in critically ill patients (46). In addition, the intense focus on SARS-CoV-2 has led to many advances in our understanding of the viral pathway that could provide new targets for developing more effective therapies against this and other viruses. The use of statins may have several benefits: the disruption of lipid raft composition (134) could reduce the various pathways of viral entry (163). In addition, statins have general anti-coagulant and anti-inflammatory effects (163); the latter could be particularly beneficial in combination with glucocorticoids in critically ill patients (46).

SUMMARY

The consequences of adopting a lifestyle, consuming excess calories with limited physical activity, are the metabolic derangements culminating in diabetes and obesity that are now at pandemic levels throughout the West. It has become clear that these conditions predispose individuals to severe COVID-19 that is caused by a virus spreading from the East, that in the majority of cases causes mild influenza-like symptoms. There are many consequences of diabetes and obesity that may accentuate the clinical response to SARS-CoV-2 infection. These include an impaired immune response, an atherothrombotic state, accumulation of AGEs activating RAGE and especially the pre-existing chronic inflammatory state. The later could prime an exaggerated cytokine response to viral infection, predisposing to the cytokine storm that triggers progression to septic shock, ARDS, and MOF.

In addition, to all of these factors that may contribute to these metabolic conditions exacerbating the clinical course of COVID-19, there are more fundamental mechanisms that may contribute to facilitating the viral infection. Infection leads to an inflammatory response and tissue damage and this results in increased metabolic activity. This is associated with an increase in the mechanisms by which cells ingest and degrade tissue debris and foreign materials. It appears that viruses have acquired the ability to exploit these mechanisms to invade cells and facilitate their own life-cycle. In obesity and diabetes these mechanisms are chronically activated due to the perturbed metabolism and this may provide an increased opportunity for a more profound and sustained viral infection.

AUTHOR CONTRIBUTIONS

All authors listed have made a substantial, direct and intellectual contribution to the work, and approved it for publication.

REFERENCES

1. Petersen E, Koopmans M, Go U, Hamer DH, Petrosillo N, Castelli F, et al. Comparing SARS-CoV-2 with SARS-CoV and influenza pandemics. *Lancet Infect Dis.* (2020) 20:E238–44. doi: 10.1016/S1473-3099(20)30484-9
2. Wang L, Gao P, Zhang M, Huang Z, Zhang D, Deng Q, et al. Prevalence and ethnic pattern of diabetes and prediabetes in China in 2013. *JAMA.* (2017) 317:2515–23. doi: 10.1001/jama.2017.7596
3. Guy RK, Di Paola RS, Romanelli F, Dutch RE. Rapid repurposing of drugs for COVID-19. *Science.* (2020) 368:829–30. doi: 10.1126/science.abb9332
4. Lippi G, Sanchis-Gomar F, Henry BM. COVID-19: unravelling the clinical progression of nature's virtually perfect biological weapon. *Ann Transl Med.* (2020) 8:693–8. doi: 10.21037/atm-20-3989
5. Fung TS, Liu DX. Human coronavirus: host-pathogen interaction. *Annu Rev Microbiol.* (2019) 73:529–57. doi: 10.1146/annurev-micro-020518-115759
6. Onder G, Rezza G, Brusaferro S. Case-fatality rate and characteristics of patients dying in relation to COVID-19 in Italy. *JAMA.* (2020) 323:1775–6. doi: 10.1001/jama.2020.4683
7. Saeedi P, Petersohn I, Salpea P, Malanda B, Karuranga S, Unwin N, et al. Global and regional diabetes prevalence estimates for 2019 and projections for 2030 and 2045: results from the international diabetes federation diabetes atlas, 9(th) edition. *Diabetes Res Clin Pract.* (2019) 157:107843. doi: 10.1016/j.diabres.2019.107843
8. Zhang Y, Leung DY, Goleva E. Vitamin D enhances glucocorticoid action in human monocytes: involvement of granulocyte-macrophage

colony-stimulating factor and mediator complex subunit 14. *J Biol Chem.* (2013) 288:14544–53. doi: 10.1074/jbc.M112.427054

9. Park JE, Pichiah PBT, Cha YS. Vitamin D and metabolic diseases: growing roles of Vitamin D. *J Obes Metab Syndr.* (2018) 27:223–32. doi: 10.7570/jomes.2018.27.4.223
10. Ghosal S, Sinha B, Majumder M, Misra A. Estimation of effects of nationwide lockdown for containing coronavirus infection on worsening of glycosylated haemoglobin and increase in diabetes-related complications: a simulation model using multivariate regression analysis. *Diabetes Metab Syndr.* (2020) 14:319–23. doi: 10.1016/j.dsx.2020.03.014
11. Stefan N, Birkenfeld AL, Schulze MB, Ludwig DS. Obesity and impaired metabolic health in patients with COVID-19. *Nat Rev Endocrinol.* (2020) 16:341–2. doi: 10.1038/s41574-020-0364-6
12. Li B, Yang J, Zhao F, Zhi L, Wang X, Liu L, et al. Prevalence and impact of cardiovascular metabolic diseases on COVID-19 in China. *Clin Res Cardiol.* (2020) 109:531–8. doi: 10.1007/s00392-020-01626-9
13. Fadini GP, Morieri ML, Longato E, Avogaro A. Prevalence and impact of diabetes among people infected with SARS-CoV-2. *J Endocrinol Invest.* (2020) 43:867–9. doi: 10.1007/s40618-020-01236-2
14. Guo W, Li M, Dong Y, Zhou H, Zhang Z, Tian C, et al. Diabetes is a risk factor for the progression and prognosis of COVID-19. *Diabetes Metab Res Rev.* (2020) 2020:e3319. doi: 10.1002/dmrr.3319
15. Wu Z, McGoogan JM. Characteristics of and important lessons from the coronavirus disease 2019. (COVID-19) outbreak in china: summary of a report of 72314 cases from the Chinese center for disease control and prevention. *JAMA.* (2020) 2020:1239–42. doi: 10.1001/jama.2020.2648
16. Guan WJ, Ni ZY, Hu Y, Liang WH, Ou CQ, He JX, et al. Clinical characteristics of coronavirus disease 2019 in China. *N Engl J Med.* (2020) 382:1708–20. doi: 10.1056/NEJMoa2002032
17. Petrilli CM, Jones SA, Yang J, Rajagopalan H, O'Donnell L, Chernyak Y, et al. Factors associated with hospital admission and critical illness among 5279 people with coronavirus disease 2019 in New York city: prospective cohort study. *BMJ.* (2020) 369:m1966. doi: 10.1136/bmj.m1966
18. CDC COVID-19 Response Team. Preliminary estimates of the prevalence of selected underlying health conditions among patients with coronavirus disease 2019 - United States, February 12-March 28, 2020. *MMWR Morb Mortal Wkly Rep.* (2020) 69:382–6. doi: 10.15585/mmwr.mm6913e2
19. Al-Sabah S, Al-Haddad M, Al-Youha S, Jamal M, Almazeedi S. COVID-19: impact of obesity and diabetes in disease severity. *medRxiv.* (2020). doi: 10.1101/2020.05.24.20111724. [Epub ahead of print].
20. Wang X, Fang X, Cai Z, Wu X, Gao X, Min J, et al. Comorbid chronic diseases and acute organ injuries are strongly correlated with disease severity and mortality among COVID-19 patients: a systemic review and meta-analysis. *Research.* (2020) 2020:2402961. doi: 10.34133/2020/2402961
21. Tian W, Jiang W, Yao J, Nicholson CJ, Li RH, Sigurslid HH, et al. Predictors of mortality in hospitalized COVID-19 patients: a systematic review and meta-analysis. *J Med Virol.* (2020) 92:1875–83. doi: 10.1002/jmv.26050
22. Kumar A, Arora A, Sharma P, Anikhindi SA, Bansal N, Singla V, et al. Is diabetes mellitus associated with mortality and severity of COVID-19? a meta-analysis. *Diabetes Metab Syndr.* (2020) 14:535–45. doi: 10.1016/j.dsx.2020.04.044
23. Huang I, Lim MA, Pranata R. Diabetes mellitus is associated with increased mortality and severity of disease in COVID-19 pneumonia - a systematic review, meta-analysis, and meta-regression. *Diabetes Metab Syndr.* (2020) 14:395–403. doi: 10.1016/j.dsx.2020.04.018
24. Simonnet A, Chetboun M, Poissy J, Raverdy V, Noulette J, Duhamel A, et al. High prevalence of obesity in severe acute respiratory syndrome coronavirus-2 (SARS-CoV-2) requiring invasive mechanical ventilation. *Obesity.* (2020) 28:1195–9. doi: 10.1002/oby.22831
25. Lighter J, Phillips M, Hochman S, Sterling S, Johnson D, Francois F, et al. Obesity in patients younger than 60 years is a risk factor for Covid-19 hospital admission. *Clin Infect Dis.* (2020) 71:896–97. doi: 10.1093/cid/ciaa415
26. Docherty AB, Harrison EM, Green CA, Hardwick HE, Pius R, Norman L, et al. Features of 20 133 UK patients in hospital with covid-19 using the ISARIC WHO clinical characterisation protocol: prospective observational cohort study. *BMJ.* (2020) 369:m1985. doi: 10.1136/bmj.m1985
27. McDonald HI, Nitsch D, Millett ER, Sinclair A, Thomas SL. New estimates of the burden of acute community-acquired infections among older people with diabetes mellitus: a retrospective cohort study using linked electronic health records. *Diabet Med.* (2014) 31:606–14. doi: 10.1111/dme.12384
28. Pearson-Stuttard J, Blundell S, Harris T, Cook DG, Critchley J. Diabetes and infection: assessing the association with glycaemic control in population-based studies. *Lancet Diabetes Endocrinol.* (2016) 4:148–58. doi: 10.1016/S2213-8587(15)00379-4
29. Louie JK, Acosta M, Samuel MC, Schechter R, Vugia DJ, Harriman K, et al. A novel risk factor for a novel virus: obesity and 2009 pandemic influenza A (H1N1). *Clin Infect Dis.* (2011) 52:301–12. doi: 10.1093/cid/ciq152
30. Morgan OW, Bramley A, Fowlkes A, Freedman DS, Taylor TH, Gargiullo P, et al. Morbid obesity as a risk factor for hospitalization and death due to 2009 pandemic influenza A(H1N1) disease. *PLoS ONE.* (2010) 5:e9694. doi: 10.1371/journal.pone.0009694
31. Yang JK, Feng Y, Yuan MY, Yuan SY, Fu HJ, Wu BY, et al. Plasma glucose levels and diabetes are independent predictors for mortality and morbidity in patients with SARS. *Diabet Med.* (2006) 23:623–8. doi: 10.1111/j.1464-5491.2006.01861.x
32. Alqahtani FY, Aleanizy FS, Ali El Hadi Mohamed R, Alanazi MS, Mohamed N, Alrasheed MM, et al. Prevalence of comorbidities in cases of Middle East respiratory syndrome coronavirus: a retrospective study. *Epidemiol Infect.* (2018) 147:1–5. doi: 10.1017/S0950268818002923
33. van Crevel R, van de Vijver S, Moore DAJ. The global diabetes epidemic: what does it mean for infectious diseases in tropical countries? *Lancet Diabetes Endocrinol.* (2017) 5:457–68. doi: 10.1016/S2213-8587(16)30081-X
34. Frydrych LM, Bian G, O'Lone DE, Ward PA, Delano MJ. Obesity and type 2 diabetes mellitus drive immune dysfunction, infection development, and sepsis mortality. *J Leukoc Biol.* (2018) 104:525–34. doi: 10.1002/JLB.5VMR0118-021RR
35. Geerlings SE, Hoepelman AI. Immune dysfunction in patients with diabetes mellitus (DM). *FEMS Immunol Med Microbiol.* (1999) 26:259–65. doi: 10.1111/j.1574-695X.1999.tb01397.x
36. Berbudi A, Rahmadika N, Tjahjadi AI, Ruslami R. Type 2 diabetes and its impact on the immune system. *Curr Diabetes Rev.* (2020) 16:442–9. doi: 10.2174/1573399815666191024085838
37. Nyambuya TM, Dludla PV, Mxinwa V, Nkambule BB. T-cell activation and cardiovascular risk in adults with type 2 diabetes mellitus: a systematic review and meta-analysis. *Clin Immunol.* (2020) 210:108313. doi: 10.1016/j.clim.2019.108313
38. Moutschen MP, Scheen AJ, Lefebvre PJ. Impaired immune responses in diabetes mellitus: analysis of the factors and mechanisms involved relevance to the increased susceptibility of diabetic patients to specific infections. *Diabete Metab.* (1992) 18:187–201.
39. Chen X, Hu W, Ling J, Mo P, Zhang Y, Jiang Q, et al. Hypertension and diabetes delay the viral clearance in COVID-19 patients. *medRxiv [preprint].* (2020). doi: 10.1101/2020.03.22.20040774
40. Chan ED, Chan MM, Chan MM, Marik PE. Use of glucocorticoids in the critical care setting: science and clinical evidence. *Pharmacol Ther.* (2020) 206:107428. doi: 10.1016/j.pharmthera.2019.107428
41. Clore JN, Thurby-Hay L. Glucocorticoid-induced hyperglycemia. *Endocr Pract.* (2009) 15:469–74. doi: 10.4158/EP08331.RAR
42. Marshall AC, Shaltout HA, Nautiyal M, Rose JC, Chappell MC, Diz DI. Fetal betamethasone exposure attenuates angiotensin-(1-7)-mas receptor expression in the dorsal medulla of adult sheep. *Peptides.* (2013) 44:25–31. doi: 10.1016/j.peptides.2013.03.018
43. Russell CD, Millar JE, Baillie JK. Clinical evidence does not support corticosteroid treatment for 2019-nCoV lung injury. *Lancet.* (2020) 395:473–5. doi: 10.1016/S0140-6736(20)30317-2
44. Shang L, Zhao J, Hu Y, Du R, Cao B. On the use of corticosteroids for 2019-nCoV pneumonia. *Lancet.* (2020) 395:683–4. doi: 10.1016/S0140-6736(20)30361-5
45. Annane D, Pastores SM, Arlt W, Balk RA, Beishuizen A, Briegel J, et al. Critical illness-related corticosteroid insufficiency (CIRCI): a narrative review from a multispecialty task force of the society of critical care medicine (SCCM) and the European society of intensive care medicine (ESICM). *Intensive Care Med.* (2017) 43:1781–92. doi: 10.1007/s00134-017-4914-x

46. Meduri GU, Chrousos GP. General adaptation in critical illness: glucocorticoid receptor-alpha master regulator of homeostatic corrections. *Front Endocrinol.* (2020) 11:161. doi: 10.3389/fendo.2020.00161
47. Meduri GU, Annane D, Chrousos GP, Marik PE, Sinclair SE. Activation and regulation of systemic inflammation in ARDS: rationale for prolonged glucocorticoid therapy. *Chest.* (2009) 136:1631–43. doi: 10.1378/chest.08-2408
48. Chen RC, Tang XP, Tan SY, Liang BL, Wan ZY, Fang JQ, et al. Treatment of severe acute respiratory syndrome with glucosteroids: the Guangzhou experience. *Chest.* (2006) 129:1441–52. doi: 10.1378/chest.129.6.1441
49. RECOVERY Collaborative Group, Horby P, Lim WS, Emberson JR, Mafham M, Bell JL, et al. Dexamethasone in hospitalized patients with Covid-19 - preliminary report. *N Engl J Med.* (2020). doi: 10.1056/NEJMoa2021436. [Epub ahead of print].
50. Ferlita S, Yegiazaryan A, Noori N, Lal G, Nguyen T, To K, et al. Type 2 diabetes mellitus and altered immune system leading to susceptibility to pathogens, especially mycobacterium tuberculosis. *J Clin Med.* (2019) 8:2219. doi: 10.3390/jcm8122219
51. Gonzalez LL, Garrie K, Turner MD. Type 2 diabetes - an autoinflammatory disease driven by metabolic stress. *Biochim Biophys Acta Mol Basis Dis.* (2018) 1864:3805–23. doi: 10.1016/j.bbadis.2018.08.034
52. Reddy P, Lent-Schochet D, Ramakrishnana N, McLaughlina M, Jialal I. Metabolic syndrome is an inflammatory disorder: a conspiracy between adipose tissue and phagocytes. *Clinica Chimica Acta.* (2019) 496:35–44. doi: 10.1016/j.cca.2019.06.019
53. Zhou F, Yu T, Du R, Fan G, Liu Y, Liu Z, et al. Clinical course and risk factors for mortality of adult inpatients with COVID-19 in Wuhan, China: a retrospective cohort study. *Lancet.* (2020) 395:1054–62. doi: 10.1016/S0140-6736(20)30566-3
54. Mehta P, McAuley DF, Brown M, Sanchez E, Tattersall RS, Manson JJ, et al. COVID-19: consider cytokine storm syndromes and immunosuppression. *Lancet.* (2020) 395:1033–4. doi: 10.1016/S0140-6736(20)30628-0
55. Xiao W, Mindrinos MN, Seok J, Cuschieri J, Cuenca AG, Gao H, et al. A genomic storm in critically injured humans. *J Exp Med.* (2011) 208:2581–90. doi: 10.1084/jem.20111354
56. Blokhin IO, Lentz SR. Mechanisms of thrombosis in obesity. *Curr Opin Hematol.* (2013) 20:437–44. doi: 10.1097/MOH.0b013e3283634443
57. Dunn EJ, Grant PJ. Type 2 diabetes: an atherothrombotic syndrome. *Curr Mol Med.* (2005) 5:323–32. doi: 10.2174/1566524053766059
58. Zhang B, Zhou X, Qiu Y, Feng F, Feng J, Jia Y, et al. *Clinical* characteristics of 82 death cases with COVID-19. *PLoS ONE.* (2020) 15:e0235458. doi: 10.1371/journal.pone.0235458
59. Ji HL, Zhao R, Matalon S, Matthay MA. Elevated plasmin(ogen) as a common risk factor for COVID-19 susceptibility. *Physiol Rev.* (2020) 100:1065–75. doi: 10.1152/physrev.00013.2020
60. Do Nascimento GP, Braz-de-Melo HA, Faria SS, Santos ID, Kobinger G, Magalhaes KG. Hypercoagulopathy and adipose tissue exacerbated inflammation may explain higher mortality in COVID-19 patients with obesity. *Front Endocrinol.* (2020) 11:530. doi: 10.3389/fendo.2020.00530
61. Liu X, Wang R, Qu G, Wang Y, Liu P, Zhu Y. et al. General observation report on systemic anatomy of cadavers who died of new coronavirus pneumonia. *Chinese J Forensic Med.* (2020) 36:21–3. doi: 10.12116/j.issn.1004-5619.2020.01.005
62. Xu Z, Shi L, Wang Y, Zhang J, Huang L, Zhang C, et al. Pathological findings of COVID-19 associated with acute respiratory distress syndrome. *Lancet Respir Med.* (2020) 8:420–2. doi: 10.1016/S2213-2600(20)30076-X
63. Dietz W, Santos-Burgoa C. Obesity and its implications for COVID-19 mortality. *Obesity.* (2020) 28:1005. doi: 10.1002/oby.22818
64. Hudson BI, Lippman ME. Targeting RAGE signaling in inflammatory disease. *Annu Rev Med.* (2018) 69:349–64. doi: 10.1146/annurev-med-041316-085215
65. Oczypok EA, Perkins TN, Oury TD. All the "RAGE" in lung disease: the receptor for advanced glycation endproducts (RAGE) is a major mediator of pulmonary inflammatory responses. *Paediatr Respir Rev.* (2017) 23:40–9. doi: 10.1016/j.prrv.2017.03.012
66. Pickering RJ, Tikellis C, Rosado CJ, Tsorotes D, Dimitropoulos A, Smith M, et al. Transactivation of RAGE mediates angiotensin-induced inflammation and atherogenesis. *J Clin Invest.* (2019) 129:406–21. doi: 10.1172/JCI99987
67. De Fracesco EM, Vella V, Belfiore A. COVID-19 and diabetes: the importance of controlling RAGE. *Front Endocrinol.* (2020) 11:526. doi: 10.3389/fendo.2020.00526
68. Rojas A, Gonzalez I, Morales MA. SARS-CoV-2-mediated inflammatory response in lungs: should we look at RAGE? *Inflamm Res.* (2020) 69:641–3. doi: 10.1007/s00011-020-01353-x
69. Yang JK, Lin SS, Ji XJ, Guo LM. Binding of SARS coronavirus to its receptor damages islets and causes acute diabetes. *Acta Diabetol.* (2010) 47:193–9. doi: 10.1007/s00592-009-0109-4
70. Ou X, Liu Y, Lei X, Li P, Mi D, Ren L, et al. Characterization of spike glycoprotein of SARS-CoV-2 on virus entry and its immune cross-reactivity With SARS-CoV. *Nat Commun.* (2020) 11:1620. doi: 10.1038/s41467-020-15562-9
71. Yan R, Zhang Y, Li Y, Xia L, Guo Y, Zhou Q. Structural basis for the recognition of SARS-CoV-2 by full-length human ACE2. *Science.* (2020) 367:1444–8. doi: 10.1126/science.abb2762
72. Letko M, Marzi A, Munster V. Functional assessment of cell entry and receptor usage for SARS-CoV-2 and other lineage B betacoronaviruses. *Nat Microbiol.* (2020) 5:562–9. doi: 10.1038/s41564-020-0688-y
73. Tikellis C, Thomas MC. Angiotensin-converting enzyme 2 (ACE2) is a key modulator of the renin angiotensin system in health and disease. *Int J Pept.* (2012) 2012:256294. doi: 10.1155/2012/256294
74. Hamming I, Timens W, Bulthuis ML, Lely AT, Navis G, van Goor H. Tissue distribution of ACE2 protein, the functional receptor for SARS coronavirus. a first step in understanding SARS pathogenesis. *J Pathol.* (2004) 203:631–7. doi: 10.1002/path.1570
75. Hikmet F, Méar L, Edvinsson A, Micke P, Uhlén M, Lindskog C. The protein expression profile of ACE2 in human tissues. *bioRxiv [preprint].* (2020).doi: 10.1101/2020.03.31.016048
76. Imai Y, Kuba K, Rao S, Huan Y, Guo F, Guan B, et al. Angiotensin-converting enzyme 2 protects from severe acute lung failure. *Nature.* (2005) 436:112–6. doi: 10.1038/nature03712
77. Zou Z, Yan Y, Shu Y, Gao R, Sun Y, Li X, et al. Angiotensin-converting enzyme 2 protects from lethal avian influenza A H5N1 infections. *Nat Commun.* (2014) 5:3594. doi: 10.1038/ncomms4594
78. Kuba K, Imai Y, Rao S, Gao H, Guo F, Guan B, et al. A crucial role of angiotensin converting enzyme 2 (ACE2) in SARS coronavirus-induced lung injury. *Nat Med.* (2005) 11:875–9. doi: 10.1038/nm1267
79. Bernardi S, Tikellis C, Candido R, Tsorotes D, Pickering RJ, Bossi F, et al. ACE2 deficiency shifts energy metabolism towards glucose utilization. *Metabolism.* (2015) 64:406–15. doi: 10.1016/j.metabol.2014.11.004
80. Niu MJ, Yang JK, Lin SS, Ji XJ, Guo LM. Loss of angiotensin-converting enzyme 2 leads to impaired glucose homeostasis in mice. *Endocrine.* (2008) 34:56–61. doi: 10.1007/s12020-008-9110-x
81. Shoemaker R, Yiannikouris F, Thatcher S, Cassis L. ACE2 deficiency reduces beta-cell mass and impairs beta-cell proliferation in obese C57BL/6 mice. *Am J Physiol Endocrinol Metab.* (2015) 309:E621–31. doi: 10.1152/ajpendo.00054.2015
82. Takeda M, Yamamoto K, Takemura Y, Takeshita H, Hongyo K, Kawai T, et al. Loss of ACE2 exaggerates high-calorie diet-induced insulin resistance by reduction of GLUT4 in mice. *Diabetes.* (2013) 62:223–33. doi: 10.2337/db12-0177
83. Bindom SM, Hans CP, Xia H, Boulares AH, Lazartigues E. Angiotensin I-converting enzyme type 2 (ACE2) gene therapy improves glycemic control in diabetic mice. *Diabetes.* (2010) 59:2540–8. doi: 10.2337/db09-0782
84. Patel VB, Parajuli N, Oudit GY. Role of angiotensin-converting enzyme 2 (ACE2) in diabetic cardiovascular complications. *Clin Sci.* (2014) 126:471–82. doi: 10.1042/CS20130344
85. Roca-Ho H, Riera M, Palau V, Pascual J, Soler MJ. Characterization of ACE and ACE2 expression within different organs of the NOD mouse. *Int J Mol Sci.* (2017) 18:563. doi: 10.3390/ijms18030563
86. Burns KD, Lytvyn Y, Mahmud FH, Daneman D, Deda L, Dunger DB, et al. The relationship between urinary renin-angiotensin system markers, renal function, and blood pressure in adolescents with type 1 diabetes. *Am J Physiol Renal Physiol.* (2017) 312:F335–42. doi: 10.1152/ajprenal.00438.2016

87. Gutta S, Grobe N, Kumbaji M, Osman H, Saklayen M, Li G, et al. Increased urinary angiotensin converting enzyme 2 and neprilysin in patients with type 2 diabetes. *Am J Physiol Renal Physiol.* (2018) 315:F263–74. doi: 10.1152/ajprenal.00565.2017
88. Liang Y, Deng H, Bi S, Cui Z, Lata A, Zheng D, et al. Urinary angiotensin converting enzyme 2 increases in patients with type 2 diabetic mellitus. *Kidney Blood Press Res.* (2015) 40:101–10. doi: 10.1159/000368486
89. Emilsson V, Gudmundsson EF, Aspelund T, Jonsson BG, Gudjonsson A, Launer LJ, et al. ACE2 levels are altered in comorbidities linked to severe outcome in COVID-19. *medRxiv [preprint].* (2020). doi: 10.1101/2020.06.04.20122044
90. Peters MC, Sajuthi S, Deford P, Christenson S, Rios CL, Montgomery MT, et al. COVID-19-related genes in sputum cells in Asthma. Relationship to demographic features and corticosteroids. *Am J Respir Crit Care Med.* (2020) 202:83–90. doi: 10.1164/rccm.202003-0821OC
91. Rao S, Lau A, So HC. Exploring diseases/traits and blood proteins causally related to expression of ACE2, the putative receptor of SARS-CoV-2: a mendelian randomization analysis highlights tentative relevance of diabetes-related traits. *Diabetes Care.* (2020) 43:1416–26. doi: 10.2337/dc20-0643
92. Gilbert RE, Caldwell L, Misra PS, Chan K, Burns KD, Wrana JL, et al. Overexpression of the SARS-CoV-2 receptor, ACE-2, in diabetic kidney disease: implications for kidney injury in Covid-19. *Can J Diab.* (2020). doi: 10.1016/j.jcjd.2020.07.003. [Epub ahead of print].
93. Soldo J, Heni M, Königsrainer A, Häring HU, Birkenfeld AL, Peter A. Increased hepatic ACE2 expression in NAFL and diabetes-a risk for COVID-19 patients? *Diabetes Care.* (2020). doi: 10.2337/dc20-1458. [Epub ahead of print].
94. Li W, Moore MJ, Vasilieva N, Sui J, Wong SK, Berne MA, et al. Angiotensin-converting enzyme 2 is a functional receptor for the SARS coronavirus. *Nature.* (2003) 426:450–4. doi: 10.1038/nature02145
95. Walls AC, Park YJ, Tortorici MA, Wall A, McGuire AT, Veesler D. Structure, function, and antigenicity of the SARS-CoV-2 spike glycoprotein. *Cell.* (2020) 181:281–92.e6. doi: 10.1016/j.cell.2020.02.058
96. Gheblawi M, Wang K, Viveiros A, Nguyen Q, Zhong JC, Turner AJ, et al. Angiotensin-converting enzyme 2: SARS-CoV-2 receptor and regulator of the renin-angiotensin system: celebrating the 20th anniversary of the discovery of ACE2. *Circ Res.* (2020) 126:1456–74. doi: 10.1161/CIRCRESAHA.120.317015
97. Liu Y, Yang Y, Zhang C, Huang F, Wang F, Yuan J, et al. Clinical and biochemical indexes from 2019-nCoV infected patients linked to viral loads and lung injury. *Sci China Life Sci.* (2020) 63:364–74. doi: 10.1007/s11427-020-1643-8
98. Hennighausen L, Lee HK. Activation of the SARS-CoV-2 receptor Ace2 by cytokines through pan JAK-STAT enhancers. *bioRxiv [preprint].* (2020). doi: 10.1101/2020.05.11.089045
99. Sajuthi SP, Deford P, Jackson ND, Montgomery MT, Everman JL, Rios CL, et al. Type 2 and interferon inflammation strongly regulate SARS-CoV-2 related gene expression in the airway epithelium. *bioRxiv [preprint].* (2020). doi: 10.1101/2020.04.09.034454
100. Wysocki J, Ye M, Soler MJ, Gurley SB, Xiao HD, Bernstein KE, et al. ACE and ACE2 activity in diabetic mice. *Diabetes.* (2006) 55:2132–9. doi: 10.2337/db06-0033
101. Zhuang MW, Cheng Y, Zhang J, Jiang XM, Wang L, Deng J. Increasing host cellular receptor-angiotensin-converting enzyme 2 expression by coronavirus may facilitate 2019-nCoV (or SARS-CoV-2) infection. *J Med Virol.* (2020). doi: 10.1002/jmv.26139. [Epub ahead of print].
102. Hoffmann M, Kleine-Weber H, Schroeder S, Kruger N, Herrler T, Erichsen S, et al. SARS-CoV-2 cell entry depends on ACE2 and TMPRSS2 and is blocked by a clinically proven protease inhibitor. *Cell.* (2020) 181:271–80.e8. doi: 10.1016/j.cell.2020.02.052
103. Heurich A, Hofmann-Winkler H, Gierer S, Liepold T, Jahn O, Pohlmann S. TMPRSS2 and ADAM17 cleave ACE2 differentially and only proteolysis by TMPRSS2 augments entry driven by the severe acute respiratory syndrome coronavirus spike protein. *J Virol.* (2014) 88:1293–307. doi: 10.1128/JVI.02202-13
104. Jacquinet E, Rao NV, Rao GV, Zhengming W, Albertine KH, Hoidal JR. Cloning and characterization of the cDNA and gene for human epitheliasin. *Eur J Biochem.* (2001) 268:2687–99. doi: 10.1046/j.1432-1327.2001.02165.x
105. Lin B, Ferguson C, White JT, Wang S, Vessella R, True LD, et al. Prostate-localized and androgen-regulated expression of the membrane-bound serine protease TMPRSS2. *Cancer Res.* (1999) 59:4180–4.
106. Mikkonen L, Pihlajamaa P, Sahu B, Zhang FP, Janne OA. Androgen receptor and androgen-dependent gene expression in lung. *Mol Cell Endocrinol.* (2010) 317:14–24. doi: 10.1016/j.mce.2009.12.022
107. Gebhard C, Regitz-Zagrosek V, Neuhauser HK, Morgan R, Klein SL. Impact of sex and gender on COVID-19 outcomes in Europe. *Biol Sex Differ.* (2020) 11:29. doi: 10.1186/s13293-020-00304-9
108. Lambert DW, Yarski M, Warner FJ, Thornhill P, Parkin ET, Smith AI, et al. Tumor necrosis factor-alpha convertase (ADAM17) mediates regulated ectodomain shedding of the severe-acute respiratory syndrome-coronavirus (SARS-CoV) receptor, angiotensin-converting enzyme-2 (ACE2). *J Biol Chem.* (2005) 280:30113–9. doi: 10.1074/jbc.M505111200
109. Jia D, Taguchi M, Otsuki M. Synthetic protease inhibitor camostat prevents and reverses dyslipidemia, insulin secretory defects, and histological abnormalities of the pancreas in genetically obese and diabetic rats. *Metabolism.* (2005) 54:619–27. doi: 10.1016/j.metabol.2004.12.005
110. Ballout RA, Sviridov D, Bukrinsky MI, Remaley AT. The lysosome: a potential juncture between SARS-CoV-2 infectivity and niemann-pick disease type C, with therapeutic implications. *FASEB J.* (2020) 34:7253–64. doi: 10.1096/fj.202000654R
111. Wang H, Yuan Z, Pavel MA, Hansen SB. The role of high cholesterol in age-related COVID19 lethality. *bioRxiv [preprint].* (2020). doi: 10.1101/2020.05.09.086249
112. Li GM, Li YG, Yamate M, Li SM, Ikuta K. Lipid rafts play an important role in the early stage of severe acute respiratory syndrome-coronavirus life cycle. *Microbes Infect.* (2007) 9:96–102. doi: 10.1016/j.micinf.2006.10.015
113. Glende J, Schwegmann-Wessels C, Al-Falah M, Pfefferle S, Qu X, Deng H, et al. Importance of cholesterol-rich membrane microdomains in the interaction of the S protein of SARS-coronavirus with the cellular receptor angiotensin-converting enzyme 2. *Virology.* (2008) 381:215–21. doi: 10.1016/j.virol.2008.08.026
114. Choi KS, Aizaki H, Lai MM. Murine coronavirus requires lipid rafts for virus entry and cell-cell fusion but not for virus release. *J Virol.* (2005) 79:9862–71. doi: 10.1128/JVI.79.15.9862-9871.2005
115. Heaton NS, Randall G. Multifaceted roles for lipids in viral infection. *Trends Microbiol.* (2011) 19:368–75. doi: 10.1016/j.tim.2011.03.007
116. Chen Y, Wang S, Yi Z, Tian H, Aliyari R, Li Y, et al. Interferon-inducible cholesterol-25-hydroxylase inhibits hepatitis C virus replication via distinct mechanisms. *Sci Rep.* (2014) 4:7242. doi: 10.1038/srep07242
117. Li C, Deng YQ, Wang S, Ma F, Aliyari R, Huang XY, et al. 25-hydroxycholesterol protects host against zika virus infection and its associated microcephaly in a mouse model. *Immunity.* (2017) 46:446–56. doi: 10.1016/j.immuni.2017.02.012
118. Liu SY, Aliyari R, Chikere K, Li G, Marsden MD, Smith JK, et al. Interferon-inducible cholesterol-25-hydroxylase broadly inhibits viral entry by production of 25-hydroxycholesterol. *Immunity.* (2013) 38:92–105. doi: 10.1016/j.immuni.2012.11.005
119. Willard KA, Eilling C, Stice SL, Brindley MA. The oxysterol 7-ketocholesterol reduces zika virus titers in vero cells and human neurons. *Viruses.* (2018) 11:20. doi: 10.3390/v11010020
120. Zhang Y, Song Z, Wang M, Lan M, Zhang K, Jiang P, et al. Cholesterol 25-hydroxylase negatively regulates porcine intestinal coronavirus replication by the production of 25-hydroxycholesterol. *Vet Microbiol.* (2019) 231:129–38. doi: 10.1016/j.vetmic.2019.03.004
121. Russo L, Muir L, Geletka L, Delproposto J, Baker N, Flesher C, et al. Cholesterol 25-hydroxylase (CH25H) as a promoter of adipose tissue inflammation in obesity and diabetes. *Mol Metab.* (2020) 39:100983. doi: 10.1016/j.molmet.2020.100983
122. Fernandez-Oliva A, Ortega-Gonzalez P, Risco C. Targeting host lipid flows: exploring new antiviral and antibiotic strategies. *Cell Microbiol.* (2019) 21:e12996. doi: 10.1111/cmi.12996

123. Chen J, Jiang Q, Xia X, Liu K, Yu Z, Tao W. Individual variation of the SARS-CoV-2 receptor ACE2 gene expression and regulation. *Aging Cell.* (2020) 19:e13168. doi: 10.1111/acel.13168
124. Wang K, Chen W, Zhou YS, Lian JQ, Zhang Z, Du P, et al. SARS-CoV-2 invades host cells via a novel route: CD147-spike protein. *BioRxiv [preprint].* (2020). doi: 10.1101/2020.03.14.988345
125. Chen Z, Mi L, Xu J, Yu J, Wang X, Jiang J, et al. Function of HAb18G/CD147 in invasion of host cells by severe acute respiratory syndrome coronavirus. *J Infect Dis.* (2005) 191:755–60. doi: 10.1086/427811
126. Muramatsu T. Basigin (CD147), a multifunctional transmembrane glycoprotein with various binding partners. *J Biochem.* (2016) 159:481–90. doi: 10.1093/jb/mvv127
127. Vanarsdall AL, Pritchard S, Wisner TW, Liu J, Jardetzky TS, Johnson DC. CD147 promotes entry of pentamer-expressing human cytomegalovirus into epithelial and endothelial cells. *mBio.* (2018) 9:e00781-18. doi: 10.1128/mBio.00781-18
128. Xiong L, Edwards CK III, Zhou L. The biological function and clinical utilization of CD147 in human diseases: a review of the current scientific literature. *Int J Mol Sci.* (2014) 15:17411–41. doi: 10.3390/ijms151017411
129. Moheimani F, Koops J, Williams T, Reid AT, Hansbro PM, Wark PA, et al. Influenza A virus infection dysregulates the expression of microRNA-22 and its targets; CD147 and HDAC4, in epithelium of asthmatics. *Respir Res.* (2018) 19:145. doi: 10.1186/s12931-018-0851-7
130. Jouneau S, Khorasani N, Souza PDE, Macedo P, Zhu J, Bhavsar PK, et al. EMMPRIN (CD147) regulation of MMP-9 in bronchial epithelial cells in COPD. *Respirology.* (2011) 16:705–12. doi: 10.1111/j.1440-1843.2011.01960.x
131. Guillot S, Delaval P, Brinchault G, Caulet-Maugendre S, Depince A, Lena H, et al. Increased extracellular matrix metalloproteinase inducer (EMMPRIN) expression in pulmonary fibrosis. *Exp Lung Res.* (2006) 32:81–97. doi: 10.1080/01902140600710512
132. Bao W, Min D, Twigg SM, Shackel NA, Warner FJ, Yue DK, et al. Monocyte CD147 is induced by advanced glycation end products and high glucose concentration: possible role in diabetic complications. *Am J Physiol Cell Physiol.* (2010) 299:C1212–9. doi: 10.1152/ajpcell.00228.2010
133. Tang W, Hemler ME. Caveolin-1 regulates matrix metalloproteinases-1 induction and CD147/EMMPRIN cell surface clustering. *J Biol Chem.* (2004) 279:11112–8. doi: 10.1074/jbc.M312947200
134. Sasidhar MV, Chevooru SK, Eickelberg O, Hartung HP, Neuhaus O. Downregulation of monocytic differentiation via modulation of CD147 by 3-hydroxy-3-methylglutaryl coenzyme a reductase inhibitors. *PLoS ONE.* (2017) 12:e0189701. doi: 10.1371/journal.pone.0189701
135. Staffler G, Szekeres A, Schutz GJ, Saemann MD, Prager E, Zeyda M, et al. Selective inhibition of T cell activation via CD147 through novel modulation of lipid rafts. *J Immunol.* (2003) 171:1707–14. doi: 10.4049/jimmunol.171.4.1707
136. Kirk P, Wilson MC, Heddle C, Brown MH, Barclay AN, Halestrap AP. CD147 is tightly associated with lactate transporters MCT1 and MCT4 and facilitates their cell surface expression. *EMBO J.* (2000) 19:3896–904. doi: 10.1093/emboj/19.15.3896
137. Su J, Gao T, Jiang M, Wu L, Zeng W, Zhao S, et al. CD147 silencing inhibits tumor growth by suppressing glucose transport in melanoma. *Oncotarget.* (2016) 7:64778–84. doi: 10.18632/oncotarget.11415
138. Huang Q, Li J, Xing J, Li W, Li H, Ke X, et al. CD147 promotes reprogramming of glucose metabolism and cell proliferation in HCC cells by inhibiting the p53-dependent signaling pathway. *J Hepatol.* (2014) 61:859–66. doi: 10.1016/j.jhep.2014.04.035
139. Ibrahim IM, Abdelmalek DH, Elshahat ME, Elfiky AA. COVID-19 spike-host cell receptor GRP78 binding site prediction. *J Infect.* (2020) 80:554–62. doi: 10.1016/j.jinf.2020.02.026
140. Chu H, Chan CM, Zhang X, Wang Y, Yuan S, Zhou J, et al. Middle East respiratory syndrome coronavirus and bat coronavirus HKU9 both can utilize GRP78 for attachment onto host cells. *J Biol Chem.* (2018) 293:11709–26. doi: 10.1074/jbc.RA118.001897
141. Lee AS. The ER chaperone and signaling regulator GRP78/BiP as a monitor of endoplasmic reticulum stress. *Methods.* (2005) 35:373–81. doi: 10.1016/j.ymeth.2004.10.010
142. Li J, Ni M, Lee B, Barron E, Hinton DR, Lee AS. The unfolded protein response regulator GRP78/BiP is required for endoplasmic reticulum integrity and stress-induced autophagy in mammalian cells. *Cell Death Differ.* (2008) 15:1460–71. doi: 10.1038/cdd.2008.81
143. Merkel A, Chen Y, George A. Endocytic trafficking of DMP1 and GRP78 complex facilitates osteogenic differentiation of human periodontal ligament stem cells. *Front Physiol.* (2019) 10:1175. doi: 10.3389/fphys.2019.01175
144. Triantafilou K, Triantafilou M. Lipid raft microdomains: key sites for coxsackievirus A9 infectious cycle. *Virology.* (2003) 317:128–35. doi: 10.1016/j.virol.2003.08.036
145. Ojha CR, Rodriguez M, Lapierre J, Muthu Karuppan MK, Branscome H, Kashanchi F, et al. Complementary mechanisms potentially involved in the pathology of zika virus. *Front Immunol.* (2018) 9:2340. doi: 10.3389/fimmu.2018.02340
146. Jindadamrongwech S, Thepparit C, Smith DR. Identification of GRP 78 (BiP) as a liver cell expressed receptor element for dengue virus serotype 2. *Arch Virol.* (2004) 149:915–27. doi: 10.1007/s00705-003-0263-x
147. Wati S, Soo ML, Zilm P, Li P, Paton AW, Burrell CJ, et al. Dengue virus infection induces upregulation of GRP78, which acts to chaperone viral antigen production. *J Virol.* (2009) 83:12871–80. doi: 10.1128/JVI.01419-09
148. Nain M, Mukherjee S, Karmakar SP, Paton AW, Paton JC, Abdin MZ. GRP78 is an important host factor for japanese encephalitis virus entry and replication in mammalian cells. *J Virol.* (2017) 91:e02274-16. doi: 10.1128/JVI.02274-16
149. Reid SP, Shurtleff AC, Costantino JA, Tritsch SR, Retterer C, Spurgers KB, et al. HSPA5 is an essential host factor for Ebola virus infection. *Antiviral Res.* (2014) 109:171–4. doi: 10.1016/j.antiviral.2014.07.004
150. Ibrahim IM, Abdelmalek DH, Elfiky AA. GRP78: a cell's response to stress. *Life Sci.* (2019) 226:156–63. doi: 10.1016/j.lfs.2019.04.022
151. Girona J, Rodriguez-Borjabad C, Ibarretxe D, Vallve JC, Ferre R, Heras M. The circulating GRP78/bip is a marker of metabolic diseases and atherosclerosis: bringing endoplasmic reticulum stress into the clinical scenario. *J Clin Med.* (2019) 8:1793. doi: 10.3390/jcm8111793
152. Vig S, Buitinga M, Rondas D, Crevecoeur I, van Zandvoort M, Waelkens E, et al. Cytokine-induced translocation of GRP78 to the plasma membrane triggers a pro-apoptotic feedback loop in pancreatic beta cells. *Cell Death Dis.* (2019) 10:309. doi: 10.1038/s41419-019-1518-0
153. Zhao YT, Qi YW, Hu CY, Chen SH, Liu Y. Advanced glycation end products inhibit testosterone secretion by rat Leydig cells by inducing oxidative stress and endoplasmic reticulum stress. *Int J Mol Med.* (2016) 38:659–65. doi: 10.3892/ijmm.2016.2645
154. Chen W, Chan Y, Wan W, Li Y, Zhang C. Abeta1-42 induces cell damage via RAGE-dependent endoplasmic reticulum stress in bEnd.3 cells. *Exp Cell Res.* (2018) 362:83–9. doi: 10.1016/j.yexcr.2017.11.005
155. van Krieken R, Mehta N, Wang T, Zheng M, Li R, Gao B, et al. Cell surface expression of 78-kDa glucose-regulated protein (GRP78) mediates diabetic nephropathy. *J Biol Chem.* (2019) 294:7755–68. doi: 10.1074/jbc.RA118.006939
156. Jiang X, Kanda T, Nakamoto S, Miyamura T, Wu S, Yokosuka O. Involvement of androgen receptor and glucose-regulated protein 78 kDa in human hepatocarcinogenesis. *Exp Cell Res.* (2014) 323:326–36. doi: 10.1016/j.yexcr.2014.02.017
157. Sheng X, Arnoldussen YJ, Storm M, Tesikova M, Nenseth HZ, Zhao S, et al. Divergent androgen regulation of unfolded protein response pathways drives prostate cancer. *EMBO Mol Med.* (2015) 7:788–801. doi: 10.15252/emmm.201404509
158. Schafer M, Granato DC, Krossa S, Bartels AK, Yokoo S, Dusterhoft S, et al. GRP78 protects a disintegrin and metalloprotease 17 against protein-disulfide isomerase A6 catalyzed inactivation. *FEBS Lett.* (2017) 591:3567–87. doi: 10.1002/1873-3468.12858
159. Bhattacharjee G, Ahamed J, Pedersen B, El-Sheikh A, Mackman N, Ruf W, et al. Regulation of tissue factor–mediated initiation of the coagulation cascade by cell surface grp78. *Arterioscler Thromb Vasc Biol.* (2005) 25:1737–43. doi: 10.1161/01.ATV.0000173419.31242.56
160. Koseler A, Sabirli R, Goren T, Turkcuer I, Kurt O. endoplasmic reticulum stress markers in SARS-COV-2 infection and pneumonia: case-control study. *In Vivo.* (2020) 34 (Suppl. 3):1645–50. doi: 10.21873/invivo.11956

161. Wambier CG, Goren A, Vano-Galvan S, Ramos PM, Ossimetha A, Nau G. Androgen sensitivity gateway to COVID-19 disease severity. *Drug Dev Res.* (2020). doi: 10.1002/ddr.21688. [Epub ahead of print].
162. Nakhleh A, Shehadeh N. Glycemic control of type 2 diabetic patients with coronavirus disease during hospitalization: a proposal for early insulin therapy. *Am J Physiol Endocrinol Metab.* (2020) 318:E835–7. doi: 10.1152/ajpendo.00163.2020
163. Rodrigues-Diez RR, Tejera- Muñoz A, Marquez-Exposito L, Rayego-Mateos S, Sanchez LS, Marchant V. Statins: could an old friend help the fight against COVID-19? *Br J Pharmacol.* (2020). doi: 10.1111/bph.15166. [Epub ahead of print].

17

Association Between Longitudinal Change in Abnormal Fasting Blood Glucose Levels and Outcome of COVID-19 Patients without Previous Diagnosis of Diabetes

Siwei Song[1†], Shujing Zhang[1†], Zhihui Wang[2†], Sufei Wang[1†], Yanling Ma[1], Pei Ma[1], Huilin Luo[3], Mengyuan Wang[4] and Yang Jin[1]*

[1] Department of Respiratory and Critical Care Medicine, NHC Key Laboratory of Pulmonary Diseases, Union Hospital, Tongji Medical College, Huazhong University of Science and Technology, Wuhan, China, [2] Department of Scientific Research, Union Hospital, Tongji Medical College, Huazhong University of Science and Technology, Wuhan, China, [3] Department of Anesthesia, Wuhan Red Cross Hospital, Wuhan, China, [4] Department of Endocrinology, Union Hospital, Tongji Medical College, Huazhong University of Science and Technology, Wuhan, China

***Correspondence:**
Yang Jin
whuhjy@126.com

†These authors have contributed equally to this work

This retrospective study examined changes in fasting blood glucose (FBG) levels during hospitalization and their effect on risk of death for Coronavirus disease 2019 (COVID-19) patients without previously diagnosed diabetes. A model with low- and high-stable pattern trajectories was established based on a longitudinal change in FBG levels. We analyzed FBG trajectory-associated clinical features and risk factors for death due to COVID-19. Of the 230 enrolled patients, 44 died and 87.83% had a low-stable pattern (average FBG range: 6.63–7.54 mmol/L), and 12.17% had a high-stable pattern (average FBG range: 12.59–14.02 mmol/L). There were statistical differences in laboratory findings and case fatality between the two FBG patterns. Multivariable logistic regression analysis showed that increased neutrophil count (odds ratio [OR], 25.43; 95% confidence interval [CI]: 2.07, 313.03), elevated direct bilirubin (OR, 5.80; 95%CI: 1.72, 19.58), elevated creatinine (OR, 26.69; 95% CI: 5.82, 122.29), lymphopenia (OR, 8.07; 95% CI: 2.70, 24.14), and high-stable FBG pattern (OR, 8.79; 95% CI: 2.39, 32.29) were independent risk factors for higher case fatality in patients with COVID-19 and hyperglycemia but no history of diabetes. FBG trajectories were significantly associated with death risk in patients with COVID-19 and no diabetes.

Keywords: fasting blood glucose trajectory, COVID-19, glycemic control, SARS-CoV-2, longitudinal change

---

Abbreviations: FBG, fasting blood glucose; COVID-19, coronavirus disease 2019; OR, odds ratio; CI, confidence interval; GBTM, group-based trajectory modeling; DBIL, direct bilirubin.

INTRODUCTION

Coronavirus disease 2019 (COVID-19), caused by severe acute respiratory syndrome coronavirus 2, has become a major threat to global health since it was first reported in December 2019. As of February 16, 2021, more than 100 million cases of COVID-19 have been confirmed worldwide, resulting in more than 2.4 million deaths (1). Pneumonia is the main clinical manifestation of COVID-19. Mild cases may have no obvious symptoms, whereas severe cases may involve severe respiratory distress syndrome, septic shock, or multiple organ dysfunction syndrome (2).

It is well-known that hyperglycemia and poor glycemic control are established risk factors for most infectious diseases (3, 4), including severe acute respiratory syndrome (5) and Middle East respiratory syndrome (6). Hyperglycemia is detrimental to the control of viremia and inflammation and aggravates morbidity and mortality in patients. Previous studies have shown that stress hyperglycemia due to an acute blood glucose disorder can occur in patients with COVID-19, even in those without a previous diagnosis of diabetes. Furthermore, it has been confirmed that hyperglycemia is an independent poor prognostic factor for COVID-19 with or without pre-existing diabetes (7, 8).

Long-term hyperglycemia may induce abnormal coagulation function, endothelial dysfunction, and inflammatory cytokine overproduction caused by abnormal immune activation (9, 10). Therefore, blood glucose control is necessary for recovery from infectious diseases. Evidence indicates that poor glycemic control in patients with COVID-19 is associated with a higher risk of complications or case fatality (11–13). However, these studies, in which fasting blood glucose (FBG) was presented in the form of an initial value at admission or as a mean value during hospitalization, have primarily focused on patients with pre-existing diabetes. Moreover, they did not consider longitudinal change in FBG related to COVID-19. Therefore, in this study, we aimed to examine the association between longitudinal change in COVID-19-related abnormal FBG and outcome for patients with COVID-19 who without a previous diagnosis of diabetes.

MATERIAL AND METHODS

Study Design and Participants

This retrospective study was conducted in three hospitals in Wuhan, China, namely, Wuhan Union Hospital, Wuhan Union West Hospital, and Wuhan Red Cross Hospital, all of which had been mandatorily designated to treat patients with COVID-19. Ethical approval was granted by the Institutional Ethics Committees of Wuhan Union Hospital (No. 0036). No patients or medical staff participated in the study design or statistical analysis.

A total of 1,474 adult patients with a laboratory-confirmed diagnosis of COVID-19 had been admitted to one of the three hospitals between January 14 and February 25, 2020. A diagnosis of COVID-19 was laboratory-confirmed in accordance with the interim guidance formulated by the World Health Organization (14). We excluded 1,244 patients based on the following exclusion criteria: (i) previous diagnosis of diabetes; (ii) admission FBG <6.1 mmol/L (impaired fasting glucose was defined as FBG >6.1 mmol/L according to the World Health Organization guidelines (15); (iii) FBG measured less than three times during hospitalization. Finally, 230 patients with COVID-19 were included in the analysis. A patient selection flowchart is presented in **Figure 1**. All patients were followed up until discharge or in-hospital death.

Data Collection

Information derived from demographic data, clinical manifestations, comorbidities, laboratory findings during hospitalization, and final outcomes (discharge or death) of all enrolled patients was acquired retrospectively from the admission records of the relevant departments. Comorbidities included chronic obstructive pulmonary disease, asthma, hypertension, chronic cardiac disease, anemia, chronic kidney disease, chronic hepatic disease, cerebrovascular disease, and malignant disease, all of which had been diagnosed using standard criteria. Laboratory findings included complete blood count, coagulation profile, renal and liver function, and inflammation markers.

Clinical management was standardized and appeared to be similar across the three hospitals, comprising antiviral therapy; symptomatic and supportive treatment; empirical antimicrobial

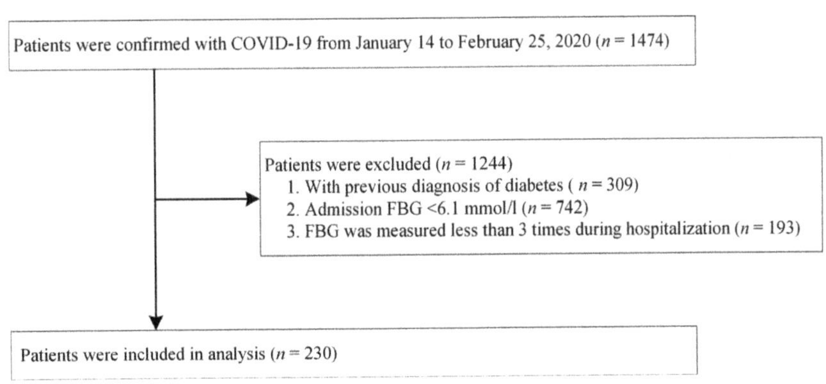

FIGURE 1 | Flowchart of patient selection.

therapy as appropriate to prevent or treat secondary infections; and oxygen support, in accordance with the Diagnosis and Treatment Plan for COVID-19 issued by the National Health Commission of People's Republic of China (6th Edition) (16). Hypoglycemic therapy included oral hypoglycemic medications and insulin injections. Patients were discharged at the discretion of the attending physician after a standard prescribed set of discharge criteria had been met, according to the aforementioned Diagnosis and Treatment Plan (16).

Measurement of FBG

The timing and frequency of FBG monitoring varied from person to person, depending on hyperglycemia severity, and patients with severe hyperglycemia had more frequent FBG surveillance accordingly. In our study, we collected FBG data on at least three occasions during hospitalization, including at admission and at discharge. All blood samplings had been conducted under fasting conditions (overnight fasting for at least 8 hours). Serum concentrations of FBG had been measured using an automatic biochemical analyzer (AU5800 Analyzer; Beckman Coulter, Brea, CA).

Statistical Analysis

FBG trajectories were modeled using group-based trajectory modeling (GBTM) for all enrolled participants with the FBG measured more than three times, using SAS Proc Traj program. GBTM, a form of finite mixed model, is applied to longitudinal data to identify sharing common potential development trajectories of group using maximum likelihood estimation, which has been increasingly applied in clinical research (17, 18). One advantage of GBTM is that its trajectories are not restricted to a single pattern since GBTM does not assume a single functional form of population, that is, it allows for group trajectories to rise, fall, or remain stable. Optimal trajectory numbers in GBTM cannot be selected and identified in advance; however, they can be identified according to superior and inferior models in the process of statistical analysis (17, 19). After exploring various numbers of potential trajectories and the polynomial orders of each trajectory, the optimal trajectory model was selected, which had the smallest Bayesian information criterion value. Moreover, the number of observed objects in each trajectory was guaranteed to account for at least 5% of the total number of cases, and the average posterior probability of each trajectory was >70% (18). Finally, two FBG trajectories were obtained in this study (**Figure 2**). The optimal FBG trajectory model was a polynomial order 2,0 model. Patients were categorized as having either "low-stable pattern" or "high-stable pattern" and two patient groups were formed accordingly.

Descriptive statistics were used to describe patient baseline data. Categorical variables are presented as numbers with percentage proportions, and continuous variables are expressed as mean ± standard deviation, if they were normally distributed, or as median (interquartile range [IQR]), if they were non-normally distributed. Proportions for categorical variables were compared using the $\chi2$ test, Cochran-Mantel-Hensel $\chi2$ test, or Fisher's exact test. All laboratory data are presented as average concentrations based on measurements during hospitalization, including at admission and at discharge. The optimal cut-off value was determined using Youden's index. In the descriptive analysis, the characteristics of the data were compared according to survival status and trajectory classes.

We conducted univariable and multivariable logistics regression analysis to identify factors correlating with case fatality, whose variables were screened using least absolute shrinkage and selection operator (LASSO) regression analysis to avoid overfitting for the large number of variables. A Kaplan-Meier survival curve was plotted to determine the relationship between the FBG patterns and the final outcomes. Linear mixed model was used to describe the relationship between changes in FBG levels and COVID-19 survivors and non-survivors. We analyzed the association between reduction in FBG level during hospitalization and prognosis using logistical regression. Pearson correlation coefficient was used to evaluate the correlation between glycemic variations and the evolution of biochemical parameters.

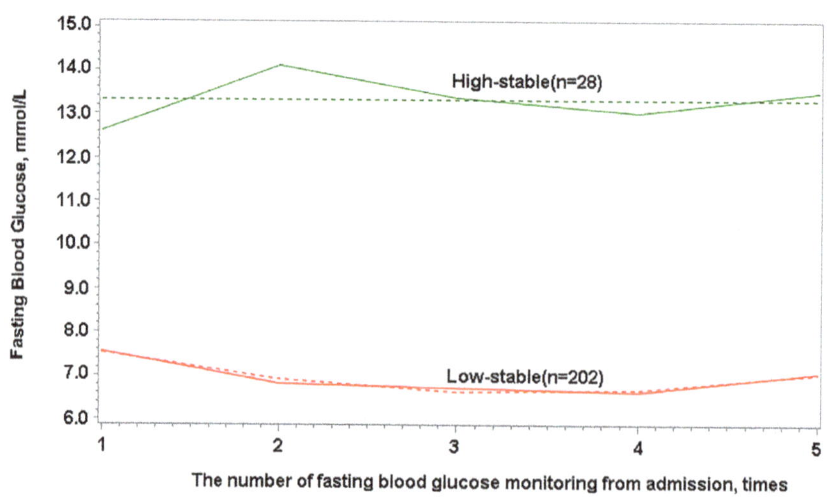

FIGURE 2 | Fasting blood glucose trajectories with low-stable and high-stable patterns based on longitudinal change in fasting blood glucose.

R software (version 3.6.3) was used to calculate Pearson's correlation coefficient, and other analyses were conducted using SAS version 9.4 software.

RESULTS

Demographics and Clinical Features of Patients

From January 14 to February 25, 2020, 1,474 patients with confirmed COVID-19 had been admitted to the aforementioned three hospitals. After excluding 309 patients with a previous diagnosis of diabetes, 742 with an FBG <6.1 mmol/L at admission, and 193 whose FBG had been measured less than three times during hospitalization, a total of 230 patients were retrospectively enrolled in final analysis (**Figure 1**). All of these patients had hyperglycemia during hospitalization (average FBG, 7.70 mmol/L).

The baseline data and clinical features of all patients are shown in **Table 1**. The median age of these patients was 63 (IQR, 54–70) years, and 139 (59.13%) were men. Among the 230 patients, 44 (19.13%) died during hospitalization. Compared with survivors, there were more elderly patients (63.64% vs. 35.48%, P = 0.0006) among non-survivors. Moreover, non-survivors were more likely to present expectoration (55.00% vs. 37.58%, P = 0.0444), have a history of malignant disease (15.00% vs. 4.46%, P = 0.0165), and require invasive mechanical ventilation (IMV) (38.64% vs. 4.84%, P < 0.0001).

In terms of treatment, the use of antibiotic (90.91% vs. 72.58%, P = 0.018), corticosteroid (59.09% vs. 36.02%, P = 0.0050), and hypoglycemic therapy (13.64% vs. 2.69%, P = 0.0022) was more common among non-survivors than survivors, whereas the use of traditional Chinese medicine (63.44% vs. 31.81, P = 0.0001) and antihypertensive medicine (23.12% vs. 6.82%, P = 0.0263) was more common in survivors than in non-survivors. There were no significant differences in the use of antiviral (P > 0.9999) and lipid-lowing therapy (P = 0.6350) between survivors and non-survivors.

The results of relevant laboratory examinations are shown in **Table 1**. We found that, compared with survivors, non-survivors were more likely to have abnormal routine blood test results, elevated hepatic and renal biochemical indicators, hypoproteinemia, and coagulation function disorders. The FBG in non-survivors (median, 9.35; IQR, 8.13–11.97) were higher than those in survivors (median, 6.49; IQR, 5.92–7.52; P < 0.0001).

FBG Trajectories of Patients

The study population was categorized based on two observed trajectories of FBG during hospitalization. These trajectories were based on FBG levels and changing patterns (**Figure 2**): 87.83% (n = 202) of patients with sustained abnormal but relatively low FBG levels (categorized as "low-stable pattern", in which the mean FBG levels ranged from 6.63 to 7.54 mmol/L during hospitalization), and 12.17% (n = 28) of patients with sustained high FBG levels (categorized as "high-stable pattern", in which the mean FBG levels ranged from 12.59 to 14.02 mmol/L during hospitalization). The proportion of non-surviving patients with a high-stable pattern was 38.64%, which was found to be considerably higher than that of survivors (5.91%; P < 0.0001) (**Table 1**).

Clinical Features Between Patients With Low- or High-Stable FBG Patterns

The clinical features concerning all patients with low- or high-stable FBG patterns are presented in **Supplementary Table 1**. Compared with patients having the low-stable pattern, those with the high-stable pattern were found to be older (median age, 69.50 vs 63.00 years; P = 0.0359) and to have a malignant disease (17.39% vs. 5.17%, P = 0.0265). There were no statistically significant differences in terms of onset symptoms and comorbidities, except for the presence of malignant disease, between the low- and the high-stable pattern groups. However, individuals with the high-stable pattern were more likely to accept IMV treatment throughout their whole course than those with the low-stable pattern (28.57% vs. 8.91%, P = 0.0021). Furthermore, in patients with the high-stable pattern, the use of corticosteroid (64.29% vs. 37.13%, P = 0.0061) and hypoglycemic therapy (39.29% vs. 0, P < 0.0001) was more common than in those with low-stable pattern.

Laboratory findings indicated several differences between the two FBG pattern groups. The high-stable pattern group had higher blood cell and neutrophil counts than the low-stable pattern group (96.43% vs. 69.31%, P = 0.0026; 96.43% vs. 54.95%, P < 0.0001, respectively), but lower platelet, lymphocyte, and monocyte counts (53.57% vs. 14.85%, P < 0.0001; 57.14% vs. 22.77%, P = 0.0001; 21.43% vs. 3.96%, P = 0.0001, respectively). Compared with patients in the low-stable pattern group, those in the high-stable pattern had a higher level of direct bilirubin (DBIL) (64.29% vs. 37.13%, P = 0.0061), a higher prothrombin time (57.14% vs. 33.85%, P = 0.0005), and a lower level of total protein (60.71% vs. 20.79%, P < 0.0001). In addition, 92.59% of patients in the high-stable pattern group had a high C-reactive protein level, which was significantly higher than in patients in the low-stable pattern group (58.88%, P = 0.0007). The survival analysis showed that the high-stable pattern was significantly associated with increased case fatality (**Figure 3**).

Factors Associated With Case Fatality

The number of deaths (n = 44) in our study was relatively low and the number of variables included in this analysis was relatively large; therefore, the LASSO model (**Supplementary Figure 1**), in combination with clinical relevance, was used to screen the variables for logistic regression analysis. Age, sex, neutrophil count, lymphocyte count, eosinophil count, DBIL, prealbumin, creatinine, uric acid, prothrombin time, and FBG trajectory patterns were selected for univariable logistic regression analysis. Univariate logistic regression analysis showed that older age; lymphopenia; eosinophilia; an increased neutrophil count; elevated DBIL, prealbumin, creatinine, and uric acid; prolonged prothrombin time; and the high-stable FBG pattern were associated with higher case fatality (**Table 2**).

Multivariable logistic regression analysis showed that increased neutrophil count (OR, 25.43; 95% CI: 2.07, 313.03; P = 0.0115), elevated DBIL (OR, 5.80; 95% CI: 1.72, 19.58; P = 0.0047), elevated

TABLE 1 | Baseline clinical characteristics and laboratory findings concerning patients with COVID-19 and hyperglycemia without previous diagnosis of diabetes.

Variables	All patients (n = 230)	Non-survivor (n = 44)	Survivor (n = 186)	*P*-value
Age, years				
Median, (IQR)	63.00 (54.00, 70.00)	69.00 (61.00, 73.50)	62.00 (52.00, 69.00)	0.0016
≤65, n (%)	136 (59.13)	16 (36.36)	120 (64.52)	0.0006
>65, n (%)	94 (40.87)	28 (63.64)	66 (35.48)	
Sex				
Female, n (%)	91 (39.57)	14 (31.82)	77 (41.40)	0.2426
Male, n (%)	139 (60.43)	30 (68.18)	109 (58.60)	
Onset symptoms				
Fever, n (%)	183/218 (83.94)	31/41 (75.61)	152/177 (85.88)	0.1067
Pharyngalgia, n (%)	8/201 (3.98)	2/38 (5.26)	6/163 (3.68)	0.6475
Fatigue, n (%)	100/206 (48.54)	21/39 (53.85)	79/167 (47.31)	0.4618
Muscular soreness, n (%)	42/203 (20.69)	12/38 (31.58)	30/165 (18.18)	0.0661
Cough, n (%)	158/210 (75.24)	27/40 (67.50)	131/170 (77.06)	0.2076
Expectoration, n (%)	84/205 (40.98)	22/40 (55.00)	62/165 (37.58)	0.0444
Hemoptysis, n (%)	6/202 (2.97)	0	6/164 (3.66)	0.5965
Dyspnea, n (%)	81/204 (39.71)	19/40 (47.50)	62/164 (37.80)	0.2612
Rhinorrhea, n (%)	3/202 (1.49)	1/40 (2.50)	2/162 (1.23)	0.4861
Nausea, n (%)	17/203 (8.37)	3/38 (7.89)	14/165 (8.48)	> 0.9999
Vomiting, n (%)	14/203 (6.90)	2/38 (5.26)	12/165 (7.27)	>0.9999
Stomach ache, n (%)	4/203 (1.97)	1/39 (2.56)	3/164 (1.83)	0.5770
Diarrhea, n (%)	29/204 (14.22)	6/40 (15.00)	23/164 (14.02)	0.8741
Poor appetite, n (%)	36/203 (17.73)	4/39 (10.26)	32/164 (19.51)	0.1738
Headache, n (%)	11/202 (5.45)	1/40 (2.50)	10/162 (6.17)	0.6964
Delirium, n (%)	0	0	0	0.3593
Chest distress, n (%)	66/204 (32.35)	17/40 (42.50)	49/164 (29.88)	0.1260
Non-symptoms, n (%)	0	0	0	0.1260
Comorbidity				
Chronic obstructive pulmonary disease, n (%)	3/198 (1.52)	1/40 (2.50)	2/158 (1.27)	0.4938
Asthma, n (%)	3/198 (1.52)	0	3/158 (1.90)	>0.9999
Hypertension, n (%)	74/202 (36.63)	15/40 (37.50)	59/162 (36.42)	0.8989
Chronic cardiac disease, n (%)	27/201 (13.43)	4/40 (10.00)	23/161 (14.29)	0.4768
Anemia, n (%)	1/197 (0.51)	1/40 (2.50)	0	0.2030
Chronic kidney disease, n (%)	9/197 (4.57)	3/40 (7.50)	6/157 (3.82)	0.3908
Chronic hepatic disease, n (%)	5/197 (2.54)	0	5/157 (3.18)	0.5852
Cerebrovascular disease, n (%)	6/197 (3.05)	2/40 (5.00)	4/157 (2.55)	0.6034
Malignant disease, n (%)	13/197 (6.60)	6/40 (15.00)	7/157 (4.46)	0.0165
Respiratory support				
Invasive mechanical ventilation, n (%)	26/230 (11.30)	17/44 (38.64)	9/186 (4.84)	<0.0001
Treatment				
Traditional Chinese medicine, n (%)	132/230 (57.39)	14/44 (31.81)	118/230 (63.44)	0.0001
Antiviral therapy, n (%)	210/230 (91.30)	40/44 (90.91)	170/186 (91.40)	<0.9999
Antibiotic therapy, n (%)	175/230 (76.09)	40/44 (90.91)	135/186 (72.58)	0.0180
Corticosteroid, n (%)	93/230 (40.43)	26/44 (59.09)	67/186 (36.02)	0.0050
Intravenous immunoglobin, n (%)	58/230 (25.22)	12/44 (27.27)	46/186 (24.73)	0.7270
Antihypertensive medicine, n (%)	46/230 (20.00)	3/44 (6.82)	43/186 (23.12)	0.0263
Lipid-lowering therapy, n (%)	11/230 (4.78)	1/44 (2.27)	10/186 (5.38)	0.6350
Hypoglycemic therapy, n (%)	11/230 (4.78)	6/44 (13.64)	5/186 (2.69)	0.0022
Laboratory findings				
Fasting blood glucose, mmol/L				
Median, (IQR)	6.79 (6.05, 8.49)	9.35 (8.13, 11.97)	6.49 (5.92, 7.52)	<0.0001
Low-stable, n (%)	202/230 (87.83)	27/44 (61.36)	175/186 (94.09)	<0.0001
High-stable, n (%)	28/230 (12.17)	17/44 (38.64)	11/186 (5.91)	
White blood cell count, $\times 10^9$ /L				0.0002
≤5.6, n (%)	63/230 (27.39)	2/44 (4.55)	61/186 (32.80)	
>5.6, n (%)	167/230 (72.61)	42/44 (95.45)	125/186 (67.20)	
Red blood cell count, $\times 10^{12}$ /L				0.1443
≤4.0, n (%)	129/230 (56.09)	29/44 (65.91)	100/186 (53.76)	
>4.0, n (%)	101/230 (43.91)	15/44 (34.09)	86/186 (46.24)	
Platelet count, $\times 10^9$ /L				<0.0001
≤136, n (%)	45/230 (19.57)	23/44 (52.27)	22/186 (11.83)	
>136, n (%)	185/230 (80.43)	21/44 (47.73)	164/186 (88.17)	
Neutrophil count, $\times 10^9$ /L				<0.0001
≤4.7, n (%)	92/230 (40.00)	2/44 (4.55)	90/186 (48.39)	

(Continued)

TABLE 1 | Continued

Variables	All patients (n = 230)	Non-survivor (n = 44)	Survivor (n = 186)	*P*-value
>4.7, n (%)	138/230 (60.00)	42/44 (95.45)	96/186 (51.61)	
Lymphocyte count, ×10^9 /L				<0.0001
≤0.7, n (%)	62/230 (26.96)	33/44 (75.00)	29/186 (15.59)	
>0.7, n (%)	168/230 (73.04)	11/44 (25.00)	157/186 (84.41)	
Monocyte count, ×10^9 /L				<0.0001
≤0.2, n (%)	14/230 (6.09)	10/44 (22.73)	4/186 (2.15)	
>0.2, n (%)	216/230 (93.91)	34/44 (77.27)	182/186 (97.85)	
Eosinophil count, ×10^9 /L				<0.0001
≤0.01, n (%)	23/230 (10.00)	13/44 (29.55)	10/186 (5.38)	
>0.01, n (%)	207/230 (90.00)	31/44 (70.45)	176/186 (94.62)	
Basophil count, ×10^9 /L				<0.0001
≤0.01, n (%)	38/230 (16.52)	7/44 (15.91)	31/186 (16.67)	
>0.01, n (%)	192/230 (83.48)	37/44 (84.09)	155/186 (83.33)	
Total bilirubin, µmol/L				<0.0001
≤12.3, n (%)	113/230 (49.13)	9/44 (20.45)	104/186 (55.91)	
>12.3, n (%)	117/230 (50.87)	35/44 (79.55)	82/186 (44.09)	
Direct bilirubin, µmol/L				<0.0001
≤4.6, n (%)	137/230 (59.57)	7/44 (15.91)	130/186 (69.89)	
>4.6, n (%)	93/230 (40.43)	37/44 (84.09)	56/186 (30.11)	
Alanine aminotransferase, U/L				0.4284
≤23.3, n (%)	25/230 (10.87)	3/44 (6.82)	22/186 (11.83)	
>23.3, n (%)	205/230 (89.13)	41/44 (93.18)	164/186 (88.17)	
Aspartate aminotransferase, U/L				0.0313
≤27.2, n (%)	61/230 (26.52)	6/44 (13.64)	55/186 (29.57)	
>27.2, n (%)	169/230 (73.48)	38/44 (86.36)	131/186 (70.43)	
Alkaline phosphatase, U/L				0.0014
≤53, n (%)	44/228 (19.30)	1/44 (2.27)	43/184 (23.37)	
>53, n (%)	184/228 (80.70)	43/44 (97.73)	141/184 (76.63)	
Glutamyl transpeptidase, U/L				0.9278
≤27.3, n (%)	53/228 (23.25)	10/44 (22.73)	43/184 (23.37)	
>27.3, n (%)	175/228 (76.75)	34/44 (77.27)	141/184 (76.63)	
Total protein, g/L				<0.0001
≤58.6, n (%)	59/230 (25.65)	23/44 (52.27)	36/186 (19.35)	
>58.6, n (%)	171/230 (74.35)	21/44 (47.73)	150/186 (80.65)	
Globulin, g/L				0.4592
≤30.5, n (%)	95/230 (41.30)	16/44 (36.36)	79/186 (42.47)	
>30.5, n (%)	135/230 (58.70)	28/44 (63.64)	107/186 (57.53)	
Prealbumin, mg/L				<0.0001
≤100.6, n (%)	37/210 (17.62)	24/44 (54.55)	13/166 (7.83)	
>100.6, n (%)	173/210 (82.38)	20/44 (45.45)	153/166 (92.17)	
Albumin, g/L				<0.0001
≤33.8, n (%)	163/230 (70.87)	44/44 (100.00)	119/186 (63.98)	
>33.8, n (%)	67/230 (29.13)	0	67/186 (36.02)	
Total bile acid, µmol/L				0.0695
≤3.5, n (%)	95/228 (41.67)	13/44 (29.55)	82/184 (44.57)	
>3.5, n (%)	133/228 (58.33)	31/44 (70.45)	102/184 (55.43)	
Creatinine, µmol/L				<0.0001
≤111, n (%)	203/230 (88.26)	24/44 (54.55)	179/186 (96.24)	
>111, n (%)	27/230 (11.74)	20/44 (45.45)	7/186 (3.76)	
Blood Urea Nitrogen, mmol/L				<0.0001
≤8.2, n (%)	174/230 (75.65)	14/44 (31.82)	160/186 (86.02)	
>8.2, n (%)	56/230 (24.35)	30/44 (68.18)	26/186 (13.98)	
Uric acid, µmol/L				0.0001
≤428, n (%)	217/230 (94.35)	36/44 (81.82)	181/186 (97.31)	
>428, n (%)	13/230 (5.65)	8/44 (18.18)	5/186 (2.69)	
Creatine kinase, U/L				0.0002
≤83, n (%)	108/214 (50.47)	11/44 (25.00)	97/170 (57.06)	
>83, n (%)	106/214 (49.53)	33/44 (75.00)	73/170 (42.94)	
D-dimer, µg/mL				<0.0001
≤0.97, n (%)	84/223 (37.67)	2/43 (4.65)	82/180 (45.56)	
>0.97, n (%)	139/223 (62.33)	41/43 (95.35)	98/180 (54.44)	
Prothrombin time, s				<0.0001
≤14.3, n (%)	158/223 (70.85)	13/43 (30.23)	145/180 (80.56)	

(Continued)

TABLE 1 | Continued

Variables	All patients (n = 230)	Non-survivor (n = 44)	Survivor (n = 186)	*P*-value
>14.3, n (%)	65/223 (29.15)	30/43 (69.77)	35/180 (19.44)	
International Normalized Ratio				<0.0001
≤1.1, n (%)	141/223 (63.23)	13/43 (30.23)	128/180 (71.11)	
>1.1, n (%)	82/223 (36.77)	30/43 (69.77)	52/180 (28.89)	
Activated partial thromboplastin time, s				<0.0001
≤40.2, n (%)	164/226 (72.57)	19/43 (44.19)	145/183 (79.23)	
>40.2, n (%)	62/226 (27.43)	24/43 (55.81)	38/183 (20.77)	
Thromboplastin time, s				0.0123
≤16.5, n (%)	164/218 (75.23)	26/43 (60.47)	138/175 (78.86)	
>16.5, n (%)	54/218 (24.77)	17/43 (39.53)	37/175 (21.14)	
Fibrinogen, g/L				0.0568
≤4.1, n (%)	124/226 (54.87)	18/43 (41.86)	106/183 (57.92)	
>4.1, n (%)	102/226 (45.13)	25/43 (58.14)	77/183 (42.08)	
C-reactive protein, mg/L				<0.0001
≤21.4, n (%)	83/224 (37.05)	0	83/180 (46.11)	
>21.4, n (%)	141/224 (62.95)	44/44 (100.00)	97/180 (53.89)	
Erythrocyte sedimentation rate, mm/h				0.6486
≤22, n (%)	10/91 (10.99)	2/14 (14.29)	8/77 (10.39)	
>22, n (%)	81/91 (89.01)	12/14 (85.71)	69/77 (89.61)	

Data are median (IQR) or n (%). P-values were calculated using χ^2 test, Cochran–Mantel–Haenszel χ^2 test, Fisher's exact test or Wilcoxon rank-sum test, as appropriate. IQR, interquartile range.

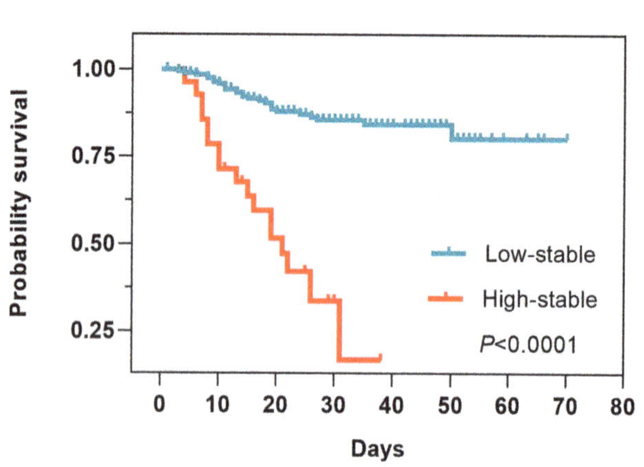

FIGURE 3 | Survival analysis between low-stable and high-stable pattern trajectories.

creatinine (OR, 26.69; 95% CI: 5.82, 122.29; $P < 0.0001$), lymphopenia (OR, 8.07; 95% CI: 2.70, 24.14; $P = 0.0002$), and high-stable FBG pattern (OR, 8.79; 95% CI: 2.39, 32.29; $P = 0.0011$) were independent risk factors for higher case fatality in patients with COVID-19 with hyperglycemia but with no history of diabetes (**Table 2**). Finally, FBG levels were higher and tended to increase during hospitalization in non-survivors more than in survivors ($P <$ 0.001, **Supplementary Figure 2**).

The Relationship Between a Reduction in the FBG Level During Hospitalization and Prognosis

Among the 230 patients, 11 (4.78%) who had been treated with hypoglycemic therapy were all in the high-stable pattern group. There were no statistically significant differences in terms of patient's outcomes for those treated with or without hypoglycemic therapy in the patients with a high-stable pattern ($P = 0.7011$). In 146 patients (63.48%), including 9 patients who died, final FBG levels prior to discharge or death decreased relative to their on-admission FBG, whereas 84 patients (36.52%), including 35 who died, had increased final FBG relative to their on-admission FBG. Patients with decreased FBG had a lower risk of death compared to those with increased FBG (OR, 0.092; 95% CI: 0.041, 0.205; $P < 0.0001$).

In **Supplementary Figure 3**, we present the results of associations between the glycemic variations and the evolution of biochemical parameters. There were several statistically significant correlations between the glycemic variations and routine blood tests, liver and kidney function, and coagulation indicators; however, Pearson's correlation coefficients (r) were all very small (all $r < 0.4$) suggesting that the strength of these relationships was weak.

DISCUSSION

In this study, we analyzed clinical characteristics and outcomes in relation to 230 patients with COVID-19 and abnormal FBG but without a previous diagnosis of diabetes. In preliminary study, we found that FBG ≥7.0 mmol/L at admission could predict the risk of 28-day mortality in patients with COVID-19 without previous diagnosis of diabetes (7). It has also been reported that at-admission hyperglycemia (at-admission glycemia ≥7.78 mmol/L) is a major and independent risk factor associated with a poor prognosis in people hospitalized for COVID-19 (20). However, much of our understanding of FBG levels in patients with COVID-19 has been derived from cross-sectional data. In this study, we investigated changes in FBG in hospitalized patients throughout the course of their treatment for COVID-19. This current study extended those findings to demonstrate that not only is at-admission glycemia

TABLE 2 | Univariable and multivariable analyses for death concerning all study patients.

		Univariable analysis OR (95% CI)	*P*-value	Multivariable analysis OR (95% CI)	*P*-value
FBG trajectories	Low-stable	Ref			
	High-stable	10.02 (4.24, 23.67)	<0.0001	8.79 (2.39, 32.29)	0.0011
Age, years	≤65	Ref			
	>65	3.18 (1.61, 6.30)	0.0009		
Sex	Female	0 (ref)			
	Male	1.51 (0.75, 3.04)	0.2447		
Neutrophil count, $\times10^9$ /L	≤4.7	0 (ref)			
	>4.7	19.69 (4.63, 83.71)	<0.0001	25.43 (2.07, 313.03)	0.0115
Direct bilirubin, μmol/L	≤4.6	0 (ref)			
	>4.6	12.27 (5.16, 29.18)	<0.0001	5.80 (1.72, 19.58)	0.0047
Creatinine, μmol/L	≤111	0 (ref)			
	>111	21.30 (8.15, 55.65)	<0.0001	26.69 (5.82, 122.29)	<0.0001
Prothrombin time, s	≤14.3	0 (ref)			
	>14.3	9.56 (4.52, 20.20)	<0.0001		
Lymphocyte count, $\times10^9$ /L	≤0.7	16.24 (7.38, 35.75)		8.07 (2.70, 24.14)	0.0002
	>0.7	1 (ref)	<0.0001		
Uric acid, μmol/L	≤428	0 (ref)			
	>428	8.04 (2.49, 26.00)	0.0005		
Prealbumin, g/L	≤100.6	14.12 (6.22, 32.07)			
	>100.6	1 (ref)	<0.0001		
Eosinophil count, $\times10^9$ /L	≤0.01	0 (ref)			
	>0.01	7.38 (2.98, 18.31)	<0.0001		

FBG, fasting blood glucose; OR, odds ratio.

important, but also that certain populations, such as patients with high-stable FBG patterns, were more likely to have consistently high FBG levels, placing them at higher risk of a poor outcome than those with low FBG levels.

We observed heterogeneous FBG patterns in patients with COVID-19 during their entire hospitalization period. We identified two distinctive trajectories, namely, low-stable and high-stable patterns. The average FBG level ranged from 6.63 mmol/L to 7.54 mmol/L in patients with the low-stable pattern, whereas the average FBG level ranged from 12.59 mmol/L to 14.02 mmol/L in patients with the high-stable pattern. This finding indicated that patients with a high-stable pattern fulfilled diagnostic criteria for diabetes, which involve a patient having classic symptoms of hyperglycemia or a hyperglycemic crisis and a random plasma glucose level ≥200 mg/dl (11.1 mmol/L) (21). Our study findings showed that corticosteroid therapy was associated with patient outcomes and the FBG trajectory. It is known that corticosteroids can induce hyperglycemia, which results from impairment of multiple pathways affecting carbohydrate metabolism. Glucocorticoids cause hepatic insulin resistance, resulting in increased hepatic glucose output and induce peripheral insulin resistance, which predominantly reflects insulin action in skeletal muscle (22). The American Diabetes Association defined stress-induced hyperglycemia as >140 mg/dl (7.77 mmol/L) in patients with no previous diagnosis of diabetes (23). Although many patients have multiple episodes of abnormal FBG during hospitalization, it remains unclear whether a patient should be diagnosed with type 2 diabetes, considering the possibility of stress hyperglycemia and the effect of medications on blood glucose. In a prospective cohort study, discrete FBG trajectories were significantly associated with subsequent risk of myocardial infarction and cancer in individuals without diabetes (24, 25). In addition to diabetes, changes in FBG may also play a key role in the development of other diseases. Moreover, the FBG data were more accessible than other laboratory indicators and the relationship between FBG trajectories and disease, except diabetes, was also more closely investigated.

Individuals with the high-stable pattern were more likely to have abnormal laboratory data in relation to including inflammatory cell counts (neutrophil, lymphocyte, and monocyte counts), serum liver and kidney function indicators, and coagulation function indicators than those with the low-stable pattern (**Supplementary Table 1**). A previous study revealed that hyperglycemia (12 mmol/L), regardless of the level of insulin, activated the coagulation cascade (13). In our study, 89.29% of the patients with the high-stable pattern had high D-dimer levels, which was consistent with the results reported in the aforementioned studies. Moreover, patients with systemic inflammatory response syndrome tend to be hyperglycemic (26). One clinical trial reported that hyperglycemia also enhanced coagulation and reduced neutrophil degranulation in patients during systemic inflammation (27). These results further support our findings.

The findings of our analysis indicated that participants with a high-stable FBG pattern had a higher risk of death. These findings provide a novel insight into the long-term patterns of FBG change and highlight that, among patients with COVID-19 without diabetes, there are heterogeneous FBG trajectories. To our knowledge, no prior study has examined the potential effect of FBG trajectories on the risk of death in patients with COVID-19 and with no prior diagnosis of diabetes. Similarly, it has been reported that severe hyperglycemia after admission is a strong predictor of death among patients with COVID-19 not requiring intensive care unit admission (28), which is consistent with our results. A recent study found that patients who had higher average glucose during their first week of hospitalization were more likely to have comorbidity and abnormal laboratory markers, and were at greater risk of severe pneumonia, acute respiratory distress syndrome, and death (29). Our data further confirmed that higher FBG during the entire hospitalization was independently correlated with death. Our findings indicate that a patient's FBG is a more sensitive marker of metabolic balance.

Results of our multivariable logistic regression analysis also showed that increased neutrophil count, elevated DBIL and creatinine, and lymphopenia were independently associated with case fatality in patients with COVID-19 and no prior diagnosis of diabetes (**Table 2**). In addition, our findings suggest that non-survivors of COVID-19 were more likely to accept IMV treatment than survivors. Moreover, a higher proportion of patients with the high-stability FBG pattern received IMV treatment than those with the low-stability FBG pattern.

Our findings provide direct evidence to support recent suggestions that regularly monitoring FBG in patients with COVID-19 is of significance in terms of public health, and for clinical diagnosis and treatment. One recent study reported that continuous glucose monitoring was more sensitive than HbA1c and fasting glucose measurements in detecting dysglycemia in a Spanish population without diabetes; therefore, continuous blood glucose monitoring could facilitate screening and prompt treatment in patients with suspected dysglycemia (27). We recommend that more attention should be paid to the trajectories of the FBG pattern throughout the disease course rather than focusing particularly on one single measurement. It has been previously reported that well-controlled blood glucose levels and maintaining glycemic variability within 3.9–10.0 mmol/L is associated with a significant reduction in composite adverse outcomes and death among patients with COVID-19 with type 2 diabetes (11). A retrospective study of 2,748 medical patients in an intensive care unit showed that blood glucose levels exceeding the upper and lower limits of the normoglycemic range (4.4–6.1 mmol/L) sustained over time, a high amplitude variation, and a high entropy of blood glucose time series were independently associated with hospital mortality (30). Therefore, these findings suggest that sustained high levels or a high amplitude variation of FBG might not be beneficial for patients with COVID-19.

Nevertheless, hypoglycemic therapy, especially insulin treatment, has remained controversial for patients with COVID-19. No significant difference was found between patients treated with hypoglycemic therapy and those who were not in the high-stable pattern group in this study, which may be due to the smaller number of patients included. However, our data showed that reducing the FBG level during hospitalization may improve prognosis, suggesting that a decreased FBG may be a protective factor. One study reported that, among 25 patients with glycemic levels >7.7 mmol/L, 10 patients treated without insulin infusion had a higher risk of severe disease, including increased mortality, compared with 15 patients treated with insulin infusion (13). However, insulin treatment has been reportedly associated with increased mortality in patients with COVID-19 and type 2 diabetes (31). However, randomized controlled studies involving tight glycemic control have reported increased incidences of hypoglycemia when targeting normoglycemia (32). Moreover, a clear association has been found between the occurrence of hypoglycemia and increased mortality in critically ill patients (32), possibly due to a lack of timely changes in medication or dose adjustment. Thus, regular FBG monitoring is vital for assisting clinicians in making treatment adjustments. For critically ill patients or those with severe sepsis, the recommended strategy for glycemic control is that insulin therapy should be started when blood glucose exceeds 180 mg/dl (10 mmol/L), with a goal of maintaining blood glucose between 144 and 180 mg/dL (8–10 mmol/L) using insulin, as necessary (33, 34). Although there are no data regarding optimal glycemic targets for inpatients with COVID-19, it is clear that extreme FBG levels can lead to poor outcomes, and that continuous blood glucose monitoring and timely and appropriate blood glucose control may contribute to positive patient outcomes.

Due to its retrospective design and the unprecedented scale of the COVID-19 pandemic, this study had several limitations. First, this was a retrospective study. Second, out study comprised a small number of participants. Because the FBG measurement time was not regular and repeat FBG examinations might have been scheduled according to the change in the patient's condition. Third, HbA1c data, used for the assessment of glycemic status before admission, were missing; therefore, we could not distinguish whether elevated FBG levels corresponded to stress hyperglycemia or to a previous history of diabetes. Fourth, the data lacked external validation.

In conclusion, in this study, we identified two FBG trajectories and found that these patterns were significantly associated with the risk of death in patients with COVID-19 without diabetes. Monitoring FBG trajectories may provide an important approach to assist clinicians in assessing disease conditions and in adjusting medication or dosages. Future research needs to explore the key risk factors associated with elevated FBG trajectories.

AUTHOR CONTRIBUTIONS

YJ designed this study. SS, SZ, YM, PM, and HL collected all the data. SS and ZW analyzed the data. SW, YM, PM, HL, and MW interpreted the data. SS and SZ drafted the initial manuscript. All authors reviewed the first draft and provided essential suggestions on revision. SS and SZ revised the final manuscript. YJ is the guarantor of this work and takes responsibility for the contents of the article. All authors contributed to the article and approved the submitted version.

ACKNOWLEDGMENTS

We heartily thank the healthcare workers who have fought COVID-19 on the front lines during this pandemic.

SUPPLEMENTARY MATERIAL

Supplementary Figure 1 | Variables selection using LASSO regression model. **(A)** Tuning parameters (λ) selection in LASSO model used 10-fold cross-validation *via* minimum criteria. **(B)** LASSO coefficient profile of 42 clinical features (age, sex, 8 treatments, and 32 laboratory indices).

Supplementary Figure 2 | Relationship between changes in fasting blood glucose levels and the monitoring time in survivors and non-survivors.

Supplementary Figure 3 | Visual correlation matrix of glycemic variations and the evolution of biochemical parameters. This figure provides a visual representation of the respective correlations as measured using Pearson's correlation coefficients (r), based on $P = 0.05$. The color-intensity signal indicates correlation strength, whereas the blue and red colors indicate strong positive and negative correlations, respectively. * <0.05. **(A)** The metrics (columns) represent biochemical parameters in blood routine test. **(B)** The metrics (columns) represent biochemical parameters in hepatic and renal function tests. **(C)** The metrics (columns) represent biochemical parameters in coagulation function test.

REFERENCES

1. WHO. *Coronavirus disease (COVID-19) pandemic.* Available at: https://www.who.int/emergencies/diseases/novel-coronavirus-2019 (Accessed 2021 February 17).
2. Wu Z, McGoogan JM. Characteristics of and Important Lessons From the Coronavirus Disease 2019 (COVID-19) Outbreak in China: Summary of a Report of 72 314 Cases From the Chinese Center for Disease Control and Prevention. *Jama* (2020) 323:1239–42. doi: 10.1001/jama.2020.2648
3. Benfield T, Jensen JS, Nordestgaard BG. Influence of diabetes and hyperglycaemia on infectious disease hospitalisation and outcome. *Diabetologia* (2007) 50:549–54. doi: 10.1007/s00125-006-0570-3
4. Rao Kondapally Seshasai S, Kaptoge S, Thompson A, Di Angelantonio E, Gao P, Sarwar N, et al. Diabetes mellitus, fasting glucose, and risk of cause-specific death. *New Engl J Med* (2011) 364:829–41. doi: 10.1056/NEJMoa1008862
5. Yang JK, Feng Y, Yuan MY, Yuan SY, Fu HJ, Wu BY, et al. Plasma glucose levels and diabetes are independent predictors for mortality and morbidity in patients with SARS. *Diabetic Med J Br Diabetic Assoc* (2006) 23:623–8. doi: 10.1111/j.1464-5491.2006.01861.x
6. Alanazi KH, Abedi GR, Midgley CM, Alkhamis A, Alsaqer T, Almoaddi A, et al. Diabetes Mellitus, Hypertension, and Death among 32 Patients with MERS-CoV Infection, Saudi Arabia. *Emerging Infect Dis* (2020) 26:166–8. doi: 10.3201/eid2601.190952
7. Wang S, Ma P, Zhang S, Song S, Wang Z, Ma Y, et al. Fasting blood glucose at admission is an independent predictor for 28-day mortality in patients with COVID-19 without previous diagnosis of diabetes: a multi-centre retrospective study. *Diabetologia* (2020) 63:2102–11. doi: 10.1007/s00125-020-05209-1
8. Zhang Y, Li H, Zhang J, Cao Y, Zhao X, Yu N, et al. The clinical characteristics and outcomes of patients with diabetes and secondary hyperglycaemia with coronavirus disease 2019: A single-centre, retrospective, observational study in Wuhan. *Diabetes Obes Metab* (2020) 22:1443–54. doi: 10.1111/dom.14086
9. Esposito K, Nappo F, Marfella R, Giugliano G, Giugliano F, Ciotola M, et al. Inflammatory cytokine concentrations are acutely increased by hyperglycemia in humans: role of oxidative stress. *Circulation* (2002) 106:2067–72. doi: 10.1161/01.CIR.0000034509.14906.AE
10. Nieuwdorp M, van Haeften TW, Gouverneur MC, Mooij HL, van Lieshout MH, Levi M, et al. Loss of endothelial glycocalyx during acute hyperglycemia coincides with endothelial dysfunction and coagulation activation in vivo. *Diabetes* (2006) 55:480–6. doi: 10.2337/diabetes.55.02.06.db05-1103
11. Zhu L, She ZG, Cheng X, Qin JJ, Zhang XJ, Cai J, et al. Association of Blood Glucose Control and Outcomes in Patients with COVID-19 and Pre-existing Type 2 Diabetes. *Cell Metab* (2020) 31:1068–77.e3. doi: 10.1016/j.cmet.2020.04.021
12. Bode B, Garrett V, Messler J, McFarland R, Crowe J, Booth R, et al. Glycemic Characteristics and Clinical Outcomes of COVID-19 Patients Hospitalized in the United States. *J Diabetes Sci Technol* (2020) 14:813–21. doi: 10.1177/1932296820924469
13. Sardu C, D'Onofrio N, Balestrieri ML, Barbieri M, Rizzo MR, Messina V, et al. Outcomes in Patients With Hyperglycemia Affected by COVID-19: Can We Do More on Glycemic Control? *Diabetes Care* (2020) 43:1408–15. doi: 10.2337/dc20-0723
14. WHO and WHO. *Laboratory testing for coronavirus disease 2019 (COVID-19) in suspected human cases* (2020). Available at: www.who.int/publications-detail/laboratory-testing-for-2019-novel-coronavirus-in-suspected-human-cases-20200117 (Accessed 2020 21 October).
15. WHO. *Definition and diagnosis of diabetes mellitus and intermediate hyperglycaemia.* Available at: https://www.who.int/publications/i/item/definition-and-diagnosis-of-diabetes-mellitus-and-intermediate-hyperglycaemia (Accessed 2020 21 Ocotober).
16. National Health Commission of the People's Republic of China. *Diagnosis and treatment plan of coronavirus disease 2019 (COVID-19) (trial version 6)* (2020). Available at: www.nhc.gov.cn/yzygj/s7653p/202002/8334a8326dd94d329df351d7da8aefc2/files/b218cfeb1bc54639af227f922bf6b817.pdf (Accessed 2020 21 October).
17. Nagin DS, Odgers CL. Group-based trajectory modeling in clinical research. *Annu Rev Clin Psychol* (2010) 6:109–38. doi: 10.1146/annurev.clinpsy.121208.131413
18. Nagin DS. Group-Based Trajectory Modeling: An Overview. In: Piquero, Weisburd, editors. *Handbook of Quantitative Criminology.* New York: Springer (2009) p. 53–67.
19. Nylund KL, Asparoutiov T, Muthen BO. Deciding on the number of classes in latent class analysis and growth mixture modeling: A Monte Carlo simulation study. *Struct Equ Modeling* (2007) 14:535–69. doi: 10.1080/10705510701575396
20. Coppelli A, Giannarelli R, Aragona M, Penno G, Falcone M, Tiseo G, et al. Hyperglycemia at Hospital Admission Is Associated With Severity of the Prognosis in Patients Hospitalized for COVID-19: The Pisa COVID-19 Study. *Diabetes Care* (2020) 43:2345. doi: 10.2337/dc20-1380
21. American Diabetes Association. 2. Classification and Diagnosis of Diabetes: Standards of Medical Care in Diabetes-2018. *Diabetes Care* (2018) 41:S13–27. doi: 10.2337/dc18-S002
22. Anjana R, Morton GB. MANAGEMENT OF ENDOCRINE DISEASE: Critical review of the evidence underlying management of glucocorticoid-induced hyperglycaemia. *Eur J Endocrinol* (2018) 179:R207–18. doi: 10.1530/EJE-18-0315
23. Moghissi ES, Korytkowski MT, DiNardo M, Einhorn D, Hellman R, Hirsch IB, et al. American Association of Clinical Endocrinologists and American Diabetes Association Consensus Statement on Inpatient Glycemic Control. *Diabetes Care* (2009) 32:1119. doi: 10.2337/dc09-9029
24. Jin C, Chen S, Vaidya A, Wu Y, Wu Z, Hu FB, et al. Longitudinal Change in Fasting Blood Glucose and Myocardial Infarction Risk in a Population Without Diabetes. *Diabetes Care* (2017) 40:1565–72. doi: 10.2337/dc17-0610
25. Feng X, Wang G, Lyu Z, Chen S, Wei L, Li X, et al. The association between fasting blood glucose trajectory and cancer risk in Chinese population without diabetes. *Int J Cancer* (2020) 147:958–66. doi: 10.1002/ijc.32858
26. Bar-Or D, Rael LT, Madayag RM, Banton KL, Tanner A,2, Acuna DL, et al. Stress Hyperglycemia in Critically Ill Patients: Insight Into Possible Molecular Pathways. *Front Med (Lausanne)* (2019) 6:54–4. doi: 10.3389/fmed.2019.00054
27. Stegenga ME, van der Crabben SN, Blümer RME, Levi M, Meijers JCM, Serlie MJ, et al. Hyperglycemia enhances coagulation and reduces neutrophil degranulation, whereas hyperinsulinemia inhibits fibrinolysis during human endotoxemia. *Blood* (2008) 112:82–9. doi: 10.1182/blood-2007-11-121723
28. Klonoff DC, Messler JC, Umpierrez GE, Peng L, Booth R, Crowe J, et al. Association Between Achieving Inpatient Glycemic Control and Clinical Outcomes in Hospitalized Patients With COVID-19: A Multicenter, Retrospective Hospital-Based Analysis. *Diabetes Care* (2021) 44:578–85. doi: 10.2337/dc20-1857
29. Chen L, Sun W, Liu Y, Zhang L, Lv Y, Wang Q, et al. Association of Early-Phase In-Hospital Glycemic Fluctuation With Mortality in Adult Patients With Coronavirus Disease 2019. *Diabetes Care* (2021) 44:865–73. doi: 10.2337/dc20-0780

30. Meyfroidt G, Keenan DM, Wang X, Wouters PJ, Veldhuis JD. and Van den Berghe, G., Dynamic characteristics of blood glucose time series during the course of critical illness: effects of intensive insulin therapy and relative association with mortality. *Crit Care Med* (2010) 38:1021–9. doi: 10.1097/CCM.0b013e3181cf710e
31. Yu B, Li C, Sun Y, Wang DW. Insulin Treatment Is Associated with Increased Mortality in Patients with COVID-19 and Type 2 Diabetes. *Cell Metab* (2021) 33:65–77.e2. doi: 10.1016/j.cmet.2020.11.014
32. Annane D, Cariou A, Maxime V, Azoulay E, D'Honneur G, Timsit JF, et al. Corticosteroid treatment and intensive insulin therapy for septic shock in adults: a randomized controlled trial. *Jama* (2010) 303:341–8. doi: 10.1001/jama.2010.2
33. American Diabetes A. Standards of medical care in diabetes–2012. *Diabetes Care* (2012) 35 Suppl 1:S11–63. doi: 10.2337/dc12-s011
34. Dellinger RP, Levy MM, Rhodes A, Annane D, Gerlach H, Opal SM, et al. Surviving Sepsis Campaign: international guidelines for management of severe sepsis and septic shock, 2012. *Intensive Care Med* (2013) 39:165–228. doi: 10.1007/s00134-012-2769-8

18

Association Between Diabetes and COVID-19: A Retrospective Observational Study with a Large Sample of 1,880 Cases in Leishenshan Hospital, Wuhan

Zeming Liu[1†], Jinpeng Li[2†], Jianglong Huang[1†], Liang Guo[1†], Rongfen Gao[3†], Kuan Luo[4], Guang Zeng[5], Tingbao Zhang[6], Meilin Yi[7], Yihui Huang[1], Jincao Chen[6], Yibin Yang[8*] and Xiaohui Wu[6*]*

[1] Department of Plastic Surgery, Zhongnan Hospital of Wuhan University, Wuhan, China, [2] Department of Thyroid and Breast Surgery, Zhongnan Hospital of Wuhan University, Wuhan, China, [3] Department of Rheumatology and Immunology, Tongji Medical College, Tongji Hospital, Huazhong University of Science and Technology, Wuhan, China, [4] Department of Neurosurgery, Wuhan Puren Hospital, Wuhan, China, [5] Department of Urology, Zhongnan Hospital of Wuhan University, Wuhan, China, [6] Department of Neurosurgery, Zhongnan Hospital of Wuhan University, Wuhan, China, [7] Department of Burn and Plastic Surgery, College of Traditional Chinese Medicine, Three Gorges University, Yichang Hospital of Traditional Chinese Medicine, Yichang, China, [8] Department of Respiratory and Critical Care Medicine, Zhongnan Hospital of Wuhan University, Wuhan, China

***Correspondence:**
Jincao Chen
chenjincao@hotmail.com
Yibin Yang
1594559173@qq.com
Xiaohui Wu
wuxiaohui1971@sina.com

† These authors have contributed equally to this work

Aims: This study aimed to investigate the clinical courses and outcomes of diabetes mellitus patients with coronavirus disease 2019 (COVID-19) in Wuhan.

Methods: This study enrolled 1,880 consecutive patients with confirmed COVID-19 in Leishenshan Hospital. We collected and analyzed their data, including demographic data, history of comorbidity, clinical symptoms, laboratory tests, chest computed tomography (CT) images, treatment options, and survival.

Results: The percentages of patients with diabetes among the severe and critical COVID-19 cases were higher than those among the mild or general cases (89.2%, 10.8 vs. 0%, $p = 0.001$). However, patients with and without diabetes showed no difference in the follow-up period ($p = 0.993$). The mortality rate in patients with or without diabetes was 2.9% ($n = 4$) and 1.1% ($n = 9$), respectively ($p = 0.114$). Univariate and multivariate Cox regression analyses and the Kaplan-Meier curves did not show any statistically significant differences between patients with and without diabetes (all $p > 0.05$).

Conclusions: Our study results suggested that diabetes had no effect on the prognosis of COVID-19 patients but had a negative association with their clinical courses. These results may be useful for clinicians in the management of diabetic patients with COVID-19.

Keywords: clinical courses, comorbidity, Coronavirus disease 2019 (COVID-19), diabetes mellitus, prognosis

INTRODUCTION

Coronavirus disease 2019 (COVID-19) cause by severe acute respiratory syndrome–coronavirus 2 (SARS-CoV-2) was first identified in Wuhan, China, and has subsequently and quickly spread to more than 70 countries, including the United States, Spain, and Italy (1, 2). SARS-CoV-2 could cause severe, even lethal pneumonia and lung failure. As of April 25, 2020, more than 2,800,000 confirmed cases and 190,000 deaths of COVID-19 have been reported worldwide (3).

As an emergency specialty field hospital hosted by the Zhongnan hospital, Leishenshan Hospital was put into use in February to provide treatment for COVID-19 patients in Wuhan, marking a milestone in China's battle against COVID-19. In Leishenshan Hospital, 1,880 patients were diagnosed with COVID-19 between February 8, 2020 and April 15, 2020. Among those patients, 139 cases had a previous diagnosis of diabetes mellitus.

Diabetes mellitus (DM) is a common endocrine disease (4) and widely known as a chronic, low-grade inflammatory disease caused by long-term immune system imbalance, metabolic syndrome, or nutrient excess (5, 6). Since the outbreak of COVID-19, several studies have been conducted to examine the relationship between diabetes and COVID-19 (1, 7, 8). However, their sample sizes were relatively small, and they did not clarify whether diabetes was a predictor of poor clinical outcomes and higher mortality of COVID-19. In this study, we investigated the association between diabetes as a comorbidity and negative clinical courses and outcomes of COVID-19 in a large sample of patients from a single hospital in Wuhan, China. The findings are expected to inform follow-up clinical treatment for patients with both diseases and COVID-19.

MATERIALS AND METHODS

Study Design and Participants

This single-center retrospective observational study was conducted on 1,880 patients diagnosed with COVID-19 at Leishenshan Hospital. After excluding cases without information about the history of diabetes, the final sample included 934 patients. Data were collected on admission or during hospitalization by attending physicians and documented in the form of electronic medical records. This study was approved by the Ethics Commission of the Zhongnan Hospital of Wuhan University (Approval number: 2020074) and carried out in accordance with the principles of the Declaration of Helsinki revised in 2008. The need for informed consent from patients was waived due to the time constraints during the COVID-19 emergency.

Data Collection

We collected data of 1,880 patients from their medical records. These data included age, sex, comorbidities, levels of illness severity (mild, moderate, severe, and critical), signs and symptoms, treatment options (i.e., antiviral therapy, antibiotic therapy, traditional Chinese medicine therapy, anticoagulation therapy, and administration of corticosteroid and Vitamin C), laboratory findings, and computed tomography (CT) images. All the data were reviewed and analyzed by two senior physicians.

Outcomes

The primary outcomes of this study included the survival of patients (alive vs. dead) and their highest level of illness severity. Another important primary outcome was the patients' CT score—a semi-quantitative scoring system—generated according to the features of CT images. Each of the CT image features, namely ground-glass opacities, reticulation or cords change, consolidation, and pleural effusions, was assigned 1 point. Score 1 was the sum of points, and score 2 ranged from 0 to 4 points based on the area of lung involvement: no involvement, 0; <25% involvement, 1; 26–50% involvement, 2; 51–75% involvement, 3; and 76–100% involvement, 4. The total score was the sum of score 1 and score 2.

Statistical Analysis

Normally distributed continuous variables are expressed as means ± standard deviations, and non-normally distributed continuous variables as medians and interquartile ranges. Meanwhile, categorical variables are described as frequencies and percentages. The independent t-test or Mann-Whitney U-test was conducted to compare continuous variables between the group of patients with diabetes (Group 2) and that of patients without diabetes (Group 1). Meanwhile, the χ^2-test or Fisher's exact test was used to analyze the associations between categorical variables. Cox regression analysis and the Kaplan-Meier survival curves were performed to explore the prognosis of patients with and without diabetes. Besides, curve fitting analysis was conducted to further evaluate the association between the CT score and the duration from symptom onset (in days) in both groups. Two-sided $p < 0{\cdot}05$ were considered as statistically significant, and all statistical analyses were performed using SPSS (version 23.0 for windows).

RESULTS

Study Participants' Demographic and Clinical Information and Laboratory Findings

Table 1 shows that Group 2 consisted of 139 patients whereas Group 1 had 795 patients. The two groups showed no differences in gender distribution (p = 0.076), means of age (p = 0.773), and the number of patients with malignancy, nervous system disease, and digestive system disease (all $p > 0.05$). However, they showed a significant difference in the number of patients with cardiovascular or pulmonary disease (both $p < 0.05$). The percentages of patients with diabetes among the severe and critical COVID-19 cases were higher than among the mild or general cases (89.2%, 10.8 vs. 0%, p = 0.001). However, no difference was observed in the follow-up period between patients with and without diabetes (p = 0.993). The mortality rate was 2.9% ($n = 4$) in Group 2 and 1.1% ($n = 9$) in Group 1 ($p = 0.114$). As shown in **Table 2**, the positive rate of IgG against SARS-CoV-2 among patients with diabetes was lower than that among those without diabetes (82.5 vs. 91.8%, $p = 0.029$).

TABLE 1 | Demographics and clinical characteristics of patients with COVID-19.

Covariate	Group 1* ($n = 795$)	Group 2# ($n = 139$)	*P*-value
Age, year	61.6 ± 14.5	64.5 ± 10.0	0.076
Sex			
Male	388 (48.8%)	66 (47.5%)	0.773
Female	407 (51.2%)	73 (52.5%)	
Comorbidity			
Cardiovascular disease	275 (34.6%)	89 (64.0%)	<0.001
Pulmonary disease	90 (11.8%)	3 (2.4%)	0.001
Malignancy	52 (6.5%)	14 (10.1%)	0.134
Nervous system disease	47 (5.9%)	12 (8.6%)	0.224
Digestive system disease	39 (4.9%)	7 (5.0%)	0.948
The highest level of severity			
Mild and general	19 (2.4%)	0 (0)	0.001
Severe	739 (93.3%)	124 (89.2%)	
Critical	34 (4.3%)	15 (10.8%)	
Status of illness when admission			
Mild	286 (38.2%)	43 (30.9%)	0.150
General	211 (28.2%)	37 (26.6%)	
Severe	235 (31.4%)	53 (38.1%)	
Critical	17 (2.3%)	6 (4.3%)	
Symptoms when admitted to the hospital			
Fever or Myalgia	559 (78.8%)	95 (76.6%)	0.577
Respiratory system symptoms	571 (80.5%)	104 (83.9%)	0.382
Digestive system symptoms	77 (10.9%)	13 (10.5%)	0.901
Nervous system symptoms	22 (3.1%)	5 (4.0%)	0.590
Antiviral therapy	449 (98.0%)	86 (97.7%)	0.693
Antibiotic therapy	297 (98.3%)	47 (97.9%)	0.590
The appliance of Vitamin C	106 (98.1%)	19 (100.0%)	1.000
Traditional Chinese medicine therapy	687 (99.7%)	118 (100.0%)	1.000
Anticoagulation treatment	98 (12.3%)	21 (15.1%)	0.364
Use of corticosteroid	82 (10.3%)	16 (11.5%)	0.671
Deaths	9 (1.1%)	4 (2.9%)	0.114
Follow-up days	22.4 ± 9.7	22.4 ± 9.3	0.993

**Group 1 for patients without diabetes.*
#Group 2 for patients with diabetes.

Survival Analysis

Figure 1 presents the distribution of the number of deaths by the level of illness severity in both groups. There were six critical COVID-19 cases in Group 2, and three cases in Group 1. Besides, no deaths were observed among the severe cases in Group 2 while there were six deaths in Group 1. As shown in **Table 3**, the difference between the prognosis of Group 2 and that of Group 1 was demonstrated using either the univariate Cox regression analysis ($p = 0.124$) or the multivariate analysis ($p = 0.256$, **Table 3**). Similarly, the Kaplan-Meier curves showed no difference between the two groups ($p = 0.111$, in **Supplemental Figure 1**).

Evaluation of Chest CT Images

Score 1 for all patients and that for patients without diabetes present the same tendency, i.e., rising and then descending (**Figures 2A–C** for all patients vs. **Figures 2D–F** for patients without diabetes). Similarly, score 1 for patients with diabetes sharply increased and significantly decreased after peaking at 2.70 points on day 23 (**Figure 2G**). However, score 2 for patients with diabetes showed an inverse tendency (**Figure 2H**), reaching its nadir of 2.30 points on day 35. This inconsistent tendency might be because the largest area of lung involvement for patients with diabetes appeared earlier than that for all patients or those without diabetes. In patients with diabetes, the total score peaked at 5.30 points after 19 days (**Figure 2I**), exceeding the peak of 4.95 points on day 20 in all patients (**Figure 2C**) and that of 4.95 points on day 19 in patients without diabetes (**Figure 2F**). Curve fitting equation for **Figure 2** and coefficients of each curve are shown in **Supplemental Table 1**.

DISCUSSION

The prevalence of diabetes mellitus is anticipated to increase substantially during the next decades worldwide and considered to be main cause of human deaths (9). People with diabetes are more susceptible to certain infectious diseases, such as staphylococcus aureus and mycobacterium tuberculosis, possibly because of their dysregulated immune system (10, 11). During the outbreak of SARS in 2003 in Guangzhou, Yang et al. reported that plasma glucose levels and diabetes were independent predictors for mortality and morbidity, and metabolic control might improve the prognosis in patients with SARS (12). Recently, COVID-19 has been a focal topic of research, and several investigations have focused on diabetes as a predictor of clinical course and prognosis of COVID-19 cases (13–16). Certain studies found that diabetes negatively affected medical complications, including mortality, in COVID-19 cases (13, 17, 18).

In our study, we collected data with a large sample from Leishenshan Hospital. We found that COVID-19 patients with DM were older and the proportion of patients with cardiovascular disease were higher among COVID-19 patients with DM than COVID-19 patients without DM. However, the latter had a higher proportion of pulmonary disease as comorbidities than the former. Furthermore, aspartate aminotransferase (AST) and platelet counts were lower in COVID-19 patients with diabetes than those without disease. In addition, non-diabetes-related comorbidities did not ameliorate the severity of illness on admission or improve survival outcomes, compared to diabetes-related ones. However, severe or critical COVID-19 cases were more prevalent among patients with diabetes than those did not suffer from this disease. A systematic review by Huang et al. revealed that diabetes was associated with mortality, severity, acute respiratory distress syndrome, and disease progression in patients with COVID-19 (19). The results of our present study differ from those of previous ones possibly because Leishenshan Hospital is a designated hospital for COVID-19, and the standard of care for patients with diabetes has become better. Further researches are needed in the future to generate more precise results.

Having assessed the association between diabetes with the severity of COVID-19, Wu et al. found out the proportion of diabetes as a comorbidity among severe COVID-19 cases was

TABLE 2 | Laboratory results in the COVID-19 patients with or without diabetes.

Covariate	Group 1 (n = 795)	Group 2 (n = 139)	P-value	Reference
Interleukin-6, pg/mL	2.16 (1.50–7.34)	3.69 (1.50–7.47)	0.133	0–7
Procalcitonin, ng/mL	0.04 (0.03–0.07)	0.05 (0.03–0.08)	0.142	<0.05
Alanine aminotransferase, U/L	23.00 (14.83–39.00)	21.00 (13.00–34.50)	0.054	9–50
Aspartate aminotransferase, U/L	21.00 (16.00–29.00)	18.00 (14.50–25.00)	<0.001	15–40
Albumin, g/L	35.95 (33.30–38.50)	35.90 (33.10–38,70)	0.880	40–55
Creatine kinase, U/L	47.00 (33.00–71.25)	49.00 (30.00–74.00)	0.817	18.0–198
Lactate dehydrogenase, U/L	197.50 (167.00–234.25)	194.00 (172.00–231.00)	0.941	125–343
Total bilirubin, μmol/L	9.10 (6.68–12.00)	9.20 (6.75–12.45)	0.420	5–21
Creatinine, μmol/L	65.90 (55.40–77.16)	66.00 (54.70–83.55)	0.545	64–104
BUN, mmol/L	4.90 (3.90–6.00)	5.20 (4.30–6.60)	0.004	2.8–7.6
Prothrombin time, s	11.40 (11.00–11.90)	11.40 (10.90–12.00)	0.784	9.4–12.5
Activated partial thromboplastin time, s	27.00 (24.20–30.40)	27.7 (24.98–30.48)	0.311	25.1–36.5
Fibrinogen, g/L	3.24 (2.58–3.99)	3.37 (2.65–4.08)	0.170	2.0–4.0
D-dimer, ng/mL	0.59 (0.27–1.42)	0.76 (0.32–1.91)	0.030	<0.50
White blood cell count, $\times 10^9/L$	5.73 (4.67–7.07)	5.68 (4.77–7.15)	0.785	3.5–9.5
Neutrophil count, $\times 10^9/L$	3.44 (2.51–4.54)	3.60 (2.51–4.86)	0.433	1.8–6.3
Lymphocyte count, $\times 10^9/L$	1.45 (1.11–1.84)	1.46 (1.10–1.81)	0.785	1.1–3.2
Monocyte count, $\times 10^9/L$	0.52 (0.41–0.67)	0.49 (0.41–0.62)	0.149	0.1–0.6
Red blood cell count, $\times 10^9/L$	4.01 (3.60–4.37)	3.94 (3.49–4.30)	0.259	4.3–5.8
Hemoglobin, g/L	122.00 (111.00–133.00)	121.00 (108.00–132.00)	0.215	130–175
Platelet count, $\times 10^9/L$	231.00 (183.00–287.75)	205.00 (163.00–259.00)	0.004	125–350
IgM (+) of SARS-CoV-2, No. (%)	101 (38.1%)	19 (29.7%)	0.209	(-)
IgG (+) of SARS-CoV-2, No. (%)	234 (91.8%)	52 (82.5%)	0.029	(-)

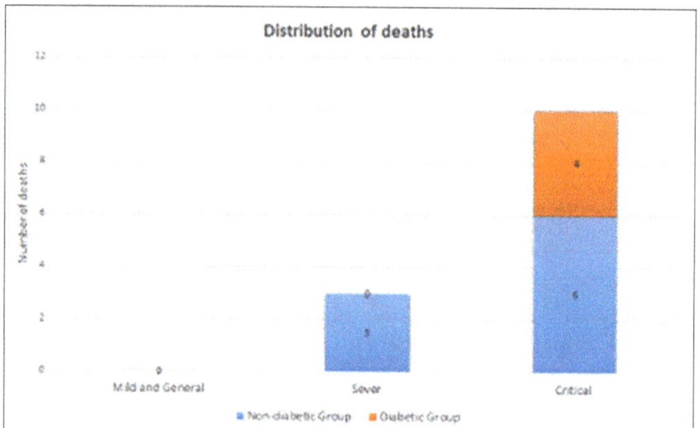

FIGURE 1 | The distribution of the number of deaths by the level of illness severity in the DM group and the non-DM group.

TABLE 3 | Univariate and multivariate Cox regression analyses of diabetes for the mortality of patients with COVID-19.

Covariate	Group	Cox regression analysis			
		HR	95 % CI		P-value
Univariate analysis	Group 1	ref			
	Group 2	2.522	0.777	8.191	0.124
Multivariate analysis*	Group 1	ref			
	Group 2	2.135	0.576	7.912	0.256

Adjust for age, the history of cardiovascular disease, D-dimer, WBC, and lymphocyte count.

significantly higher than that among mild cases (14). Similarly, our data supported that the proportion of severe or critical COVID-19 cases among patients with diabetes was higher than that among those without diabetes. This means the clinical course of COVID-19 in patients with diabetes may be more severe than that in those without diabetes. Currently, the mechanisms behind this phenomenon remain unknown; however, high glucose levels may play a certain role in the impaired antibacterial neutrophil function and complications caused by chronic diabetes (9). In addition, the comorbidity with cardiovascular diseases, such as ischemic heart disease and heart failure, was reported to have an association with higher mortality due to COVID-19 (20). In our study population, 64.0% of patients with diabetes suffered from cardiovascular diseases, higher than that of those without diabetes. This may partly explain that the group of patients with diabetes had a higher proportion of COVID-19 cases in severe or critical conditions than the group of those without diabetes.

In our present study, biochemical laboratory test results showed that the increased AST level, an indicator of liver injury, was not observed in the blood of all patients, regardless of

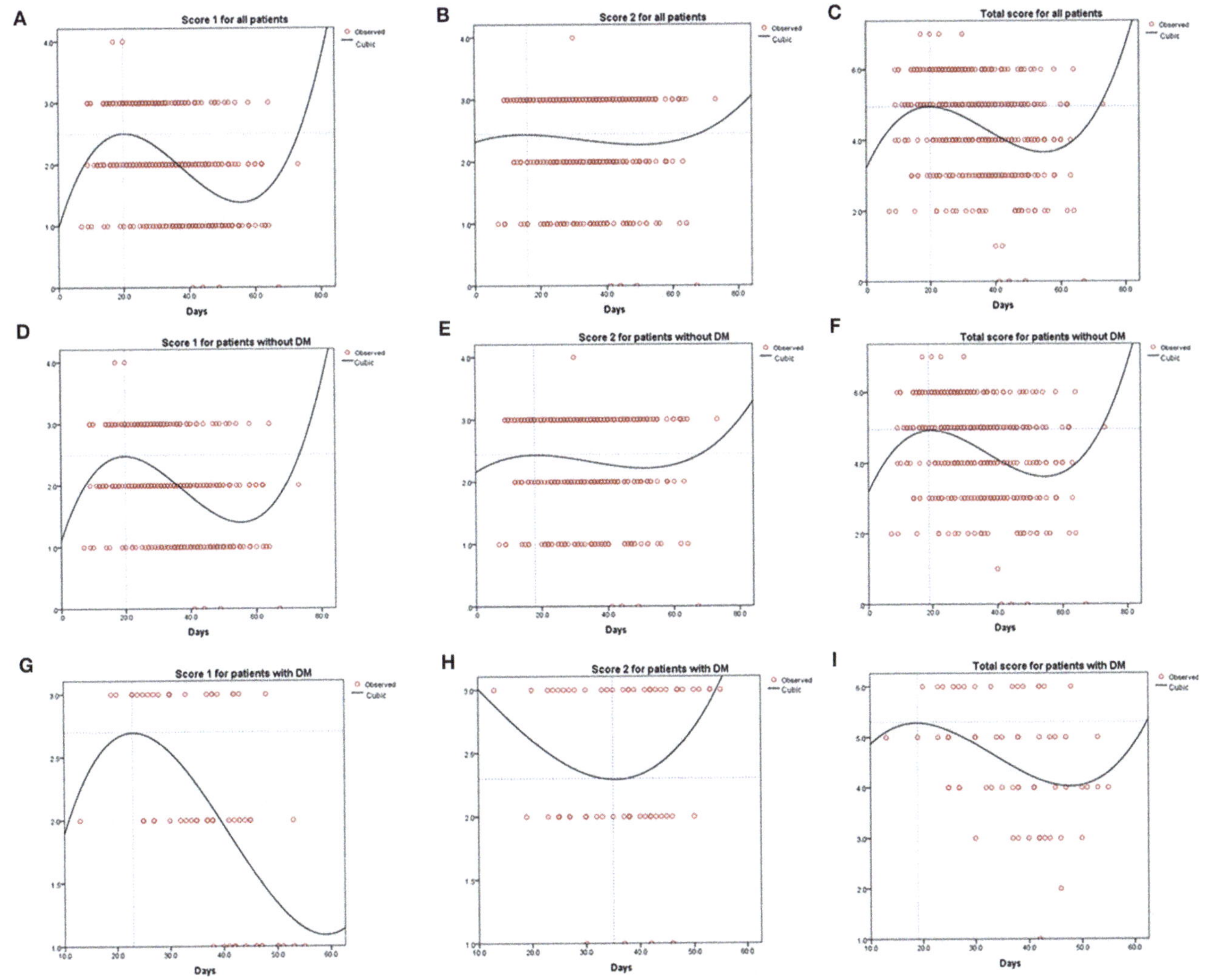

FIGURE 2 | Curve fitting analysis for all the COVID-19 patients **(A–C)**, patients without diabetes mellitus **(D–F)**, and patients with diabetes mellitus **(G–I)**.

their status of diabetes. Furthermore, the two groups showed no difference in the levels of albumin and hemoglobin, suggesting that both groups had similar nutritional status. Having analyzed 138 COVID-19 patients, Wang et al. found that cytokine storms, sustained inflammatory response, and acute kidney injury might be associated with the mortality of COVID-19 patients (21). Cytokine storms also proved to be the main cause of eventual deaths among many patients with Ebola virus infections (13). In our study, however, patients with diabetes shared similar lymphocyte and neutrophil counts than patients without diabetes, the inflammation-related biomarkers (e.g., IL-6). These results indicate that the inflammatory response of patients with diabetes was not different from that of those without diabetes, resulting in similar rates of mortality due to COVID-19.

The use of angiotensin-converting enzyme 2 (ACE2) inhibitors and Angiotensin II Receptor Antagonists (ARBs) for COVID-19 patients has been of great controversy. ACE2 is the surface receptor for SARS-CoV-2 that directly interacts with the spike glycoprotein (22). Wrapp et al. has recently suggested that the affinity between ACE2 and the receptor binding domain of SARS-CoV-2 is much higher than that between ACE2 and the RBC of SARS-CoV (23). The expression of ACE2 in various organs, including the cardiovascular system, lungs, kidneys, and brain might explain why some COVID-19 patients died of multiple organ failure (24, 25). ACE inhibitors and ARBs may play a protective role in the treatment of COVID-19 cases (26). However, Cure et al. demonstrated that SARS-CoV-2 could enter cells by attaching to ACE2 enzymes and then cause infection. Furthermore, ACE inhibitors enhanced the sympathetic activity via the central stimulation and then increased pulmonary capillary leaking, possibly resulting in the development of ARDS. The authors suggested that the morbidity and mortality of COVID-19 among patients with diabetes would be higher if they used ACE inhibitors and ARBs (27). Our primary findings showed that as a comorbidity, diabetes did not increase the risk of mortality but negatively regulated the clinical course of COVID-19. Therefore, the treatment for COVID-19 patients should be appropriately adjusted.

Our study has serval limitations that need to be addressed. First, the retrospective, non-randomized nature led to sample heterogeneity. Second, we were not able to collect and analyze the characteristic data of patients with diabetes, such as the type of diabetes, glucose level, HbA1c and treatment options for diabetes due to the time limitation; hence, we could not analyze the data on anti-DM treatment although they could affect the clinical course and treatment outcome of COVID-19. Third, we did not examine the relative mechanism behind the effect of diabetes on COVID-19 in this study. Finally, the difference in disease progress and prognosis between the COVID-19 patients with or without diabetes may change with a longer follow-up period.

CONCLUSION

Our findings which were contradictory to those of previous studies with large sample sizes, suggested that diabetes did not significantly impact the prognosis of COVID-19 patients but negatively affect their clinical course. This may be helpful for clinicians in managing COVID-19 patients with diabetes. However, future prospective studies with larger sample sizes should focus on examining whether patients with diabetes are more at risk of COVID-19.

AUTHOR CONTRIBUTIONS

ZL: conceptualization, writing—review, and editing. JH: formal analysis and writing—original draft preparation. JL, LG, and RG: investigation and data curation. KL and GZ: methodology and software. TZ, MY, and YH: software, visualization, and validation. JC, YY, and XW: supervision and project administration. All authors: contributed to the article and approved the submitted version.

REFERENCES

1. Wu C, Chen X, Cai Y, Xia J, Zhou X, Xu S, et al. Risk factors associated with acute respiratory distress syndrome and death in patients with coronavirus disease 2019 pneumonia in Wuhan, China. *JAMA Intern Med.* (2020) e200994. doi: 10.1001/jamainternmed.2020.0994. [Epub ahead of print].
2. Huang Y, Tu M, Wang S, Chen S, Zhou W, Chen D, et al. Clinical characteristics of laboratory confirmed positive cases of SARS-CoV-2 infection in Wuhan, China: a retrospective single center analysis. *Travel Med Infect Dis.* (2020) 101606. doi: 10.1016/j.tmaid.2020.101606. [Epub ahead of print].
3. Chen N, Zhou M, Dong X, Qu J, Gong F, Han Y, et al. Epidemiological and clinical characteristics of 99 cases of 2019 novel coronavirus pneumonia in Wuhan, China: a descriptive study. *Lancet.* (2020) 395:507–13. doi: 10.1016/S0140-6736(20)30211-7
4. Ingelfinger JR, Jarcho JA. Increase in the Incidence of Diabetes and Its Implications. *N Engl J Med.* (2017) 376:1473–4. doi: 10.1056/NEJMe1616575
5. Guzman-Flores JM, Lopez-Briones S. Cells of innate and adaptive immunity in type 2 diabetes and obesity. *Gac Med Mex.* (2012) 148:381–9.
6. Shu CJ, Benoist C, Mathis D. The immune system's involvement in obesity-driven type 2 diabetes. *Semin Immunol.* (2012) 24:436–42. doi: 10.1016/j.smim.2012.12.001
7. Bhatraju PK, Ghassemieh BJ, Nichols M, Kim R, Jerome KR, Nalla AK, et al. Covid-19 in critically ill patients in the seattle region - case series. *N Engl J Med.* (2020) 382:2012–22. doi: 10.1056/NEJMoa2004500
8. Roncon L, Zuin M, Rigatelli G, Zuliani G. Diabetic patients with COVID-19 infection are at higher risk of ICU admission and poor short-term outcome. *J Clin Virol.* (2020) 127:104354. doi: 10.1016/j.jcv.2020.104354
9. Knapp S. Diabetes and infection: is there a link?–a mini-review. *Gerontology.* (2013) 59:99–104. doi: 10.1159/000345107
10. Muller LM, Gorter KJ, Hak E, Goudzwaard WL, Schellevis FG, Hoepelman AI, et al. Increased risk of common infections in patients with type 1 and type 2 diabetes mellitus. *Clin Infect Dis.* (2005) 41:281–8. doi: 10.1086/431587
11. Hodgson K, Morris J, Bridson T, Govan B, Rush C, Ketheesan N. Immunological mechanisms contributing to the double burden of diabetes and intracellular bacterial infections. *Immunology.* (2015) 144:171–85. doi: 10.1111/imm.12394
12. Yang JK, Feng Y, Yuan MY, Yuan SY, Fu HJ, Wu BY, et al. Plasma glucose levels and diabetes are independent predictors for mortality and morbidity in patients with SARS. *Diabet Med.* (2006) 23:623–8. doi: 10.1111/j.1464-5491.2006.01861.x
13. Guo W, Li M, Dong Y, Zhou H, Zhang Z, Tian C, et al. Diabetes is a risk factor for the progression and prognosis of COVID-19. *Diabetes Metab Res Rev.* (2020) e3319. doi: 10.1002/dmrr.3319. [Epub ahead of print].
14. Wu J, Li W, Shi X, Chen Z, Jiang B, Liu J, et al. Early antiviral treatment contributes to alleviate the severity and improve the prognosis of patients with novel coronavirus disease (COVID-19). *J Intern Med.* (2020). doi: 10.1111/joim.13063. [Epub ahead of print].
15. John TJ, John K. What is the role of angiotensin-converting enzyme 2 (ACE2) in COVID-19 infection in hypertensive patients with diabetes? *Can J Cardiol.* (2020) 36:969.e3. doi: 10.1016/j.cjca.2020.03.049
16. Gentile S, Strollo F, Ceriello A. COVID-19 infection in Italian people with diabetes: lessons learned for our future (an experience to be used). *Diabetes Res Clin Pract.* (2020) 162:108137. doi: 10.1016/j.diabres.2020.108137
17. Hill MA, Mantzoros C, Sowers JR. Commentary: COVID-19 in patients with diabetes. *Metabolism.* (2020) 107:154217. doi: 10.1016/j.metabol.2020.154217
18. Klonoff DC, Umpierrez GE. COVID-19 in patients with diabetes: risk factors that increase morbidity. *Metabolism.* (2020). doi: 10.1016/j.metabol.2020.154224. [Epub ahead of print].
19. Huang I, Lim MA, Pranata R. Diabetes mellitus is associated with increased mortality and severity of disease in COVID-19 pneumonia - a systematic review, meta-analysis, and meta-regression. *Diabetes Metab Syndr.* (2020) 14:395–403. doi: 10.1016/j.dsx.2020.04.018
20. Zhou F, Yu T, Du R, Fan G, Liu Y, Liu Z, et al. Clinical course and risk factors for mortality of adult inpatients with COVID-19 in Wuhan, China: a retrospective cohort study. *Lancet.* (2020) 395:1054–62. doi: 10.1016/S0140-6736(20)30566-3
21. Wang D, Hu B, Hu C, Zhu F, Liu X, Zhang J, et al. Clinical characteristics of 138 hospitalized patients with 2019 novel coronavirus-infected pneumonia in Wuhan, China. *JAMA.* (2020). doi: 10.1001/jama.2020.1585. [Epub ahead of print].

22. Kuba K, Imai Y, Rao S, Gao H, Guo F, Guan B, et al. A crucial role of angiotensin converting enzyme 2 (ACE2) in SARS coronavirus-induced lung injury. *Nat Med.* (2005) 11:875–9. doi: 10.1038/nm1267
23. Wrapp D, Wang N, Corbett KS, Goldsmith JA, Hsieh CL, Abiona O, et al. Cryo-EM structure of the 2019-nCoV spike in the prefusion conformation. *Science.* (2020) 367:1260–3. doi: 10.1126/science.abb2507
24. Patel VB, Zhong JC, Grant MB, Oudit GY. Role of the ACE2/angiotensin 1-7 axis of the renin-angiotensin system in heart failure. *Circ Res.* (2016) 118:1313–26. doi: 10.1161/CIRCRESAHA.116.307708
25. Tipnis SR, Hooper NM, Hyde R, Karran E, Christie G, Turner AJ. A human homolog of angiotensin-converting enzyme. Cloning and functional expression as a captopril-insensitive carboxypeptidase. *J Biol Chem.* (2000) 275:33238–43. doi: 10.1074/jbc.M002615200
26. Kuster GM, Pfister O, Burkard T, Zhou Q, Twerenbold R, Haaf P, et al. SARS-CoV2: should inhibitors of the renin-angiotensin system be withdrawn in patients with COVID-19? *Eur Heart J.* (2020) 41:1801–3. doi: 10.1093/eurheartj/ehaa235
27. Cure E, Cumhur Cure M. Angiotensin-converting enzyme inhibitors and angiotensin receptor blockers may be harmful in patients with diabetes during COVID-19 pandemic. *Diabetes Metab Syndr.* (2020) 14:349–50. doi: 10.1016/j.dsx.2020.04.019

19

Severity of COVID-19 and Treatment Strategy for Patient with Diabetes

Shi Jin[1] *and Weina Hu*[2*]

[1] Department of Endocrinology, The Fourth Affiliated Hospital of China Medical University, Shenyang, China, [2] Department of Cardiology, The Fourth Affiliated Hospital of China Medical University, Shenyang, China

Correspondence:
Weina Hu
cmu4h_huweina@163.com

Coronavirus disease 2019 (COVID-19), which was named by the World Health Organization (WHO) in February 2020, has quickly spread to more than 200 countries around the world and was declared as a global pandemic in March 2020. The severity of the disease makes it more prone to severe symptoms and higher mortality rates in patients, especially those who are with comorbidities, including high blood pressure, cardiovascular disease, obesity, and diabetes, increases the concern over the consequences of this pandemic. However, initial reports do not clearly describe whether diabetes itself or associated comorbidities or treatment strategies contribute to the severe prognosis of COVID-19 infections. Various clinical trials are being conducted on glucose-lowering agents but to date, there is no standard treatment protocol approved for COVID-19 cases with pre-existing diabetes. This review is aimed to decipher the potential risk factors of COVID-19 involved from existing evidence. Identification of a novel therapeutic strategy could be beneficial for combating SARS-CoV-2, which might be dreadful to debilitating people who have diabetes.

Keywords: Diabetes mellitus, COVID-19, SARS-CoV-2, cytokine storm, glycemic control

INTRODUCTION

Severe acute respiratory syndrome coronavirus 2 (SARS-CoV-2), the cause for coronavirus disease 2019 (COVID-19), has infected more than 126 million people in the world and over 2.76 million deaths have been reported worldwide at the time this review was written (1). This virus is a new enveloped beta-coronavirus with a single stand that shares 82% of genomic similarities with human SARS-CoV, the virus responsible for the SARS pandemic in 2003 (2). SARS-CoV-2 has a higher reproduction rate compared to other beta-coronaviruses such as SARS-CoV and Middle East Respiratory Syndrome (MERS-CoV), indicating a greater risk for global health (3). The COVID-19 outbreak has caused a much higher number of deaths (2.76 million total deaths until March 28th, 2021) than the other coronavirus respiratory syndromes (8096 cases with 774 total deaths for 2003 SARS outbreak while the 2012 MERS outbreak has 2519 confirmed cases with 866 total deaths) (1, 4, 5). As the number of confirmed cases and death increasing exponentially, using epidemiological data to characterize COVID-19 patients could help to control the spread and also for the development of interventions for the disease. The characteristic of a respiratory virus is multi-organ damage and lungs, heart and kidneys are often the major affected organs.

Studies found that having one or more comorbidities is linked to the increased severity of COVID-19. In a systematic review and meta-analysis with a total number of 46248 confirmed cases, data showed that hypertension and diabetes are the most common comorbidities among COVID-19 patients (6). Generally, personal history of diabetes or newly diagnosed diabetes was ascertained in medical records or a self-reported diagnosis with the defined diagnostic criteria according to the WHO diagnostic criteria: fasting plasma glucose ≥ 7.0 mmol/L (≥126 mg/dL) or 2-h plasma glucose ≥ 11.1 mmol/L (≥ 200 mg/dL) or HbA1c ≥ 48 mmol/mol (6.5%) (7, 8). Studies also found that older age, hypertension, obesity, diabetes, cardiovascular disease, and chronic obstructive pulmonary disease are most commonly observed in patients with severe COVID-19 and those who died (9, 10). People with diabetes have a higher risk of viral infection in previous respiratory disease (11). Although diabetes does not seem to increase the risk for COVID-19 in some regions in Europe such as Italy (12), the risk for COVID-19 associated with diabetes is increased in most parts of the world as well as the mortality rates.

However, whether diabetes per se or together with the concomitant comorbidities contribute to the worse prognosis remains to be fully uncovered. Therefore, this review aims to highlight potential risk factors in patients with COVID-19 comorbid with diabetes. We will also discuss the specific therapeutic strategies being used for people who have both COVID-19 and diabetes.

POTENTIAL RISK FACTORS OF COVID-19

Age and Gender

COVID-19 morbidity and mortality are higher in older and male individuals. In a systematic literature review and meta-analysis of 13 studies including a total number of 3027 COVID-19 patients and in aged patients over 65, Zheng et al. reported a greater risk of mortality and more comorbidities such as hypertension, diabetes also greatly affecting the prognosis of the COVID-19 (13). Data from an Israeli study of 5769 recovered patients showed that younger individuals, not only are less likely to have severe COVID-19 requiring ICU and hospitalization but have an average faster recovery rate from SARS-CoV-2 infection (14). In a large Chinese case study of a total of 72314 patients, the fatality rate of the overall case is 2.3% but it was increased by up to 14.8% in patients aged 80 and older (15). The prevalence of diabetes is increased with age both in the general population and in patients with COVID-19. Patients with COVID-19 and diabetes have an older average age than those without diabetes. In one retrospective study involving 904 patients with COVID-19 (136 with diabetes), patients with diabetes were at least more than 10 years older compared to that of non-diabetic patients (7). Another study including a matched population of patients with and without diabetes found that survivors were much younger than non-survivors and older age (more than 70 years) is an independent predictor of severity of COVID-19 such as in-hospital death (16).

A preliminary study showed an overall even distribution of SARS-CoV-2 infections between men and women (51% versus 47%, respectively) (17). However, the fatality rates are 2-fold higher in males than females (18). What's more, the sex distribution of recovering cases was 36% and 65% for males and females, respectively (19). Another study concluded that male and age serve as risk factors for poorer outcomes in COVID-19. There was a 12-fold higher risk in patients aged 80 years and older than those 50-59 years old and men have twice the risk as women (20). In a recent risk assessment for the COVID-19 confirmed cases from European Union/European Economic Area (EU/EEA) countries and the United Kingdom (UK), data described that the male-to-female ratio overall was 0.9, with more males than females admitted to hospital, requiring intensive care or respiratory support and also dying (21).

High Blood Pressure

High blood pressure (hypertension) is the most common comorbidity in severe COVID-19 patients (22). Studies speculated that SARS-CoV-2 might directly bind to angiotensin-converting enzyme 2 (ACE2) to enter target cells (23). ACE2 is widely expressed in the upper airways, lung, heart, liver, kidney, ileum, testis and brain and it plays an important role in anti-inflammatory responses (24–26). Recent studies have investigated the link between disease severity in COVID-19 patients with hypertension and their medical therapy. In a clinical trial of 3017 hospitalized COVID-19 patients, data showed that 53% were hypertensive. Besides, the mortality rates among patients on angiotensin-converting enzyme inhibitors (ACEI) and angiotensin receptor blockers (ARBs) treatment were lower compared to other anti-hypertensive drugs. These results were supported by another Chinese study that there was a lower rate of severe diseases and a lower rate of the inflammatory response in COVID-19 patients treated with ACEI and ARBs versus patients treated with other antihypertensive agents (27). However, some *in vitro* and animal studies have demonstrated that ACEI and ARBs increased the expression of ACE2, and those drugs could facilitate the infection of target organs and exacerbate COVID-19 disease progression (28, 29). Moreover, the detailed relationship between ACEI and the renin-angiotensin system (RAS) in humans is not yet clearly understood (30). In recent systematic reviews and meta-analysis studies, data showed that hypertension is one of the major comorbidities in COVID-19 fatal cases (31) and COVID-19 patients with hypertension have a significantly increased mortality risk (32) and also a higher risk of ICU admission (33).

Cardiovascular Disease

A high prevalence of the cardiovascular disease has been observed in patients with COVID-19 (34) and clinical studies have also reported the association between COVID-19 and cardiovascular disease (35). Pre-existing cardiovascular disease was believed to be linked with poorer outcomes and increased risk of death in COVID-19 patients. Other studies have also observed higher troponin concentration in patients with more severe COVID-19 (36). Although the predominant clinical symptoms of COVID-19 is viral pneumonia (37–39), COVID-19 can also cause cardiovascular complications such as myocardial injury, myocarditis, acute coronary syndrome

(ACS), heart failure, arrhythmias, sudden cardiac arrest, coagulation abnormalities and thrombosis (40–43). A case study in South Korea reported that a COVID-19 patient was diagnosed as acute myocarditis and this patient presented very high levels of cardiac troponin I and N-terminal (NT) pro B-type natriuretic peptide (NTproBNP), the two most sensitive clinical biomarkers for myocardial injury (44), although no SRAS-Cov-2 genomes from myocardial biopsy samples were observed (45).

Recently, several cases of stress-induced cardiomyopathy with COVID-19 have been reported, while the past medical histories of these patients were unremarkable (45–47). The postulated underlying mechanism is that COVID-19 pneumonia decreased systemic oxygenation supply and while it inversely increased cardiac demand, immune dysregulation and electrolyte imbalance (48).

In summary, these findings suggest that cardiovascular disease is not only a common symptom of COVID-19 but also a risk factor for poor prognosis. Although we do not understand the mechanisms underlying COVID-19-related cardiovascular disease, this could be largely attributable to systemic inflammation based on the available clinical findings.

Obesity

Obesity is now being recognized as a risk factor for severe outcomes and the death of COVID-19. Evidence from around the world suggesting obese people are at greater risk of becoming seriously ill from COVID-19, means there must be an extra reason to take on obesity (49, 50). Importantly, a study of 4103 patients with COVID-19 disease in New York reported that the most important clinical features leading to hospital admission were aged (over 65 years) and obesity itself, more than hypertension, cardiovascular disease or diabetes (51). In this study, body mass index (BMI, >40 kg/m^2) is one of the strongest hospitalization risks for COVID-19 positive patients. This finding was consistent with the results from the CORONADO study. It was found that in people with diabetes hospitalized for COVID-19, BMI (>40 kg/m^2) was independently associated with the severity of COVID-19 but not long-term glycemic control assessed by HbA1c (8). Multiple underlying mechanisms are accounted for this association. Firstly, the alteration of respiratory performance and impaired lung perfusion may be due to abdominal fat (52) and intravascular disseminated coagulation (53). Secondly, pre-existing comorbidities such as hypertension and diabetes are prothrombotic conditions (54, 55) that contribute to worse prognosis in COVID-19 patients. This was supported by a Germany autopsy study that found that deep venous thromboembolism was observed in 7 of 12 patients and pulmonary embolism was the direct cause of death for 4 patients (56). Finally, obesity is often linked with inadequate and excessive immunological responses and chronic inflammation which could rapidly mediate disease progression to multi-organ failure in severe COVID-19 patients (57).

Furthermore, another explanation is based on the findings that SARS-CoV-2 has a high affinity for human ACE2. And ACE2 is much highly expressed in adipose tissue compared to that in the lung, major SARS-CoV-2 target tissue and obese individuals have more adipose tissue, therefore an increased ACE2-expressing cell numbers and consequently a larger amount of ACE2 (58). ACE2 was believed to be the receptor for the entry of SARS-CoV-2 into host cells (59).

Inflammation

Higher levels of inflammatory markers in the blood (such as C-reactive protein and ferritin), an increased neutrophil-to-lymphocyte ratio and increased serum levels of inflammatory cytokines and chemokines have been associated with COVID-19 disease severity and death (51, 60). The cytokine profiles in severe COVID-19 patients are similar to those in cytokine release syndromes, with increased production of cytokines such as interleukin (IL)-6, IL-7 and tumor necrosis factor (TNF) and also CXC-chemokine ligand 10 (CXCL10) (61). Studies have reported that inflammatory infiltration was observed in the lung, heart, kidney, spleen, and lymph nodes (62–64). Several reports have also observed higher concentrations of C-reactive protein, IL-6, IL-10, ferritin, leukocytes and lower lymphocyte percentage in severe COVID-19 patients compared to that of non-severe patients (65, 66). A low-grade systemic and chronic inflammation was often observed in diabetes. Thus, a dysregulated inflammatory innate and an adaptive impaired immune response consequently occur in diabetic patients. Therefore, a more severe disease in COVID-19 patients with diabetes may be the result of a cytokine storm, in which the patient's immune system fights against SARS-CoV-2 and inflicts compromised damage on its organs. Several studies have reported that COVID-19 patients with diabetes have higher lymphopenia incidence and increased proinflammatory biomarkers than those without diabetes (67, 68). Moreover, increased inflammation such as elevated IL-6 and TNF levels were also observed in obese patients, thus favors COVID-19 disease progression, and worsens the lung and heart functions (69). Therefore, obesity is also an important predisposing factor for this phenomenon.

Hyperglycemia-the Importance of Glycemic Control

Diabetes is characterized by impaired glucose homeostasis resulting from insulin resistance or deficiency. As we know, diabetes is a well-established risk factor and predictor for elevated morbidity and mortality in various diseases such as cardiovascular diseases, cancer, and infection diseases (70–73).

In a cohort of 1561 patients with COVID-19 in two hospitals from Wuhan, those with diabetes are more likely to require an intensive care unit (ICU) admission or to die (16). In a centered, retrospective study, Yang et al. demonstrated that among cases with a poor outcome, in a group of 32 non-survivors of 52 ICU patients, 7 (22%) had diabetes (74). Data from a British hospital including 10926 COVID-19 related death in a cohort of 17278392 adults showed that the risk of death is much higher in those with uncontrolled diabetes (20). Other studies also described that there was a worse outcome in COVID-19 patients is diabetes (75), therefore, result in more hospitalizations, more admission for ICU and more death (33).

As we know, the virulence of some pathogens is increased during the hyperglycemic environment. It was reported that phagocytosis and chemotaxis are impaired and the production of T cells and neutrophils in response to infection is also reduced in diabetes (76). Generally, the immune response is damaged in diabetic COVID-19 patients with poor blood glucose control. Among the COVID-19 patients with diabetes, higher incidences of neutrophilia and lymphopenia are observed in those with higher levels of blood glucose concentration (67). Recently, several studies have shown that impaired pulmonary function significantly correlates with blood glucose levels (77, 78). Therefore, the vulnerability to respiratory infections is increased along with reduced pulmonary capacity. This might be another factor that diabetes is more commonly observed in severe COVID-19 patients. Moreover, in a total of 663 COVID-19 patients' study, type 2 diabetes was found to be associated with no improvement in patients with COVID-19 and type 2 diabetes patients were prone to developing into severe and critical condition of COVID-19 and having a poorer therapeutic effect. Furthermore, having a severe and critical condition and decreased lymphocyte count were independent risk factors associated with poor therapeutic effects in COVID-19 patients with type 2 diabetes (79). Interestingly, in a population-based cohort study with diagnosed type 1 and type 2 diabetes in England, Holman found that increased COVID-19-related mortality was associated not only with cardiovascular and renal complications of both types of diabetes but also independently with glycemic control and BMI (80).

A recent study reported that COVID-19 patients with diabetes and uncontrolled hyperglycemia (defined as two or more blood glucose > 180 mg/dL within any 24-hour period with an HbA1C < 6.5% or no HbA1C testing during hospitalization) were associated with longer hospitalization and higher mortality (81). Studies also found that higher blood glucose concentration at admission was associated with the poorer primary outcome. In a retrospective analysis of 85 COVID-19 patients, Iacobellis et al. reported that hyperglycemia on the first day of admission is the best predictor of radiographic imaging, regardless of pre-existing diabetes (82). Furthermore, hyperglycemia during treatment was a risk factor for death in patients with severe COVID-19 (83). In a retrospective multi-center study including COVID-19 patients hospitalized in Spain, it was found that hyperglycaemia (>180 mg/dL) is a strong predictor of all-cause mortality in non-critically hospitalized COVID-19 patients regardless of diabetes history (84). Thus, glucose testing and glycemic control are important to all COVID-19 patients even without pre-existing diabetes, as most COVID-19 patients are prone to glucose metabolic disorders. This is because the ACE receptors where SARS-CoV-2 binds to enter target cells are also expressed in pancreatic β cells (24). This could induce acute impairment of insulin secretion and β cell destruction resulting in *de novo* diabetes development.

In summary, uncontrolled glycemic at admission and hospitalization exacerbate poor outcomes of COVID-19 patients. In COVID-19 patients with hyperglycemia, therapeutic strategies combined with glycemic control should be considered to reduce the risk of severe outcomes and mortality.

THERAPEUTICS-TREATMENT SPECIFIC TO PATIENTS HAVING BOTH COVID-19 AND DIABETES

Medical teams should ensure sufficient glycemic control in COVID-19 patients with diabetes. This requires full consideration of all potential complications the therapies may generate which will be used for those patients.

Insulin treatment is a general therapy for both types of diabetes. However, insulin therapy should be decided based on the severity of COVID-19 and those patients should be intensely monitored, although this treatment has been recommended in severe COVID-19 patients with diabetes (85). One study found that poorer clinical outcomes in patients treated with insulin compared with those under metformin treatment (7). Despite better outcomes reported in diabetic patients with COVID-19 on metformin, this drug should be discontinued if patients with respiratory distress, renal dysfunction, or heart failure due to acidosis (85). In the CORONADO study, Cariou et al. reported that the use of metformin was lower in patients who died and other therapies such as insulin treatment, renin–angiotensin–aldosterone system (RAAS) blockers, β-blockers and loop diuretics were associated with death on day 7. They believed this finding could be attributed to the underling comorbidities and diabetic complications in people who died because these patients were received more frequent treatment including insulin and other multiples drugs (8). A recent study reported significantly higher postprandial glycemic fluctuations and exposure to hyperglycemia were observed among patients with COVID-19 followed by continuous glucose monitoring (86). Thus, continuous blood glucose monitoring should also be included during the treatment process.

Sodium-glucose transporter 2 inhibitors should also be treated with caution due to their adverse effects such as ketoacidosis and impaired fat metabolism (87). Besides, Care should also be taken with the use of glucagon-like receptor-1 (GLP-1R) analogues since they may cause diarrhea, nausea, vomiting and headaches (88). In a recent multicenter, case-control, retrospective, and observational study, sitagliptin, an oral and highly selective dipeptidyl peptidase 4 (DPP4) inhibitor, was used as an add-on therapy to the standard of care in patients with type 2 diabetes and COVID-19. Sitagliptin treatment was found to be associated with reduced mortality, an improved clinical outcome and a greater number of hospital discharges in this study (89). These beneficial effects may be attributed to the shared disease pathophysiology pathways in coronavirus infections and type 2 diabetes. DPP4 and ACE2, two major coronavirus receptor proteins, are well-established transducers of metabolic signals and pathways regulating inflammation, cardiorenal physiology, and glucose homeostasis. Moreover, glucose-lowering drugs such as the DPP4 inhibitors, widely used in type 2 diabetes patients, are known to modify the biological activities of multiple immunomodulatory substrates (90).

As we know, it is a multistep process for virus infection. Researchers have proposed several targets to treat COVID-19.

The beneficial effects of ACEI and ARBs for kidney and heart in diabetes have already been proven (91). However, as stated above, for COVID-19 patients with diabetes, the use of ACEI and ARBs for those patients should be carefully discussed based on the context of the individuals.

Glucocorticoids are known to cause hyperglycemia in patients with or without pre-existing diabetes. However, it has been used for the treatment of severely ill patients to suppress the very high levels of cytokines and c-reactive peptides which are often observed in those patients, although they can exacerbate insulin resistance, reduce insulin sensitivity and cause severe hyperglycemia. No studies have found that they could decrease mortality or slow viral clearance in clinical.

CONCLUSIONS

Patients with COVID-19 and diabetes are at greater risk for more severe infections, poorer prognosis and much higher mortality compared to those patients without diabetes. The grave prognosis and the risk factors for patients with diabetes are well linked with older age, sex, high blood pressure, cardiovascular disease, obesity, inflammation and hyperglycemia. All those factors contribute to the increased risk of getting severely ill in those individuals. It is a great challenge for blood glucose management in COVID-19 patients because it requires more detailed strategies for medical team integration and fully considerations of all possible complications and death.

It is also clear that the relationship between diabetes and COVID-19 is tightly linked together and it requires more research to fully uncover the specific mechanisms of SARS-CoV-2 such as how SARS-CoV-2 impairs the pancreatic islets, deteriorates insulin homeostasis and induce *de novo* diabetes development.

AUTHOR CONTRIBUTIONS

SJ and WH wrote different sections of the manuscript. WH revised, wrote, and prepared the manuscript. All authors contributed to the article and approved the submitted version.

REFERENCES

1. World Health Organization. *Coronavirus Disease (COVID-2019) Situation Reports* (2021). Available at: https://www.who.int/emergencies/diseases/novel-coronavirus-2019/situation-reports/.
2. Lu R, Zhao X, Li J, Niu P, Yang B, Wu H, et al. Genomic Characterisation and Epidemiology of 2019 Novel Coronavirus: Implications for Virus Origins and Receptor Binding. *Lancet* (2020) 395:565–74. doi: 10.1016/S0140-6736(20)30251-8
3. Hellewell J, Abbott S, Gimma A, Bosse NI, Jarvis CI, Russell TW, et al. Feasibility of Controlling COVID-19 Outbreaks by Isolation of Cases and Contacts. *Lancet Glob Health* (2020) 8:e488–96. doi: 10.1016/S2214-109X(20)30074-7
4. World Health Organization. *Middle East Respiratory Syndrome Coronavirus (MERS-Cov)* (2020). Available at: https://www.who.int/health-topics/middle-east-respiratory-syndrome-coronavirus-mers#tab=tab_1.
5. World Health Organization. *Severe Acute Respiratory Syndrome (Sars)* (2020). Available at: https://www.who.int/health-topics/severe-acute-respiratory-syndrome#tab=tab_1.
6. Yang J, Zheng Y, Gou X, Pu K, Chen Z, Guo Q, et al. Prevalence of Comorbidities and its Effects in Patients Infected With SARS-CoV-2: A Systematic Review and Meta-Analysis. *Int J Infect Dis IJID Off Publ Int Soc Infect Dis* (2020) 94:91–5. doi: 10.1016/j.ijid.2020.03.017
7. Chen Y, Yang D, Cheng B, Chen J, Peng A, Yang C, et al. Clinical Characteristics and Outcomes of Patients With Diabetes and COVID-19 in Association With Glucose-Lowering Medication. *Diabetes Care* (2020) 43:1399–407. doi: 10.2337/dc20-0660
8. Cariou B, Hadjadj S, Wargny M, Pichelin M, Al-Salameh A, Allix I, et al. Phenotypic Characteristics and Prognosis of Inpatients With COVID-19 and Diabetes: The CORONADO Study. *Diabetologia* (2020) 63:1500–15. doi: 10.1007/s00125-020-05180-x
9. Wu Z, McGoogan JM. Characteristics of and Important Lessons From the Coronavirus Disease 2019 (Covid-19) Outbreak in China: Summary of a Report of 72314 Cases From the Chinese Center for Disease Control and Prevention. *Jama* (2020) 323:1239–42. doi: 10.1001/jama.2020.2648
10. Huang C, Wang Y, Li X, Ren L, Zhao J, Hu Y, et al. Clinical Features of Patients Infected With 2019 Novel Coronavirus in Wuhan, China. *Lancet* (2020) 395:497–506. doi: 10.1016/S0140-6736(20)30183-5
11. Booth CM, Matukas LM, Tomlinson GA, Rachlis AR, Rose DB, Dwosh HA, et al. Clinical Features and Short-Term Outcomes of 144 Patients With SARS in the Greater Toronto Area. *Jama* (2003) 289:2801–9. doi: 10.1001/jama.289.21.JOC30885
12. Orioli L, Hermans MP, Thissen JP, Maiter D, Vandeleene B, Yombi JC. Covid-19 in Diabetic Patients: Related Risks and Specifics of Management. *Ann Endocrinol (Paris)* (2020) 81:101–9. doi: 10.1016/j.ando.2020.05.001
13. Zheng Z, Peng F, Xu B, Zhao J, Liu H, Peng J, et al. Risk Factors of Critical & Mortal COVID-19 Cases: A Systematic Literature Review and Meta-Analysis. *J Infect* (2020) 81:e16–25. doi: 10.1016/j.jinf.2020.04.021
14. Voinsky I, Baristaite G, Gurwitz D. Effects of Age and Sex on Recovery From COVID-19: Analysis of 5769 Israeli Patients. *J Infect* (2020) 81:e102–3. doi: 10.1016/j.jinf.2020.05.026
15. Cdc Weekly C. The Epidemiological Characteristics of an Outbreak of 2019 Novel Coronavirus Diseases (Covid-19) — China, 2020. *China CDC Weekly* (2020) 2:113–22. doi: 10.46234/ccdcw2020.032
16. Shi Q, Zhang X, Jiang F, Zhang X, Hu N, Bimu C, et al. Clinical Characteristics and Risk Factors for Mortality of COVID-19 Patients With Diabetes in Wuhan, China: A Two-Center, Retrospective Study. *Diabetes Care* (2020) 43:1382–91. doi: 10.2337/dc20-0598
17. World Health Organization. *Gender and COVID-19* (2020). Available at: https://www.who.int/publications/i/item/gender-and-covid-19.
18. Klein SL, Dhakal S, Ursin RL, Deshpande S, Sandberg K, Mauvais-Jarvis F. Biological Sex Impacts COVID-19 Outcomes. *PloS Pathog* (2020) 16:e1008570. doi: 10.1371/journal.ppat.1008570
19. Zeng F, Dai C, Cai P, Wang J, Xu L, Li J, et al. A Comparison Study of SARS-CoV-2 Igg Antibody Between Male and Female COVID-19 Patients: A Possible Reason Underlying Different Outcome Between Sex. *J Med Virol* (2020) 92:2050–4. doi: 10.1101/2020.03.26.20040709
20. Williamson EJ, Walker AJ, Bhaskaran K, Bacon S, Bates C, Morton CE, et al. Factors Associated With COVID-19-related Death Using Opensafely. *Nature* (2020) 584:430–6. doi: 10.1038/s41586-020-2521-4
21. European Centre for Disease prevention and Control. *Coronavirus Disease 2019 (COVID-19) in the EU/EEA and the UK – Eleventh Update: Resurgence of Cases* (2020). Available at: https://www.ecdc.europa.eu/en/publications-data/rapid-risk-assessment-coronavirus-disease-2019-covid-19-eueea-and-uk-eleventh.

22. Guan WJ, Liang WH, Zhao Y, Liang HR, Chen ZS, Li YM, et al. Comorbidity and its Impact on 1590 Patients With COVID-19 in China: A Nationwide Analysis. *Eur Respir J* (2020) 55:2000547. doi: 10.1183/13993003.01227-2020
23. Cheng Y, Luo R, Wang K, Zhang M, Wang Z, Dong L, et al. Kidney Disease is Associated With in-Hospital Death of Patients With COVID-19. *Kidney Int* (2020) 97:829–38. doi: 10.1016/j.kint.2020.03.005
24. Hamming I, Timens W, Bulthuis ML, Lely AT, Navis G, van Goor H. Tissue Distribution of ACE2 Protein, the Functional Receptor for SARS Coronavirus. A First Step in Understanding SARS Pathogenesis. *J Pathol* (2004) 203:631–7. doi: 10.1002/path.1570
25. Gheblawi M, Wang K, Viveiros A, Nguyen Q, Zhong JC, Turner AJ, et al. Angiotensin-Converting Enzyme 2: SARS-CoV-2 Receptor and Regulator of the Renin-Angiotensin System: Celebrating the 20th Anniversary of the Discovery of ACE2. *Circ Res* (2020) 126:1456–74. doi: 10.1161/CIRCRESAHA.120.317015
26. Xu X, Chen P, Wang J, Feng J, Zhou H, Li X, et al. Evolution of the Novel Coronavirus From the Ongoing Wuhan Outbreak and Modeling of its Spike Protein for Risk of Human Transmission. *Sci China Life Sci* (2020) 63:457–60. doi: 10.1007/s11427-020-1637-5
27. Meng J, Xiao G, Zhang J, He X, Ou M, Bi J, et al. Renin-Angiotensin System Inhibitors Improve the Clinical Outcomes of COVID-19 Patients With Hypertension. *Emerg Microbes Infect* (2020) 9:757–60. doi: 10.1080/22221751.2020.1746200
28. Arendse LB, Danser AHJ, Poglitsch M, Touyz RM, Burnett JC Jr, Llorens-Cortes C, et al. Novel Therapeutic Approaches Targeting the Renin-Angiotensin System and Associated Peptides in Hypertension and Heart Failure. *Pharmacol Rev* (2019) 71:539–70. doi: 10.1124/pr.118.017129
29. Igase M, Strawn WB, Gallagher PE, Geary RL, Ferrario CM. Angiotensin II AT1 Receptors Regulate ACE2 and Angiotensin-(1-7) Expression in the Aorta of Spontaneously Hypertensive Rats. *American Journal of Physiology. Heart Circulatory Physiol* (2005) 289:H1013–1019. doi: 10.1152/ajpheart.00068.2005
30. Takimoto-Ohnishi E, Murakami K. Renin-Angiotensin System Research: From Molecules to the Whole Body. *J Physiol Sci* (2019) 69:581–7. doi: 10.1007/s12576-019-00679-4
31. Chen Y, Gong X, Wang L, Guo J. Effects of Hypertension, Diabetes and Coronary Heart Disease on COVID-19 Diseases Severity: A Systematic Review and Meta-Analysis. *medRxiv* (2020) 2020:2003.2025.20043133. doi: 10.1101/2020.03.25.20043133
32. Zuin M, Rigatelli G, Zuliani G, Rigatelli A, Mazza A, Roncon L. Arterial Hypertension and Risk of Death in Patients With COVID-19 Infection: Systematic Review and Meta-Analysis. *J Infect* (2020) 81:e84–6. doi: 10.1016/j.jinf.2020.03.059
33. Roncon L, Zuin M, Rigatelli G, Zuliani G. Diabetic Patients With COVID-19 Infection are At Higher Risk of ICU Admission and Poor Short-Term Outcome. *J Clin Virol Off Publ Pan Am Soc Clin Virol* (2020) 127:104354. doi: 10.1016/j.jcv.2020.104354
34. Li B, Yang J, Zhao F, Zhi L, Wang X, Liu L, et al. Prevalence and Impact of Cardiovascular Metabolic Diseases on COVID-19 in China. *Clin Res Cardiol* (2020) 109:531–8. doi: 10.1007/s00392-020-01626-9
35. Nishiga M, Wang DW, Han Y, Lewis DB, Wu JC. Covid-19 and Cardiovascular Disease: From Basic Mechanisms to Clinical Perspectives. *Nat Rev Cardiol* (2020) 17:543–58. doi: 10.1038/s41569-020-0413-9
36. Li JW, Han TW, Woodward M, Anderson CS, Zhou H, Chen YD, et al. The Impact of 2019 Novel Coronavirus on Heart Injury: A Systematic Review and Meta-Analysis. *Prog Cardiovasc Dis* (2020) 63:518–24. doi: 10.1016/j.pcad.2020.04.008
37. Wu F, Zhao S, Yu B, Chen YM, Wang W, Song ZG, et al. A New Coronavirus Associated With Human Respiratory Disease in China. *Nature* (2020) 579:265–9. doi: 10.1038/s41586-020-2008-3
38. Bhatraju PK, Ghassemieh BJ, Nichols M, Kim R, Jerome KR, Nalla AK, et al. Covid-19 in Critically Ill Patients in the Seattle Region - Case Series. *New Engl J Med* (2020) 382:2012–22. doi: 10.1056/NEJMoa2004500
39. Onder G, Rezza G, Brusaferro S. Case-Fatality Rate and Characteristics of Patients Dying in Relation to COVID-19 in Italy. *Jama* (2020) 323:1775–6. doi: 10.1001/jama.2020.4683
40. Madjid M, Safavi-Naeini P, Solomon SD, Vardeny O. Potential Effects of Coronaviruses on the Cardiovascular System: A Review. *JAMA Cardiol* (2020) 5:831–40. doi: 10.1001/jamacardio.2020.1286
41. Clerkin KJ, Fried JA, Raikhelkar J, Sayer G, Griffin JM, Masoumi A, et al. Covid-19 and Cardiovascular Disease. *Circulation* (2020) 141:1648–55. doi: 10.1161/CIRCULATIONAHA.120.046941
42. Driggin E, Madhavan MV, Bikdeli B, Chuich T, Laracy J, Biondi-Zoccai G, et al. Cardiovascular Considerations for Patients, Health Care Workers, and Health Systems During the COVID-19 Pandemic. *J Am Coll Cardiol* (2020) 75:2352–71. doi: 10.1016/j.jacc.2020.03.031
43. Zheng YY, Ma YT, Zhang JY, Xie X. Covid-19 and the Cardiovascular System. *Nat Rev Cardiol* (2020) 17:259–60. doi: 10.1038/s41569-020-0360-5
44. Kim IC, Kim JY, Kim HA, Han S. Covid-19-related Myocarditis in a 21-Year-Old Female Patient. *Eur Heart J* (2020) 41:1859. doi: 10.1093/eurheartj/ehaa288
45. Sala S, Peretto G, Gramegna M, Palmisano A, Villatore A, Vignale D, et al. Acute Myocarditis Presenting as a Reverse Tako-Tsubo Syndrome in a Patient With SARS-CoV-2 Respiratory Infection. *Eur Heart J* (2020) 41:1861–2. doi: 10.1093/eurheartj/ehaa286
46. Tsao CW, Strom JB, Chang JD, Manning WJ. Covid-19-Associated Stress (Takotsubo) Cardiomyopathy. *Circ Cardiovasc Imaging* (2020) 13:e011222. doi: 10.1161/CIRCIMAGING.120.011222
47. Minhas AS, Scheel P, Garibaldi B, Liu G, Horton M, Jennings M, et al. Takotsubo Syndrome in the Setting of COVID-19. *JACC Case Rep* (2020) 2:1321–5. doi: 10.1016/j.jaccas.2020.04.023
48. Babapoor-Farrokhran S, Gill D, Walker J, Rasekhi RT, Bozorgnia B, Amanullah A. Myocardial Injury and COVID-19: Possible Mechanisms. *Life Sci* (2020) 253:117723. doi: 10.1016/j.lfs.2020.117723
49. Scheen AJ. Obesity and Risk of Severe COVID-19. *Rev medicale suisse* (2020) 16:1115–9.
50. Kassir R. Risk of COVID-19 for Patients With Obesity. *Obes Rev an Off J Int Assoc Study Obes* (2020) 21:e13034. doi: 10.1111/obr.13034
51. Petrilli CM, Jones SA, Yang J, Rajagopalan H, O'Donnell LF, Chernyak Y, et al. Factors associated with hospital admission and critical illness among 5279 people with coronavirus disease 2019 in New York City: prospective cohort study. *BMJ* (2020) 369:m1966. doi: 10.1136/bmj.m1966
52. Sattar N, McInnes IB, McMurray JJV. Obesity Is a Risk Factor for Severe Covid-19 Infection: Multiple Potential Mechanisms. *Circulation* (2020) 142:4–6. doi: 10.1161/CIRCULATIONAHA.120.047659
53. Connors JM, Levy JH. Covid-19 and its Implications for Thrombosis and Anticoagulation. *Blood* (2020) 135:2033–40. doi: 10.1182/blood.2020006000
54. Nadar S, Lip GY. The Prothrombotic State in Hypertension and the Effects of Antihypertensive Treatment. *Curr Pharm Design* (2003) 9:1715–32. doi: 10.2174/1381612033454559
55. Ghosh K. Chapter 16. In: CC Kartha, S Ramachandran, RM Pillai, editors. *Mechanisms of Vascular Defects in Diabetes Mellitus*. Cham, Switzerland: Springer International Publishing (2017) 361–76. doi: 10.1007/978-3-319-60324-7_16
56. Wichmann D, Sperhake JP, Lutgehetmann M, Steurer S, Edler C, Heinemann A, et al. Autopsy Findings and Venous Thromboembolism in Patients With Covid-19: A Prospective Cohort Study. *Ann Internal Med* (2020) 173:268–77. doi: 10.7326/L20-1206
57. Yang L, Liu S, Liu J, Zhang Z, Wan X, Huang B, et al. Covid-19: Immunopathogenesis and Immunotherapeutics. *Signal Transduct Target Ther* (2020) 5:128. doi: 10.1038/s41392-020-00243-2
58. Jia X, Yin C, Lu S, Chen Y, Liu Q, Bai J, et al. Two Things About COVID-19 Might Need Attention. *Preprints* (2020). doi: 10.20944/preprints202002.0315.v1
59. Zhou P, Yang XL, Wang XG, Hu B, Zhang L, Zhang W, et al. A Pneumonia Outbreak Associated With a New Coronavirus of Probable Bat Origin. *Nature* (2020) 579:270–3. doi: 10.1038/s41586-020-2012-7
60. Zhou F, Yu T, Du R, Fan G, Liu Y, Liu Z, et al. Clinical Course and Risk Factors for Mortality of Adult Inpatients With COVID-19 in Wuhan, China: A Retrospective Cohort Study. *Lancet* (2020) 395:1054–62. doi: 10.1016/S0140-6736(20)30566-3
61. Merad M, Martin JC. Pathological Inflammation in Patients With COVID-19: A Key Role for Monocytes and Macrophages. *Nat Rev Immunol* (2020) 20:355–62. doi: 10.1038/s41577-020-0331-4
62. Xu Z, Shi L, Wang Y, Zhang J, Huang L, Zhang C, et al. Pathological Findings of COVID-19 Associated With Acute Respiratory Distress Syndrome. *Lancet Respir Med* (2020) 8:420–2. doi: 10.1016/S2213-2600(20)30076-X

63. Chen Y, Feng Z, Diao B, Wang R, Wang G, Wang C, et al. The Novel Severe Acute Respiratory Syndrome Coronavirus 2 (SARS-Cov-2) Directly Decimates Human Spleens and Lymph Nodes. *medRxiv* (2020). 2020.2003.2027.20045427. doi: 10.1101/2020.03.27.20045427
64. Diao B, Wang C, Wang R, Feng Z, Tan Y, Wang H, et al. Human Kidney is a Target for Novel Severe Acute Respiratory Syndrome Coronavirus 2 (Sars-CoV-2) Infection. *medRxiv* (2020). 2020.2003.2004.20031120. doi: 10.1101/2020.03.04.20031120
65. Henry BM, de Oliveira MHS, Benoit S, Plebani M, Lippi G. Hematologic, Biochemical and Immune Biomarker Abnormalities Associated With Severe Illness and Mortality in Coronavirus Disease 2019 (COVID-19): A Meta-Analysis. *Clin Chem Lab Med* (2020) 58:1021–8. doi: 10.1515/cclm-2020-0369
66. Zhang JJ, Dong X, Cao YY, Yuan YD, Yang YB, Yan YQ, et al. Clinical Characteristics of 140 Patients Infected With SARS-CoV-2 in Wuhan, China. *Allergy* (2020) 75:1730–41. doi: 10.1111/all.14238
67. Zhu L, She ZG, Cheng X, Qin JJ, Zhang XJ, Cai J, et al. Association of Blood Glucose Control and Outcomes in Patients With COVID-19 and Pre-existing Type 2 Diabetes. *Cell Metab* (2020) 31:1068–77.e1063. doi: 10.1016/j.cmet.2020.04.021
68. Guo W, Li M, Dong Y, Zhou H, Zhang Z, Tian C, et al. Diabetes is a Risk Factor for the Progression and Prognosis of COVID-19. *Diabetes/Metab Res Rev* (2020) 36:e3319. doi: 10.1002/dmrr.3319
69. Bhattacharya I, Ghayor C, Pérez Dominguez A, Weber FE. From Influenza Virus to Novel Corona Virus (SARS-Cov-2)-the Contribution of Obesity. *Front Endocrinol* (2020) 11:556962. doi: 10.3389/fendo.2020.556962
70. Wang S, Ma P, Zhang S, Song S, Wang Z, Ma Y, et al. Fasting Blood Glucose At Admission is an Independent Predictor for 28-Day Mortality in Patients With COVID-19 Without Previous Diagnosis of Diabetes: A Multi-Centre Retrospective Study. *Diabetologia* (2020) 63:2102–11. doi: 10.1007/s00125-020-05209-1
71. Gregg EW, Cheng YJ, Srinivasan M, Lin J, Geiss LS, Albright AL, et al. Trends in Cause-Specific Mortality Among Adults With and Without Diagnosed Diabetes in the USA: An Epidemiological Analysis of Linked National Survey and Vital Statistics Data. *Lancet* (2018) 391:2430–40. doi: 10.1016/S0140-6736(18)30314-3
72. Pearson-Stuttard J, Blundell S, Harris T, Cook DG, Critchley J. Diabetes and Infection: Assessing the Association With Glycaemic Control in Population-Based Studies. *Lancet Diabetes Endocrinol* (2016) 4:148–58. doi: 10.1016/S2213-8587(15)00379-4
73. Rao Kondapally Seshasai S, Kaptoge S, Thompson A, Di Angelantonio E, Gao P, Sarwar N, et al. Diabetes Mellitus, Fasting Glucose, and Risk of Cause-Specific Death. *New Engl J Med* (2011) 364:829–41. doi: 10.1056/NEJMoa1008862
74. Yang X, Yu Y, Xu J, Shu H, Xia J, Liu H, et al. Clinical Course and Outcomes of Critically Ill Patients With SARS-CoV-2 Pneumonia in Wuhan, China: A Single-Centered, Retrospective, Observational Study. *Lancet Respir Med* (2020) 8:475–81. doi: 10.1016/S2213-2600(20)30079-5
75. Fadini GP, Morieri ML, Longato E, Avogaro A. Prevalence and Impact of Diabetes Among People Infected With SARS-Cov-2. *J Endocrinol Invest* (2020) 43:867–9. doi: 10.1007/s40618-020-01236-2
76. Peleg AY, Weerarathna T, McCarthy JS, Davis TM. Common Infections in Diabetes: Pathogenesis, Management and Relationship to Glycaemic Control. *Diabetes/Metab Res Rev* (2007) 23:3–13. doi: 10.1002/dmrr.682
77. Yeh HC, Punjabi NM, Wang NY, Pankow JS, Duncan BB, Cox CE, et al. Cross-Sectional and Prospective Study of Lung Function in Adults With Type 2 Diabetes: The Atherosclerosis Risk in Communities (ARIC) Study. *Diabetes Care* (2008) 31:741–6. doi: 10.2337/dc07-1464
78. Shah SH, Sonawane P, Nahar P, Vaidya S, Salvi S. Pulmonary Function Tests in Type 2 Diabetes Mellitus and Their Association With Glycemic Control and Duration of the Disease. *Lung India Off Organ Indian Chest Soc* (2013) 30:108–12. doi: 10.4103/0970-2113.110417
79. Wang X, Liu Z, Li J, Zhang J, Tian S, Lu S, et al. Impacts of Type 2 Diabetes on Disease Severity, Therapeutic Effect, and Mortality of Patients With Covid-19. *J Clin Endocrinol Metab* (2020) 105:dgaa535. doi: 10.1210/clinem/dgaa535
80. Holman N, Knighton P, Kar P, O'Keefe J, Curley M, Weaver A, et al. Risk Factors for COVID-19-related Mortality in People With Type 1 and Type 2 Diabetes in England: A Population-Based Cohort Study. *Lancet Diabetes Endocrinol* (2020) 8:823–33. doi: 10.1016/S2213-8587(20)30271-0
81. Bode B, Garrett V, Messler J, McFarland R, Crowe J, Booth R, et al. Glycemic Characteristics and Clinical Outcomes of COVID-19 Patients Hospitalized in the United States. *J Diabetes Sci Technol* (2020) 14:813–21. doi: 10.1177/1932296820924469
82. Iacobellis G, Penaherrera CA, Bermudez LE, Bernal Mizrachi E. Admission Hyperglycemia and Radiological Findings of SARS-CoV2 in Patients With and Without Diabetes. *Diabetes Res Clin Pract* (2020) 164:108185. doi: 10.1016/j.diabres.2020.108185
83. Li X, Xu S, Yu M, Wang K, Tao Y, Zhou Y, et al. Risk Factors for Severity and Mortality in Adult COVID-19 Inpatients in Wuhan. *J Allergy Clin Immunol* (2020) 146:110–8. doi: 10.1016/j.jaci.2020.04.006
84. Carrasco-Sánchez FJ, López-Carmona MD, Martínez-Marcos FJ, Pérez-Belmonte LM, Hidalgo-Jiménez A, Buonaiuto V, et al. Admission Hyperglycaemia as a Predictor of Mortality in Patients Hospitalized With COVID-19 Regardless of Diabetes Status: Data From the Spanish Semi-COVID-19 Registry. *Ann Med* (2021) 53:103–16. doi: 10.1080/07853890.2020.1836566
85. Bornstein SR, Rubino F, Khunti K, Mingrone G, Hopkins D, Birkenfeld AL, et al. Practical Recommendations for the Management of Diabetes in Patients With COVID-19. *Lancet Diabetes Endocrinol* (2020) 8:546–50. doi: 10.1016/S2213-8587(20)30152-2
86. Shen Y, Zhang L, Fan X, Zhou J. Glycemic Fluctuations Caused by COVID-19: Results From Continuous Glucose Monitoring. *Obes Med* (2021) 22:100328. doi: 10.1016/j.obmed.2021.100328
87. Hsia DS, Grove O, Cefalu WT. An Update on Sodium-Glucose Co-Transporter-2 Inhibitors for the Treatment of Diabetes Mellitus. *Curr Opin Endocrinol Diabetes Obes* (2017) 24:73–9. doi: 10.1097/MED.0000000000000311
88. Filippatos TD, Panagiotopoulou TV, Elisaf MS. Adverse Effects of GLP-1 Receptor Agonists. *Rev Diabetic Stud RDS* (2014) 11:202–30. doi: 10.1900/RDS.2014.11.202
89. Solerte SB, D'Addio F, Trevisan R, Lovati E, Rossi A, Pastore I, et al. Sitagliptin Treatment At the Time of Hospitalization was Associated With Reduced Mortality in Patients With Type 2 Diabetes and COVID-19: A Multicenter, Case-Control, Retrospective, Observational Study. *Diabetes Care* (2020) 43:2999–3006. doi: 10.2337/dc20-1521
90. Drucker DJ. Coronavirus Infections and Type 2 Diabetes-Shared Pathways With Therapeutic Implications. *Endocrine Rev* (2020) 41:bnaa011. doi: 10.1210/endrev/bnaa011
91. Gillespie EL, White CM, Kardas M, Lindberg M, Coleman CI. The Impact of ACE Inhibitors or Angiotensin II Type 1 Receptor Blockers on the Development of New-Onset Type 2 Diabetes. *Diabetes Care* (2005) 28:2261–6. doi: 10.2337/diacare.28.9.2261

20

Impact of Diabetes in Patients Diagnosed with COVID-19

Mohamed Abu-Farha[1†], Fahd Al-Mulla[2†], Thangavel Alphonse Thanaraj[2†], Sina Kavalakatt[1], Hamad Ali[2,3], Mohammed Abdul Ghani[4] and Jehad Abubaker[1*]*

[1] Department of Biochemistry and Molecular Biology, Dasman Diabetes Institute, Dasman, Kuwait, [2] Department of Genetics and Bioinformatics, Dasman Diabetes Institute, Dasman, Kuwait, [3] Department of Medical Laboratory Sciences, Faculty of Allied Health Sciences, Health Sciences Center, Kuwait University, Jabriya, Kuwait, [4] Diabetes Division, University of Texas Health Science Center at San Antonio, San Antonio, TX, United States

***Correspondence:**
Fahd Al-Mulla
fahd.almulla@dasmaninstitute.org
Jehad Abubaker
jehad.abubakr@dasmaninstitute.org

†These authors have contributed equally to this work

COVID-19 is a disease caused by the coronavirus SARS-CoV-2 (Severe Acute Respiratory Syndrome Coronavirus-2), known as a highly contagious disease, currently affecting more than 200 countries worldwide. The main feature of SARS-CoV-2 that distinguishes it from other viruses is the speed of transmission combined with higher risk of mortality from acute respiratory distress syndrome (ARDS). People with diabetes mellitus (DM), severe obesity, cardiovascular disease, and hypertension are more likely to get infected and are at a higher risk of mortality from COVID-19. Among elderly patients who are at higher risk of death from COVID-19, 26.8% have DM. Although the reasons for this increased risk are yet to be determined, several factors may contribute to type-2 DM patients' increased susceptibility to infections. A possible factor that may play a role in increasing the risk in people affected by diabetes and/or obesity is the impaired innate and adaptive immune response, characterized by a state of chronic and low-grade inflammation that can lead to abrupt systemic metabolic alteration. SARS patients previously diagnosed with diabetes or hyperglycemia had higher mortality and morbidity rates when compared with patients who were under metabolic control. Similarly, obese individuals are at higher risk of developing complications from SARS-CoV-2. In this review, we will explore the current and evolving insights pertinent to the metabolic impact of coronavirus infections with special attention to the main pathways and mechanisms that are linked to the pathophysiology and treatment of diabetes.

Keywords: coronavirus disease (COVID-19), type 2 diabetes, angiotensin converting enzyme2 (ACE2), Furin, transmembrane protease, serine 2 (TMPRSS2), metformin, interferon induced membrane (IFITM3)

Abbreviations: SARS-CoV-2, severe acute respiratory syndrome coronavirus-2; ARDS, acute respiratory distress syndrome; DM, diabetes mellitus; MERS-CoV, middle east respiratory syndrome coronavirus; COPD, chronic obstructive pulmonary disease; CVD, cardiovascular disease; CKD, chronic kidney disease; ACE2, angiotensin-converting enzyme 2; T2DM, type-2 dm; TNF-α, tumor necrosis factor alpha; MCP-1, monocyte chemoattractant protein-1; IL-6, interleukin-6; rhACE2, recombinant angiotensin-converting enzyme 2; TCZ, tocilizumab; IFITM, interferon-induced transmembrane; ADAM17, a disintegrin and metallopeptidase domain 17; GRP78, glucose regulated protein 78; SBDβ, GRP78 substrate binding domain; βDKA, Diabetic Ketoacidosis; DPP-4i, Dipeptidyl peptidase 4 inhibitor; AICAR, 5-Aminoimidazole-4-carboxamide ribonucleotide.

WORSE OUTCOMES IN COVID-19 PATIENTS AFFECTED BY OBESITY AND DIABETES

COVID-19 is caused by the coronavirus SARS-CoV-2 and has emerged as a fast-spreading contagious disease affecting most countries across the globe (1). SARS-CoV-2 is the third coronavirus appearance in human history following severe acute respiratory syndrome coronavirus (SARS-CoV) and the Middle East respiratory syndrome coronavirus (MERS-CoV) (2, 3). Coronaviruses are a family of enveloped viruses encoded by a single-stranded positive-sense RNA genome and named for the crown-like appearance of their virions under the electron microscope. The key feature of SARS-CoV-2 that differentiates it from other viruses is its transmissibility combined with a greater risk of mortality due to the acute respiratory distress syndrome (ARDS). Signs and symptoms of SARS-CoV-2 infections range from mild/asymptomatic infections (20-86% of all infections), restricted to the upper respiratory tract (20–86% of all infections), to severe respiratory distress characterized by the spread of infection to the lower airways leading to regional inflammation and pneumonia. This is manifested particularly in patients with comorbidities such as chronic obstructive pulmonary disease (COPD), asthma, diabetes, hypertension, and cardiovascular disease (CVD) (4, 5). Significantly, Maddaloni et al. suggested an increased prevalence of COPD and of chronic kidney disease (CKD) in Covid-19 patients with diabetes (6).

People with diabetes mellitus (DM), severe obesity, CVD, and hypertension are at a higher risk of poor outcome from COVID-19 (4, 7–10). The reasons underlying this increased risk have not been determined. However, a panoply of factors may contribute to type-2 DM (T2DM) patient increased risk of poor outcomes of COVID-19 disease (**Figure 1**). Individuals affected by diabetes and/or obesity generally have an impaired innate and adaptive immune response, characterized by a state of chronic low-grade inflammation (11), which can lead to abrupt systemic metabolic alteration, characterized by higher levels of leptin (a proinflammatory adipokine) and lower adiponectin (an anti-inflammatory adipokine) (12–16). An unfavorable hormone environment also contributes to dysregulation of the immune response (17). Typically, obese people have defective innate immunity manifested by enhanced production of several proinflammatory cytokines, such as tumor necrosis factor alpha (TNF-α), monocyte chemoattractant protein-1 (MCP-1), and interleukin-6 (IL-6) (18). Upon antigen exposure, obesity-related chronic inflammation reduces the activation of macrophages and dampens proinflammatory cytokine production (19). This exceptional obesogenic state may partly

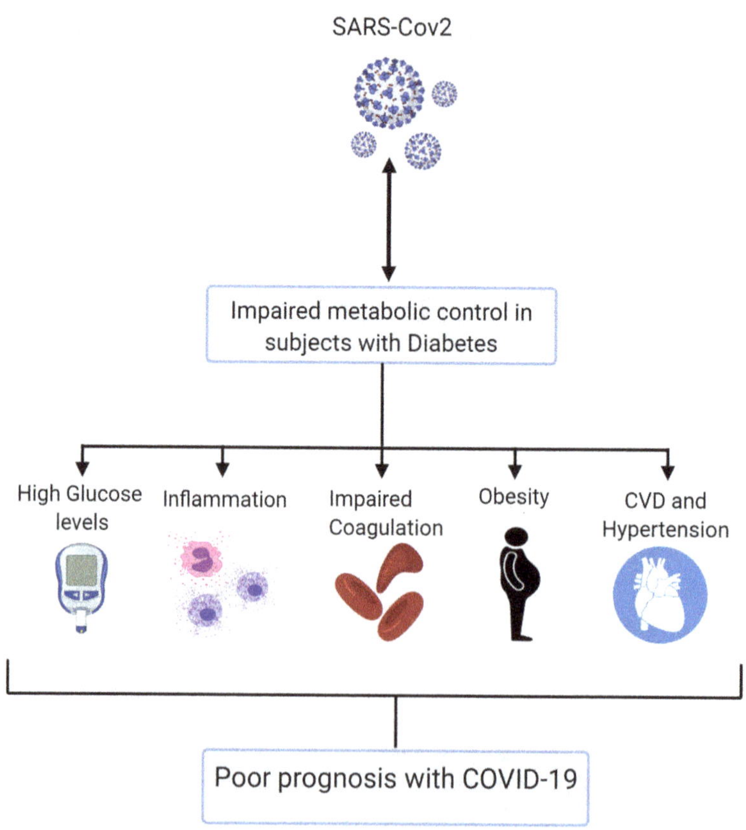

FIGURE 1 | A schematic model summarizing the various mechanisms by which diabetes can impact on COVID-19 poor outcome.

explain the presence of antiviral-resistance and vaccine-escape deviations in the obese population (19, 20). Moreover, B- and T-cell responses are weakened in obese patients and even more so in obese patients with diabetes (21). After analyzing a case cohort of 70,000 individuals infected with COVID-19, the Chinese Centre for Disease Control and Prevention reported augmented mortality in individuals with diabetes, increasing from 2.3% in the general population to 7.3% in people with diabetes (22). Interestingly, earlier studies demonstrated that individuals with diabetes exhibit a similar high risk for SARS and MERS (23, 24). Among patients infected with the SARS virus, it has been shown that histories of diabetes and hyperglycemia are independent predictors of mortality and morbidity and that metabolic control might improve their prognosis (24). Moreover, hyperglycemia is a strong prognostic predictor of outcome in hospitalized patients with COVID-19. Earlier studies showed that hyperglycemic patients with COVID-19 displayed higher cumulative incidence of severe disease than normoglycemic controls (25, 26). Possible mechanisms for this increased mortality include hyperglycemia-induced changes in the immune system and increases in inflammatory cytokines (27). Furthermore, among elderly individuals who were at higher risk of death from COVID-19, 26.8% had diabetes (4). In the United States, 10.5% of the total population has diabetes (4). Similarly, obese individuals are at higher risk of developing complications from SARS-CoV-2 (28, 29).

In this review, we will discuss current and growing perceptions pertinent to the metabolic impact of coronavirus infections while paying special attention to the main pathways and mechanisms that are connected to the pathophysiology and treatment of diabetes.

Hypertension is another predictor of poor outcomes in COVID-19 patients. This may be due to the SARS-CoV-2 binding to the angiotensin-converting enzyme 2 (ACE2) in human epithelial lung cells, potentially involved in ARDS. Ace2 KO mice display severe pathology of ARDS (30). An earlier report has shown that recombinant angiotensin-converting enzyme 2 (rhACE2) can attenuate arterial hypoxemia and pulmonary blood flow in a piglet model of lipopolysaccharide-induced ARDS (31). ACE2 exerts its functions through cleaving either Angiotensin I or Angiotensin II into inactive Angiotensin (1–9) and Angiotensin (1–7) respectively. Angiotensin (1–9) gets further metabolized into Angiotensin (1–7). Angiotensin (1–7) is a vasodilator. Hence, ACE2 counteracts the vasoconstrictor effects of the ACE-Angiotensin II axis. Angiotensin-converting enzyme inhibitors (ACEi) and/or angiotensin receptor blockers (ARBs) may interfere with angiotensin-converting enzyme 2 expression and/or activity. Thus, as recommended by several medical associations, and in light of more scientific evidence supporting their beneficial/non-harmful impact, ACEis/ARBs should be continued in COVID-19 patients (32–34). Moreover, the impact of metabolic syndrome (MS) and its comorbidities on COVID-19 prognosis must be considered. Yet, MS by definition is a set of metabolic disorders that include insulin resistance, dyslipidemia, central obesity and hypertension. All are risk factors for the development of type-2 diabetes and cardiovascular diseases (35). In 2017, it was estimated that MS affected 20% of North American population, 25% of European population and approximately 15% of Chinese population (36). Considering the presence of MS across different ethnicities and continents, more future studies focusing on the effect of MS on COVID-19 outcomes are needed.

Studies from different countries have demonstrated a varying prevalence of diabetes, other comorbidities, and mortality among patients infected with COVID-19. **Table 1** summarizes the

TABLE 1 | Prevalence (%) of comorbidities in COVID-19 infected patients.

Study	Sample size (n)	Diabetes (%)	CVD (%)	HTN (%)	CKD (%)	Ref
Li B et al.	1,527	9.7	16.4	17.1	NR	(5)
Covid-19 group, Italy	481	33.9	30.1	73.8	20.2	(37)
Onder et al.	355	35.5	42.5	NR	NR	(7)
Zhou et al.	191	19	8	30	1	(8)
Wu C et al.	201	10.9	4	19.4	1	(9)
Guan et al.	1,099	7.4	3.8	15	0.7	(10)
Bhatraju et al.	24	58	NR	NR	21	(38)
CDC, USA	7,162	10.9	9	NR	3	(39)
Zhang et al.	140	12.1	8.6	30	1.4	(40)
Liu J et al.	61	8.2	1.6	19.7	NR	(41)
Guo et al.	187	15	11.2	32.6	3.2	(42)
Huang et al.	41	19.5	15	14.6	NR	(43)
Chen N et al.	99	12.1	40	NR	NR	(44)
Wang et al.	138	10.1	19.6	31.2	2.9	(45)
Yang J et al.	Meta-analysis of eight studies n = 46,248	0.08	0.05	0.17	NR	(46)
Yang X et al.	52	17	23	NR	NR	(47)
Liu K et al.	137	10.2	7.3	9.5	NR	(41)
Chen T et al.	274	17	8	34	1	(48)
CDC China	20,982	5.3	4.2	12.8	NR	(49)
Singh et al.	Meta-analysis of 10 studies = 2,209	0.11	0.07	0.21	NR	(50)
Hu Y et al.	Meta-analysis of 21 studies n = 47,344	7.7	4.7	15.6	2.1	(37)

CVD, cardiovascular disease; HTN, hypertension; CKD, chronic kidney disease; NR, not reported; CDC, Centers for Disease Control and Prevention.

TABLE 2 | Prevalence of diabetes amongst non-severe and severe COVID-19 infected patients.

Study	Sample size(n)	DM (%)	ICU admission (Severe/ Critical) (%)*	Significance p value of non-severe *vs* severe COVID	Ref.
Wu et al.	201	10.90%	19.00%	0.002	(9)
Guan et al.	1,099	7.40%	16.20%	NR	(10)
CDC, USA	7,162	10.90%	32.00%	NR	(39)
Zhang et al.	140	12.10%	13.80%	0.615	(40)
Huang et al.	41	15%	25.00%	0.160	(43)
Wang et al.	138	10.10%	22.20%	0.009	(45)
Liu J et al.	61	8.20%	17.60%	0.094	(41)
Hu Y et al.	Meta-analysis of 21 studies n = 47,344	7.70%	44.50%	NR	(37)

DM, diabetes mellitus; Ref., references; CDC, Centers for Disease Control and Prevention.
**% is calculated from total population with COVID-19.*

prevalence of comorbidities among patients with COVID-19, and **Tables 2** and **3** summarize the prevalence of diabetes and other comorbidities among patients with severe *versus* mild COVID-19 symptoms and among survivors *versus* non-survivors of COVID-19. Overall, it was reported that the proportion of people affected by diabetes among COVID-19 patients was from 5.3% to 20%. Although the COVID-19 surveillance group in Italy showed a higher prevalence of comorbidities such as hypertension and diabetes (73% and 34%, respectively), other studies from China showed a 9 to 15% prevalence rate. Bhatraju et al. (38). reported that US patients had morbidity rates similar to patients in Italy. However, it is important to note that Bhatraju et al. included only critically ill patients from the Seattle area. Differences in the characteristics of patients included in the studies could explain the difference in the prevalence of comorbidities among various cohorts. Data also show that the presence of diabetes is associated with a high risk of severe to critical illness in 14 to 32% of patients with COVID-19 (39, 40). Other studies showed higher rate of admission into the intensive care unit (ICU) among people who were diagnosed with diabetes or other comorbidities when compared with non-ICU patients (22.2 *vs* 5.9%) (45). Furthermore, mortality rates among COVID-19 patients with various comorbidities when compared to those without any comorbidities were 15 *vs* 2.3%, respectively (43–45). Notably, several studies showed that diabetes is strongly associated with increased risk of mortality due to COVID-19 as compared with COVID-19 patients without diabetes and other comorbidities (22–31 *vs* 2–4%) (8, 10, 47). Zhou et al. also showed that the mortality rate among COVID-19 patients with diabetes was higher than the overall mortality rate with the viral infection (8). Wu et al. showed that diabetes was associated with a hazard ratio of 2.3 for ARDS (9). Other studies associated diabetes to the severity of COVID-19 (51). Hence, it was proposed that the course of treatment and prognosis should be stratified based on occurrence or absence of comorbidities (52).

In Italy, patients with diabetes showed high prevalence, severity of disease and mortality during SARS-COV-2 infection as well as higher rates of ICU admission. They frequently reported respiratory symptoms and were at increased risk of numerous pulmonary diseases, such as COPD, bronchial severe asthma and idiopathic pulmonary fibrosis (53, 54). Thus, we speculate that the complicated alveolar-capillary network of lungs could be targeted by diabetes micro-vascular injury. Recently, continuous experimental therapy with monoclonal antibody against the IL-6 receptor (tocilizumab, TCZ) in Italy seems to have positive effects on severe lung disease and prognosis in patients with COVID-19. Hence, TCZ could be administered to patients with diabetes during the SARS-COV-2 infection (55). However, an earlier study showed that at admission, hyperglycemic (n = 31) *vs.* normoglycemic (n = 47) patients had fivefold higher IL-6 levels, which persisted even after TCZ administration ($P < 0.05$) (56). Interestingly, in a risk-adjusted Cox regression analysis, TCZ in hyperglycemic patients failed to reduce risk of severe outcomes as it did in normoglycemic patients ($P < 0.009$). Thus, hyperglycemia could result in an unfavorable effect on hospital admission, clinical outcomes and drug therapy (25, 26, 56). It is possible that comorbidities associated with diabetes (*e.g.*, obesity, hypertension, and CVD) contribute to increased morbidity and mortality due to COVID-19. Diabetes was associated with COVID-19 poor outcomes (51) and with increased time required for viral clearance (4). Increased expression of ACE2, furin, and IL-6 and impaired T-cell function are several factors that were associated with the risk and severity of SARS-CoV2 infection in individuals with diabetes (57).

COVID-19 could cause endothelial dysfunction and a hyper-coagulation state. This condition is intensified by hypoxia, which augments thrombosis by both increasing blood viscosity and hypoxia-inducible transcription factors (HIF) (58, 59). Consequently, these could lead to pulmonary embolism with occlusion and micro-thrombosis in pulmonary vessels, as detected in critically ill COVID-19 patients (59). It is also

TABLE 3 | Prevalence of diabetes among non-survivor and survivor COVID-19 infected patients.

Study	Sample size (n)	DM in entire cohort (%)	DM (%) in non-survivors	DM (%) in survivors	Mortality rate	Ref.
Zhou et al.	191	19%	31.00%	14.00%	OR 2.8(1.35 to 6.05) p < 0.001	(8)
Wu et al.	88	18.2%	25.00%	12.50%	HR 1.58(0.80 to 3.13), p = 0.19	(22)
Guan et al.	1,099	7.4%	26.90%	6.10%	NR	(10)
Yang X et al.	52	17%	22%	10%	NR	(47)
Chen N et al.	274	17%	21.00%	14.00%	NR	(44)

reported that COVID-19 is associated with increased incidence of coagulation as well as thrombotic and inflammatory events (60), which was responsible, at least in part, for the severe morbidity and mortality. This suggests that COVID-19 activates yet another unidentified mechanism, which is involved in the coagulation process. Interestingly, it is well established that diabetes is a state of increased coagulability; where increased plasminogen activator inhibitor-1 is a consistent finding in patients with diabetes. Thus, increased coagulability in diabetes may be a possible mechanism that links diabetes to severity of COVID-19.

POSSIBLE MECHANISMS THAT PREDISPOSE COVID-19 PATIENTS WITH DIABETES AND/OR OBESITY TO POOR OUTCOMES

Considering the high incidence of obesity, hypertension, and CVD in patients with diabetes, it remains unclear whether diabetes is an independent contributor to the higher morbidity and mortality associated with COVID-19 (7–10). Maddaloni et al. have shown that patients with cardiometabolic multimorbidity, and not diabetes or CVD alone, experience worse COVID-19 outcomes (61). Nevertheless, plasma glucose levels and diabetes are independent predictors of mortality and morbidity in patients with SARS (24, 62). Mechanisms that likely increase the vulnerability for COVID-19 in DM patients comprise increased binding affinity and efficient virus entry, reduced viral clearance, weakened T-cell role, increased susceptibility to cytokine storm disorder, and the existence of CVD. Lung cells, including pneumocytes, are the main cellular sites for coronavirus entrance and inflammation (63). They express key proteins that enable coronavirus entry into cells, such as ACE2, transmembrane protease serine 2 (TMPRSS2), furin, and dipeptidyl peptidase-4 (DPP4). ACE2 and DPP4 also have established multiple metabolic activities linked to the pharmacologic and physiologic control of cardiovascular and glucose homeostasis and DPP4 inhibitors are used extensively in diabetes therapy (28).

Increased ACE2 expression in pulmonary cells, kidney, myocardium, and pancreas may mediate increased cellular binding of SARS-CoV-2 (64–66). The increased expression of ACE2 in these tissues is well documented in animal models of diabetes (67, 68). Although insulin administration downregulates ACE2 expression (46, 68), other hypoglycemic agents such as glucagon-like peptide-1 (GLP-1) agonists and thiazolidinediones (pioglitazone), anti-hypertensive drugs such as statins, and ACE inhibitors increase ACE2 expression (69–73). Recently, Rao et al. investigated illnesses or traits that may be connected to increased ACE2 expression in the lung. Using a phenome-wide Mendelian randomization analyses, they identified the association between diabetes and higher lung ACE2 expression (74). Moreover, circulating levels of furin (cellular protease) were found to be higher in patients with type-2 diabetes (75). The findings of these studies support the hypothesis that COVID-19 patients with diabetes are predisposed to poor outcomes. Furthermore, a recent study stated that clearance of SARS-CoV-2 was delayed in patients with diabetes (76). However, more extensive studies are needed to confirm this finding.

HOW ARE THE DIFFERENT HOST-CELLULAR PROTEINS INVOLVED IN SARS-COV-2 INFECTION ASSOCIATED WITH DIABETES?

Apart from ACE2, a number of other host-cellular protein components are thought to have the ability to regulate the entry of SARS-COV-2; such components are known to be involved in the pathogenesis of diabetes, as illustrated in **Figure 2** and as described below.

ACE2

ACE2 acts as the receptor for the binding of SARS-CoV-2 with the host cell. It is already known that the binding of the SARS coronavirus to its receptor damages islets and causes acute diabetes (77). Clinical data, which includes patients with mild and severe COVID-19, established the existence of mild pancreatitis (78). Diabetes and hypertension (common comorbidities associated with COVID-19) are often treated with ACE inhibitors and angiotensin II type-I receptor blockers. Studies have reported that the expression of ACE2 is elevated in people with diabetes treated with these medications (79, 80). The higher levels of ACE2 can thus facilitate critical illness in COVID-19 patients (81).

Furin

Furin cleaves cell surface proteins. The SARS-CoV-2 S-protein S1/S2 cleavage site is the target for furin during infection. This cleavage is critical, as it allows the fusion sequences on the COVID-19 spike protein to be exposed for the fusion of the virus with the host cell membranes (1, 65, 82). Thus, high levels of furin enhance the ability of the virus to enter the host cell. It is known that individuals with high plasma furin concentrations have a pronounced dysmetabolic phenotype and elevated risk of diabetes and premature mortality (75, 83). A point mutation at the furin cleavage site in the insulin pro-receptor was seen in an individual with extreme insulin-resistant diabetes (84). Furthermore, variations in the furin gene have been associated with decreased triglyceride and increased high-density lipoprotein cholesterol levels (85). Furin has an impact on the pancreas, as verified by previous studies, which demonstrated that furin controls the growth of pancreatic β-cells (86). It also plays a role in granular acidification in the endocrine pancreas *via* impaired processing of Ac45 (87). We have previously identified a higher proportion of damaging variations in the furin gene in the Arab population as compared with Europeans (88), which is a population with high rates of diabetes that requires special attention during this pandemic (89).

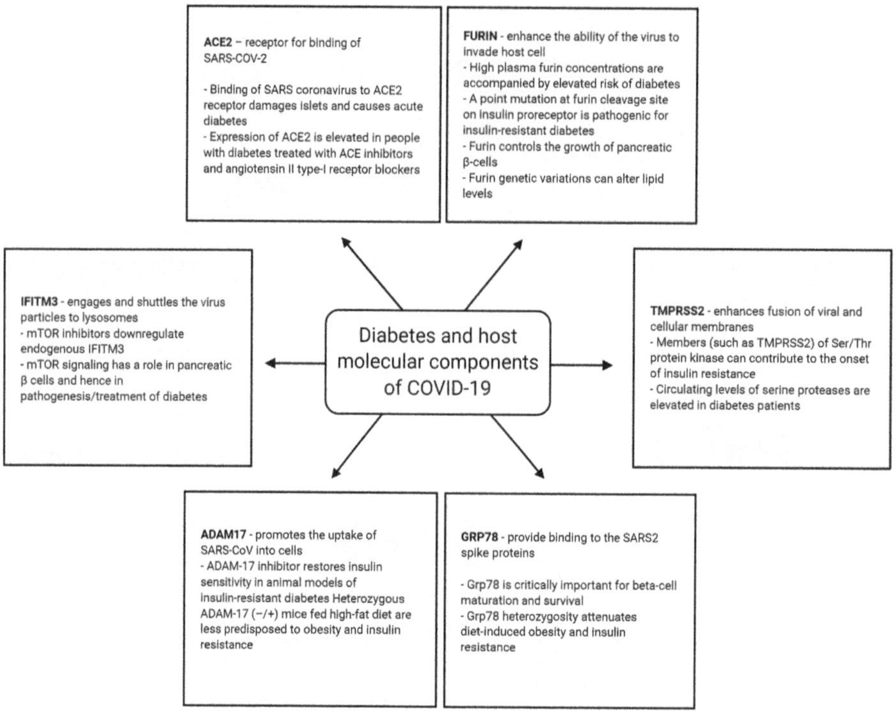

FIGURE 2 | Illustration of association of the different host-cellular proteins involved in SARS-COV-2 infection with diabetes.

TMPRSS2

SARS-CoV-2 uses the SARS-CoV receptor ACE2 for entry, and the serine protease TMPRSS2 is required for S-protein priming, which entails S-protein cleavage at the S1/S2 and the S2′ site and allows fusion of viral and cellular membranes. TMPRSS2 belongs to the family of serine proteases. It is now known that ser/thr protein kinases contribute to the onset of insulin resistance *via* the introduction of phosphorylation-based negative feedback control mechanisms, which disengage the insulin receptor from its downstream effectors (90). Circulating levels of serine proteases, such as granzyme B, are elevated in diabetes patients (91). Hence, it can be assumed that the increased activity of TMPRSS2 can increase the viral entry in the host.

IFITM3

Interferon-induced transmembrane (IFITM) proteins are important effectors that inhibit viral infections. IFITM3 directly engages and shuttles the incoming virus particles to lysosomes. It is known that the MERS-CoV entry into host cells is sensitive to inhibition by IFITM proteins (particularly IFITM3) and that the cellular context and/or IFITM expression levels can affect the efficiency of inhibition (92, 93). IFITM3 is now indicated as a novel entry site in the SARS-CoV-2 domain as well (94, 95). Inhibitors of the mammalian target of rapamycin (mTOR), such as rapamycin, downregulate endogenous IFITM3 through a lysosomal degradation pathway in hematopoietic and non-hematopoietic cells (96). Interestingly, mTOR signaling has a role in pancreatic β cells and immune cells, and hence it is also involved in the pathogenesis and treatment of diabetes (97).

Adam17

In the context of SARS-CoV infection, it has been proposed that SARS-S binding to ACE2 triggers shedding of ACE2 *via* the disintegrin and metallopeptidase domain 17 (ADAM17) protein to release the extracellular domain of ACE2 into the extracellular space. This process promotes the uptake of SARS-CoV into cells (98, 99). It is now further proposed that the inhibition of ADAM17 may exert a protective effect on COVID-19 (100). ADAM17 is a metalloprotease and disintegrin that lodges in the plasma membrane in several cell types and can cleave a wide variety of cell surface proteins. In this way, ADAM17 can influence several physiological and pathological processes (101). In animal models of insulin-resistant diabetes, the intraperitoneal injection of ADAM-17 inhibitor, restored insulin sensitivity through the inhibition of TNF-α (102). Consistent with these findings, Serino et al. demonstrated that heterozygous ADAM-17 (−/+) mice fed a high-fat diet were less predisposed to obesity and insulin resistance than their wild-type littermates (103).

Other Players: GRP78 and CD147

It appears that apart from the ACE2 receptor entry mode, SARS-CoV-2 may use the protease called TMPRSS2 to enter the cells; some researchers speculate that there can be at least 8 other different proteases. It is also proposed that other receptors such as glucose regulated protein 78 (GRP78 receptors) may provide binding to the SARS-CoV-2 spike proteins. Protein–protein docking studies revealed that four regions of the spike protein can fit tightly in the GRP78 substrate binding domain β (SBDβ) (104). Grp78 is critically important for β-cell maturation and survival; it is demonstrated that Grp78 heterozygosity attenuates diet-induced obesity and insulin resistance (105). It is also possible that other receptors mediate the entry of SARS-CoV-2, such as CD147 into T cells. Also called Basigin or EMMPRIN, CD147 is a transmembrane glycoprotein that belongs to the immunoglobulin superfamily on the surface of T lymphocytes (106). A recent study reported that it is a novel invasive route for SARS-CoV-2 entry (106, 107). CD147 is essential for diabetes-associated recombinant tissue-plasminogen activator (rt-PA)-induced hemorrhagic transformation, and reduced CD147 glycosylation is an encouraging therapy for neurovascular-unit repair following rt-PA treatment of diabetes patients (108).

USE OF GLUCOSE-LOWERING THERAPIES IN COVID-19 PATIENTS WITH DIABETES

Lack of specific and effective therapeutics is the major challenge in dealing with COVID-19 patients that are suffering from severe comorbidities such as diabetes. In the absence of specific medication for COVID-19 patients, it is essential to evaluate the applicability of drugs in practice for various comorbidities. Diabetes is one of the major comorbidities of COVID-19 patients who developed ARDS (43). It was originally thought that some anti-diabetes treatment (such as metformin, PPARs, DPP4 inhibitors, GLP-1R agonists, SGLT2 inhibitors and insulin therapy) could influence the course of COVID-19; however, no convincing evidence has emerged to support this view.

GLP-1R Agonists

GLP-1R agonists target many anti-inflammatory pathways in animals and lessen systemic inflammation in individuals affected by diabetes and obesity (109). These drugs decrease pulmonary type-2 immune cytokine reactions and the degree of lung injury in mice after respiratory viral infection (110). Thus, GLP-1-based drugs possess strong anti-inflammatory effects in lungs and could become possible repurposed drugs, useful to treat COVID-19 patients with ARDS (111). However, the beneficial effects of these drugs remain to be convincingly established in COVID-19.

SGLT2 Inhibitors

Based on the findings that showed the organ-protective effects of SGLT-2 inhibitors (112), in addition to their glycemic benefits, these drugs were proposed to provide benefits in COVID-19 settings. However, these inhibitors were also known to lead to risk of dehydration and euglycemic Diabetic Ketoacidosis (DKA) (112). Though SGLT2 inhibitors may be potentially beneficial as organ protective agents in COVID-19, there is no completed clinical trial to assess the risk/benefit balance of using these inhibitors in COVID-19 patients. Thus, caution needs to be exercised when these inhibitors are used (113). It is advisable to re-evaluate or discontinue SGLT2 inhibitors upon hospital admission of unstable patients with severe SARS-CoV-2 infection.

Insulin Therapy

Given that insulin therapy has an optimal glucose-lowering effect in patients affected by diabetes, it is suggested that insulin is the treatment of choice in hospitalized COVID-19 patients with diabetes (114, 115). As stated in the American Diabetes Association guidelines, basal insulin or a basal plus bolus correction insulin regimen is the favorite treatment for noncritically ill hospitalized patients. Continuous intravenous insulin infusion is preferred in critically ill patients. A target glucose range of 7.8–10.0 mmol/L is recommended for both critically and noncritically ill patients (114). Moreover, a recent study examined the effects of optimal glycemic control using insulin therapy in patients with hyperglycemia affected by COVID-19 (25). Fifty-nine patients with COVID-19 hospitalized with moderate disease were stratified into hyperglycemic and normoglycemic groups based on glycemia measure of >7.77 mmol/L at the time of hospital admission. Their data showed that patients with hyperglycemia treated with insulin infusion had a lower risk of severe disease outcome than patients without insulin infusion. Accordingly, insulin infusion may be an effective method for reaching glycemic control and improving outcomes in patients with COVID-19 (25). Consistently, Bornstein et al. recommended insulin treatment for diabetic patients with severe COVID-19 (116). However, a recent study examining the effects of insulin therapy in hospitalized diabetic patients with COVID-19 reported a greater than threefold risk of mortality and severe outcome in treated patients (117). Thus, it remains unclear whether insulin therapy worsens COVID-19 outcomes or if these results were caused by a patient selection bias (note: patients with diabetes receiving insulin tend to have longer duration of disease with a higher rate of comorbidities).

ACE2 and DPP4

DPP4 (CD26), a transmembrane ectopeptidase, acts as a co-receptor for a subset of coronaviruses including MERS-CoV. Its activity can potentially modulate the levels and activity of many immunomodulatory cytokines and chemokines (118). Although ACE2 and DPP4 are crucial modulators of glucose homeostasis, there is no convincing evidence to propose that medications regulating the ACE2- or DPP4-linked pathways yield obvious benefit or harm during coronavirus infections. Several studies have evaluated whether DPP4i are associated to improved Covid-19 outcomes, with apparently opposing results. Some groups have shown that patients with COVID-19 who were on Dipeptidyl peptidase 4 inhibitor (DPP-4is) had a similar disease outcome as those who were not (119–121). Instead, Solerte et al. have found that sitagliptin (DPP-4i) treatment at the time of admission was associated with improved clinical outcomes and reduced mortality, compared to standard-of-care treatment (122). ACE2 decoy receptors or antibodies targeting ACE2 can be promising tools to block the viral cell-entry. However, the impact of these drugs on metabolic parameters has not been sensibly investigated and requires further investigation (123).

CONCLUSION

Evidence implies that obesity and diabetes are leading risk factors that affect the severity of disease caused by coronaviruses infections, such as COVID-19. Among patients infected with the SARS-CoV-2, history has shown that diabetes and hyperglycemia are independent predictors for mortality and morbidity, and that glycemic control might improve patient prognosis. The risk seen among people with diabetes may be due to insulin resistance, inflammation, or hypercoagulation, or owed to underlying obesity, which may lead to adverse outcome.

Several classes of anti-obesity and anti-diabetes medications (such as metformin, 5-Aminoimidazole-4-carboxamide ribonucleotide (AICAR), and PPARγ agonists) are known to modulate the immune system and result in improved insulin sensitivity. Hence, further investigations are warranted to address their use alone or in combination with other antiviral/ immunomodulatory drugs in the treatment of COVID-19. Moreover, GLP-1R agonists and DPP4 inhibitors are known to mediate anti-inflammatory effects in human patients, while controlling glucose levels in hospitalized patients (124) Nevertheless, there is no convincing evidence advocating the use of these drugs as replacements for insulin in severely ill COVID-19 patients. The fast-growing medical information pertaining to the COVID-19 pandemic entails continuing scrutiny to assess the practical use, risks, and advantages of these anti-hyperglycemic drugs and any other associated medications generally used to treat diabetic people, who are at higher risk of coronavirus infections.

AUTHOR CONTRIBUTIONS

MA-F, FA-M, TT, SK, HA, MA, and JA contributed to the design, writing, and planning of the manuscript. All authors contributed to the article and approved the submitted version.

REFERENCES

1. Walls AC, Park YJ, Tortorici MA, Wall A, Mcguire AT, Veesler D. Structure, Function, and Antigenicity of the SARS-CoV-2 Spike Glycoprotein. *Cell* (2020) 181(2):281–292.e6. doi: 10.1016/j.cell.2020.02.058
2. Zhou J, Chu H, Chan JF, Yuen KY. Middle East respiratory syndrome coronavirus infection: virus-host cell interactions and implications on pathogenesis. *Virol J* (2015) 12:218. doi: 10.1186/s12985-015-0446-6
3. Chan JF, Lau SK, To KK, Cheng VC, Woo PC, Yuen KY. Middle East respiratory syndrome coronavirus: another zoonotic betacoronavirus causing SARS-like disease. *Clin Microbiol Rev* (2015) 28(2):465–522. doi: 10.1128/CMR.00102-14
4. Muniyappa R, Gubbi S. COVID-19 pandemic, coronaviruses, and diabetes mellitus. *Am J Physiol Endocrinol Metab* (2020) 318(5):E736–e741. doi: 10.1152/ajpendo.00124.2020
5. Li B, Yang J, Zhao F, Zhi L, Wang X, Liu L, et al. Prevalence and impact of cardiovascular metabolic diseases on COVID-19 in China. *Clin Res Cardiol* (2020) 109(5):531–8. doi: 10.1007/s00392-020-01626-9
6. Maddaloni E, D'onofrio L, Alessandri F, Mignogna C, Leto G, Pascarella, et al. Clinical features of patients with type 2 diabetes with and without Covid-19: a case control study (CoViDiab I). *Diabetes Res Clin Pract* (2020) p:108454. doi: 10.1016/j.diabres.2020.108454
7. Onder G, Rezza G, Brusaferro S. Case-Fatality Rate and Characteristics of Patients Dying in Relation to COVID-19 in Italy. *JAMA* (2020) 323 (18):1775–6. doi: 10.1001/jama.2020.4683
8. Zhou F, Yu T, Du R, Fan G, Liu Y, Liu Z, et al. Clinical course and risk factors for mortality of adult inpatients with COVID-19 in Wuhan, China: a retrospective cohort study. *Lancet* (2020) 395(10229):1054–62. doi: 10.1016/ S0140-6736(20)30566-3
9. Wu C, Chen X, Cai Y, Xia J, Zhou X, Xu S, et al. Risk Factors Associated With Acute Respiratory Distress Syndrome and Death in Patients With Coronavirus Disease 2019 Pneumonia in Wuhan, China. *JAMA Intern Med* (2020) 180(7):934–43. doi: 10.1001/jamainternmed.2020.0994
10. Guan WJ, Ni ZY, Hu Y, Liang WH, Ou. Clinical Characteristics of Coronavirus Disease 2019 in China. *N Engl J Med* (2020) 382(18):1708–20. doi: 10.1056/NEJMoa2002032
11. Andersen CJ, Murphy KE, Fernandez ML. Impact of Obesity and Metabolic Syndrome on Immunity. *Adv Nutr* (2016) 7(1):66–75. doi: 10.3945/ an.115.010207
12. Francisco V, Ruiz-Fernández C, Pino J, Mera A, González-Gay MA, Gómez, et al. Adipokines: Linking metabolic syndrome, the immune system, and arthritic diseases. *Biochem Pharmacol* (2019) 165:196–206. doi: 10.1016/ j.bcp.2019.03.030
13. Francisco V, Pino J, Campos-Cabaleiro V, Ruiz-Fernández C, Mera A, Gonzalez-Gay MA, et al. Obesity, Fat Mass and Immune System: Role for Leptin. *Front Physiol* (2018) 9:640. doi: 10.3389/fphys.2018.00640
14. Andrade-Oliveira V, Câmara NO. Adipokines as drug targets in diabetes and underlying disturbances. *J Diabetes Res* (2015) 2015:681612. doi: 10.1155/ 2015/681612
15. Bremer AA, Jialal I. Adipose tissue dysfunction in nascent metabolic syndrome. *J Obes* (2013) 2013:393192. doi: 10.1155/2013/393192
16. Faber DR, de Groot PG, Visseren FL. Role of adipose tissue in haemostasis, coagulation and fibrinolysis. *Obes Rev* (2009) 10(5):554–63. doi: 10.1111/ j.1467-789X.2009.00593.x
17. Ouchi N, Parker JL, Lugus JJ, Walsh K. Adipokines in inflammation and metabolic disease. *Nat Rev Immunol* (2011) 11(2):85–97. doi: 10.1038/ nri2921
18. Richard C, Wadowski M, Goruk S, Cameron L, Sharma AM, Field CJ. Individuals with obesity and type 2 diabetes have additional immune dysfunction compared with obese individuals who are metabolically healthy. *BMJ Open Diabetes Res Care* (2017) 5(1):e000379. doi: 10.1136/ bmjdrc-2016-000379
19. Luzi L, Radaelli MG. Influenza and obesity: its odd relationship and the lessons for COVID-19 pandemic. *Acta Diabetol* (2020) 57(6):759–64. doi: 10.1007/s00592-020-01522-8
20. Karlsson EA, Hertz T, Johnson C, Mehle A, Krammer F, Schultz-Cherry S, et al. Obesity Outweighs Protection Conferred by Adjuvanted Influenza Vaccination. *mBio* (2016) 7(4):e01144-16. doi: 10.1128/ mBio.01144-16
21. Magdy Beshbishy A, Hetta HF. Factors Associated with Increased Morbidity and Mortality of Obese and Overweight COVID-19 Patients. *Biol (Basel)* (2020) 9(9):280. doi: 10.3390/biology9090280
22. Wu Z, McGoogan JM. Characteristics of and Important Lessons From the Coronavirus Disease 2019 (COVID-19) Outbreak in China: Summary of a Report of 72 314 Cases From the Chinese Center for Disease Control and Prevention. *Jama* (2020) 323(13):1239–42. doi: 10.1001/jama.2020.2648
23. Kulcsar KA, Coleman CM, Beck SE, Frieman MB. Comorbid diabetes results in immune dysregulation and enhanced disease severity following MERS-CoV infection. *JCI Insight* (2019) 4(20):e131774. doi: 10.1172/ jci.insight.131774
24. Yang JK, Zheng Y, Gou X, Pu K, Chen Z, Guo Q, et al. Plasma glucose levels and diabetes are independent predictors for mortality and morbidity in

patients with SARS. *Diabetes Med* (2006) 23(6):623–8. doi: 10.1111/j.1464-5491.2006.01861.x
25. Sardu C, D'onofrio N, Balestrieri ML, Barbieri M, Rizzo MR, Messina V, et al. Outcomes in Patients With Hyperglycemia Affected by COVID-19: Can We Do More on Glycemic Control? *Diabetes Care* (2020) 43(7):1408–15. doi: 10.2337/dc20-0723
26. Sardu C, D'onofrio N, Balestrieri ML, Barbieri M, Rizzo MR, Messina V, et al. Hyperglycaemia on admission to hospital and COVID-19. *Diabetologia* (2020) 63(11):2486–7. doi: 10.1007/s00125-020-05216-2
27. Schuetz P, Castro P, Shapiro NI. Diabetes and sepsis: preclinical findings and clinical relevance. *Diabetes Care* (2011) 34(3):771–8. doi: 10.2337/dc10-1185
28. Drucker DJ. Coronavirus Infections and Type 2 Diabetes-Shared Pathways with Therapeutic Implications. *Endocr Rev* (2020) 41(3):bnaa011. doi: 10.1210/endrev/bnaa011
29. Ryan DH, Ravussin E. COVID 19 and the Patient with Obesity - The Editors Speak Out. *Obesity* (2020) 28(5):847. doi: 10.1002/oby.22808
30. Imai Y, Kuba K, Rao S, Huan Y, Guo F, Guan B, et al. Angiotensin-converting enzyme 2 protects from severe acute lung failure. *Nature* (2005) 436(7047):112–6. doi: 10.1038/nature03712
31. Treml B, Neu N, Kleinsasser A, Gritsch C, Finsterwalder T, Geiger R, et al. Recombinant angiotensin-converting enzyme 2 improves pulmonary blood flow and oxygenation in lipopolysaccharide-induced lung injury in piglets. *Crit Care Med* (2010) 38(2):596–601. doi: 10.1097/CCM.0b013e3181c03009
32. Bosso M, Thanaraj TA, Abu-Farha M, Alanbaei M, Abubaker J, Al-Mulla F. The Two Faces of ACE2: The Role of ACE2 Receptor and Its Polymorphisms in Hypertension and COVID-19. *Mol Ther Methods Clin Dev* (2020) 18:321–7. doi: 10.1016/j.omtm.2020.06.017
33. Vaduganathan M, Vardeny O, Michel T, Mcmurray JJV. Renin-Angiotensin-Aldosterone System Inhibitors in Patients with Covid-19. *N Engl J Med* (2020) 382(17):1653–9. doi: 10.1056/NEJMsr2005760
34. Sardu C, Maggi P, Messina V, Iuliano P, Sardu A, Iovinella V, et al. Could Anti-Hypertensive Drug Therapy Affect the Clinical Prognosis of Hypertensive Patients With COVID-19 Infection? Data From Centers of Southern Italy. *J Am Heart Assoc* (2020) 9(17):e016948. doi: 10.1161/JAHA.120.016948
35. Grundy SM, Cleeman JI, Daniels SR, Donato KA, Eckel RH, Franklin BA, et al. Diagnosis and management of the metabolic syndrome: an American Heart Association/National Heart, Lung, and Blood Institute Scientific Statement. *Circulation* (2005) 112(17):2735–52. doi: 10.1161/CIRCULATIONAHA.105.169404
36. Costa FF, Rosário WR, Ribeiro Farias AC, De Souza RG, Duarte GondimRS, Barroso WA. Metabolic syndrome and COVID-19: An update on the associated comorbidities and proposed therapies. *Diabetes Metab Syndr* (2020) 14(5):809–14. doi: 10.1016/j.dsx.2020.06.016
37. Hu Y, Sun J, Dai Z, Deng H, Li X, Huang Q, et al. Prevalence and severity of corona virus disease 2019 (COVID-19): A systematic review and meta-analysis. *J Clin Virol* (2020) 127:104371. doi: 10.1016/j.jcv.2020.104371
38. Bhatraju PK, Ghassemieh BJ, Nichols M, Kim R, Jerome, KR, Nalla, et al. Covid-19 in Critically Ill Patients in the Seattle Region - Case Series. *N Engl J Med* (2020) 382(21):2012–22. doi: 10.1056/NEJMoa2004500
39. CDC Covid-19 response team. Preliminary Estimates of the Prevalence of Selected Underlying Health Conditions Among Patients with Coronavirus Disease 2019 - United States, February 12-March 28, 2020. *MMWR Morb Mortal Wkly Rep* (2020) 69(13):382–6. doi: 10.15585/mmwr.mm6913e2
40. Zhang JJ, Dong X, Cao YY, Yuan YD, Yang YB, Yan YQ, et al. Clinical characteristics of 140 patients infected with SARS-CoV-2 in Wuhan, China. *Allergy* (2020) 75(7):1730–41. doi: 10.1111/all.14238
41. Liu K, Fang YY, Deng Y, Liu W, Wang MF, Ma JP, et al. Clinical characteristics of novel coronavirus cases in tertiary hospitals in Hubei Province. *Chin Med J (Engl)* (2020) 133(9):1025–31. doi: 10.1097/CM9.0000000000000744
42. Guo T, Fan Y, Chen M, Wu X, Zhang L, He T, et al. Cardiovascular Implications of Fatal Outcomes of Patients With Coronavirus Disease 2019 (COVID-19). *JAMA Cardiol* (2020) 5(7):811–8. doi: 10.1001/jamacardio.2020.1017
43. Huang C, Wang Y, Li X, Ren L, Zhao J, Hu Y, et al. Clinical features of patients infected with 2019 novel coronavirus in Wuhan, China. *Lancet* (2020) 395(10223):497–506. doi: 10.1016/S0140-6736(20)30183-5
44. Chen N, Zhou M, Dong X, Qu J, Gong F, Han Y, et al. Epidemiological and clinical characteristics of 99 cases of 2019 novel coronavirus pneumonia in Wuhan, China: a descriptive study. *Lancet* (2020) 395(10223):507–13. doi: 10.1016/S0140-6736(20)30211-7
45. Wang D, Hu B, Hu C, Zhu F, Liu X, Zhang J, et al. Clinical Characteristics of 138 Hospitalized Patients With 2019 Novel Coronavirus-Infected Pneumonia in Wuhan, China. *Jama* (2020) 323(11):1061–9. doi: 10.1001/jama.2020.1585
46. Yang J, Zheng Y, Gou X, Pu K, Chen Z, Guo Q, et al. Prevalence of comorbidities and its effects in patients infected with SARS-CoV-2: a systematic review and meta-analysis. *Int J Infect Dis* (2020) 94:91–5. doi: 10.1016/j.ijid.2020.03.017
47. Yang X, Yu Y, Xu J, Shu H, Xia J, Liu H, et al. Clinical course and outcomes of critically ill patients with SARS-CoV-2 pneumonia in Wuhan, China: a single-centered, retrospective, observational study. *Lancet Respir Med* (2020) 8(5):475–81. doi: 10.1016/S2213-2600(20)30079-5
48. Chen T, Wu D, Chen H, Yan W, Yang D, Chen G, et al. Clinical characteristics of 113 deceased patients with coronavirus disease 2019: retrospective study. *BMJ* (2020) 368:m1091. doi: 10.1136/bmj.m1091
49. Disease control and prevention. The epidemiological characteristics of an outbreak of 2019 novel coronavirus diseases (COVID-19) in China. *Zhonghua Liu Xing Bing Xue Za Zhi* (2020) 41(2):145–51. doi: 10.3760/cma.j.issn.0254-6450.2020.02.003
50. Singh AK, Gupta R, Ghosh A, Misra A. Diabetes in COVID-19: Prevalence, pathophysiology, prognosis and practical considerations. *Diabetes Metab Syndr* (2020) 14(4):303–10. doi: 10.1016/j.dsx.2020.04.004
51. Ali H, Alshukry A, Bu Abbas M, Ali Y, Alahmad B, Al-Shammari AA, et al. Clinical Characteristics and Outcomes of Diabetic COVID-19 patients in Kuwait. *medRxiv* (2020) p:2020.08.20.20178525.
52. Wang T, Du Z, Zhu F, Cao Z, An Y, Gao Y, et al. Comorbidities and multi-organ injuries in the treatment of COVID-19. *Lancet* (2020) 395(10228):e52. doi: 10.1016/S0140-6736(20)30558-4
53. Carsana L, Sonzogni A, Nasr A, Rossi RS, Pellegrinelli A, Zerbi P, et al. Pulmonary post-mortem findings in a series of COVID-19 cases from northern Italy: a two-centre descriptive study. *Lancet Infect Dis* (2020) 20 (10):1135–40. doi: 10.1016/S1473-3099(20)30434-5
54. Poletti V, Capozzolo A. Respiratory Rehabilitation in the COVID-19 Era. *Respiration* (2020) 99(6):461–2. doi: 10.1159/000509558
55. Sardu C, Gargiulo G, Esposito G, Paolisso G, Marfella R. Impact of diabetes mellitus on clinical outcomes in patients affected by Covid-19. *Cardiovasc Diabetol* (2020) 19(1):76. doi: 10.1186/s12933-020-01047-y
56. Marfella R, Paolisso P, Sardu C, Bergamaschi L, D'angelo EC, Barbieri, et al. Negative impact of hyperglycaemia on tocilizumab therapy in Covid-19 patients. *Diabetes Metab* (2020). 46(5):403–405. doi: 10.1016/j.diabet.2020.05.005
57. Feng SQ, Chen XD, Xia T, Gan L, Qiu H, Dai MH, et al. Cloning, chromosome mapping and expression characteristics of porcine ANGPTL3 and -4. *Cytogenet Genome Res* (2006) 114(1):44–9. doi: 10.1159/000091927
58. Gupta N, Zhao YY, Evans CE. The stimulation of thrombosis by hypoxia. *Thromb Res* (2019) 181:77–83. doi: 10.1016/j.thromres.2019.07.013
59. Sardu C, Gambardella J, Morelli MB, Wang, X, Marfella R, Santulli G. Hypertension, Thrombosis, Kidney Failure, and Diabetes: Is COVID-19 an Endothelial Disease? A Comprehensive Evaluation of Clinical and Basic Evidence. *J Clin Med* (2020) 9(5):1417. doi: 10.3390/jcm9051417
60. Alshukry A, Ali H, Ali Y, Al-Taweel T, Abu-Farha M, Abubaker J, et al. Clinical characteristics of Coronavirus Disease 2019 (COVID-19) patients in Kuwait. *medRxiv* (2020) p:2020.06.14.20131045. doi: 10.1101/2020.10.11.20210740
61. Maddaloni E, D'onofrio L, Alessandri F, Mignogna C, Leto G, Pascarella G, et al. Cardiometabolic multimorbidity is associated with a worse Covid-19 prognosis than individual cardiometabolic risk factors: a multicentre retrospective study (CoViDiab II). *Cardiovasc Diabetol* (2020) 19(1):164. doi: 10.1186/s12933-020-01140-2
62. Alahmad B, Al-Shammari AA, Bennakhi A, Al-Mulla F, Ali H. Fasting Blood Glucose and COVID-19 Severity: Nonlinearity Matters. *Diabetes Care* (2020) dc201941. doi: 10.2337/dc20-1941
63. Hamming I, Timens W, Bulthuis ML, Lely AT, Navis G, Van Goor H. Tissue distribution of ACE2 protein, the functional receptor for SARS coronavirus.

A first step in understanding SARS pathogenesis. *J Pathol* (2004) 203 (2):631–7. doi: 10.1002/path.1570
64. Verdecchia P, Cavallini C, Spanevello A, Angeli F. The pivotal link between ACE2 deficiency and SARS-CoV-2 infection. *Eur J Intern Med* (2020) 76:14–20. doi: 10.1016/j.ejim.2020.04.037
65. Lukassen S, Chua RL, Trefzer T, Kahn NC, Schneider MA, Muley T, et al. SARS-CoV-2 receptor ACE2 and TMPRSS2 are primarily expressed in bronchial transient secretory cells. *EMBO J* (2020) 39(10):e105114. doi: 10.15252/embj.20105114
66. Zou X, Chen K, Zou J, Han P, Hao J, Han Z. Single-cell RNA-seq data analysis on the receptor ACE2 expression reveals the potential risk of different human organs vulnerable to 2019-nCoV infection. *Front Med* (2020) 14(2):185–92. doi: 10.1007/s11684-020-0754-0
67. Roca-Ho H, Riera M, Palau V, Pascual J, Soler MJ. Characterization of ACE and ACE2 Expression within Different Organs of the NOD Mouse. *Int J Mol Sci* (2017) 18(3):563. doi: 10.3390/ijms18030563
68. Wysocki J, Ye M, Soler MJ, Gurley SB, Xiao HD, BernsteinKE, et al. ACE and ACE2 activity in diabetic mice. *Diabetes* (2006) 55(7):2132–9. doi: 10.2337/db06-0033
69. Romaní-Pérez M, Outeiriño-Iglesias V, Moya CM, Santisteban P, González-Matípas LC, Vigo E, et al. Activation of the GLP-1 Receptor by Liraglutide Increases ACE2 Expression, Reversing Right Ventricle Hypertrophy, and Improving the Production of SP-A and SP-B in the Lungs of Type 1 Diabetes Rats. *Endocrinology* (2015) 156(10):3559–69. doi: 10.1210/en.2014-1685
70. Tikoo K, Patel G, Kumar S, Karpe PA, Sanghavi M, Malek V, et al. Tissue specific up regulation of ACE2 in rabbit model of atherosclerosis by atorvastatin: role of epigenetic histone modifications. *Biochem Pharmacol* (2015) 93(3):343–51. doi: 10.1016/j.bcp.2014.11.013
71. Zhang W, Xu YZ, Liu B, Wu R, Yang YY, Xiao XQ, et al. Pioglitazone upregulates angiotensin converting enzyme 2 expression in insulin-sensitive tissues in rats with high-fat diet-induced nonalcoholic steatohepatitis. *ScientificWorldJournal* (2014) 2014:603409. doi: 10.1155/2014/603409
72. Wösten-van Asperen RM, Lutter R, Specht PA, Moll GN, Van Woensel JB, Van Der Loos, et al. Acute respiratory distress syndrome leads to reduced ratio of ACE/ACE2 activities and is prevented by angiotensin-(1-7) or an angiotensin II receptor antagonist. *J Pathol* (2011) 225(4):618–27. doi: 10.1002/path.2987
73. Ferrario CM, Jessup J, Chappell MC, Averill DB, Brosnihan KB, Tallant EA, et al. Effect of angiotensin-converting enzyme inhibition and angiotensin II receptor blockers on cardiac angiotensin-converting enzyme 2. *Circulation* (2005) 111(20):2605–10. doi: 10.1161/CIRCULATIONAHA.104.510461
74. Rao S, Lau A, So HC. Exploring Diseases/Traits and Blood Proteins Causally Related to Expression of ACE2, the Putative Receptor of SARS-CoV-2: A Mendelian Randomization Analysis Highlights Tentative Relevance of Diabetes-Related Traits. *Diabetes Care* (2020) 43(7):1416–26. doi: 10.2337/dc20-0643
75. Fernandez C, Rysä J, Almgren P, Nilsson J. Plasma levels of the proprotein convertase furin and incidence of diabetes and mortality. *J Intern Med* (2018) 284(4):377–87. doi: 10.1111/joim.12783
76. Chen X, Hu W, Ling J, Mo P, Zhang Y, Jiang Q, et al. Hypertension and Diabetes Delay the Viral Clearance in COVID-19 Patients. *medRxiv* (2020) p:2020.03.22.20040774. doi: 10.1101/2020.03.22.20040774
77. Yang JK, Lin SS, Ji XJ, Guo LM. Binding of SARS coronavirus to its receptor damages islets and causes acute diabetes. *Acta Diabetol* (2010) 47(3):193–9. doi: 10.1007/s00592-009-0109-4
78. Liu F, Long X, Zou W, Fang M, Wu W, Li W, et al. Highly ACE2 Expression in Pancreas May Cause Pancreas Damage After SARS-CoV-2 Infection. *medRxiv* (2020) p:2020.02.28.20029181. doi: 10.1101/2020.02.28.20029181
79. Wan Y, Shang J, Graham R, Baric RS, Li F. Receptor Recognition by the Novel Coronavirus from Wuhan: an Analysis Based on Decade-Long Structural Studies of SARS Coronavirus. *J Virol* (2020) 94(7):e00127-20. doi: 10.1128/JVI.00127-20
80. Li XC, Zhang J, Zhuo JL. The vasoprotective axes of the renin-angiotensin system: Physiological relevance and therapeutic implications in cardiovascular, hypertensive and kidney diseases. *Pharmacol Res* (2017) 125(Pt A):21–38. doi: 10.1016/j.phrs.2017.06.005
81. Fang L, Karakiulakis G, Roth M. Are patients with hypertension and diabetes mellitus at increased risk for COVID-19 infection? *Lancet Respir Med* (2020) 8(4):e21. doi: 10.1016/S2213-2600(20)30116-8
82. Braun E, Sauter D. Furin-mediated protein processing in infectious diseases and cancer. *Clin Transl Immunol* (2019) 8(8):e1073. doi: 10.1002/cti2.1073
83. Harlid S, Myte R, Van Guelpen B. The Metabolic Syndrome, Inflammation, and Colorectal Cancer Risk: An Evaluation of Large Panels of Plasma Protein Markers Using Repeated, Prediagnostic Samples. *Mediators Inflammation* (2017) 2017:4803156. doi: 10.1155/2017/4803156
84. Bravo DA, Gleason JB, Sanchez RI, Roth RA, Fuller RS. Accurate and efficient cleavage of the human insulin proreceptor by the human proprotein-processing protease furin. Characterization and kinetic parameters using the purified, secreted soluble protease expressed by a recombinant baculovirus. *J Biol Chem* (1994) 269(41):25830–7.
85. Ueyama C, Horibe H, Yamase Y, Fujimaki T, Oguri M, Kato K, et al. Association of FURIN and ZPR1 polymorphisms with metabolic syndrome. *BioMed Rep* (2015) 3(5):641–7. doi: 10.3892/br.2015.484
86. Kayo T, Sawada Y, Suda M, Konda Y, Izumi T, Tanaka S, et al. Proprotein-processing endoprotease furin controls growth of pancreatic beta-cells. *Diabetes* (1997) 46(8):1296–304. doi: 10.2337/diabetes.46.8.1296
87. Louagie E, Taylor NA, Flamez D, Roebroek AJ, Bright NA, Meulemans S, et al. Role of furin in granular acidification in the endocrine pancreas: identification of the V-ATPase subunit Ac45 as a candidate substrate. *Proc Natl Acad Sci U S A* (2008) 105(34):12319–24. doi: 10.1073/pnas.0800340105
88. Al-Mulla F, Mohammad A, Al Madhoun A, Haddad D, Ali H, Eaaswarkhanth M, et al. A comprehensive germline variant and expression analyses of ACE2, TMPRSS2 and SARS-CoV-2 activator FURIN genes from the Middle East: Combating SARS-CoV-2 with precision medicine. *bioRxiv* (2020) p:2020.05.16.099176. doi: 10.1101/2020.05.16.099176
89. Flint SW, Tahrani AA. COVID-19 and obesity-lack of clarity, guidance, and implications for care. *Lancet Diabetes Endocrinol* (2020) 8(6):474–5. doi: 10.1016/S2213-8587(20)30156-X
90. Zick Y. Role of Ser/Thr kinases in the uncoupling of insulin signaling. *Int J Obes Relat Metab Disord* (2003) 27 Suppl 3:S56–60. doi: 10.1038/sj.ijo.0802503
91. El Mesallamy HO, Hamdy NM, Mostafa DM, Amin AI. The serine protease granzyme B as an inflammatory marker, in relation to the insulin receptor cleavage in human obesity and type 2 diabetes mellitus. *J Interferon Cytokine Res* (2014) 34(3):179–86. doi: 10.1089/jir.2013.0059
92. Spence JS, He R, Hoffmann HH, Das T, Thinon E, Rice CM, et al. IFITM3 directly engages and shuttles incoming virus particles to lysosomes. *Nat Chem Biol* (2019) 15(3):259–68. doi: 10.1038/s41589-018-0213-2
93. Wrensch F, Winkler M, Pöhlmann S. IFITM proteins inhibit entry driven by the MERS-coronavirus spike protein: evidence for cholesterol-independent mechanisms. *Viruses* (2014) 6(9):3683–98. doi: 10.3390/v6093683
94. Thevarajan I, Nguyen THO, Koutsakos M, Druce J, Caly L, Van De Sandt CE, et al. Breadth of concomitant immune responses prior to patient recovery: a case report of non-severe COVID-19. *Nat Med* (2020) 26: (4):453–5. doi: 10.1038/s41591-020-0819-2
95. Hoffmann M, Kleine-Weber H, Schroeder S, Krüger N, Herrler T, Erichsen S, et al. SARS-CoV-2 Cell Entry Depends on ACE2 and TMPRSS2 and Is Blocked by a Clinically Proven Protease Inhibitor. *Cell* (2020) 181(2):271–280.e8. doi: 10.1016/j.cell.2020.02.052
96. Shi G, Ozog S, Torbett BE, Compton AA. mTOR inhibitors lower an intrinsic barrier to virus infection mediated by IFITM3. *Proc Natl Acad Sci U S A* (2018) 115: (43):E10069–e10078. doi: 10.1073/pnas.1811892115
97. Tuo Y, Xiang M. mTOR: A double-edged sword for diabetes. *J Leukoc Biol* (2018) 106(2):385–95. doi: 10.1002/JLB.3MR0317-095RR
98. Haga S, Nagata N, Okamura T, Yamamoto N, Sata T, Yamamoto N, et al. TACE antagonists blocking ACE2 shedding caused by the spike protein of SARS-CoV are candidate antiviral compounds. *Antiviral Res* (2010) 85 (3):551–5. doi: 10.1016/j.antiviral.2009.12.001
99. Haga S, Yamamoto N, Nakai-Murakami C, Osawa Y, Tokunaga K, Sata T, et al. Modulation of TNF-alpha-converting enzyme by the spike protein of SARS-CoV and ACE2 induces TNF-alpha production and facilitates viral entry. *Proc Natl Acad Sci U S A* (2008) 105(22):7809–14. doi: 10.1073/pnas.0711241105

100. Palau V, Riera M, Soler MJ. ADAM17 inhibition may exert a protective effect on COVID-19. *Nephrol Dial Transplant* (2020) 35(6):1071–2. doi: 10.1093/ndt/gfaa093
101. Xu J, Mukerjee S, Silva-Alves CR, Carvalho-Galvão A, Cruz JC, Balarini, et al. A Disintegrin and Metalloprotease 17 in the Cardiovascular and Central Nervous Systems. *Front Physiol* (2016) 7:469. doi: 10.3389/fphys.2016.00469
102. Togashi N, Ura N, Higashiura K, Murakami H, Shimamoto K. Effect of TNF-alpha–converting enzyme inhibitor on insulin resistance in fructose-fed rats. *Hypertension* (2002) 39(2 Pt 2):578–80. doi: 10.1161/hy0202.103290
103. Serino M, Menghini R, Fiorentino L, Amoruso R, Mauriello A, Lauro D, et al. Mice heterozygous for tumor necrosis factor-alpha converting enzyme are protected from obesity-induced insulin resistance and diabetes. *Diabetes* (2007) 56(10):2541–6. doi: 10.2337/db07-0360
104. Ibrahim IM, Abdelmalek DH, Elshahat ME, Elfiky AA. COVID-19 spike-host cell receptor GRP78 binding site prediction. *J Infect* (2020) 80(5):554–62. doi: 10.1016/j.jinf.2020.02.026
105. Ye R, Jung DY, Jun JY, Li J, Luo S, Ko HJ, et al. Grp78 heterozygosity promotes adaptive unfolded protein response and attenuates diet-induced obesity and insulin resistance. *Diabetes* (2010) 59(1):6–16. doi: 10.2337/db09-0755
106. Koch C, Staffler G, Hüttinger R, Hilgert I, Prager E, Cerný J, et al. T cell activation-associated epitopes of CD147 in regulation of the T cell response, and their definition by antibody affinity and antigen density. *Int Immunol* (1999) 11(5):777–86. doi: 10.1093/intimm/11.5.777
107. Ulrich H, Pillat MM. CD147 as a Target for COVID-19 Treatment: Suggested Effects of Azithromycin and Stem Cell Engagement. *Stem Cell Rev Rep* (2020) 16(3):434–40. doi: 10.1007/s12015-020-09976-7
108. Xie Y, Wang Y, Ding H, Guo M, Wang X, Dong Q, et al. Highly glycosylated CD147 promotes hemorrhagic transformation after rt-PA treatment in diabetes: a novel therapeutic target? *J Neuroinflammation* (2019) 16(1):72. doi: 10.1186/s12974-019-1460-1
109. Drucker DJ. Mechanisms of Action and Therapeutic Application of Glucagon-like Peptide-1. *Cell Metab* (2018) 27(4):740–56. doi: 10.1016/j.cmet.2018.03.001
110. Bloodworth MH, Rusznak M, Pfister CC, Zhang J, Bastarache L, Calvillo SA, et al. Glucagon-like peptide 1 receptor signaling attenuates respiratory syncytial virus-induced type 2 responses and immunopathology. *J Allergy Clin Immunol* (2018) 142(2):683–7.e12. doi: 10.1016/j.jaci.2018.01.053
111. Jin T, Liu M. Letter to the editor: Comment on GLP-1-based drugs and COVID-19 treatment. *Acta Pharm Sin B* (2020) 10(7):1249–50. doi: 10.1016/j.apsb.2020.05.006
112. Chatterjee S. SGLT-2 inhibitors for COVID-19 - A miracle waiting to happen or just another beat around the bush? *Prim Care Diabetes* (2020) 14(5):564–5. doi: 10.1016/j.pcd.2020.05.013
113. Fernandez-Fernandez B, D Marco L. Exploring Sodium Glucose Co-Transporter-2 (SGLT2) Inhibitors for Organ Protection in COVID-19. *J Clin Med* (2020) 9(7):2030. doi: 10.3390/jcm9072030
114. American diabetes association15. Diabetes Care in the Hospital: Standards of Medical Care in Diabetes-2020. *Diabetes Care* (2020) 43(Suppl 1):S193–s202. doi: 10.2337/dc20-S015
115. Papadokostaki E, Tentolouris N, Liberopoulos E. COVID-19 and diabetes: What does the clinician need to know? *Prim Care Diabetes* (2020) 14(5):558–63. doi: 10.1016/j.pcd.2020.06.010
116. Bornstein SR, Rubino F, Khunti K, Mingrone G, Hopkins D, Birkenfeld AL, et al. Practical recommendations for the management of diabetes in patients with COVID-19. *Lancet Diabetes Endocrinol* (2020) 8(6):546–50. doi: 10.1016/S2213-8587(20)30223-0
117. Chen Y, Yang D, Cheng B, Chen J, Peng A, Yang C, et al. Clinical Characteristics and Outcomes of Patients With Diabetes and COVID-19 in Association With Glucose-Lowering Medication. *Diabetes Care* (2020) 43 (7):1399–407. doi: 10.2337/dc20-0660
118. Mulvihill EE, Drucker DJ. Pharmacology, physiology, and mechanisms of action of dipeptidyl peptidase-4 inhibitors. *Endocr Rev* (2014) 35(6):992–1019. doi: 10.1210/er.2014-1035
119. Fadini GP, Morieri ML, Longato E, Bonora BM, Pinelli S, Selmin E, et al. Exposure to dipeptidyl-peptidase-4 inhibitors and COVID-19 among people with type 2 diabetes: A case-control study. *Diabetes Obes Metab* (2020). doi: 10.1111/dom.14097
120. Strollo R, Maddaloni E, Dauriz M, Pedone C, Buzzetti R, Pozzilli P, et al. Use of DPP4 inhibitors in Italy does not correlate with diabetes prevalence among COVID-19 deaths. *Diabetes Res Clin Pract* (2020), 108444. doi: 10.1016/j.diabres.2020.108444
121. Cariou B, Hadjadj S. Phenotypic characteristics and prognosis of inpatients with COVID-19 and diabetes: the CORONADO study. *Diabetologia* (2020) 63(8):1500–15. doi: 10.1007/s00125-020-05180-x
122. Solerte SB, D'addio F, Trevisan R, Lovati E, Rossi A, Pastore I, et al. Sitagliptin Treatment at the Time of Hospitalization Was Associated With Reduced Mortality in Patients With Type 2 Diabetes and COVID-19: A Multicenter, Case-Control, Retrospective, Observational Study. *Diabetes Care* (2020) dc201521. doi: 10.2337/dc20-1521
123. Monteil V, Kwon H, Prado P, Hagelkrüys A, Wimmer RA, Stahl M, et al. Inhibition of SARS-CoV-2 Infections in Engineered Human Tissues Using Clinical-Grade Soluble Human ACE2. *Cell* (2020) 181(4):905–913.e7. doi: 10.1016/j.cell.2020.04.004
124. Mozafari N, Azadi S, Mehdi-Alamdarlou S, Ashrafi H, et al. Inflammation: A bridge between diabetes and COVID-19, and possible management with sitagliptin. *Med Hypotheses* (2020) 143:110111. doi: 10.1016/j.mehy.2020.110111

21

Factors Behind the Higher COVID-19 Risk in Diabetes

Amany Magdy Beshbishy[1†], *Victor B. Oti*[2], *Diaa E. Hussein*[3], *Ibrahim F. Rehan*[4], *Oluyomi S. Adeyemi*[5], *Nallely Rivero-Perez*[6], *Adrian Zaragoza-Bastida*[6], *Muhammad Ajmal Shah*[7], *Khaled Abouelezz*[8], *Helal F. Hetta*[8], *Natália Cruz-Martins*[9,10,11*] *and Gaber El-Saber Batiha*[12*†]

[1] National Research Center for Protozoan Diseases, Obihiro University of Agriculture and Veterinary Medicine, Obihiro, Japan, [2] Department of Microbiology, Nasarawa State University, Keffi, Nigeria, [3] Researcher, Department of Food Hygiene, Agricultural Research Center, Animal Health Research Institute, Port of Alexandria, Egypt, [4] Department of Husbandry and Development of Animal Wealth, Faculty of Veterinary Medicine, Menofa University, Shebin Alkom, Egypt, [5] Medicinal Biochemistry, Infectious Diseases, Nanomedicine & Toxicology Laboratory, Department of Biochemistry, Landmark University, Omu-Aran, Nigeria, [6] Área Académica de Medicina Veterinaria y Zootecnia, Instituto de Ciencias Agropecuaria, Universidad Autónoma del Estado de Hidalgo, Tulancingo, Mexico, [7] Department of Pharmacognosy, Faculty of Pharmaceutical Sciences, Government College University, Faisalabad, Pakistan, [8] Department of Medical Microbiology and Immunology, Faculty of Medicine, Assiut University, Assiut, Egypt, [9] Faculty of Medicine, University of Porto, Porto, Portugal, [10] Institute for Research and Innovation in Health (i3S), University of Porto, Porto, Portugal, [11] Laboratory of Neuropsychophysiology, Faculty of Psychology and Education Sciences, University of Porto, Porto, Portugal, [12] Department of Pharmacology and Therapeutics, Faculty of Veterinary Medicine, Damanhour University, Damanhour, Egypt

***Correspondence:**
Natália Cruz-Martins
ncmartins@med.up.pt
Gaber El-Saber Batiha
gaberbatiha@gmail.com

† These authors have contributed equally to this work*

Diabetes mellitus (DM) and coronavirus disease 2019 (COVID-19) are public health issues worldwide, and their comorbidities trigger the progress to severe disease and even death in such patients. Globally, DM has affected an estimated 9.3% adults, and as of April 18, 2021, the World Health Organization (WHO) has confirmed 141,727,940 COVID-19 confirmed cases. The virus is spread via droplets, aerosols, and direct touch with others. Numerous predictive factors have been linked to COVID-19 severity, including impaired immune response and increased inflammatory response, among others. Angiotensin receptor blockers and angiotensin converting enzyme 2 have also been identified as playing a boosting role in both susceptibility and severity to severe acute respiratory syndrome coronavirus 2 (SARS-CoV-2). Specifically, in DM patients, both their control and management during this pandemic is herculean as the restriction periods have markedly hampered the maintenance of means to control glycemia, hypertension, and neuroendocrine and kidney diseases. In addition, as a result of the underlyin cardio-metabolic and immunological disorders, DM patients are at a higher risk of developing the severe form of COVID-19 despite other comorbidities, such as hypertension, also potentially boosting the development of higher COVID-19 severity. However, even in non-DM patients, SARS-CoV-2 may also cause transient hyperglycemia through induction of insulin resistance and/or pancreatic β-cell injury. Therefore, a strict glucose monitoring of DM patients with COVID-19 is mandatory to prevent life-threatening complications.

Keywords: diabetes, COVID-19, SARS-CoV-2, comorbidities, mortality

INTRODUCTION

COVID-19 Disease: An Overview

Coronavirus disease 2019, named COVID-19, discovered in Wuhan, China, is being quickly transmitted to the worldwide population. The viral agent, known as severe acute respiratory syndrome coronavirus 2 (SARS-CoV-2) is capable of inducing severe to acute pneumonia, lethal lung failure, and even death in susceptible hosts (1). Genetically, this virus differs from the closely related SARS members and is classified into the group of *beta coronavirus* infecting humans (2). Despite having a negative impact on the respiratory tract, clinical features range from asymptomatic to moderate-to-serious or critical disease. Currently, the viral infection case fatality rate is <5%, but 15–18% of infected patients may develop the severe form of the disease, even becoming critically ill, and others may need mechanical ventilation and intensive care unit (ICU) admission (3).

Declared a worldwide pandemic on March 11, 2020, by the World Health Organization (WHO) (4), the SARS-CoV-2 infection triggers various clinical manifestations, including respiratory tract disorders, severe pneumonia, septic shock, and multiorgan failure (4). However, clinical data available so far reveal that children aged <10 years usually remain asymptomatic and has a low case fatality rate (5). The median incubation period is 4 days, ranging from 2 to 14 days maximum (5, 6). The viral agent is shown to be spread via droplets, aerosols, and through direct contact with infected individuals. Concerning the virus dissemination via droplets, it can happen if a respiratory droplet is generated when an infected individual sneezes or coughs, and it is ingested or inhaled by close people (about 6 feet away). Thus, an individual may become infected by mere touching of surfaces or objects that harbor the viral agent and subsequently touching the nose, mouth, or eyes (7). Increased viral loads have been reported as soon as the symptoms start to appear, which suggests that viral transmission is more likely to occur early in viral infection (8). The duration of viral shedding differs based on the disease severity. For instance, Liu et al. (9) report that mild symptoms were found in 90% of COVID-19 patients who show a negative virus RNA test with swabs from the nasopharyngeal region by day 10 post-onset. Meanwhile, for a long time, the test remained positive in all severe cases. A study by Zou et al. (8) found that the detected viral load in patients without symptoms was similar to those that show symptoms. Indeed, there is evidence of spread of the viral agent during the incubation period of patients without symptoms (10).

Diabetes: An Overview

Diabetes mellitus (DM) is among the world's greatest causes of morbidity with a high anticipation of exponential increase in the coming decades (11). The condition has several macro and microvascular complications as its predictors, which negatively affect the patient's overall survival (12). Globally, DM has affected about 9.3% of adults, there is a likelihood of it skyrocketing to 10.2% by the year 2030, and it might reach 10.9% by the year 2045 (13). In the last three decades, China has seen DM rise 17-fold, giving it the controversial slogan the "Diabetes World Capital" (14). Several metabolic predictors have been listed as triggers for metabolic disorders (DM and obesity, inclusive), such as chronic inflammation, oxidative stress, subclinical atherosclerosis, endothelial dysfunction, insulin resistance, glucose metabolism, and changed lipid, among others (14).

DIABETES AND INFECTIOUS DISEASES

The interlink between DM and infectious diseases has been underlined by several clinical studies (15, 16). DM patients are more prone to infections as compared with those without DM as a result of impaired immunity (16, 17). Scientific evidence has found a greater rate of susceptibility to infectious diseases in DM individuals (**Figure 1**), such as those triggered by *Mycobacterium tuberculosis* and *Staphylococcus aureus* (18), directly attributed a dysregulated immune system (17). There is a general perception that DM patients can have higher morbidity and death rates by infectious diseases, and there is a paucity of epidemiologic data that would make it evident. There are reports that try to look at DM as a predisposing factor to some infection that can lead to death (19, 20). In this way, different viral infections are reported to increase the vulnerability of DM patients (21), such as those deriving from SARS-CoV (19), Middle East respiratory syndrome coronavirus (MERS-CoV) (21), and the 2009 influenza A (H1N1) infection (20). A recent review summarizing the clinical features linked to a higher risk of acquiring infectious diseases among DM individuals underlined that poorly controlled DM is a major risk factor, including for SARS-CoV-2 infection (22).

CORONA VIRUS RECEPTORS

SARS-CoV-2, similarly to SARS-CoV, uses angiotensin converting enzyme 2 (ACE2) as a cellular receptor (**Figure 2**),

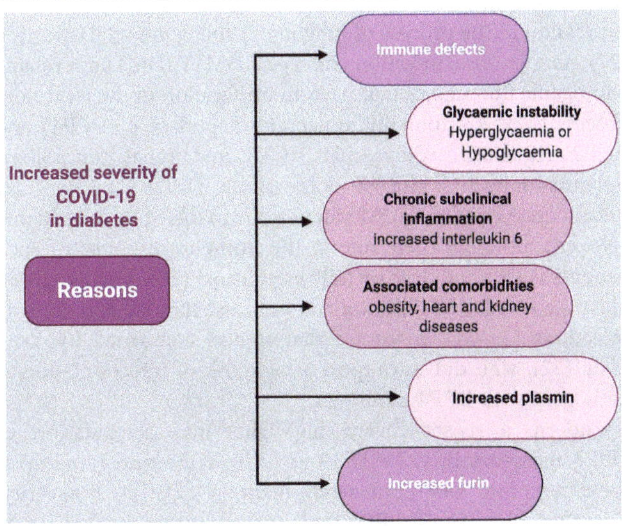

FIGURE 1 | Viral entry mechanism to the host.

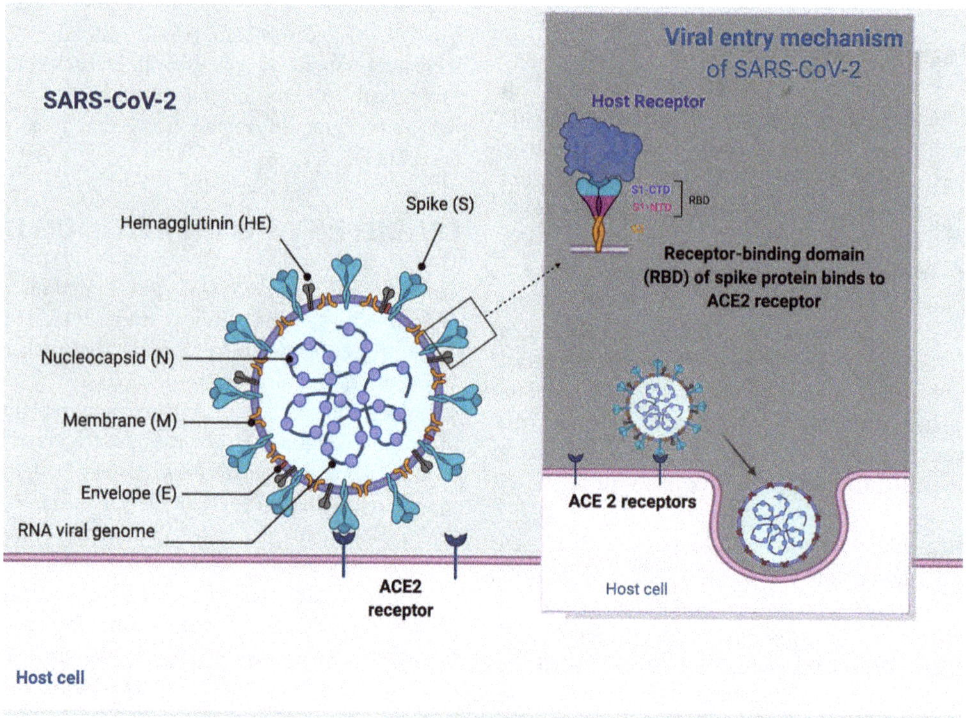

FIGURE 2 | Diabetes as a risk factor for COVID-19.

interacting directly with the spike glycoprotein (23). Wrapp et al. (24) report that the interaction between ACE2 and receptor-binding domain (RBD) is 10 to 20 times higher than the enzyme found in other coronaviruses. The enzyme has been found in myriad organ systems, including the heart, kidneys, brain, and lungs, among others (25). Indeed, there is evidence that the counter-regulatory enzyme ACE2, which metabolizes angiotensin II (Ang II), can enhance SARS-CoV-2 entry and replication (26). Many reports implicate the role of renin-angiotensin system (RAS) activation and reduced ACE2 expression in the process of lung injury following viral infection (27). As such, viral infection and type 2 DM (T2DM) have related pathogenic flow charts that have an implication in the treatment process (27). Additionally, dipeptidyl peptidase 4 (DPP4) and ACE2 regulate cardiovascular (CV) and renal physiology, inflammation, and glucose homeostasis. DPP4 inhibitors are greatly functional in T2DM patients due to their role in reducing glycemia although their role in the immune response of such patients is still not clear or fully established (28). Meta-analyses illustrate that DPP4 inhibitors do not raise the risk of acquiring infections (29–31), a feature that is also confirmed by Yang et al. (32), who did not report a high risk of infections due to pathogens with DPP4 inhibitors.

Indeed, a recent review highlights that deregulation of DPP4 receptors in COVID-19 as well as the upregulation of these receptors may be a determinant in COVID-19 severity. Therefore, the use of DPP4 inhibitors (gliptins) in COVID-19 management should be better exploited to improve the overall knowledge on how DPP4 may be useful to design novel therapies to block SARS-CoV-2 entry (33).

Other receptors on the human cell surface have been reported to facilitate the penetration of the viral agent, including transmembrane serine protease 2 (TMPRSS2) (34), extracellular matrix metalloproteinase inducer (35), and sialic acid receptors (36). Furthermore, cathepsins L and B have been reported to be key penetrating factors in the COVID-19 pathogenesis (34).

DIABETOGENIC VIRUSES

Data from animal and human studies postulate that there are diabetogenic viral agents, but they are few (37). Two different studies found two DM patients who depend on acute insulin for a short and transient period following chicken pox infection (38). Guo et al. (26) recommend that viral infection could induce fast changes in blood glucose levels of DM patients, playing a negative role in such patients' recovery. Yang et al. (19) report an increase in fasting blood sugar (FBS), even in patients with non-severe SARS, who did not receive glucocorticoid therapy.

Briefly, coronavirus can trigger DM by inducing damage to the islets. This assertion is backed by the strong nature of immunostained ACE2 protein and its weak nature in exocrine tissues (39). Findings obtained so far show that DM and SARS-CoV-2 pneumonia can be entangled, and this may be detrimental to the COVID-19 prognosis.

MORBIDITY OF SARS-COV-2 INFECTION IN DIABETIC PATIENTS

Yang et al. (19) reveal that DM and plasma glucose levels are independent probable factors for morbimortality in SARS-CoV-2 infected patients. In China (Wuhan), a retrospective study showed that out of the 41 SARS-CoV-2 infected individuals, about 32% presented with other underlying diseases, 20% of them diabetic (40, 41). Research conducted in 8,910 patients with COVID-19 infection revealed that 14.3% had DM (42). Similarly, in a study performed in China with 1,099 hospitalized patients with novel coronavirus cases, 81 had DM, and about 34.6% had a serious ailment related to the 41/165 that had hypertension, 10/27 with coronary artery disorder, 67/261 with some coexisting disease, and 106/838 did not have any coexisting disease (43). Tentolouris et al. (44) carried out a study with 30,000 individuals in Greece and found a 6.6% incidence rate of DM. DM patients presented a higher incidence of comorbidities, including kidney, heart, and lung diseases. In addition, in the United States, CDC found that in 7,162 cases with incomplete data, above 50% of them were hospitalized, 10.9% had DM and 148 (18.9%) need admission into the intensive care unit (ICU) (45). The authors also found that the number of patients needing ICU admission did not differ from that with CV disease (20.4%) although it was higher than that with chronic lung disease (14.3%) or at an immuno-compromised status (15.5%). A report in Kuwait states that individuals with DM and obesity are more prone to ICU admission as the COVID-19 pandemic continues (46).

DM: RISK FACTOR FOR COVID-19

Studies conducted in recent times show that the elderly or individuals with underlying comorbidities, such as CV disease, DM, and hypertension, are more susceptible to complications and possibly death as a result of COVID-19 (45). DM has also been found to be an important predictor for the severe form of COVID-19 due to respiratory tract infections (47). Also, DM has been reported to be linked to higher mortality following MERS-CoV and SARS-CoV infections by different studies (21, 47), and the level of FBS has been considered an independent probable factor for fatality in SARS infected patients (19). Diabetes is a possible predictor of infection, more so in those aged >60 years old and in those with poor glycemic control (48). Currently, there are no public findings, but obviously, there is a higher likelihood that DM patients will get SARS-CoV-2 infection (49). Moreover, it is known that DM and obesity are associated with the synthesis and clearance of dysregulated lipids that can trigger lung inflammation and injury (50, 51). In DM patients, the risk of pneumonia or lower and upper respiratory tract infections is greater than that of general population (52). Another study found that COVID-19 patients who have DM not only have a greater risk to severe pneumonia, but also spread inflammatory biomarkers excessively (25). However, DM patients might be at greater risk for hospitalization and development of complications due to COVID-19 (53).

Thus, the presence of patients with DM underlying viral infection is associated with two-fold heightened risk of death and also two-fold greater risk of COVID-19 severity (51). The main possible predictors include uncontrolled blood glucose levels before infection with the new coronavirus, shorter contact with DM healthcare experts, and unusual discontinuation of ACE2 inhibitor. The latter aspect mentioned is stated because reports show that the virus connects to cells via ACE2; therefore, these drugs can heighten the ACE2 level with the ability theoretically that there is a higher pickup of the viral agent. However, halting these medications can cause more damage in most cases (49). Indeed, related studies and reports have reported danger in DM individuals for the two new coronavirus infections discovered, SARS starts in 2002 in Asia and the Middle East, affecting more than 8,000 individuals (54) and MERS in 2012, mostly in Saudi Arabia, which affected more than 2,000 individuals (55).

COMORBIDITY OF DIABETES

DM is a comorbidity usually reported by COVID-19 patients (56, 57). Indeed, about 7% of COVID-19 patients have DM. Zhou et al. (47) state a recovery rate of 14% for COVID-19 patients with DM although a higher rate was stated (31%) for patients who were non-survivors. In a new published meta-analysis, it is found that DM incidence in ICU patients with viral infection increased twice in comparison with non-ICU patients (58). SARS-CoV-2 infection in DM patients can facilitate increased stress conditions with high release of hyperglycemic hormones, including catecholamines and glucocorticoids, ultimately resulting in high blood sugar levels and abnormalities in glucose levels (59). Recently, in the United States, the Centers for Disease Control and Prevention (CDC) reported that the incidence of DM was 10.9% in 7,162 patients who had all data on their health status on March 28, 2020 (58). Anyway, data published so far underline that DM patients and severe SARS-CoV-2 infection are older and have comorbidities when compared with non-DM patients (60).

MORTALITY RATES OF DM PATIENTS WITH COVID-19

A recent study revealed that, among 191 Chinese COVID-19 patients hospitalized, 19% had DM with 54 deaths being recorded (45). The Chinese Center for Disease Control and Prevention (CCDC) registered a case fatality rate (CFR) of 2.3% in a detailed study with 44,672 COVID-19 patients. However, the rate increased to 10.5% in those with CV disease, 7.3% in those with DM, and 6.0% in those with hypertension (61). A fatality rate of 35% was also reported for those with DM as compared with 20% in the general population (62). Indeed, much research has reported that DM patients suffering from comorbidities have higher mortality rates due to complicated hyperglycemia and myocardial infarction because blood glucose plays a distinct role (63, 64). In addition, a recent multicenter retrospective study provides clinical evidence that correlate better blood glucose control with good clinical outcomes in COVID-19 patients and preexisting T2DM (65).

Regarding viral agent transmission, it occurs at a high efficiency, which impacts not only healthy individuals, but majorly the elderly, with higher complication rates than other pandemics (66). In several countries, these high rates of disease and death are often found in individuals of older ages and in those with comorbidities (67) although it is not certain if there are variations in the severity of infection between men and women with DM and if it differs between DMT1 and T2 (68). However, men are more prone to develop a severe form of COVID-19 due to underlying cardiometabolic risk factors, hormonal changes, ACE2 expression, inflammatory status, and exaggerated immune response (69). Also, Shahid et al. (70) illustrate that older subjects are at higher risk of death by COVID-19.

Additionally, a study shows that individuals who take corticosteroids for no obvious justification are at high risk (63). Thus, these patients are overrepresented in those at a high death risk from the virus: elderly people and those with comorbidities (5). Also worth noting is that it has been suggested that ACE2 can raise both viral infection susceptibility and severity through enzyme upregulation, which explains the overrepresentation of hypertensive patients in COVID-19 death causes (71). Finally, diabetic kidney disease (DKD) is also a leading factor that triggers disease and death in DM patients with estimations reporting that 30–40% of DM patients may die from DKD.

DIABETES AND IMMUNE RESPONSE

Several abnormal immune system changes have been seen in DM patients, well-describing the relationship between immune dysfunction and hyperglycemia, involving weakening of the polymorphonuclear and monocytic white blood cell chemotaxis phagocytosis, complementary role and cytokine dysregulation (72). T2DM is generally recognized by a reduced level of chronic inflammatory disorder, triggered by a prolonged immune system imbalance, metabolic syndrome, and obesity (73). DM leads to proinflammatory homeostatic interactions of the immune system that is geared toward T helper 1 (Th1) and T17 cells and a decline in T-cell regulation (Treg) (17). Indeed, immune system dysfunction due to DM or infection has been observed in a variety of immune cells, not only $CD4^+$ T cells, but also monocytes and macrophages (17). A recent study reported that the total number of $CD8^+$ and $CD4^+$ T cells lessens drastically and is functionally drained in SARS-CoV-2 infected patients, particularly in geriatric and in those critically ill who need ICU admission (74). Kulcsar et al. (75) found that DM mice had a long-term serious disease phase and postponed healing from MERS-CoV infection due to immune response dysregulation with lower rates of inflammatory $CD4^+$ T cells and monocytes/macrophages. Moreover, several research studies found a greater risk of severe COVID-19 in DM patients with the increased risk of respiratory infections being linked to a compromised innate immune function. Nonetheless, temporary hyperglycemia may also partially alter the innate immune response to infection (76). Anyway, it is doubtless that DM patients are more prone to develop infectious diseases due to impaired immune system function (77). Moreover, DM patients with DKD have a chronic systemic inflammation resulting from a reduced immune system status that can lead to infectious complications, and together these may determine the risk of disease and death (78).

DIABETES COMPLICATIONS

Increasing evidence states that DM-derived complications not only depict the disease severity, but also that such patients often have enhanced death rates that further justify the fact that DM is a key predictor in COVID-19 prognosis with DM severity being directly related to a bad prognosis (25). Reports also show that bad glycemic control, for example, evidenced by an increase in HbA1c, is importantly related to a higher risk to different infections (79, 80). Nonetheless, hyperosmolar hyperglycemic state (HHS) and DKA are still considered the most acute metabolic complications of DM, which are generally triggered by infection. Moreover, it is known that viral infection is tagged to precipitate the acute hyperglycemic issues in uncontrolled DM patients, but there is still a paucity of scientific evidence regarding this association (81). Zhang et al. (82) state that COVID-19 patients with DM are more prone to generate severe subtypes, including acute respiratory disease (ARDS) complications and acute cardiac injury that occurs due to mechanical ventilation and antibiotic treatment.

Diabetes and Hypertension

Globally, hypertension is viewed as one of the most generalized diseases and comorbidities in DM patients and considered as a silent killer (83). Published 2020 studies from China's Wuhan province show that patients with hypertension and DM are overrepresented among the sickest COVID-19 patients and those susceptible to the disease (5, 63). The increased rate of hypertensive patients with SARS-CoV-2 is reported in a study with 41 patients found in Wuhan hospital (84) although a larger analysis of 138 hospitalized patients also report a similar outcome (40). Similarly, a study conducted in Jinyintan Hospital and Wuhan Pulmonary Hospital among 191 patients with the novel coronavirus found hypertension in 58 (30%) patients, 26 (48%) did not survive the viral infection, and 32 (23%) survived (45). Another study performed in Switzerland found that hypertensive patients (23.7%) with cerebrovascular disorders (22%) and diabetes (22%) were the most striking comorbidities (65). Recent findings also point out that the CV system is the second target system of the virus besides the lungs. Therefore, hypertension is linked to poor clinical outcomes in COVID-19 patients, and current ACEIs or ARBs should not be discontinued (85, 86).

Diabetes and Endothelial Dysfunction

DM is typically characterized by endothelial dysfunction apart from hyperglycemia and microcirculatory impairment (87). More than one third of newly diagnosed T2DM patients may have microvascular disease (88). The bad blow of endothelial impairment involves fibrinolysis, vasodilation dysregulation, and anti-aggregation, which typically leads to macrovascular disorders (81). Nevertheless, the evidence of microvascular impairment in one organ is a key indicator of systemic damage. There is evidence that such complications derive from microvascular lung diseases of DM ("diabetic lung") (89). Furthermore, atherosclerosis, endothelial impairment, and vascular inflammation are also involved in the pathogenicity of other chronic disorders, such as CV diseases and hypertension (90). Indeed, endothelial dysfunction in DM patients with COVID-19 might be due to direct invasion of vascular endothelial cells by SARS-CoV-2 through endothelial ACE2 (91). As well, the high levels of pro-inflammatory cytokines and the development of cytokine storm (CS) in severe COVID-19 patients may cause endothelial injury and boost the development of endothelial dysfunctions (92).

Diabetes and Thrombosis

Coagulation dysfunction is also reported in severe COVID-19 patients (93) with fatal cases presenting diffuse microvascular thrombosis, which is suggestive of a thrombogenic microangiopathy (94), In T2DM, aside from the marked inflammatory stage, an imbalance also exists between coagulation and fibrinolysis and also enhances clotting factor levels and relative fibrinolytic system stoppage (72). T2DM and insulin resistance are known to be related to endothelial cell dysfunction and increased platelet activation and aggregation. These abnormal changes foster the generation of hypercoagulable pro-thrombosis. Guo et al. (25) posit that, during the inflammatory storm, the D-dimer rises geometrically. It is an outcome of inflammation activating plasmin during the early stage. However, as inflammation goes on in hypoxia-induced molecules, which can trigger direct thrombin and activate monocyte-macrophages, which can also emit tissue factors in masses and open the pathway of exogenous coagulation, this results in a general state of hypercoagulability. For example, Guo et al. (25) found that the level of FIB and D-dimer increased greatly in DM patients, which is an indicator of prone hypercoagulable state as compared to non-DM patients. McFadyen et al. (95) reveal that SARS-CoV-2-induced endothelial dysfunction may lead to immune-related thrombosis due to both platelet and complement activations so that the use of anti-thrombotic agents, such as heparin and dipyridamole, may prevent these complications in COVID-19 patients.

Diabetes and Kidney Disease

Acute kidney injury (AKI) has been found in <20% of critically sick and COVID-19 patients with this finding being supported by data from China (63), Italy (96), and the United States (97). A study carried out in 2020 found that kidneys have an increased vulnerability to ACE2 expression-based destruction (98), and in addition, kidney disease is a common DM-related clinical complication. Worldwide, more than 2 million individuals receive dialysis therapy, and up to half a million individuals are receiving maintenance dialysis in the United States, which poses a greater danger for the acquisition of SARS-CoV-2 infection. The CDC and the American Society of Nephrology (ASN) have compiled best practices for in-center dialysis (99). Marked changes in immune system function have been stated in patients with kidney-related problems; nonetheless, despite immune system impairment, meticulous attention should be paid on the uremic state because the excessive oxidative stress status caused by excess toxin retention and gathering of synthesized products of oxidation can exacerbate the clinical status in infected patients (72). A study recorded that endothelial damage is normal in 26 patients with SARS-CoV-2 renal histopathology without interstitial inflammatory infiltration (100). However, so far, there are still not certain reports with respect to the kidneys. The direct mechanism in viral infection includes syndrome of CS via targeted viral renal tubular cell destruction, and sepsis pathways have been investigated (101). Presently, the major expression of renal destruction in SARS-CoV-2-infected patients looks to be acute although certain conditions of proteinuria/hematuria and macroalbuminuria may be interrelated to endothelial cell impairment found in such patients (102).

Chest Tomography (CT) Imaging and Biochemical Tests of Diabetic Patients

In DM patients, a chest CT scan usually depicts ground-glass opacifications with abnormalities that are united or not. Involvement in normal lobes can also be seen bilaterally with peripheral features of COVID-19 (103). Moreover, although normal CT images can also be found in some confirmed cases (104), abnormal images have also been seen in asymptomatic patients. For instance, Guo et al. (25) report that the DM patients' group had an increase in the CT image score when compared with those non-DM who have COVID-19 pneumonia with clinical status being also more serious than in those without DM. Into the bargain, the retrospective study by Wang et al. (105), involving 307 COVID-19 patients, shows that early definitive diagnosis could be grasped by age-related clinical and CT scan findings. Moreover, lung CT scan findings were correlated with COVID-19 severity and development of acute ischemic stroke in T2DM patients with COVID-19 (106).

Regarding biochemical outcomes in such patients, some authors have already stated that few enzymes serving as indicators are raised aberrantly in the blood of viral pneumonia patients, including α-hydroxybutyrate dehydrogenase (HBDH), gamma glutamyltransferase (GGT), lactate dehydrogenase (LDH), and alanine aminotransferase (ALT), which shows myocardium, liver, and kidney injury. This outcome is in consonance with the excessive frequency of viral receptors (ACE2) and may partly explain why death occurred in some patients with multiple organ failure (107, 108).

Blood Picture of Diabetic Patients With COVID-19

SARS-CoV-2-infected patients commonly depict lymphocytopenia on entry and, to a limited degree, leukopenia and thrombocytopenia, more conspicuous in those with severe disease status (5). Elevated pro-inflammatory cytokine levels, which include, among others, C-reactive protein (CRP), interleukin (IL)-6, and enhanced coagulation activity, shown by higher d-dimer concentrations, have also been correlated with disease severity (45). Furthermore, DM patients had greater neutrophils, IL-6, white cells, LDH, IL-2R, CRP, IL-8, D-dimer, and N-terminal pro-B-type natriuretic peptide (NT-proBNP) levels and lower lymphocyte counts. Taken together, these outcomes indicate an increased response to pro-inflammatory cytokines compared with non-DM patients (58). Moreover, the serum levels of some inflammation-related biomarkers are higher in DM when compared with non-DM individuals, such as IL-6, ESR, CRP, and serum ferritin. Additionally, a pronounced raise in serum ferritin levels is an indicator of monocyte-macrophage activation, a crucial part of the inflammatory storm. Taken together, these results show that patients with an inflammatory storm are more prone to rapid destruction by COVID-19 (25).

Inflammatory Storm in Diabetic Patients With SARS-CoV-2 Infection

A recently published report, analyzing 138 hospitalized SARS-CoV-2 infected patients, observed that CS-associated neutrophilia triggered by virus invasion and coagulation opening similar to the longer response of inflammation and acute kidney injury has a similar negative impact on SARS-CoV-2, which may be related to the death rate of infected patients (40). A study report that severe SARS-CoV-2 infected patients with pneumonia have a significantly reduced lymphocyte count with high levels of inflammatory factors, especially IL-6 (78). Guo et al. (25) report that, compared with non-DM patients, in DM individuals, the total absolute lymphocyte count in peripheral blood is greatly reduced, and the neutrophil absolute count shows a remarkable increase. Therefore, a high neutrophil–lymphocyte ratio (NLR) in DM patients may increase COVID-19 severity because high NLR is regarded as a poor prognostic factor linked to COVID-19 severity and mortality (109).

CONTROL OF DM PATIENTS WITH COVID-19

Regarding the management of DM patients with COVID-19, Guo et al. (25) in their study suggest that, whether there is interference or not from other comorbidities, DM patients with viral pneumonia present a more serious status when compared with non-DM ones, stated through organ destruction and inflammatory factor evaluation, that can lead to a complicated prognosis. In the face of such findings, more intensive care should be given to DM patients in case of rapid deterioration. Nevertheless, careful attention should be given to those with nephropathic DM because such patients are at greater risk of viral infection, serious complications, and even death (110, 111).

Current CDC guidance for preventing SARS-CoV-2 infection in DM individuals reveals no differences from the general population, but awareness that DM can lead to a high risk of serious illness should make it easier for healthcare providers to monitor such patients with symptoms of viral infection (i.e., fever and breath shortness) (112). Thus, the role of doctors who give suggestions to DM patients is of crucial importance as they should provide information on extra precaution measures, including social distancing and hand washing toward preventing them from SARS-CoV-2 infection (97). In addition, there should be improved surveillance in DM outpatients for the viral agent, and the starting point for testing this viral infection in such patients should be reduced (64). For instance, Whyte et al. (113) conclude that endothelial dysfunction and microvascular disease may depict as absent a pathophysiological relationship that indicates susceptible populations and may involve specific therapy. Moreover, Zhang et al. (76) postulate that more intensive vigilance and therapy should be considered in DM patients infected with the viral agent, most especially in geriatric ones and in those with preexisting comorbidities. In addition, DM patients are associated with increased mortality and higher disease severity. In a systematic review, Huang et al. (76) show that DM is linked to higher COVID-19 severity, high mortality, disease progression, and development of ARDS.

Glycemic Control of DM Patients With COVID-19

So far, only a small percentage of experimental studies have addressed the role of hyperglycemia in the respiratory system of individuals with COVID-19 (59). However, studies have reported that hyperglycemia can heighten the glucose concentrations in airway secretions (54). In addition, hyperglycemia can also have a negative impact on pulmonary activity so that respiratory dysfunction triggered by the influenza virus is exacerbated in DM patients (64). DM is related to many changes in lung structure, and these include supplemented vasculature permeability and a relaxed alveolar epithelium in animal models with the disease (114). Glycemic regulation may have a relevant impact on clinical outcomes in individuals with coexistent viral respiratory diseases and DM, such as COVID-19 (65). It has been shown that hyperglycemia and SARS-CoV-2 infection interact in a vicious cycle, in which hyperglycemia induces ACE2 glycation that increases affinity to the SARS-CoV-2. Thus, severe SARS-CoV-2 infection-induced insulin resistance and pancreatic β-cell damage by high levels of pro-inflammatory cytokines can also lead to hyperglycemia (115). Thus, strict control of blood glucose in DM patients with COVID-19 is mandatory to prevent life-threatening complications.

Control of Hypertension in DM Patients With COVID-19

The coexistence of DM and hypertension requires judicious control of blood pressure increases. A distinct caveat in hypertension therapy in such patients shows that coronaviruses can bind to cells via ACE2, which means that patients who receive therapy with drugs of pharmacological origin that rise ACE2 levels may be put in jeopardy (65). The prevalence of hypertension and CV diseases is clinically relevant in COVID-19 patients, particularly in the elderly with DM. Based on animal models, some concerns have been raised on RAS inhibitors, particularly ARBs, as they can affect ACE2 expression despite there being no clinical evidence that they should be restricted or momentarily obsolete in COVID-19 patients (53). Thus, the European Society of Cardiology (ESC), the American College of Cardiology, the American Heart Association and the Heart Failure Society of America (ACC/AHA-HFSA), and the American Society of Hypertension (ASH) have issued policy statements that strongly recommend

DM patients continue therapy with their usual antihypertensive treatment as no empirical reports exist suggesting that therapy with ACE inhibitors or ARBs should be stopped due to SARS-CoV-2 infection. Nonetheless, the issues that cannot be recognized in relation to COVID-19 and DM are significant and numerous (64).

Control of Neuroendocrine Diseases in COVID-19 Patients With DM

A study by Kaiser et al. (116) found that, in COVID-19 patients, those with pituitary or other neuroendocrine disorders need to be addressed. Patients that have a shortage of primary adrenaline may develop DM insipidus, which further complicate both electrolyte and fluid disorders. Thus, close control and judicious replacement of water and electrolytes to avoid hyponatremia or hypernatremia is crucial to block the high loss of insensitive fluid linked to fever and tachypnea, combined with impaired fluid intake and altered levels of consciousness (117). Indeed, DDP4 inhibitors reduce mortality and COVID-19 severity in DM patients through attenuation of SARS-CoV-2 entry and associated pro-inflammatory cytokine release (118).

Control of Kidney Diseases in Diabetic Patients With COVID-19

ACEi/ARB therapy use has no have negative impact on COVID-19 morbimortality in synergy with CV disorders (119). D'Marco et al. (72), testing a hypothetical assertion, showed a worsening of DKD that could result in the progression of a serious CKD stage, need for renal replacement, and even death. The authors also postulate that the actual observations support the assertion that reduced immune system defenses and other kidney-associated factors make DM patients more susceptible to infections by certain infectious agents (72).

Clinical Medication of DM Patients With COVID-19

Recent studies raise the hypothesis that both the treatment course and prognosis of COVID-19 should be grouped, depending on the presence or absence of comorbidities into types A, B, and C. Type A refers to patients with the virus and pneumonia and without comorbidities, type B patients with the virus and pneumonia and comorbidities, and type C represents COVID-19 patients with pneumonia and multiorgan dysfunction (120). In China, Yan et al. (121) studied the clinical features and outcomes in 48 patients with extreme DM and SARS-CoV-2 and compared them with 145 severe COVID-19 patients hospitalized but without DM. As main findings, the authors show that DM patients with serious viral infection had a more severe response due to inflammation and were more prone to require mechanical ventilation and experience death (and survival delay) when compared with non-DM. Regarding clinical medication, the authors state that the insulin dose increased after the patient was infected with SARS-CoV-2, which depicts that the viral agent plays a direct role in glucose metabolism of such patients. Consequently, glucose metabolic dysfunction triggers DM and then impacts pneumonia severity, acting as an amplification loop (25). A study carried out in more than 500 COVID-19 patients revealed that hyperglycemia has often been temporary and usually addressed in most patients after hospital discharge (63). For such hospitalized patients, it is imperative to ensure an excellent glycemic control and look for blood sugar results of 4–10 mmol/L to halt bad results (65, 66). Thus, when reacting to the novel coronavirus pandemic, policies and actions need to involve DM when health inequities are not triggered (49). Indeed, it is reported that uncontrolled or poorly regulated hyperglycemia for any reason, including DM or stress hyperglycemia, is linked to poor outcomes in COVID-19 patients (122). Therefore, strict glucose monitoring and control is advisable in severely affected COVID-19 patients even in non-DM ones (123, 124). For example, in India, the T2DM treatment with hydroxychloroquine has been approved as an alternative for patients with a non-controlled DM with other hypoglycemic agents (i.e., stable-dose insulin therapy with metformin and glimepiride) (125). Moreover, despite inflammation being linked to impaired glucose regulation, the underlying mechanism of the hypoglycemic effect of hydroxychloroquine is still not clear (106).

Micallef et al. (126) indicated that corticosteroid therapy could worsen a patient's condition and that non-steroidal anti-inflammatory drugs, such as ibuprofen, might increase the risk of developing a complicated type of the disease. Indeed, according to the updated clinical guideline, the WHO recommends the use of corticosteroids in severe cases of SARS-CoV-2 infection (127). It is reported that respiratory viral infections are linked to development of DM due to autoimmune pancreatic β-cells injury (128). Specifically, in COVID-19 patients, SARS-CoV-2 may trigger development of DM due to direct pancreatic β-cell injury of SARS-CoV-2 due to a higher expression of ACE2, a receptor for this virus, or indirectly through induction of insulin resistance triggered by SARS-CoV-2-induced oxidative stress (129). Likewise, acute pancreatitis and secondary DM have been reported as an adverse effect of ritonavir and lopinavir, commonly used drugs for the treatment of COVID-19 (130). Likewise, the constant use of ARBs and ACEIs are associated with immunomodulatory properties and reduced pulmonary and systemic inflammatory reactions due to delayed cytokines (131, 132). SARS-CoV-2 may have a direct effect on endothelial cells so that other drugs may also be successful in the treatment of COVID-19 patients via their positive impact on endothelial cells, including α1-adrenergic receptor blockers (e.g., doxazosin) (133), modulators of Sigma receptors (134), metformin (135), indomethacin (136), endothelin receptor antagonists (e.g., bosentan) (137), and heparin and low-molecular weight heparin (LMWH) (138). These drugs, which are often used by DM patients, particularly metformin, reduces endothelial dysfunction and associated complications.

APN01 is a recombinant human ACE2 produced by APEIRON to treat ARDS, pulmonary arterial hypertension, and acute lung injury; briefly, it works by delaying the virus entry and spread and, therefore, may be of high benefit although the clinical trials are still ongoing (100). Indeed, recombinant human ACE2 increases metabolism of vasoconstrictor Ang II to vasodilator Ang1-7, which attenuates development of ARDS (139).

In this sense, the optimal therapy for these patients should derive from an approach involving a consortium of multidisciplinary members, including specialists in infectious diseases, emergency medicine, endocrinology, and respiratory function. Furthermore, backup from exercise rehabilitation specialists and nutritionists may be needed during a longer period of recovery and hospital stay (140). Finally, and regarding therapy, although there are different clinical trials and studies ongoing to assess the efficacy and safety of possible therapeutic alternatives, such as the use of chloroquine phosphate, lopinavir/ritonavir, remdesivir, interferon, tocilizumab, ribavirin, and arbidol, among others (110), no drug against SARS-CoV-2 has been developed and officially approved so far (141).

CONCLUSION

In short, DM patients are at a higher risk of developing the severe form of COVID-19 as a consequence of the presence of cardio-metabolic and immunological disorder, including insulin resistance, prolonged hyperglycemia, and hyperinflammation despite other comorbidities, such as hypertension, also maybe boosting the risk. However, and noteworthy, SARS-CoV-2 may cause transient hyperglycemia even in non-DM patients as it is able to induce insulin resistance and/or damage to pancreatic β-cells. Thus, it is essential to ensure strict glucose monitoring in COVID-19 patients with DM to prevent the occurrence of life-threatening complications. Regarding pharmacotherapy in DM, the use of DDP4 inhibitors, mainly sitagliptin, have demonstrated noteworthy anti-inflammatory and anti-SARS-CoV-2 activity, so their use seems to be extremely useful in the management of DM patients with COVID-19.

AUTHOR CONTRIBUTIONS

AM, VO, DH, IR, OA, NR-P, AZ-B, MS, HH, NC-M, and GB wrote and revised the paper. All authors have read and agreed to the published version of the manuscript.

ACKNOWLEDGMENTS

NC-M acknowledges the Portuguese Foundation for Science and Technology under the Horizon 2020 Program (PTDC/PSI-GER/28076/2017).

REFERENCES

1. Al-Kuraishy HM, Al-Gareeb AI. From SARS-CoV to nCoV-2019: ruction and argument. *Arch Clin Infect Dis.* (2020) 15:1–2. doi: 10.5812/archcid.102624
2. Andersen KG, Rambaut A, Lipkin WI, Holmes EC, Garry RF. The proximal origin of SARS-CoV-2. *Nat Med.* (2020) 26:450–2. doi: 10.1038/s41591-020-0820-9
3. Al-kuraishy HM, Al-Maiahy TJ, Al-Gareeb AI, Musa RA, Ali ZH. COVID-19 pneumonia in an Iraqi pregnant woman with preterm delivery. *Asian Pac J Reprod.* (2020) 9:156. doi: 10.4103/2305-0500.282984
4. Becerra-Flores M, Cardozo T. SARS-CoV-2 viral spike G614 mutation exhibits higher case fatality rate. *Int J Clin Pract.* (2020) 74:e13525. doi: 10.1111/ijcp.13525
5. Al-Kuraishy HM, Al-Naimi MS, Lungnier CM, Al-Gareeb AI. Macrolides and COVID-19: An optimum premise. *Biomed Biotechnol Res J.* (2020) 4:189. doi: 10.4103/bbrj.bbrj_103_20
6. Lugnier C, Al-Kuraishy HM, Rousseau E. PDE4 inhibition as a therapeutic strategy for improvement of pulmonary dysfunctions in Covid-19 and cigarette smoking. *Biochem Pharmacol.* (2021) 185:114431. doi: 10.1016/j.bcp.2021.114431
7. Adhikari SP, Meng S, Wu Y-J, Mao Y-P, Ye R-X, Wang Q-Z, et al. Epidemiology, causes, clinical manifestation and diagnosis, prevention and control of coronavirus disease (COVID-19) during the early outbreak period: a scoping review. *Infect Dis Poverty.* (2020) 9:1–12 doi: 10.1186/s40249-020-00646-x
8. Zou L, Ruan F, Huang M, Liang L, Huang H, Hong Z, et al. SARS-CoV-2 viral load in upper respiratory specimens of infected patients. *N Engl J Med.* (2020) 382:1177–9. doi: 10.1056/NEJMc2001737
9. Liu Y, Yan L-M, Wan L, Xiang T-X, Le A, Liu J-M, et al. Viral dynamics in mild and severe cases of COVID-19. *Lancet Infect Dis.* (2020) 20:656–7. doi: 10.1016/S1473-3099(20)30232-2
10. Rothe C, Schunk M, Sothmann P, Bretzel G, Froeschl G, Wallrauch C, et al. Transmission of 2019-nCoV infection from an asymptomatic contact in Germany. *N Engl J Med.* (2020) 382:970–1. doi: 10.1056/NEJMc2001468
11. Al-Kuraishy HM, Sami OM, Hussain NR, Al-Gareeb AI. Metformin and/or vildagliptin mitigate type II diabetes mellitus induced-oxidative stress: the intriguing effect. *J Adv Pharm Technol Res.* (2020) 11:142. doi: 10.4103/japtr.JAPTR_18_20
12. Rasheed HA, Al-Kuraishy HM, Al-Gareeb AI, Hussien NR, Al-Nami MS. Effects of diabetic pharmacotherapy on prolactin hormone in patients with type 2 diabetes mellitus: Bane or Boon. *J Adv Pharm Technol Res.* (2019) 10:163. doi: 10.4103/japtr.JAPTR_65_19
13. Al-Kuraishy HM, Al-Gareeb AI, Shams HA, Al-Mamorri F. Endothelial dysfunction and inflammatory biomarkers as a response factor of concurrent coenzyme Q10 add-on metformin in patients with type 2 diabetes mellitus. *J Lab Phys.* (2019) 11:317. doi: 10.4103/JLP.JLP_123_19
14. Muralidharan G, Rao GH. Oxygen as a therapeutic drug: hyperbaric oxygen therapy. *Biomed Pharmacol J.* (2020) 13:521–8. doi: 10.13005/bpj/1913
15. Pearson-Stuttard J, Blundell S, Harris T, Cook DG, Critchley J. Diabetes and infection: assessing the association with glycaemic control in population-based studies. *Lancet Diabetes Endocrinol.* (2016) 4:148–58. doi: 10.1016/S2213-8587(15)00379-4
16. Xia C, Rao X, Zhong J. Role of T lymphocytes in type 2 diabetes and diabetes-associated inflammation. *J Diabetes Res.* (2017) 2017:6494795. doi: 10.1155/2017/6494795
17. Hodgson K, Morris J, Bridson T, Govan B, Rush C, Ketheesan N. Immunological mechanisms contributing to the double burden of diabetes and intracellular bacterial infections. *Immunology.* (2015) 144:171–85. doi: 10.1111/imm.12394
18. Muller L, Gorter K, Hak E, Goudzwaard W, Schellevis F, Hoepelman A, et al. Increased risk of common infections in patients with type 1 and type 2 diabetes mellitus. *Clin Infect Dis.* (2005) 41:281–8. doi: 10.1086/431587
19. Yang J, Feng Y, Yuan M, Yuan S, Fu H, Wu B, et al. Plasma glucose levels and diabetes are independent predictors for mortality and morbidity in patients with SARS. *Diabetic Med.* (2006) 23:623–8. doi: 10.1111/j.1464-5491.2006.01861.x
20. Schoen K, Horvat N, Guerreiro NF, de Castro I, de Giassi KS. Spectrum of clinical and radiographic findings in patients with diagnosis of H1N1 and correlation with clinical severity. *BMC Infect Dis.* (2019) 19:1–8 doi: 10.1186/s12879-019-4592-0
21. Banik GR, Alqahtani AS, Booy R, Rashid H. Risk factors for severity and mortality in patients with MERS-CoV: analysis of publicly available data from Saudi Arabia. *Virol Sin.* (2016) 31:81–4. doi: 10.1007/s12250-015-3679-z
22. Erener S. Diabetes, infection risk and COVID-19. *Mol Metab.* (2020) 39:101044. doi: 10.1016/j.molmet.2020.101044

23. Kuba K, Imai Y, Rao S, Gao H, Guo F, Guan B, et al. A crucial role of angiotensin converting enzyme 2 (ACE2) in SARS coronavirus-induced lung injury. *Nat Med.* (2005) 11:875–9. doi: 10.1038/nm1267
24. Wrapp D, Wang N, Corbett KS, Goldsmith JA, Hsieh C-L, Abiona O, et al. Cryo-EM structure of the 2019-nCoV spike in the prefusion conformation. *Science.* (2020) 367:1260–3. doi: 10.1126/science.abb2507
25. Patel VB, Zhong J-C, Grant MB, Oudit GY. Role of the ACE2/angiotensin 1-7 axis of the renin-angiotensin system in heart failure. *Circ Res.* (2016) 118:1313–26. doi: 10.1161/CIRCRESAHA.116.307708
26. Guo W, Li M, Dong Y, Zhou H, Zhang Z, Tian C, et al. Diabetes is a risk factor for the progression and prognosis of COVID-19. *Diabetes Metab Res Rev.* (2020) 36:1–9. doi: 10.1002/dmrr.3319
27. Sommerstein R, Kochen MM, Messerli FH, Gräni C. Coronavirus Disease 2019 (COVID-19): do angiotensin-converting enzyme inhibitors/angiotensin receptor blockers have a biphasic effect? *J Am Heart Assoc.* (2020) 9:e016509. doi: 10.1161/JAHA.120.016509
28. Drucker DJ. Coronavirus infections and type 2 diabetes-shared pathways with therapeutic implications. *Endocr Rev.* (2020) 41:bnaa011. doi: 10.1210/endrev/bnaa011
29. Iacobellis G. COVID-19 and diabetes: can DPP4 inhibition play a role? *Diabetes Res Clin Pract.* (2020) 162:108125. doi: 10.1016/j.diabres.2020.108125
30. Karagiannis T, Paschos P, Paletas K, Matthews DR, Tsapas A. Dipeptidyl peptidase-4 inhibitors for treatment of type 2 diabetes mellitus in the clinical setting: systematic review and meta-analysis. *BMJ.* (2012) 344:e1369. doi: 10.1136/bmj.e1369
31. Amori RE, Lau J, Pittas AG. Efficacy and safety of incretin therapy in type 2 diabetes: systematic review and meta-analysis. *JAMA.* (2007) 298:194–206. doi: 10.1001/jama.298.2.194
32. Yang W, Cai X, Han X, Ji L. DPP-4 inhibitors and risk of infections: a meta-analysis of randomized controlled trials. *Diabetes Metab Res Rev.* (2016) 32:391–404. doi: 10.1002/dmrr.2723
33. Bassendine MF, Bridge SH, McCaughan GW, Gorrell MD. COVID-19 and comorbidities: a role for dipeptidyl peptidase 4 (DPP4) in disease severity?. *J Diabetes.* (2020) 12:649–58. doi: 10.1111/1753-0407.13052
34. Zhou P, Yang X-L, Wang X-G, Hu B, Zhang L, Zhang W, et al. A pneumonia outbreak associated with a new coronavirus of probable bat origin. *Nature.* (2020) 579:270–3. doi: 10.1038/s41586-020-2012-7
35. Matsuyama S, Nao N, Shirato K, Kawase M, Saito S, Takayama I, et al. Enhanced isolation of SARS-CoV-2 by TMPRSS2-expressing cells. *Proc Natl Acad Sci.* (2020) 117:7001–3. doi: 10.1073/pnas.2002589117
36. Sungnak W, Huang N, Bécavin C, Berg M, Queen R, Litvinukova M, et al. SARS-CoV-2 entry factors are highly expressed in nasal epithelial cells together with innate immune genes. *Nat Med.* (2020) 26:681–7. doi: 10.1038/s41591-020-0868-6
37. Chen Z, Mi L, Xu J, Yu J, Wang X, Jiang J, et al. Function of HAb18G/CD147 in invasion of host cells by severe acute respiratory syndrome coronavirus. *J Infect Dis.* (2005) 191:755–60. doi: 10.1086/427811
38. Tortorici MA, Walls AC, Lang Y, Wang C, Li Z, Koerhuis D, et al. Structural basis for human coronavirus attachment to sialic acid receptors. *Nat Struct Mol Biol.* (2019) 26:481–9. doi: 10.1038/s41594-019-0233-y
39. Jaeckel E, Manns M, Von Herrath M. Viruses and diabetes. *Ann N Y Acad Sci.* (2002) 958:7–25. doi: 10.1111/j.1749-6632.2002.tb02943.x
40. Jali M, Shankar P. Transient diabetes following chicken pox. *J Assoc Phys India.* (1990) 38:663–4.
41. Yang J-K, Lin S-S, Ji X-J, Guo L-M. Binding of SARS coronavirus to its receptor damages islets and causes acute diabetes. *Acta Diabetol.* (2010) 47:193–9. doi: 10.1007/s00592-009-0109-4
42. Wang D, Hu B, Hu C, Zhu F, Liu X, Zhang J, et al. Clinical characteristics of 138 hospitalized patients with 2019 novel coronavirus-infected pneumonia in Wuhan, China. *JAMA.* (2020) 323:1061–9. doi: 10.1001/jama.2020.1585
43. Mehra MR, Desai SS, Kuy S, Henry TD, Patel AN. Cardiovascular disease, drug therapy, and mortality in COVID-19. *N Engl J Med.* (2020) 382:e102. doi: 10.1056/NEJMoa2007621
44. Tentolouris A, Eleftheriadou I, Athanasakis K, Kyriopoulos J, Tsilimigras DI, Grigoropoulou P, et al. Prevalence of diabetes mellitus as well as cardiac and other main comorbidities in a representative sample of the adult Greek population in comparison with the general population. *Hellenic J Cardiol.* (2018) 61:15–22. doi: 10.1016/j.hjc.2018.04.008
45. Covid C, Team R. Severe outcomes among patients with coronavirus disease 2019 (COVID-19)-United States, February 12-March 16, 2020. *MMWR Morb Mortal Wkly Rep.* (2020) 69:343–6. doi: 10.15585/mmwr.mm6912e2
46. Al-Sabah SK, Al-Haddad M, Al Youha S, Jamal MH, AlMazeedi S. COVID-19: impact of obesity and diabetes in disease severity. *medRxiv.* (2020) 10:e12414. doi: 10.1111/cob.12414
47. Zhou F, Yu T, Du R, Fan G, Liu Y, Liu Z, et al. Clinical course and risk factors for mortality of adult inpatients with COVID-19 in Wuhan, China: a retrospective cohort study. *The lancet.* (2020) 395:1054–62. doi: 10.1016/S0140-6736(20)30566-3
48. Klekotka RB, Mizgała E, Król W. The etiology of lower respiratory tract infections in people with diabetes. *Adv Respir Med.* (2015) 83:401–8. doi: 10.5603/PiAP.2015.0065
49. Choi WS, Kang C-I, Kim Y, Choi J-P, Joh JS, Shin H-S, et al. Clinical presentation and outcomes of Middle East respiratory syndrome in the Republic of Korea. *Infect Chemother.* (2016) 48:118–26. doi: 10.3947/ic.2016.48.2.118
50. Carey IM, Critchley JA, DeWilde S, Harris T, Hosking FJ, Cook DG. Risk of infection in type 1 and type 2 diabetes compared with the general population: a matched cohort study. *Diabetes Care.* (2018) 41:513–21. doi: 10.2337/dc17-2131
51. Coppell KJ, Hall RM, Downie M, Fraser SK, Garrett M, Jefferies CA, et al. Diabetes and COVID-19-the meeting of two pandemics: what are the concerns? *N Z Med J.* (2020) 133:85–7.
52. Al Heialy S, Hachim MY, Senok A, Abou Tayoun A, Hamoudi R, Alsheikh-Ali A, et al. Regulation of angiotensin converting enzyme 2 (ACE2) in obesity: implications for COVID-19. *Front Physiol.* (2020) 11:555039 doi: 10.1101/2020.04.17.046938
53. Muniyappa R, Gubbi S. COVID-19 pandemic, coronaviruses, and diabetes mellitus. *Am J Physiol Endocrinol Metab.* (2020) 318:E736–41. doi: 10.1152/ajpendo.00124.2020
54. Kumar A, Arora A, Sharma P, Anikhindi SA, Bansal N, Singla V, et al. Is diabetes mellitus associated with mortality and severity of COVID-19? A meta-analysis. *Diabetes Metab Syndrome Clin Res Rev.* (2020) 14:535–45. doi: 10.1016/j.dsx.2020.04.044
55. Huang Y-T, Lee Y-C, Hsiao C-J. Hospitalization for ambulatory-care-sensitive conditions in Taiwan following the SARS outbreak: a population-based interrupted time series study. *J Formosan Med Assoc.* (2009) 108:386–94. doi: 10.1016/S0929-6646(09)60082-6
56. Chan-Yeung M, Xu RH. SARS: epidemiology. *Respirology.* (2003) 8:S9–S14. doi: 10.1046/j.1440-1843.2003.00518.x
57. Morra ME, Van Thanh L, Kamel MG, Ghazy AA, Altibi AM, Dat LM, et al. Clinical outcomes of current medical approaches for Middle East respiratory syndrome: a systematic review and meta-analysis. *Rev Med Virol.* (2018) 28:e1977. doi: 10.1002/rmv.1977
58. Li B, Yang J, Zhao F, Zhi L, Wang X, Liu L, et al. Prevalence and impact of cardiovascular metabolic diseases on COVID-19 in China. *Clin Res Cardiol.* (2020) 109:531–8. doi: 10.1007/s00392-020-01626-9
59. Wang A, Zhao W, Xu Z, Gu J. Timely blood glucose management for the outbreak of 2019 novel coronavirus disease (COVID-19) is urgently needed. *Diabetes Res Clin Pract.* (2020) 162:108118. doi: 10.1016/j.diabres.2020.108118
60. Chow N, Fleming-Dutra K, Gierke R, Hall A, Hughes M, Pilishvili T, et al. Preliminary estimates of the prevalence of selected underlying health conditions among patients with coronavirus disease 2019-United States, February 12-March 28, 2020. *MMWR Morb Mortal Wkly Rep.* (2020) 69:382–6. doi: 10.15585/mmwr.mm6913e2
61. Shenoy A, Ismaily M, Bajaj M. Diabetes and Covid-19: a global health challenge. *BMJ Spec J.* (2020) 8:1–2. doi: 10.1136/bmjdrc-2020-001450
62. Wu Z, McGoogan JM. Characteristics of and important lessons from the coronavirus disease 2019 (COVID-19) outbreak in China: summary of a report of 72 314 cases from the Chinese Center for Disease Control and Prevention. *JAMA.* (2020) 323:1239–42. doi: 10.1001/jama.2020.2648
63. Umpierrez GE, Isaacs SD, Bazargan N, You X, Thaler LM, Kitabchi AE. Hyperglycemia: an independent marker of in-hospital mortality in patients with undiagnosed diabetes. *J Clin Endocrinol Metab.* (2002) 87:978–82. doi: 10.1210/jcem.87.3.8341
64. Van den Berghe G, Wouters PJ, Bouillon R, Weekers F, Verwaest C, Schetz M, et al. Outcome benefit of intensive insulin therapy in the critically

ill: Insulin dose versus glycemic control. *Crit Care Med.* (2003) 31:359–66. doi: 10.1097/01.CCM.0000045568.12881.10

65. Zhu L, She ZG, Cheng X, Qin JJ, Zhang XJ, Cai J, et al. Association of blood glucose control and outcomes in patients with COVID-19 and pre-existing type 2 diabetes. *Cell Metab.* (2020) 31:1068–77. doi: 10.1016/j.cmet.2020.04.021
66. Gates B. Responding to Covid-19-a once-in-a-century pandemic? *N Engl J Med.* (2020) 382:1677–9. doi: 10.1056/NEJMp2003762
67. Yang X, Yu Y, Xu J, Shu H, Liu H, Wu Y, et al. Clinical course and outcomes of critically ill patients with SARS-CoV-2 pneumonia in Wuhan, China: a single-centered, retrospective, observational study. *Lancet Respir Med.* (2020) 8:475–81. doi: 10.1016/S2213-2600(20)30079-5
68. Tsoukas MA, Farr OM, Mantzoros CS. Leptin in congenital and HIV-associated lipodystrophy. *Metabolism.* (2015) 64:47–59. doi: 10.1016/j.metabol.2014.07.017
69. Marik PE, DePerrior SE, Ahmad Q, Dodani S. Gender-based disparities in COVID-19 patient outcomes. *J Invest Med.* (2021) 69:814–8. doi: 10.1136/jim-2020-001641
70. Shahid Z, Kalayanamitra R, McClafferty B, Kepko D, Ramgobin D, Patel R, et al. COVID-19 and older adults: what we know. *J Am Geriatr Soc.* (2020) 68:926–9 doi: 10.1111/jgs.16472
71. Fang L, Karakiulakis G, Roth M. Are patients with hypertension and diabetes mellitus at increased risk for COVID-19 infection? *Lancet Respir Med.* (2020) 8:e21. doi: 10.1016/S2213-2600(20)30116-8
72. Bode B, Garrett V, Messler J, McFarland R, Crowe J, Booth R, et al. Glycemic characteristics and clinical outcomes of COVID-19 patients hospitalized in the United States. *J Diabetes Sci Technol.* (2020) 14:813–21. doi: 10.1177/1932296820924469
73. Guzmán-Flores JM, López-Briones S. Cells of innate and adaptive immunity in type 2 diabetes and obesity. *Gac Med Mex.* (2012) 148:381–9.
74. Diao B, Wang C, Tan Y, Chen X, Liu Y, Ning L, et al. Reduction and functional exhaustion of T cells in patients with coronavirus disease 2019 (COVID-19). *Front Immunol.* (2020). 11:827. doi: 10.3389/fimmu.2020.00827
75. Kulcsar KA, Coleman CM, Beck SE, Frieman MB. Comorbid diabetes results in immune dysregulation and enhanced disease severity following MERS-CoV infection. *JCI Insight.* (2019) 4:e131774. doi: 10.1172/jci.insight.131774
76. Huang I, Lim MA, Pranata R. Diabetes mellitus is associated with increased mortality and severity of disease in COVID-19 pneumonia-a systematic review, meta-analysis, and meta-regression. *Diabetes Metab Syndrome Clin Res Rev.* (2020) 14:395–403.73. doi: 10.1016/j.dsx.2020.04.018
77. Tang N, Bai H, Chen X, Gong J, Li D, Sun Z. Anticoagulant treatment is associated with decreased mortality in severe coronavirus disease 2019 patients with coagulopathy. *J Thromb Haemost.* (2020) 18:1094–9. doi: 10.1111/jth.14817
78. D'Marco L, Puchades MJ, Romero-Parra M, Gorriz JL. Diabetic kidney disease and COVID-19: the crash of two pandemics. *Front Med.* (2020) 7:199. doi: 10.3389/fmed.2020.00199
79. Critchley JA, Carey IM, Harris T, DeWilde S, Hosking FJ, Cook DG. Glycemic control and risk of infections among people with type 1 or type 2 diabetes in a large primary care cohort study. *Diabetes Care.* (2018) 41:2127–35. doi: 10.2337/dc18-0287
80. Mor A, Dekkers OM, Nielsen JS, Beck-Nielsen H, Sørensen HT, Thomsen RW. Impact of glycemic control on risk of infections in patients with type 2 diabetes: a population-based cohort study. *Am J Epidemiol.* (2017) 186:227–36. doi: 10.1093/aje/kwx049
81. Kim N-y, Ha E, Moon JS, Lee Y-H, Choi EY. Response: acute hyperglycemic crises with coronavirus disease-19: case reports (Diabetes Metab J (2020) 44:349–53). *Diabetes Metab J.* (2020) 44:484–5. doi: 10.4093/dmj.2020.0129
82. Zhang Y, Cui Y, Shen M, Zhang J, Liu B, Dai M, et al. Comorbid diabetes mellitus was associated with poorer prognosis in patients with COVID-19: a Retrospective Cohort Study. *medRxiv [Preprint].* (2020). doi: 10.1101/2020.03.24.20042358
83. Williams B, Mancia G, Spiering W, Agabiti Rosei E, Azizi M, Burnier M, et al. 2018 ESC/ESH Guidelines for the management of arterial hypertension: the Task Force for the management of arterial hypertension of the European Society of Cardiology (ESC) and the European Society of Hypertension (ESH). *Eur Heart J.* (2018) 39:3021–104. doi: 10.1093/eurheartj/ehy339
84. Huang C, Wang Y, Li X, Ren L, Zhao J, Hu Y, et al. Clinical features of patients infected with 2019 novel coronavirus in Wuhan, China. *Lancet.* (2020) 395:497–506. doi: 10.1016/S0140-6736(20)30183-5
85. Deftereos SG, Siasos G, Giannopoulos G, Vrachatis DA, Angelidis C, Giotaki SG, et al. The GReek study in the Effects of Colchicine in COvid-19 complications prevention (GRECCO-19 study): rationale and study design. *Hellenic J Cardiol.* (2020) 61:42–5. doi: 10.1016/j.hjc.2020.03.002
86. Schiffrin EL, Flack JM, Ito S, Muntner P, Webb RC. Hypertension and COVID-19. *Am J Hypertens.* (2020) 33:373–74. doi: 10.1093/ajh/hpaa057
87. Avogaro A, Albiero M, Menegazzo L, de Kreutzenberg S, Fadini GP. Endothelial dysfunction in diabetes: the role of reparatory mechanisms. *Diabetes Care.* (2011) 34(Suppl. 2):S285–S90. doi: 10.2337/dc11-s239
88. Palladino R, Tabak AG, Khunti K, Valabhji J, Majeed A, Millett C, et al. Association between pre-diabetes and microvascular and macrovascular disease in newly diagnosed type 2 diabetes. *BMJ Open Diabetes Res Care.* (2020) 8:e001061. doi: 10.1136/bmjdrc-2019-001061
89. Chance WW, Rhee C, Yilmaz C, Dane DM, Pruneda ML, Raskin P, et al. Diminished alveolar microvascular reserves in type 2 diabetes reflect systemic microangiopathy. *Diabetes Care.* (2008) 31:1596–601. doi: 10.2337/dc07-2323
90. Petrie JR, Guzik TJ, Touyz RM. Diabetes, hypertension, and cardiovascular disease: clinical insights and vascular mechanisms. *Can J Cardiol.* (2018) 34:575–84. doi: 10.1016/j.cjca.2017.12.005
91. Bernard I, Limonta D, Mahal LK, Hobman TC. Endothelium infection and dysregulation by SARS-CoV-2: evidence and caveats in COVID-19. *Viruses.* (2021) 13:29. doi: 10.3390/v13010029
92. Sims JT, Krishnan V, Chang CY, Engle SM, Casalini G, Rodgers GH, et al. Characterization of the cytokine storm reflects hyperinflammatory endothelial dysfunction in COVID-19. *J Allergy Clin Immunol.* (2021) 147:107–11. doi: 10.1016/j.jaci.2020.08.031
93. Ciceri F, Beretta L, Scandroglio AM, Colombo S, Landoni G, Ruggeri A, et al. Microvascular COVID-19 lung vessels obstructive thromboinflammatory syndrome (MicroCLOTS): an atypical acute respiratory distress syndrome working hypothesis. *Crit Care Resusc.* (2020) 22:95–7.
94. Dunn E, Grant P. Type 2 diabetes: an atherothrombotic syndrome. *Curr Mol Med.* (2005) 5:323–32. doi: 10.2174/1566524053766059
95. McFadyen JD, Stevens H, Peter K. The emerging threat of (micro) thrombosis in COVID-19 and its therapeutic implications. *Circ Res.* (2020) 127:571–87. doi: 10.1161/CIRCRESAHA.120.317447
96. Fanelli V, Fiorentino M, Cantaluppi V, Gesualdo L, Stallone G, Ronco C, et al. Acute kidney injury in SARS-CoV-2 infected patients. *Critical Care.* (2020) 24:1–3. doi: 10.1186/s13054-020-02872-z
97. Richardson S, Hirsch J, Narasimhan M, Crawford J, McGinn T, Davidson K, et al. Presenting characteristics, comorbidities, and outcomes among 5700 patients hospitalized with Covid-19 in the New York City area. *JAMA.* (2020) 323:2052–9. doi: 10.1001/jama.2020.6775
98. Zou X, Chen K, Zou J, Han P, Hao J, Han Z. Single-cell RNA-seq data analysis on the receptor ACE2 expression reveals the potential risk of different human organs vulnerable to 2019-nCoV infection. *Front Med.* (2020) 14:185–92. doi: 10.1007/s11684-020-0754-0
99. Kliger AS, Silberzweig J. Mitigating risk of COVID-19 in dialysis facilities. *Clin J Am Soc Nephrol.* (2020) 15:707–9. doi: 10.2215/CJN.0334 0320
100. Su H, Yang M, Wan C, Yi L-X, Tang F, Zhu H-Y, et al. Renal histopathological analysis of 26 postmortem findings of patients with COVID-19 in China. *Kidney Int.* (2020) 98:219–27. doi: 10.1016/j.kint.2020.04.003
101. Saraladevi N, Chih-Wei Y, Shang-Jyh H, Bi-Cheng L, Jiang-Hua C, Vivekanand J. The Novel Coronavirus 2019 epidemic and kidneys. *Kidney Int.* (2020) 97:824–8. doi: 10.1016/j.kint.2020.03.001
102. Li Z, Wu M, Yao J, Guo J, Liao X, Song S, et al. Caution on kidney dysfunctions of COVID-19 patients (2020). doi: 10.2139/ssrn.3559601
103. Shi H, Han X, Jiang N, Cao Y, Alwalid O, Gu J, et al. Radiological findings from 81 patients with COVID-19 pneumonia in Wuhan, China: a descriptive study. *Lancet Infect Dis.* (2020) 20:425–34. doi: 10.1016/S1473-3099(20)30086-4
104. Guo Y-R, Cao Q-D, Hong Z-S, Tan Y-Y, Chen S-D, Jin H-J, et al. The origin, transmission and clinical therapies on coronavirus disease 2019

(COVID-19) outbreak-an update on the status. *Mil Med Res.* (2020) 7:1–10. doi: 10.1186/s40779-020-00240-0
105. Wang J, Zhu X, Xu Z, Yang G, Mao G, Jia Y, et al. Clinical and CT findings of COVID-19: differences among three age groups. *BMC Infect Dis.* (2020) 20:1. doi: 10.1186/s12879-020-05154-9
106. Al-Kuraishy HM, Al-Gareeb AI, Alblihed M, Cruz-Martins N, Batiha GE. COVID-19 and risk of acute ischemic stroke and acute lung injury in patients with Type II diabetes mellitus: the anti-inflammatory role of metformin. *Front Med.* (2021) 8:110 doi: 10.3389/fmed.2021.644295
107. Tang ML, Li YQ, Chen X, Lin H, Jiang ZC, Gu DL, et al. Co-infection with common respiratory pathogens and SARS-CoV-2 in patients with COVID-19 pneumonia and laboratory biochemistry findings: a retrospective cross-sectional study of 78 patients from a single center in China. *Med Sci Monit Int Med J Exp Clin Res.* (2021) 27:e929783–1. doi: 10.12659/MSM.929783
108. Marjot T, Webb GJ, Barritt AS, Moon AM, Stamataki Z, Wong VW, et al. COVID-19 and liver disease: mechanistic and clinical perspectives. *Nat Rev Gastroenterol Hepatol.* (2021) 18:348–64. doi: 10.1038/s41575-021-00426-4
109. Eid M, Al-Kaisy M, Regeia W, Jiwa Khan H. The prognostic accuracy of neutrophil-lymphocyte ratio in COVID-19 patients. *Front Emerg Med.* (2021) 5:e8.
110. Abdel-Moneim A. COVID-19-associated pancreatic dysfunction. *Hong Kong Med J.* (2021) 27:157–9. doi: 10.12809/hkmj209056
111. Zhang J-j, Dong X, Cao Y-y, Yuan Y-d, Yang Y-b, Yan Y-q, et al. Clinical characteristics of 140 patients infected with SARS-CoV-2 in Wuhan, China. *Allergy.* (2020) 75:1730–41. doi: 10.1111/all.14238
112. Gupta R, Ghosh A, Singh AK, Misra A. Clinical considerations for patients with diabetes in times of COVID-19 epidemic. *Diabetes Metab Syndrome.* (2020) 14:211. doi: 10.1016/j.dsx.2020.03.002
113. Whyte CS, Morrow GB, Mitchell JL, Chowdary P, Mutch NJ. Fibrinolytic abnormalities in acute respiratory distress syndrome (ARDS) and versatility of thrombolytic drugs to treat COVID-19. *J Thromb Haemost.* (2020) 18:1548–55. doi: 10.1111/jth.14872
114. Philips BJ, Meguer J-X, Redman J, Baker EH. Factors determining the appearance of glucose in upper and lower respiratory tract secretions. *Intens Care Med.* (2003) 29:2204–10. doi: 10.1007/s00134-003-1961-2
115. Al-kuraishy H, Al-Gareeb AI, Guerreiro SG, Cruz-Martins N, Batiha GE. COVID-19 in relation to hyperglycemia and diabetes mellitus. *Front Cardiovasc Med.* (2021) 8:335. doi: 10.3389/fcvm.2021.644095
116. Kaiser UB, Mirmira RG, Stewart PM. *Our Response to COVID-19 as Endocrinologists and Diabetologists.* Washington, DC: Oxford University Press US (2020).
117. Baldeweg S, Ball S, Brooke A, Gleeson H, Levy M, Prentice M, et al. SOCIETY FOR ENDOCRINOLOGY CLINICAL GUIDANCE: inpatient management of cranial diabetes insipidus. *Endocr Connect.* (2018) 7:G8–G11. doi: 10.1530/EC-18-0154
118. Solerte SB, D'Addio F, Trevisan R, Lovati E, Rossi A, Pastore I, et al. Sitagliptin treatment at the time of hospitalization was associated with reduced mortality in patients with type 2 diabetes and COVID-19: a multicenter, case-control, retrospective, observational study. *Diabetes Care.* (2020) 43:2999–3006. doi: 10.2337/dc20-1521
119. Peng Y, Meng K, Guan H, Leng L, Zhu R, Wang B, et al. Clinical characteristics and outcomes of 112 cardiovascular disease patients infected by 2019-nCoV. *Zhonghua Xin Xue Guan Bing Za Zhi.* (2020) 48:450–5. doi: 10.3760/cma.j.cn112148-20200220-00105
120. Wang T, Du Z, Zhu F, Cao Z, An Y, Gao Y, et al. Comorbidities and multi-organ injuries in the treatment of COVID-19. *Lancet.* (2020) 395:e52. doi: 10.1016/S0140-6736(20)30558-4
121. Yan Y, Yang Y, Wang F. Clinical characteristics and outcomes of severe COVID-19 patients with diabetes. *BMJ Open Diabetes Res Care.* (2020) 8:1–9. doi: 10.1136/bmjdrc-2020-001343
122. Singh AK, Singh R. Does poor glucose control increase the severity and mortality in patients with diabetes and COVID-19? *Diabetes Metab Syndrome Clin Res Rev.* (2020) 14:725–7. doi: 10.1016/j.dsx.2020.05.037
123. Rekedal LR, Massarotti E, Garg R, Bhatia R, Gleeson T, Lu B, et al. Changes in glycosylated hemoglobin after initiation of hydroxychloroquine or methotrexate treatment in diabetes patients with rheumatic diseases. *Arthritis Rheum.* (2010) 62:3569–73. doi: 10.1002/art.27703
124. Gerstein HC, Thorpe KE, Taylor DW, Haynes RB. The effectiveness of hydroxychloroquine in patients with type 2 diabetes mellitus who are refractory to sulfonylureas-a randomized trial. *Diabetes Res Clin Pract.* (2002) 55:209–19. doi: 10.1016/S0168-8227(01)00325-4
125. Kumar V, Singh M, Singh AP, Pandey MS, Kumar S, Kumar S. Efficacy and safety of hydroxychloroquine when added to stable insulin therapy in combination with metformin and glimepiride in patients with type 2 diabetes compare to sitagliptin. *Int J Basic Clin Pharmacol.* (2018) 7:1959–64. doi: 10.18203/2319-2003.ijbcp20183930
126. Micallef J, Soeiro T, Annie-Pierre JB. Non-steroidal anti-inflammatory drugs, pharmacology, and COVID-19 infection. *Therapies.* (2020) 75:355–62. doi: 10.1016/j.therap.2020.05.003
127. Prescott HC, Rice TW. Corticosteroids in COVID-19 ARDS: evidence and hope during the pandemic. *JAMA.* (2020) 324:1292–5. doi: 10.1001/jama.2020.16747
128. Xuan X, Gao F, Ma X, Huang C, Wang Y, Deng H, et al. Activation of ACE2/angiotensin (1-7) attenuates pancreatic β cell dedifferentiation in a high-fat-diet mouse model. *Metabolism.* (2018) 81:83–96. doi: 10.1016/j.metabol.2017.12.003
129. Henry C, Zaizafoun M, Stock E, Ghamande S, Arroliga AC, White HD, editors. Impact of angiotensin-converting enzyme inhibitors and statins on viral pneumonia. In: *Baylor University Medical Center Proceedings.* Dallas: Taylor & Francis (2018).
130. Magro P, Zanella I, Pescarolo M, Castelli F, Quiros-Roldan E. Lopinavir/ritonavir: repurposing an old drug for HIV infection in COVID-19 treatment. *Biomed J.* (2020) 44:43–53. doi: 10.1016/j.bj.2020.11.005
131. Gullestad L, Aukrust P, Ueland T, Espevik T, Yee G, Vagelos R, et al. Effect of high-versus low-dose angiotensin converting enzyme inhibition on cytokine levels in chronic heart failure. *J Am Coll Cardiol.* (1999) 34:2061–7. doi: 10.1016/S0735-1097(99)00495-7
132. Mortensen E, Pugh M, Copeland L, Restrepo M, Cornell J, Anzueto A, et al. Impact of statins and angiotensin-converting enzyme inhibitors on mortality of subjects hospitalised with pneumonia. *Eur Respir J.* (2008) 31:611–7. doi: 10.1183/09031936.00162006
133. Sardu C, Gambardella J, Morelli MB, Wang X, Marfella R, Santulli G. Is COVID-19 an endothelial disease? *Clin Basic Evid.* (2020) 9:1417. doi: 10.3390/jcm9051417
134. Ciccarelli M, Santulli G, Campanile A, Galasso G, Cervero P, Altobelli G, et al. Endothelial α1-adrenoceptors regulate neo-angiogenesis. *Br J Pharmacol.* (2008) 153:936–46. doi: 10.1038/sj.bjp.0707637
135. Amer MS, McKeown L, Tumova S, Liu R, Seymour VA, Wilson LA, et al. Inhibition of endothelial cell Ca^{2+} entry and transient receptor potential channels by Sigma-1 receptor ligands. *Br J Pharmacol.* (2013) 168:1445–55. doi: 10.1111/bph.12041
136. Shishavan MH, Henning RH, Van Buiten A, Goris M, Deelman LE, Buikema H. Metformin improves endothelial function and reduces blood pressure in diabetic spontaneously hypertensive rats independent from glycemia control: comparison to vildagliptin. *Sci Rep.* (2017) 7:1–12. doi: 10.1038/s41598-017-11430-7
137. Bolz S-S, Pohl U. Indomethacin enhances endothelial NO release-evidence for a role of PGI2 in the autocrine control of calcium-dependent autacoid production. *Cardiovasc Res.* (1997) 36:437–44. doi: 10.1016/S0008-6363(97)00197-1
138. Sfikakis P, Papamichael C, Stamatelopoulos K, Tousoulis D, Fragiadaki K, Katsichti P, et al. Improvement of vascular endothelial function using the oral endothelin receptor antagonist bosentan in patients with systemic sclerosis. *Arthritis Rheum.* (2007) 56:1985–93. doi: 10.1002/art.22634
139. Lee E, Pavy M, Young N, Freeman C, Lobigs M. Antiviral effect of the heparan sulfate mimetic, PI-88, against dengue and encephalitic flaviviruses. *Antiviral Res.* (2006) 69:31–8. doi: 10.1016/j.antiviral.2005.08.006
140. Gurwitz D. Angiotensin receptor blockers as tentative SARS-CoV-2 therapeutics. *Drug Dev Res.* (2020) 81:537–40. doi: 10.1002/ddr.21656

22

Insulin Treatment May Increase Adverse Outcomes in Patients with COVID-19 and Diabetes

*Yan Yang†, Zixin Cai† and Jingjing Zhang**

National Clinical Research Center for Metabolic Diseases, Metabolic Syndrome Research Center, Key Laboratory of Diabetes Immunology, Ministry of Education, and Department of Metabolism and Endocrinology, The Second Xiangya Hospital of Central South University, Changsha, China

Correspondence:
Jingjing Zhang
Doctorzhangjj@csu.edu.cn

†These authors have contributed equally to this work

Background and Objective: Recently, insulin treatment has been found to be associated with increased mortality and other adverse outcomes in patients with coronavirus disease 2019 (COVID-19) and diabetes, but the results remain unclear and controversial, therefore, we conducted this meta-analysis.

Methods: Four databases, namely, PubMed, Web of Science, EMBASE and the Cochrane Library, were used to identify all studies concerning insulin treatment and the adverse effects of COVID-19, including mortality, incidence of severe/critical complications, in-hospital admission and hospitalization time. To assess publication bias, funnel plots, Begg's tests and Egger's tests were used. The odds ratios (ORs) with 95% confidence intervals (CIs) were used to access the effect of insulin therapy on mortality, severe/critical complications and in-hospital admission. The association between insulin treatment and hospitalization time was calculated by the standardized mean difference (SMD) with 95% CIs.

Results: Eighteen articles, involving a total of 12277 patients with COVID-19 and diabetes were included. Insulin treatment was significantly associated with an increased risk of mortality (OR=2.10; 95% CI, 1.51-2.93) and incidence of severe/critical COVID-19 complications (OR=2.56; 95% CI, 1.18-5.55). Moreover, insulin therapy may increase in-hospital admission in patients with COVID-19 and diabetes (OR=1.31; 95% CI, 1.06-1.61). However, there was no significant difference in the hospitalization time according to insulin treatment (SMD=0.21 95% CI, -0.02-0.45).

Conclusions: Insulin treatment may increase mortality and severe/critical complications in patients with COVID-19 and diabetes, but more large-scale studies are needed to confirm and explore the exact mechanism.

Keywords: insulin treatment, COVID-19, adverse outcomes, diabetes, mortality, complications

INTRODUCTION

Since the rapid outbreak of coronavirus disease 2019 (COVID-19) in 2019, the worldwide fight against the epidemic is still ongoing. As of January 30, 2021, the number of confirmed cases and deaths reached 114140104 and 2535520, respectively (1). The concomitant occurrence of two worldwide epidemic diseases, COVID-19 and diabetes, has introduced a series of problems. Diabetes is known as among the most serious comorbidities of COVID-19 to deteriorate disease development and outcomes. Recently, mechanisms underlying why diabetic COVID-19 patients are more prone to severe outcomes include higher glucose levels, impaired innate and adaptive immune response, impaired coagulation, obesity and hypertension (2).

Good glucose control has been demonstrated to exert a protective effect in the context of the development and outcomes of COVID-19 (3–5), and strict glucose management on admission for COVID-19 cases has been suggested regardless of diabetes status (6). The role of glycemic control strategies, such as several antidiabetic drugs including metformin and DPP-4 inhibitors in the efficacy and safety of COVID-19 and diabetes has been established (7, 8). However, whether insulin injection has some effect on the development of COVID-19 remains inconsistent. Notably, early research found that insulin treatment may be associated with adverse outcomes such as death (9) and intensive care unit (ICU) admission (10); however, evidence regarding the relationship between insulin treatment and COVID-19 remains inadequate and unconvincing. Therefore, we conducted a systematic review and meta-analysis to determine the association between insulin injection and the outcomes of COVID-19 to provide certain clinical information for these patients.

METHODS

This meta-analysis was conducted according to the Preferred Reporting Items for Systematic Reviews and Meta-Analyses (PRISMA) statement guidelines, as previously described (11).

Article Search Strategy

We searched for eligible articles from January 25, 2021 and to February 20, 2021. The PubMed (2013-2020, 20 February), Cochrane Library (1960-2020, 20 February), EMBASE (1960-2020, 20 February) and Web of Science (1950-2020, 20 February) databases were searched in this study. Searches for all published articles related to both insulin treatment and COVID-19 were performed. The following search terms were used: "Insulin", "Insulin treatment", "COVID-19", "SARS-CoV-2", and "2019 novel coronavirus". The search strategy was as follows: [(insulin) OR (insulin treatment)] AND [(COVID-19) OR (SARS Cov-2) OR (coronavirus) OR (2019 novel coronavirus)]. Additional papers were identified by performing manual searches of the references of relevant articles and tracking citations to obtain more relevant studies. All articles published by February 20, 2021 with no language restrictions were included.

Selection Criteria

Two reviewers (YY and ZC) independently reviewed all eligible studies and selected those suitable for inclusion. Disagreements were settled by reaching a consensus or with the help of a third reviewer (JZ). All articles included in this meta-analysis met the following criteria: (1) population: the subjects were patients with both COVID-19 and diabetes; (2) intervention: insulin treatment; (3) comparator/control: the control group involved non-insulin treatment, including oral antidiabetic medications, no treatment or diet control; (4) importantly, the outcomes of our study refer to the mortality and other complications of COVID-19, and the form of the outcomes must be original data of COVID-19 deaths and complications or calculated adjusted/unadjusted odds ratios (ORs) or risk ratios (RRs); and (5) study design: clinical studies. Articles were excluded if they met the following criteria: (1) articles lacking information or data necessary for the purpose of this meta-analysis and (2) articles published as letters, reviews, editorials, or conference abstracts.

Data Extraction

All relevant articles were imported into EndNote X9 software and reviewed independently by two authors (YY and ZC). Discrepancies between the authors were resolved with the help of a third reviewer (JZ). The following information was extracted from the selected studies by the two independent investigators: author, publication year, country, study design, mean or median age, sample size, population and COVID-19 outcomes. All extracted data were then imported into Excel.

The severity of the disease was classified into 4 categories according to the Guidelines for the Diagnosis and Treatment of New Coronavirus Pneumonia (fifth edition) as follows (12): 1) *mild type*: patients with mild clinical symptoms and no pulmonary changes on CT imaging, 2) *common type*: patients with symptoms of fever and signs of respiratory infection, with pneumonia changes on CT imaging, 3) *severe type*: patients presenting with any of the following items: (a) respiratory distress, respiratory rate≥30/min, (b) oxygen saturation of finger ≤ 93% in resting condition, and (c) arterial partial pressure of oxygen ($PaO2$)/oxygen concentration ($FiO2$)≤300 mmHg (1 mmHg=0.133 kPa) or 4) *critical type*: patients meeting any of the following criteria: (a) respiratory failure requiring mechanical ventilation, (b) shock and (c) ICU admission requirement due to multiple organ failure. Since only 32 mild cases were available and these cases would normally not be hospitalized, these cases were removed from the analysis (**Figure 1**).

Quality Assessment of Studies

The quality of the included studies was assessed by the Newcastle-Ottawa Scale (NOS) (13). We assessed the quality of all relevant studies based on the type of study, sample size, participant selection, representativeness of the sample, adequacy of follow-up, comparability (exposed-unexposed or case-control), and method of ascertaining the cases and controls. The possible range of NOS scores is from 0 to 9; studies that scored 4-6 represent a modest risk of bias, and those that scored <3 indicate the highest risk of bias. A study with a score of 6 or higher was defined as a high-quality study.

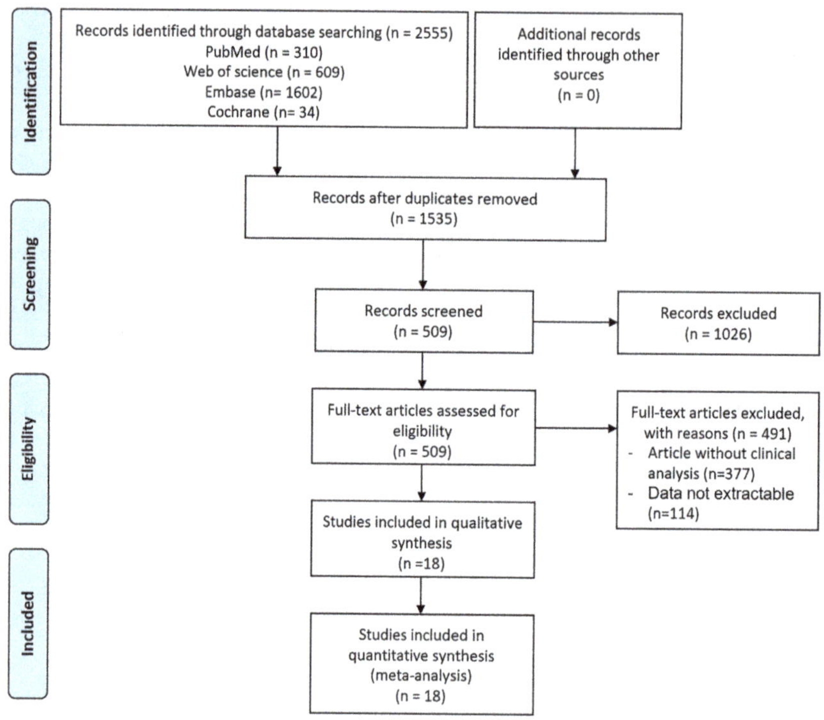

FIGURE 1 | Flow diagram of the study selection process.

Statistical Analysis

All analyses were performed using Stata (Version 13.0). The correlation between insulin treatment and mortality or incidence of complications of COVID-19 was expressed as the pooled ORs and 95% confidence interval (CI). ORs > 1 represented a direct association, and those < 1 represented an inverse association. Regarding the hospitalization time, the standardized mean difference (SMD) and 95% CI were used to analyze the results. A random-effects model was used for all results of our meta-analysis. I^2 statistics were used to assess the degree of heterogeneity as follows: 25%, 50%, and 75% represented low, moderate, and high degrees of heterogeneity, respectively. Subgroup analyses were performed using the following variables to analyze the heterogeneity: sample size (>80 or <80), period of insulin treatment (before and after admission), type of diabetes (T1DM, T2DM and Diabetes), and control groups (with or without antidiabetic drugs). Additionally, Begg's and Egger's tests and funnel plots were used to detect potential publication bias, with a p-value <0.05 suggesting the presence of bias.

RESULTS

Search Results and Study Characteristics

A flowchart of the study selection process is shown in **Figure 1**. After a preliminary search of the selected electronic databases, in total, 2555 studies were identified. After 1020 duplicates were eliminated, 1535 studies were selected by screening the titles and abstracts. After further excluding 1026 studies based on the titles and abstracts, 509 articles remained. Of these 509 articles, 491 were excluded for the following reasons after the full text was read: (1) not enough participant information was provided (n=377); and (2) the original data regarding insulin use were not provided (n=114). Finally, 18 articles (9, 10, 14–29) related to the use of insulin treatment and COVID-19 were included in this meta-analysis. The basic characteristics of the studies are presented in **Table 1**. Among the 18 studies included in this analysis, 2 studies were performed in France, 4 studies were performed in China, 5 studies were performed in the USA, 2 studies were performed in Italy, 1 in Russia, 1in Spain, 1 in Saudi Arabia, 1 in Iran and 1 in Iraq (**Table 1**). All included studies were published in 2020 or 2021. Additionally, as the different outcomes of COVID-19 were analyzed in our study, information regarding the association between insulin treatment and mortality is included in **Table 2**, and the outcomes of severe/critical complications or in-hospital admission are shown in **Table 3**.

Quality Assessment

NOS mainly consist of the following three aspects: sample selection, comparability of cases and controls, and exposure. All included studies had NOS scores higher than 6, indicating the high quality of our studies. The details of the risk of bias are described in **Table 1**.

TABLE 1 | Description of eligible studies reporting the association between insulin treatment and the outcomes of COVID-19.

No.	Author	Country	Age	Type of study	Sample size	NOS	Population
1	Bo Yu (14)	China	66 (57–73)	a retrospective study	689	8	patients with COVID-19 and T2DM
2	Cariou (15)	France	69.8 ± 13.0	a nationwide multicentre observational study	1317	7	patients with COVID-19 and diabetes
3	Yuchen Chen (16)	China	56.0 (39.0–67.0)	a retrospective study	904	8	patients with COVID-19 and diabetes (mostly T2DM)
4	Shayan Riahi (9)	USA	66.42 ± 12.67	a retrospective cohort	166	7	patients with COVID-19 and diabetes
5	Luis M. Pérez (10)	Spain	74.9 ± 8.4	a nationwide cohort study	2666	7	patients with COVID-19 and T2DM
6	Shivani Agarwal (18)	USA	68	cohort	1126	8	patients with COVID-19 and diabetes
7	Marina V (19)	Russia	NA	a retrospective study	309	7	patients with COVID-19 and T2DM
8	Marco Mirani (20)	Italy	71 (64–78)	cohort	90	8	patients with COVID-19 and T2DM
9	Shayesteh Khalili (21)	Iran	65.7 ± 12.51	cohort	127	7	patients with COVID-19 and diabetes
10	Justin J (22)	USA	65.7 ± 15.5	a retrospective study	46	8	patients with COVID-19 and diabetes
11	Huadong Yan (23)	China	49.18 (14.16)	Case-Control Study	717	8	patients with COVID-19 and T2DM
12	Ayman A (24)	Saudi Arabia	57.6 ± 13.9	cohort	806	8	patients with COVID-19 and T2DM
13	Achille Cernigliaro (25)	Italy	NA	a retrospective study	172	7	patients with COVID-19 and diabetes
14	Hussein Nafakhi (26)	Iraq	60 ± 10	a retrospective study	67	7	patients with COVID-19 and diabetes
15	Adèle Lasbleiz (27)	France	62.1 ± 14.0	cohort	2168	8	patients with COVID-19 and diabetes (mostly T2DM)
16	Michelle A (30)	USA	75.6 (10.8)	retrospective cohort study	775	8	patients with COVID-19 and T2DM
17	Grenye O'Malley (28)	USA	NA	cross-sectional study	113	7	patients with COVID-19 and T1DM
18	Ting Guo (29)	China	62.1 (42-76)	a retrospective study	19	7	patients with COVID-19 and diabetes

NA, data not available.

TABLE 2 | Description of studies reporting the association between insulin treatment and the mortality of COVID-19.

No.	Study	Sample size	Period of insulin treatment	Type of diabetes	Control groups	or	ci1	ci2
1	Bo Yu 2021 (14)	689	after admission	T2DM	with or without antidiabetic drugs	5.38	2.75	10.54
2	Cariou 2020 (15)	1317	before admission	diabetes	antidiabetic drugs	1.71	1.2	2.43
3	Yuchen Chen 2020 (16)	904	before admission	diabetes	with or without antidiabetic drugs	4.461	1.223	16.266
4	Shayan Riahi 2020 (9)	166	before admission	diabetes	antidiabetic drugs	2.486	1.204	5.134
5	Luis M. Pérez 2020 (10)	2666	after admission	T2DM	antidiabetic drugs	1.45	1.11	1.88
6	Shivani Agarwal 2020 (18)	1126	before admission	diabetes	without antidiabetic drugs	2.3	1.32	4.01
7	Marina V 2020 (19)	309	before admission	T2DM	antidiabetic drugs	2.67	1.42	5.02
8	Marco Mirani 2020 (20)	90	before admission	T2DM	antidiabetic drugs	3.05	1.57	5.95
9	Shayesteh Khalili 2020 (21)	127	before admission	diabetes	antidiabetic drugs	0.242	0.061	0.967
10	Justin J 2020 (22)	46	before admission	diabetes	with or without antidiabetic drugs	11.873	2.218	63.555
11	Achille Cernigliaro 2020 (25)	172	before admission	diabetes	antidiabetic drugs	1.87	0.89	3.89
12	Michelle A 2020 (30)	775	before admission	T2DM	with or without antidiabetic drugs	1.197	0.731	1.962

Primary Outcomes

Insulin Treatment and COVID-19 Mortality

The results of this meta-analysis of the use of insulin and COVID-19 mortality are shown in **Figure 2**. In general, the use of insulin is associated with increased mortality due to COVID-19 (OR=2.10 95% CI, 1.51-2.93); high heterogeneity was observed (I^2 statistic=71.5%, p<0.001) (**Figure 2**). The results of Egger's (p = 0.2) and Begg's tests (p = 0.193) and inspection of the funnel plots showed that there was no publication bias among the studies (**Figure 3A**). A sensitivity analysis was conducted by omitting one study at a time and showed that the results were stable (**Figure 4A**).

Insulin Treatment and COVID-19 Severe/Critical Complications

The overall analysis included 8 studies that reported quantitative data regarding severe/critical COVID-19 illness. All extracted data were divided according to the severe/critical illness status based on the standard illness severity level (12). The overall risk of severe/critical COVID-19 illness was higher in the insulin treatment group than the control group (OR = 2.56, 95% CI, 1.18–5.55, I^2 = 85.5%, p<0.001) (**Figure 5**). Begg's test (p = 0.902), Egger's test (p = 0.308) and the symmetric distribution funnel plots (**Figure 3B**) indicated that publication bias did not exist. The results of the sensitivity analysis conducted by excluding one study at a time did not change (**Figure 4B**).

Insulin Treatment and In-Hospital Admission for COVID-19

Overall, insulin therapy was not associated with in-hospital admission for COVID-19 (OR=1.23; 95% CI, 0.65-2.33) (**Figure 6A**). Strong heterogeneity existed among the 5 included articles (I^2 statistic=87.6%, p<0.001). Interestingly, the subgroup based on the type of diabetes significantly decreased

TABLE 3 | Description of studies reporting the association between insulin treatment and the severe/critical complications or in-hospital admission of COVID-19.

No.	Study	Sample size	Complications	Period of insulin treatment	Type of diabetes	Control groups	or	ci1	ci2
1	Bo Yu (14)	689	ICU admission	after admission	T2DM	with or without antidiabetic drugs	11.47	3.4	38.66
2	Bo Yu (14)	689	Invasive mechanical ventilation	after admission	T2DM	with or without antidiabetic drugs	6.73	3.39	13.37
3	Yuchen Chen (16)	904	Poor prognosis	before admission	Diabetes	with or without antidiabetic drugs	3.58	1.37	9.35
4	Luis M. Pérez (10)	2666	ICU admission;	after admission	T2DM	antidiabetic drugs	1.32	1.02	1.71
5	Huadong Yan (23)	717	severity	before admission	T2DM	antidiabetic drugs	2.71	1.6	5.5
6	Hussein Nafakhi (26)	67	extensive lung injury	before admission	Diabetes	antidiabetic drugs	0.4	0.3	5
7	Hussein Nafakhi (26)	67	Partial recovery with persistent symptoms	before admission	Diabetes	antidiabetic drugs	0.3	0.2	4
8	Ting Guo (29)	19	ICU admission	before admission	Diabetes	without antidiabetic drugs	115	4.115	3213.5
No.	**Study**	**Sample size**	**Complications**	**Period of insulin treatment**	**Type of diabetes**	**Control groups**	**or**	**ci1**	**ci2**
1	Luis M. Pérez (10)	2666	In-hospital admission	after admission	T2DM	antidiabetic drugs	1.23	0.95	1.6
2	Ayman A (24)	806	In-hospital admission	before admission	T2DM	antidiabetic drugs	1.46	1.03	2.07
3	Achille Cernigliaro (25)	172	In-hospital admission	before admission	Diabetes	antidiabetic drugs	2.13	1.01	4.49
4	Adèle Lasbleiz (27)	2168	In-hospital admission	before admission	Diabetes	antidiabetic drugs	3.8	1.9	8.1
5	Grenye O'Malley (28)	113	In-hospital admission	after admission	T1DM	without antidiabetic drugs	0.137	0.053	0.352

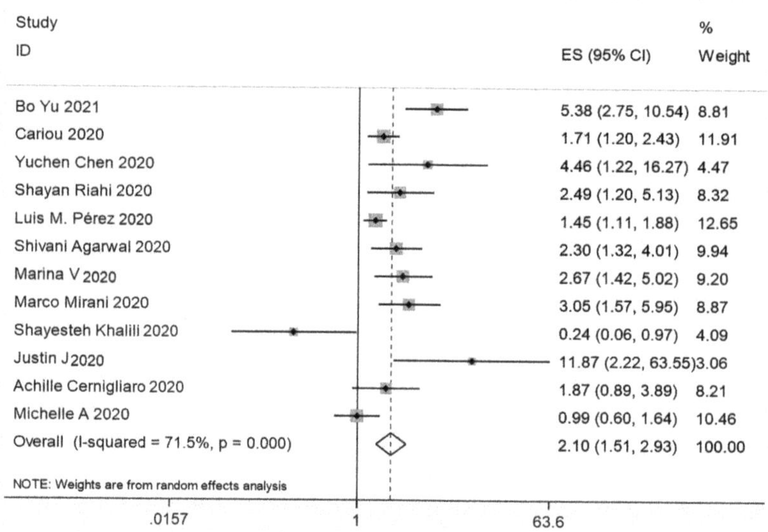

FIGURE 2 | Forest plots of OR for the association between the insulin treatment and the mortality of COVID-19.

the heterogeneity in each subgroup (**Figure 6B**). In the T2DM and Diabetes subgroups (patients with diabetes of which type was not clear in the extracted study), insulin treatment significantly increased in-hospital admission for COVID-19 (T2DM, OR=1.31; 95% CI, 1.06-1.61; Diabetes, OR=2.86; 95% CI, 1.62-5.05), which was the opposite of the results in the T1DM subgroup (OR=0.14; 95% CI, 0.05-0.35). However, due to the limited number of included T1DM studies, the effects of insulin treatment on patients with COVID-19 and T1DM require further solid evidence. According to the results of the funnel analysis (**Figure 3C**), Begg's test (p = 1.000), and Egger's test (p = 0.861), publication bias could be excluded. The sensitivity analysis also indicated the stability of our results (**Figure 4C**).

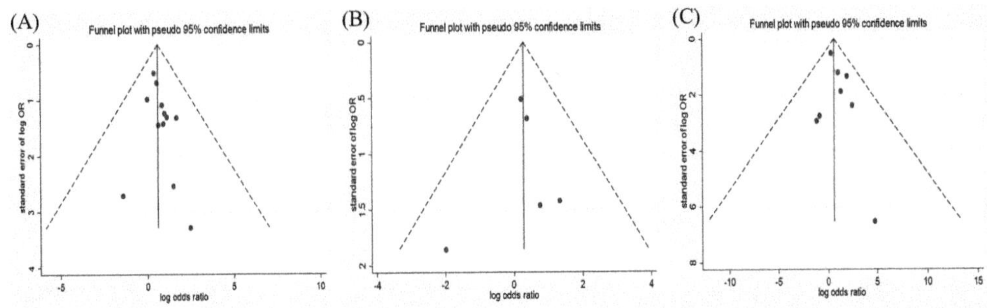

FIGURE 3 | Funnel plot of the association between the insulin treatment and the mortality **(A)**, complications **(B)**, and the in-hospital admission **(C)** of COVID-19.

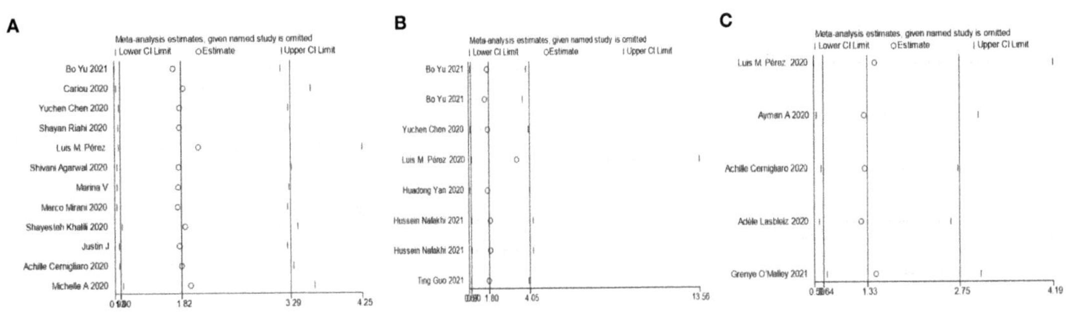

FIGURE 4 | Sensitivity analysis for the effect insulin treatment on the mortality **(A)**, complications **(B)**, and the in-hospital admission **(C)** of COVID-19.

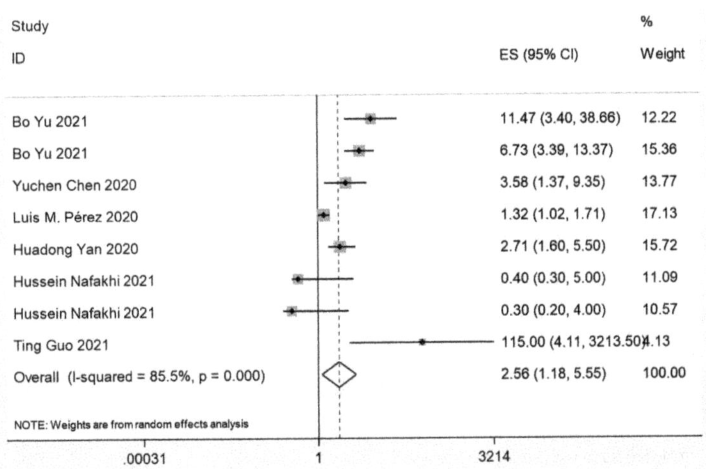

FIGURE 5 | Forest plots of OR for the association between the insulin treatment and the complications of COVID-19.

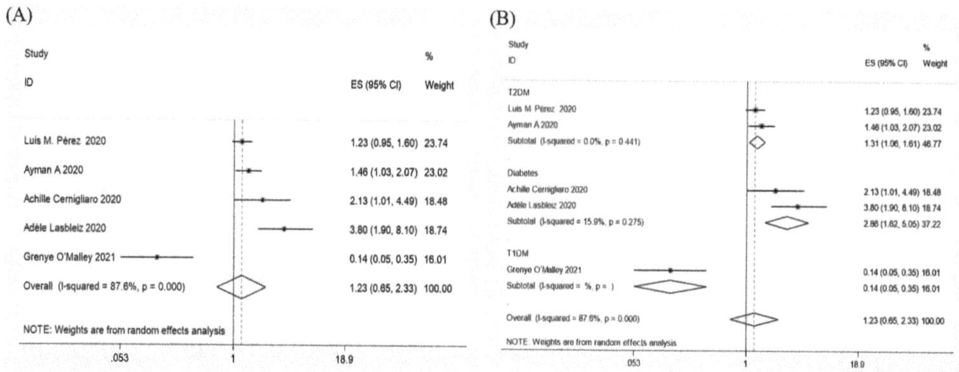

FIGURE 6 | Forest plots of OR for the overall result **(A)** and subgroup analysis based on type of diabetes **(B)** of the association between the insulin treatment and the in-hospital admission of COVID-19.

Insulin Treatment and COVID-19 Hospitalization Time

Only 2 studies mentioned the association between insulin treatment and COVID-19 hospitalization time (SMD=0.21 95% CI, -0.02-0.45). In general, insulin use did not affect the hospitalization time of COVID-19 patients (**Figure 7**). However, additional studies are needed to support this conclusion. Due to the limited number of included studies, further funnel plots or sensitivity analyses were not conducted.

Secondary Outcomes

The overall data showed that insulin treatment led to increased adverse COVID-19 outcomes, including higher mortality, with moderate heterogeneity ($I^2 = 69.2\%$, $p<0.001$) (**Figure 2**). To eliminate heterogeneity, further prespecified subgroup analyses based on the sample size, period of insulin treatment, type of diabetes and type of control group, were conducted (**Tables 2, 3**). However, moderate/high heterogeneity remained in all subgroups (**Figures S1A–D**).

High heterogeneity also existed in the analysis of the effect of insulin treatment on severe/critical complications ($I^2 = 85.5\%$, $p<0.001$) (**Figure 5**). We conducted further subgroup analyses based on the sample size (**Figure S2A**), period of insulin treatment (**Figure S2B**), and type of diabetes (**Figure S2C**), but moderate/high heterogeneity remained in all subgroups. Additionally, in the subgroup analysis based on the type of control group, heterogeneity was also present in the antidiabetic drug group ($I^2 = 74.3\%$ $p=0.002$), while there was decreased heterogeneity in the with and without antidiabetic drug groups ($I^2 = 12.9\%$ $p=0.317$) (**Figure S2D**). Overall, this

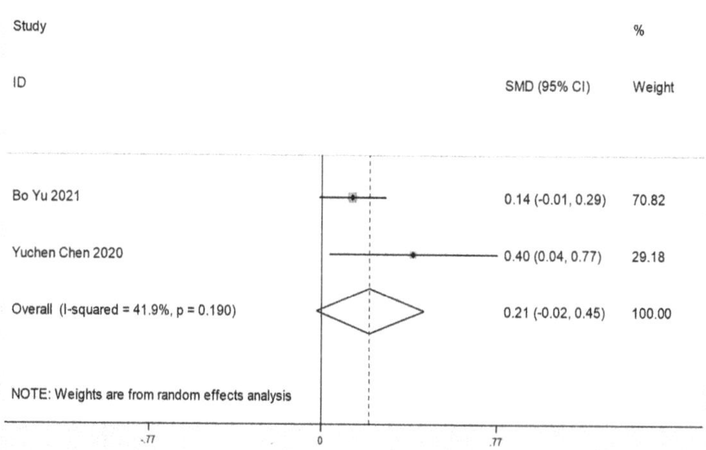

FIGURE 7 | Forest plots of SMD for the association between the insulin treatment and the hospitalization time of COVID-19.

meta-analysis still showed moderate/high heterogeneity after the subgroup analysis, indicating that the included articles failed to provide reliable information for further analysis.

DISCUSSION

Diabetes has been demonstrated to be among the most common comorbidities and is significantly associated with the mortality and severity of COVID-19 (16). Glucose-lowering medications have been proposed as a treatment for COVID-19. In contrast to preconception, insulin treatment has been demonstrated to be related to increased mortality and ICU admission for COVID-19 (14). In the current study, insulin treatment was associated with increased mortality and incidence of severe/critical complications in patients with COVID-19 and diabetes. Our study may provide evidence of the adverse effect of insulin treatment among patients with COVID-19 and diabetes, especially among those with type 2 diabetes (T2DM), as the subjects in most included studies suffered from T2DM. However, considering the limited number of studies concerning type 1 diabetes (T1DM) in our meta-analysis, the association between insulin treatment and adverse outcomes in patients with COVID-19 and T1DM are needed to be investigated in more large-scale clinical studies.

Association Between Insulin Treatment and COVID-19

Our meta-analysis mainly indicates that insulin treatment may be associated with increased mortality (**Figure 2**) and severe/critical complications in T2DM and COVID-19 patients (**Figure 5**). Insulin treatment may also increase in-hospital admission of patients with T2DM and COVID-19 (**Figure 6B**), while there may be no significant relationship between insulin treatment and hospitalization time (**Figure 7**). The patients in the included studies of this meta-analysis had used insulin before catching COVID 19, so the results in our meta-analysis should be interpreted with caution as insulin is usually given to patients in a late stage of diabetes, since it is difficult to rule out the negative effect of advanced diabetes on the poor outcome.

Mechanism Underlying the Relationship Between Insulin Treatment and Worse COVID-19 Outcomes

Although the mechanism underlying the association between insulin use and the poor outcome of COVID-19 remains unclear, there are several possible explanations for these results. First of all, diabetes itself contributed to a low grade of chronic inflammation, which characterized by impaired innate and adaptive inflammation system. This disorder of inflammation would lead to the dysregulation of the immune response with higher level of proinflammatory factors and lower anti-inflammatory cytokines. Insulin treatment was demonstrated to increase macrophage-produced inflammatory cytokine levels in the context of lipopolysaccharide-induced sepsis (31). Additionally, insulin was associated with increased lung inflammation in a sepsis model of diabetic rats (32), while lung cells are the main locations for COVID-19 inflammation. Therefore, we speculate that insulin treatment may participate in the development of COVID-19 by promoting proinflammatory system to aggravate inflammation disorder and pulmonary disease.

Moreover, insulin, an anabolic hormone to improve energy storage, is to increase appetite and weight gain, which contributed to obesity with inhibited lipolysis in adipose and muscle tissues (33, 34). Obesity people is characterized by chronic inflammation and impaired innate immunity with ample production of proinflammatory factors including tumor necrosis factor (TNF-α) and interleukin-6 (IL-6), which also comprised one of risk factors for COVID-19. Consistent with this, obesity and its impaired inflammatory imbalance contributed by insulin treatment may also be one of the mechanisms underlying the relationship between insulin use and COVID-19 outcomes.

Furthermore, hypoglycemia is among the most common adverse effects of insulin treatment, especially in the context of intensive care (35, 36). Insulin treatment increased the incidence of hypoglycemia in patients with COVID-19 and type 2 diabetes mellitus (T2DM) (14), which may impair the glucose homeostasis and glucose control to affect the COVID-19 outcomes. However, there must be other unknown mechanisms underlying the effect of insulin treatment on the outcomes of COVID-19, as the effect still remains in patients without hypoglycemia during hospitalization.

Although the potential mechanisms of the deleterious effect of insulin treatment on COVID-19 progress are discussed above, considering the irreplaceable role of insulin in controlling glucose and diabetes complications, it may be not advisable to give up insulin therapy before finding better or safer hypoglycemic agents for COVID-19 and T2DM patients. Moreover, Critical unwell patients with COVID-19 and diabetes have high insulin requirements and poorer time in optimal target range for blood glucose during peak inflammatory response (37), which indicating the insulin treatment is necessary during the late stage of COVID-19 disease. Additionally, the effects of insulin usage in COVID-19 progression are also affected by the blood glucose level and severity of diabetes (16, 17). Therefore, the results from the current meta-analysis should be interpreted with caution as the complicated situation during different stages of diabetes and insulin effectively in controlling glycemic levels, and more convinced well-designed randomized controlled trials are required to provide more precise conclusions for insulin usage in COVID-19 progression.

Theoretical and Practical Significance

Our study is to summarize the effects of insulin therapy and clinical in outcomes of patients with COVID-19 and diabetes. Additionally, we raised an interesting and significant question regarding the mechanism underlying the relationship between insulin and the development of COVID-19, as there are no reasonable explanations. Therefore, the timing or dose of insulin treatment in patients with COVID-19 and diabetes may be an urgent public problem that must be addressed to control the development of COVID-19.

Limitations of the Study

There are several limitations in our study. First, the high heterogeneity in the results cannot be ignored, and most of the study included was observational study, many biases could not be controlled. Second, the type of diabetes was unclear in several included studies, potentially rendering our conclusion not generalizable to all types of diabetes. Notably, one report focusing on the protective effect of insulin treatment on COVID-19 outcomes involved patients with T1DM and, revealed the opposite conclusion from our results (including mostly T2DM patients), indicating that a different approach to insulin therapy may be needed according to the type of diabetes. Therefore, our study is more likely to be applicable to T2DM patients, while guidance for insulin treatment in COVID-19 patients with different types of diabetes, especially T1DM, needs more clinical research. Third, the causal relationship between insulin treatment and COVID-19 outcomes remains vague due to the limited amount of prospective data in our included studies. Moreover, this systematic review and meta-analysis was not registered in PROSPERO, representing another limitation of our study. Last but not least, the results from this study are only based on observational studies which have many confounders, therefore the evidence generated from this study is not strong enough. More randomized clinical trials are still needed to confirm the results from this study.

Conclusion

In summary, our study revealed that insulin treatment is associated with increased mortality and other severe/critical complications of COVID-19. Our findings could provide clinical guidance for insulin treatment in patients with COVID-19 and diabetes. Further randomized controlled trial was needed to confirm this finding.

AUTHOR CONTRIBUTIONS

Conceptualization, YY. Methodology, ZC, JZ and YY. Software, YY. Validation, JZ, YY and ZC. Formal analysis, YY and ZC. Investigation, YY. Resources, JZ. Data curation, ZC. Writing—original draft preparation, YY. Writing—review and editing, JZ. Visualization, JZ. Supervision, ZC and JZ. Project administration, JZ. Funding acquisition, JZ. All authors contributed to the article and approved the submitted version.

SUPPLEMENTARY MATERIAL

Supplementary Figure 1 | Outcomes of the subgroup analysis of the sample size **(A)**, period of insulin treatment **(B)**, type of diabetes **(C)**, kind of control groups **(D)** of the insulin treatment with mortality in patients with T2DM by forest plots.

Supplementary Figure 2 | Outcomes of the subgroup analysis of the sample size **(A)**, period of insulin treatment **(B)**, type of diabetes **(C)**, kind of control groups **(D)** of the insulin treatment with sever/critical complications in patients with T2DM by forest plots.

Supplementary Figure 3 | Outcomes of the subgroup analysis of the period of insulin treatment **(A)**, kind of control groups **(B)** of the insulin treatment with the in-hospital admission by forest plots.

REFERENCES

1. Bhadade R, Harde M, deSouza R, Kasbe A, Deshpande C, Dave S, et al. Appraisal of Critically Ill COVID-19 Patients at a Dedicated COVID Hospital The Effects of Type 2 Diabetes Mellitus on Organ Metabolism and the Immune System. *J Assoc Phys India* (2020) 68(9):14–9. doi: 10.1016/s2213-8587(20)30271-0
2. Abu-Farha M, Al-Mulla F, Thanaraj TA, Kavalakatt S, Ali H, Abdul Ghani M, et al. Impact of Diabetes in Patients Diagnosed With COVID-19. *Front Immunol* (2020) 11:576818. doi: 10.3389/fimmu.2020.576818
3. Zhu L, She ZG, Cheng X, Qin JJ, Zhang XJ, Cai J, et al. Association of Blood Glucose Control and Outcomes in Patients With COVID-19 and Pre-Existing Type 2 Diabetes. *Cell Metab* (2020) 31(6):1068–77.e1063. doi: 10.1016/j.cmet.2020.04.021
4. Wang S, Ma P, Zhang S, Song S, Wang Z, Ma Y, et al. Fasting Blood Glucose at Admission is an Independent Predictor for 28-Day Mortality in Patients With COVID-19 Without Previous Diagnosis of Diabetes: A Multi-Centre Retrospective Study. *Diabetologia* (2020) 63(10):2102–11. doi: 10.1007/s00125-020-05209-1
5. Lee MH, Wong C, Ng CH, Yuen DCW, Lim AYL, Khoo CM. Effects of Hyperglycaemia on Complications of COVID-19: A Meta-Analysis of Observational Studies. *Diabetes Obes Metab* (2021) 23(1):287–9. doi: 10.1111/dom.14184
6. Alahmad B, Al-Shammari AA, Bennakhi A, Al-Mulla F, Ali H. Fasting Blood Glucose and COVID-19 Severity: Nonlinearity Matters. *Diabetes Care* (2020) 43(12):3113–6. doi: 10.2337/dc20-1941
7. Hariyanto TI, Kurniawan A. Metformin Use Is Associated With Reduced Mortality Rate From Coronavirus Disease 2019 (COVID-19) Infection. *Obes Med* (2020) 19:100290. doi: 10.1016/j.obmed.2020.100290
8. Hariyanto TI, Kurniawan A. Dipeptidyl Peptidase 4 (DPP4) Inhibitor and Outcome From Coronavirus Disease 2019 (COVID-19) in Diabetic Patients: A Systematic Review, Meta-Analysis, and Meta-Regression. *J Diabetes Metab Disord* (2021) 20(1):1–8. doi: 10.1007/s40200-021-00777-4
9. Riahi S, Sombra LRS, Lo KB, Chacko SR, Neto AGM, Azmaiparashvili Z, et al. Insulin Use, Diabetes Control, and Outcomes in Patients With COVID-19. *Endocr Res* (2020) 46(2):1–6. doi: 10.1080/07435800.2020.1856865
10. Pérez-Belmonte LM, Torres-Peña JD, López-Carmona MD, Ayala-Gutiérrez MM, Fuentes-Jiménez F, Huerta LJ, et al. Mortality and Other Adverse Outcomes in Patients With Type 2 Diabetes Mellitus Admitted for COVID-19 in Association With Glucose-Lowering Drugs: A Nationwide Cohort Study. *BMC Med* (2020) 18(1):359. doi: 10.1186/s12916-020-01832-2
11. Moher D, Liberati A, Tetzlaff J, Altman DG. Preferred Reporting Items for Systematic Reviews and Meta-Analyses: The PRISMA Statement. *PLoS Med* (2009) 6(7):e1000097. doi: 10.1371/journal.pmed.1000097
12. Umpierrez G, Rushakoff R, Seley JJ, Zhang JY, Shang T, Han J, et al. Hospital Diabetes Meeting 2020a Territory-Wide Study on the Impact of COVID-19 on Diabetes-Related Acute Care. *J Diabetes Sci Technol* (2020) 14(5):928–44. doi: 10.1136/bcr-2020-23672010.1177/1932296820939626
13. Stang A. Critical Evaluation of the Newcastle-Ottawa Scale for the Assessment of the Quality of Nonrandomized Studies in Meta-Analyses. *Eur J Epidemiol* (2010) 25(9):603–5. doi: 10.1007/s10654-010-9491-z

14. Yu B, Li C, Sun Y, Wang DW. Insulin Treatment Is Associated With Increased Mortality in Patients With COVID-19 and Type 2 Diabetes. *Cell Metab* (2021) 33(1):65–77.e62. doi: 10.1016/j.cmet.2020.11.014
15. Cariou B, Hadjadj S, Wargny M, Pichelin M, Al-Salameh A, Allix I, et al. Phenotypic Characteristics and Prognosis of Inpatients With COVID-19 and Diabetes: The CORONADO Study. *Diabetologia* (2020) 63(8):1500–15. doi: 10.1007/s00125-020-05180-x
16. Chen Y, Yang D, Cheng B, Chen J, Peng A, Yang C, et al. Clinical Characteristics and Outcomes of Patients With Diabetes and COVID-19 in Association With Glucose-Lowering Medication. *Diabetes Care* (2020) 43 (7):1399–407. doi: 10.2337/dc20-0660
17. Sardu C, D'Onofrio N, Balestrieri ML, Barbieri M, Rizzo MR, Messina V, et al. Outcomes in Patients With Hyperglycemia Affected by COVID-19: Can We Do More on Glycemic Control? *Diabetes Care* (2020) 43(7):1408–15. doi: 10.2337/dc20-0723
18. Agarwal S, Schechter C, Southern W, Crandall JP, Tomer Y. Preadmission Diabetes-Specific Risk Factors for Mortality in Hospitalized Patients With Diabetes and Coronavirus Disease 2019. *Diabetes Care* (2020) 43(10):2339–44. doi: 10.2337/dc20-1543
19. Shestakova MV, Vikulova OK, Isakov M, Dedov II. [Diabetes and COVID-19: Analysis of the Clinical Outcomes According to the Data of the Russian Diabetes Registry]. *Problemy Endokrinol* (2020) 66(1):35–46. doi: 10.14341/probl12458
20. Mirani M, Favacchio G, Carrone F, Betella N, Biamonte E, Morenghi E, et al. Impact of Comorbidities and Glycemia at Admission and Dipeptidyl Peptidase 4 Inhibitors in Patients With Type 2 Diabetes With COVID-19: A Case Series From an Academic Hospital in Lombardy, Italy. *Diabetes Care* (2020) 43(12):3042–9. doi: 10.2337/dc20-1340
21. Khalili S, Moradi O, Kharazmi AB, Raoufi M, Sistanizad M, Shariat M. Comparison of Mortality Rate and Severity of Pulmonary Involvement in Coronavirus Disease-2019 Adults Patients With and Without Type 2 Diabetes: A Cohort Study. *Can J Diabetes* (2020) S1499-2671(20):30426-3. doi: 10.1016/j.jcjd.2020.10.014
22. Turcotte JJ, Meisenberg BR, MacDonald JH, Menon N, Fowler MB, West M, et al. Risk Factors for Severe Illness in Hospitalized Covid-19 Patients at a Regional Hospital. *PLoS One* (2020) 15(8):e0237558. doi: 10.1371/journal.pone.0237558
23. Yan H, Valdes AM, Vijay A, Wang S, Liang L, Yang S, et al. Role of Drugs Used for Chronic Disease Management on Susceptibility and Severity of COVID-19: A Large Case-Control Study. *Clin Pharmacol Ther* (2020) 108 (6):1185–94. doi: 10.1002/cpt.2047
24. Al Hayek AA, Robert AA, Matar AB, Algarni A, Alkubedan H, Alharbi T, et al. Risk Factors for Hospital Admission Among COVID-19 Patients With Diabetes. *A Study Saudi Arabia Saudi Med J* (2020) 41(10):1090–7. doi: 10.15537/smj.2020.10.25419
25. Cernigliaro A, Allotta AV, Scondotto S. [Can Diabetes and its Related Hypoglycemic Drug Treatment be Considered Risk Factors for Health Outcomes in COVID-19 Patients? The Results of a Study in the Population Residing in Sicily Region (Southern Italy)]. *Epidemiol e Prevenzione* (2020) 44 (5-6 Suppl 2):315–22. doi: 10.19191/ep20.5-6.S2.132
26. Nafakhi H, Alareedh M, Al-Buthabhak K, Shaghee F, Nafakhi A, Kasim S. Predictors of Adverse in-Hospital Outcome and Recovery in Patients With Diabetes Mellitus and COVID-19 Pneumonia in Iraq. *Diabetes Metab Syndr* (2021) 15(1):33–8. doi: 10.1016/j.dsx.2020.12.014
27. Lasbleiz A, Cariou B, Darmon P, Soghomonian A, Ancel P, Boullu S, et al. Phenotypic Characteristics and Development of a Hospitalization Prediction Risk Score for Outpatients With Diabetes and COVID-19: The DIABCOVID Study. *J Clin Med* (2020) 9(11):3726. doi: 10.3390/jcm9113726
28. O'Malley G, Ebekozien O, Desimone M, Pinnaro CT, Roberts A, Polsky S, et al. COVID-19 Hospitalization in Adults With Type 1 Diabetes: Results From the T1D Exchange Multicenter Surveillance Study. *J Clin Endocrinol Metab* (2021) 106(2):e936–42. doi: 10.1210/clinem/dgaa825
29. Guo T, Shen Q, Ouyang X, Guo W, Li J, He W, et al. Clinical Findings in Diabetes Mellitus Patients With COVID-19. *J Diabetes Res* (2021) 2021:7830136. doi: 10.1155/2021/7830136
30. Lally MA, Tsoukas P, Halladay CW, O'Neill E, Gravenstein S, Rudolph JL. Metformin is Associated With Decreased 30-Day Mortality Among Nursing Home Residents Infected With SARS-Cov2. *J Am Med Directors Assoc* (2021) 22(1):193–8. doi: 10.1016/j.jamda.2020.10.031
31. Brundage SI, Kirilcuk NN, Lam JC, Spain DA, Zautke NA. Insulin Increases the Release of Proinflammatory Mediators. *J Trauma* (2008) 65(2):367–72. doi: 10.1097/TA.0b013e3181801cc0
32. Filgueiras LR, Capelozzi VL, Martins JO, Jancar S. Sepsis-Induced Lung Inflammation is Modulated by Insulin. *BMC Pulm Med* (2014) 14:177. doi: 10.1186/1471-2466-14-177
33. Jacob S, Hauer B, Becker R, Artzner S, Grauer P, Löblein K, et al. Lipolysis in Skeletal Muscle is Rapidly Regulated by Low Physiological Doses of Insulin. *Diabetologia* (1999) 42(10):1171–4. doi: 10.1007/s001250051288
34. Kolb H, Kempf K, Röhling M, Martin S. Insulin: Too Much of a Good Thing Is Bad. *BMC Med* (2020) 18(1):224. doi: 10.1186/s12916-020-01688-6
35. Gerstein HC, Miller ME, Byington RP, Goff DCJr., Bigger JT, Buse JB, et al. Effects of Intensive Glucose Lowering in Type 2 Diabetes. *N Engl J Med* (2008) 358(24):2545–59. doi: 10.1056/NEJMoa0802743
36. Hypoglycemia in the Diabetes Control and Complications TrialThe Diabetes Control and Complications Trial Research Group. *Diabetes* (1997) 46(2):271–86. doi: 10.2337/diabetes.46.2.271
37. Wu L, Girgis CM, Cheung NW. COVID-19 and Diabetes: Insulin Requirements Parallel Illness Severity in Critically Unwell Patients. *Clin Endocrinol (Oxf)* (2020) 93(4):390–3. doi: 10.1111/cen.14288

23

Diabetes and COVID-19: A Bidirectional Interplay

*Paraskevi Kazakou [1], Vaia Lambadiari[2], Ignatios Ikonomidis[3], Aikaterini Kountouri[2], Georgios Panagopoulos [1], Stavros Athanasopoulos [1], Eleni Korompoki[4], Ioannis Kalomenidis[5], Meletios A. Dimopoulos[6] and Asimina Mitrakou [1]**

[1] Diabetes Centre, Department of Clinical Therapeutics, Alexandra Hospital, School of Medicine, National and Kapodistrian University of Athens, Athens, Greece, [2] Second Department of Internal Medicine, Attikon University Hospital, National and Kapodistrian University of Athens, Medical School, Athens, Greece, [3] Laboratory of Preventive Cardiology, Second Cardiology Department, Attikon University Hospital National and Kapodistrian University of Athens, Medical School, Athens, Greece, [4] Department of Clinical Therapeutics, Alexandra Hospital, School of Medicine, National and Kapodistrian University of Athens, Athens, Greece, [5] 1st Department of Intensive Care, Evangelismos Hospital, National and Kapodistrian University of Athens, Medical School, Athens, Greece, [6] Unit of Hematology and Oncology, Department of Clinical Therapeutics, Alexandra Hospital, School of Medicine, National and Kapodistrian University of Athens, Athens, Greece

***Correspondence:**
Asimina Mitrakou
minamitrakou@gmail.com

There seems to be a bidirectional interplay between Diabetes mellitus (DM) and coronavirus disease 2019 (COVID-19). On the one hand, people with diabetes are at higher risk of fatal or critical care unit-treated COVID-19 as well as COVID-19 related health complications compared to individuals without diabetes. On the other hand, clinical data so far suggest that the severe acute respiratory syndrome coronavirus 2 (SARS-CoV-2) may result in metabolic dysregulation and in impaired glucose homeostasis. In addition, emerging data on new onset DM in previously infected with SARS-CoV-2 patients, reinforce the hypothesis of a direct effect of SARS-CoV-2 on glucose metabolism. Attempting to find the culprit, we currently know that the pancreas and the endothelium have been found to express Angiotensin-converting enzyme 2 (ACE2) receptors, the main binding site of the virus. To move from bench to bedside, understanding the effects of COVID-19 on metabolism and glucose homeostasis is crucial to prevent and manage complications related to COVID-19 and support recovering patients. In this article we review the potential underlying pathophysiological mechanisms between COVID-19 and glucose dysregulation as well as the effects of antidiabetic treatment in patients with diabetes and COVID-19.

Keywords: diabetes, COVID-19, endothelial (dys)function, new onset diabetes, antidiabetic medication

INTRODUCTION

Since the outbreak of COVID-19 pandemic, diabetes has been in the epicenter of identified risk factors. Epidemiological data have indicated that older adults with co-morbidities are at highest risk to develop severe COVID-19 and subsequent complications including death. Such comorbidities include DM, obesity, respiratory and cardiovascular disease - including hypertension and coronary artery disease (1–3). Based on early clinical data on 122.653 COVID-19 cases reported by the United States Centre for Disease Control and Prevention (CDC) one third of infected patients had at least one of the above conditions. Furthermore, individuals with an underlying condition account for

78% of intensive care unit (ICU) admissions and 94% of deaths. Among the comorbidities, DM was the most frequently reported (10,9% of cases) condition (4). In a recent summary report by the Chinese CDC of 72314 cases, people with DM had the second highest fatality rate (7,3%) after cardiovascular disease (10,5%) compared to a rate of 2,3% in the general population (5). Further studies from China, Europe and the USA have also shown that when people with DM get COVID-19 they are at higher risk to develop COVID-19 related complications, to require ICU admission or to die from the disease (6–8). Supporting these findings, a large UK cohort study facilitating a health analytics platform, confirmed the role of uncontrolled diabetes as a risk factor (adjusted HR 1.95) (9)

In a recent publication, we reported the early and late endocrine complications of COVID-19 (10). SARS-CoV-2 infection affects several pathophysiological pathways, during the disease course, eventually leading to late complications. From that review, it was already clear that more data are about to emerge which would unravel the pathophysiology that partners these two conditions and would evince the most effective among the available anti-diabetic arsenal.

And even though the underlying elaborate pathophysiological mechanisms between COVID-19 and diabetes are still under investigation, the fact that there is a bidirectional interplay involving stress-induced pathways commonly shared by COVID-19 and diabetes is more than clear.

Our aim is to report the rapidly accumulating evidence that sheds light not only into the causal relationship of diabetes and COVID-19 severity and vice versa, but also to the best available anti-diabetic treatments easing recovery from COVID-19 severity, details not previously reported in our own or similar reviews. To that end, we will present a narrative review of the most cited publications on COVID-19 and diabetes, putting the spot on endothelium and β-cell function and their potential to be the common ground in these two devastating diseases.

HOW DOES DM WORSEN COVID-19 CLINICAL OUTCOMES?

Epidemiological studies have rendered COVID-19 severity attributable to several diabetes complications or comorbidities as risk factors. Coexisting microvascular and macrovascular complications of DM such as cardiovascular disease, heart failure, retinopathy and reduced renal function may be responsible for the increased poor COVID-19 outcomes and mortality following infection (11–13). Obesity, a prevalent diabetes comorbidity, affects the immune system by means of adipose tissue. Adipose tissue, all along with the liver and the stressed β-cells, induce synthesis of pro-inflammatory cytokines and adhesion molecules and activate many metabolic and hemodynamic pathways, growth factors, as well as intracellular signals that mediate generalized vasculopathy and systemic inflammation (14). Obesity highly correlates with T cell immune signatures that are unique for severe COVID-19, highlighting a potential contributing mechanism (15). However, if one tries to search for mechanisms attributable to diabetes per se, endothelium and chronic inflammation are the two main conceptual approaches, as we describe next.

Endothelium is considered a major player in multiple physiological processes, supporting homeostasis of healthy individuals. Particularly, it regulates the tone of vascular smooth muscle by the release of vasodilators and vasoconstrictors, controls vascular permeability and is an important mediator of inflammation and coagulation by regulating the adhesion of leucocytes and platelets (16–18). Endothelial glycocalyx is an endothelial surface layer which consists of proteoglycans and glycoproteins and prevents the direct contact of blood cells with the endothelial surface (19). DM is associated with chronic endothelial dysfunction and endothelial glycocalyx damage which increase leucocyte and circulating inflammatory cells adhesion and promote vascular permeability and coagulation (20–23). Hyperglycemia and insulin resistance have been suggested as possible mechanisms which lead to the impairment of the endothelial micromilieu in patients with DM. Acute and long-term hyperglycemia affects sorbitol, protein kinase C, and pentose phosphate pathways and this leads to increased oxidative stress and promotes endothelial cells apoptosis contributing to endothelial dysfunction. The decreased availability of NO is another mechanism through which hyperglycemia leads to endothelial dysfunction (24). Adequate glycaemic control has been associated with improved endothelial function. Our group recently reported a study in one hundred patients with type 2 DM (T2DM). We have shown that 12-months of intensified antidiabetic treatment improves arterial stiffness, endothelial glycocalyx and markers of oxidative stress. We found that high values of hemoglobin A1c (HbA1c) are positively corelated with the perfused boundary region (PBR), a marker of glycocalyx thickness. This finding indicates that hyperglycemia may lead to the impairment of glycocalyx integrity (25). Regarding the contribution of insulin resistance in endothelial dysfunction, a case-control study showed that Matsuda Index and insulin sensitivity index (ISI) are correlated with PBR. This implies that insulin resistance induces glycocalyx damage in first-degree relatives of diabetic patients (26). Chronic endothelial dysfunction predisposes to severe COVID-19 infection by inducing alterations to the glycocalyx and endothelial cells. This leads to increases in leucocyte adhesion and promotes a procoagulant and antifibrinolytic state. DM induced chronic endothelial dysfunction in combination with the direct damage of endothelial cells by SARS-CoV-2 results in endothelial and microcirculation impairment which in turn contribute to the pathogenesis of acute respiratory syndrome and multi-organ failure.

Diabetes, even at the stages of prediabetes, is characterized by a chronic inflammatory and prothrombotic state with multiple metabolic, vascular, immune, and hematological abnormalities which may affect adversely the response to infections (27–29). The glucotoxicity of diabetes coincides with impaired immunity; inhibition of lymphocyte proliferation, reduced natural killer cell activity, monocyte/macrophage and neutrophil dysfunction (28, 30, 31). In addition to the chronic endothelial effects of diabetes and the resulting susceptibility to severe COVID-19, hyperglycemia on admission and during hospitalization results in worse prognosis, severity, and mortality of COVID-19, irrespectively of prior diabetes status. Retrospective studies from China have demonstrated that elevated glucose levels on admission were an independent risk factor of progression to critical cases and in-hospital mortality (32, 33). Similarly, an observational study of more than 1,000 inpatients with COVID-19 at US hospitals showed that 40% of the subjects had diabetes or uncontrolled hyperglycemia on admission and inpatient mortality was fourfold greater for patients with DM. Another noteworthy finding of the same study was that mortality was sevenfold higher for those without pre-existing DM who developed hyperglycemia in hospital (34). A recent meta-analysis of 14502 patients confirmed these findings further and proved a nonlinear relationship between admission fasting blood glucose and severity: each increase in glucose level by one mmol/L, increased the risk of severity by 33% (35). Similar retrospective studies of hospitalized COVID-19 patients from China revealed that disease severity was correlated with active inflammatory markers as IL-6 and lactate dehydrogenase and that patients with DM had greater inflammatory response with higher IL-6, CRP, ESR and relative neutrophilia with lymphopenia as well as higher incidence of coagulopathy with higher D-dimer levels and longer prothrombin times (36, 37). Apart from the increased inflammatory response, DM induced hyperglycemia and increased glycolysis, promoted SARS-CoV-2 replication and increased the viral load. This increased viral replication is achieved through a mitochondrial ROS/hypoxia-inducible factor-1a dependent pathway, resulting in T cell dysfunction and epithelial cell death (38). Interestingly enough, in one retrospective study, hyperglycemia halted the beneficial effects of Tocilizumab which targets interleukin-6 receptor and reduces cytokine storm (39).

Such evidence coincides with earlier coronavirus outbreaks, where it was likely to see higher rates of hyperglycemia on admission, irrespective of pre-existing glycaemic status, disease severity or glucocorticoid use (40, 41). In a Chinese study, SARS-CoV, was shown to bind to ACE2 in pancreatic islet cells, damage them and cause acute hyperglycemia, even among people without DM. Approximately 50% of SARS patients without diabetes or steroid treatment developed DM during hospitalization, and after 3 years, 5% of the patients still had DM. These findings generated the hypothesis of chronic β-cell damage, as we present later on this review (41).

HOW DOES COVID-19 WORSEN ENDOTHELIAL FUNCTION AND GLUCOSE HOMEOSTASIS

SARS-CoV-2 can have an acute effect on the endothelium which as we have presented is already affected by diabetes as a chronic disease. SARS-CoV-2 affects the vascular system directly by targeting endothelial cells leading to severe endothelial derangement and inflammation. ACE2 receptors which are the main targets of SARS-CoV-2 are expressed in various human tissues including the endothelium, allowing the direct invasion of endothelial cells (42–44). In addition, the overproduction of pro-inflammatory cytokines during COVID-19 promotes endothelial dysfunction (45). Indeed, Chen et al., showed that patients with severe COVID-19 disease displayed increased levels of pro-inflammatory cytokines including soluble interleukin-2 receptor (IL-2R), interleukin-6 (IL-6), and tumor necrosis factor-α (TNF-a) (46). IL-6 promotes endothelial derangement and contribute to procoagulability (47, 48). Furthermore, inflammatory-mediated damage of glycocalyx by IL-6, or TNF-α increases vascular permeability inducing interstitial fluid shift and generalized oedema (49). Our group recently showed that SARS-CoV-2 may cause endothelial and vascular dysfunction linked to impaired cardiac performance four months following infection (50). To further support the role of pro-inflammatory cytokines in COVID-19 pathophysiology, another recent study showed that the inhibition of IL-6 by tocilizumab reverses lymphopenia in critically ill ventilated COVID-19 patients (51). Similarly, a randomized clinical trial, including 389 hospitalized patients with COVID-19 pneumonia, showed that treatment with tocilizumab reduces the risk for adverse clinical outcomes including mechanical ventilation or death (52). The infected endothelial cells release increased levels of proinflammatory cytokines which induce immune-mediated damage of lungs and other organs. This results in acute respiratory distress syndrome (ARDS) and multi-organ failure (53). Histological studies showed that endothelial cells damage by SARS-CoV-2 results in vasculitis and endothelitis in multiple organs (54–56). Post-mortem histological evidence of three patients were the first reports to highlight the role of endothelium in the pathogenesis of COVID-19 disease and provided evidence of endothelitis during infection. This suggests that the clinical presentation of COVID-19 might be worse in vulnerable patients with pre-existing endothelial dysfunction (54). Copin et al. showed that endothelial derangement induces vascular damage of small to medium-sized pulmonary arteries contributing to lung injury in severe COVID-19 (56).

On regards to glucose homeostasis, as we previously reported, severe COVID -19 with the accompanying cytokine storm and dysregulated counterbalancing hormonal responses, potentially contributes to insulin resistance and hyperglycemia (10, 57, 58). Similarly, viral respiratory infections have the potential to provoke a raised-interferon-γ-mediated insulin resistance in skeletal muscles (59). Experience from Severe Acute Respiratory Syndrome (SARS) and Middle East Respiratory Syndrome (MERS) suggests that inflammatory cells can affect the liver, impairing insulin-mediated glucose uptake, with hyperinsulinemia and hyperglycemia as a result (60, 61). Thus, in COVID-19 the viral inflammatory and immune responses can impair insulin sensitivity and dysregulate glucose metabolism, leading to a vicious cycle of hyperglycemia and inflammatory response that destroys tissue integrity and physiological function during the critical stages of infection. Of notable mention, drugs often used in the treatment of COVID-19, such as corticosteroids or antiviral agents, can aggravate hyperglycemia and result in lipodystrophy and insulin resistance (62, 63).

Acting together, glucotoxicity with its consequences in conjunction with the inflammatory cytokine storm of COVID-19 infection, and along with the increased oxidative stress, the immune dysfunction and the endothelial damage result in further metabolic complications, as increased risk of thromboembolism and multiorgan damage in individuals with DM (64–66).

SARS-CoV-2 INFECTION AND NEW-ONSET DM

As it has already been mentioned, based on existing data, COVID-19 affects glucose homeostasis even in the absence of DM in one's past medical history (10). Recent findings have suggested a direct effect of SARS-CoV-2 on glucose metabolism as new presentations of DM with diabetic ketoacidosis (DKA), hyperosmolarity and unusually high requirements of insulin to achieve glycaemic control have been reported (67–72). Based on our established experience on critical conditions, this amplified insulin resistance is unprecedented. Additionally, a COVID -19 infection has been found to precipitate acute hyperglycemic crises and to worsen prognosis for poorly controlled patients with DM (73). Therefore, in order to reduce the risk of metabolic complications, severe outcomes, and mortality during a Covid infection, it is crucial to achieve glycaemic control (67, 74).

A direct link on how SARS-CoV-2 might cause or worsen DM has not yet been established. Reports from Germany and Italy, including data from nationwide pediatric diabetes centers, have described higher frequency of DKA and severe DKA in children and youth with new-onset Type 1 DM (T1DM) during the pandemic, while the incidence of new-onset T1DM did not change (75–77). Higher frequency of DKA diagnosis might be attributed to postponed hospital visits and diagnosis of T1DM due to the overall overload in public healthcare services. Fear of contracting COVID-19 resulted in reduced visits to public health services and hindered access to routine clinical care (78). On the other hand, the postulation that COVID-19 could precipitate or accelerate the onset of T1DM is a fascinating-yet-plausible hypothesis. In favor of this notion, a Northwest London Study, described an 80% increase of new T1DM cases for children infected or exposed to SARS-CoV-2 among those that were assessed (79). Another case report presented a 19-year-old German male who was hospitalized with DKA and insulin-dependent diabetes in the absence of typical T1DM autoantibodies 5 to 7 weeks after asymptomatic SARS-CoV-2 infection (80). A plausible explanation is that SARS-CoV-2 infection might have damaged β-cells in the pancreas through direct cytolytic effect of the virus. Additionally, autoantibody negativity -although not rare- coexisting with a rare genetic variant, has raised suspicions favoring a new type of insulin-dependent diabetes. Caution is needed though, as the hyperglycemic state might be a pre-existing condition that had not yet been diagnosed, as it is implied by the HbA1c (16,8%) upon diagnosis. Two other reports however, demonstrated DKA with high HbA1c irrespective of the duration of DM (80, 81). As we previously reported briefly, the magnified psychological stress during the extended lockdowns, could in turn be an exacerbating factor in genetically susceptible individuals, and it is a factor not to be neglected (10). Currently, a global registry of COVID-19-related diabetes has been launched to shed light into the extent and characteristics of such new cases.

SARS-CoV-2 INTERACTION WITH THE PANCREAS: THE ROLE OF ACE2

There seem to exist some possible underlying mechanisms which could explain the acute damage of the pancreatic islets by SARS-CoV-2 and the subsequent loss of insulin secretory capacity. An immune response *via* the release of chemokines and cytokines mediated by the virus, might also kill pancreatic cells and impair their ability to sense glucose and release insulin. Furthermore, the immune response of the virus may further impair the ability of the liver and muscles to identify alterations (67, 82).

Whether ACE2 is the main culprit for β-cell dysfunction has been a matter of scientific debate. A recent functional study has revealed that ACE2 is the main binding receptor for the SARS-CoV-2 spike glycoprotein, easing host cell entry (83). This receptor apart from the respiratory system is also expressed in key metabolic organs and tissues, including pancreatic β-cells, adipose tissue, the small intestine, and the kidneys (42). SARS-CoV-2 enters host cells after binding to ACE2 receptor, and both SARS-CoV-2 and ACE2 are internalized by endocytosis, so that surface ACE2 is then downregulated (84). This SARS-CoV-2 induced ACE2 under-expression and inflammatory injury seem to be extended in all cells with ACE2 activity, including pancreatic islets (85, 86). Elevated pancreatic enzymes that have been reported in COVID-19 are indicative of such damage (87–89). A study on organoids confirmed that the β-cell ACE2 expression results in SARS-CoV-2 tolerance which in turn leads to cytokine inflammation, β-cell apoptosis and eventually reduced insulin secretion (90). Another study that used human islet cell cultures and post-mortem examinations from SARS-CoV-2 infected individuals, confirmed the viral presence and replication in the islets, as well as a reduction of insulin-secretory granules and the impaired glucose dependent insulin secretion (91). Two more recent studies in autopsy samples showed a binary effect on β-cells, leading to either the death of β-cells or transdifferentiation of the surviving ones (92, 93). Preclinical studies also support the role of ACE2 in β-cell homeostasis; in high fat diet mice β-cell de-differentiation is characterized by reduction of ACE2; deletion of ACE2 in diabetic mice induces hyperglycemia, β-cell oxidative stress and decrease of insulin secretion (94, 95). Finally, ACE2 deletion in obese mice impairs β-cell proliferation, decreases β-cell mass and results in β-cell dysfunction (96, 97).

However, this might not describe the whole picture, as new evidence accumulates. What has already been established is the role of ACE2 and TMPRSS2 (transmembrane serine proteases 2) for the entry of SARS-Cov-2 in epithelial cells. Evidence from immunohistochemistry surveys suggests that they are expressed in microvasculature and ducts and only rarely -and at low levels- they are found in islet cells. (98, 99). Other investigators report an *in vitro* study where a preferential expression of ACE2 in β-cells, together with ACE2 upregulation, is observed during inflammation (100). Additional factors, namely HMBG1 (High-mobility group box 1) and NRP1 (neuropilin1), are crucial for SARS-CoV-2 infection and have been found to be also expressed in β-cells. HMGB1, a chromatin regulator, is critical in ACE2 expression, and is minimally expressed in COVID-19 patient's islets compared to controls (101, 102). NRP1, which binds furin-cleaved substrates and potentiates SARS-CoV-2 infectivity has been detected in islets (101, 103). Since an intact microvasculature is a prerequisite for full islet functionality, the vascular damage facilitated by ACE2, seems to be the main culprit in β-cell dysfunction, potentially reinforced by additional factors.

If ACE2 is not the main receptor for SARS-CoV-2 to affect islets, and several others emerge among studies, a series of other underlying mechanisms render ACE2 crucial factor to understand the impairment of β-cell function. Acute hyperglycemia provokes ACE2 expression on cells and increases urinary ACE2 activity which may lead to an increase of viral load. Urinary ACE2 activity and protein levels are elevated in patients with T1DM as well as T2DM and urinary ACE2/Creatinine is positively correlated with fasting blood glucose and HbA1c (104, 105). Furthermore, chronic hyperglycemia in diabetes counteracts ACE2 expression perpetuating the inflammation and the severity of the infection (106). In patients with DM, SARS-CoV-2 through reducing ACE2 expression results in decreased degradation of angiotensin II and increased secretion of aldosterone and renal potassium loss (107). Hypokalemia can further blunt insulin secretion (63). Of special mention, dipeptyl peptidase 4 (DPP4), important in glucose homeostasis, is another functional coronavirus receptor, interacting with MERS-CoV (108–110). Although ACE2 is recognized as the main receptor, DPP4 could also bind to SARS-CoV-2, as suggested by viral modelling, but this is yet to be confirmed experimentally (111, 112).

HOW MAY ANTIDIABETIC TREATMENT INFLUENCE SARS-CoV-2 INFECTION IN PEOPLE WITH DM

Given all the valuable information from existing research it becomes apparent that glycaemic control can be crucial as a preventive measure of adverse COVID-19 related outcomes. However, when looking for the optimal therapeutic modalities both benefits and risks of glucose lowering agents should be taken into account.

Sodium-glucose cotransporter-2 inhibitors (SGLT2is) are used to treat T2DM by promoting urinary excretion of glucose and inducing osmotic diuresis. They are well tolerated and highly cardioprotective in the context of cardiac failure, and they also exhibit anti-inflammatory properties (113). Nevertheless, despite this being rare, patients with DM using SGLT2is are at increased risk for dehydration and euglycemic DKA (euDKA), during acute illness, especially in a setting of anorexia and vomiting (114, 115). The risk for euDKA seems even more enhanced during COVID-19. A case series of euDKA in patients with T2DM and COVID-19 while on SGLT2is has been reported recently (116). Specific precipitating factors for euDKA with the use of SGLT2is during COVID-19, apart from volume depletion due to vomiting and anorexia, may include a direct cytolytic effect of the virus on β-cells with consequent decreased endogenous insulin secretion and an increased inflammatory response with elevated IL-6 levels (117). Nonetheless, a hypothetical neutralizing effect of SGLT2is on COVID-19 infection has been suggested. This can occur by two distinct mechanisms. Firstly, SGLT2is might reduce viral load by increasing lactate concentrations and by decreasing intracellular pH. Secondly, they have known anti-inflammatory effects, especially on endothelial function (64). It is therefore hypothesized that SGLT2is could play a protective role in organ failure during COVID-19. However, in a recent double-blind placebo-controlled trial (DARE-19) of dapagliflozin in patients hospitalized with COVID-19 and having one or more cardiometabolic risk factors, the SGLT-2 did not confer a significant reduction in organ dysfunction or death, nor improved clinical recovery, regardless of its safety profile (118).

Thiazolidinediones are agonists of the peroxisome proliferator- activated receptor- γ (PPARγ), a nuclear receptor that regulates the transcription of various genes involved in glucose and lipid metabolism (119). They have been shown to improve insulin resistance and to possess anti-inflammatory and anti-atherosclerotic effects (120). However, they are not suitable for critically ill patients because they have been associated with fluid retention, oedema, and heart failure aggravation (121).

DPP4 inhibitors (DPP4is) are widely used in the treatment of T2DM as they have a negligible risk of hypoglycemia and are well tolerated. DPP4 is a transmembrane glycoprotein which is known to have a vital role in glucose homeostasis. It is expressed in the spleen, lung, liver, kidney, and immune cells. Furthermore, it can also be found in the circulation as soluble DPP4 (122). It is suggested that DPP4is could be of therapeutic benefit in mild or even in severe COVID-19 (123). The role of DPP-4 inhibition as a mitigator of inflammation and a potent anti-fibrotic agent, is supported by various experimental studies (122, 124). It is compelling to presume that such medication could reduce pro-inflammatory cytokine production during COVID-19. It has been shown after all that in ARDS they managed to reduce histological lung injury (125). DPP4 is also a known coreceptor for the MERS spike protein, and mice with higher DPP4 expression had more severe disease (109, 111). In addition, plasma levels of DPP4 in patients with MERS- CoV were significantly reduced, suggesting a protective role of DPP4 (126). Nevertheless, it is not known if SARS-CoV-2 uses DPP4 for cell entry and therefore it is unclear whether DPP4is interfere with this binding, and whether they reduce virulence (112). An interaction between DPP4 and SARS-CoV-2 spike protein has been shown, suggesting that DPP4 receptor binding domain could be a potential key for treating infection by SARS- CoV-2 (111, 127). In an *in vitro* study, treatment with DPP4is did not stop the entry of coronavirus into cells (109). In a retrospective case–control study from Italy, sitagliptin use during hospitalization was associated with reduced mortality and improved clinical outcomes in patients with T2DM and COVID-19 (128). Furthermore, another Italian case series found a significantly reduced mortality in eleven patients with DPP4is treatment while in another study DPP4i treatment was associated with worse outcomes in twenty-seven patients with T2DM compared to forty-nine treated with other glucose-lowering medications (129, 130). More detailed clinical trials are needed to fully evaluate the role of DPP4is in patients with T2DM and COVID-19.

Glucagon-like peptide-1 receptor agonists (GLP-1 RA) have been shown to reduce major cardiac events in patients with T2DM in clinical trials. They have also been found to exert anti-inflammatory actions in low-grade inflammation conditions such as atherosclerosis and non-alcoholic fatty liver disease (131, 132). In addition, they contribute to weight reduction in obesity, another state of chronic inflammation and compromised immune response (133). Of note, experimental studies have shown that they can reduce cytokine production and mediate pulmonary inflammation in mice (55). It could thus be hypothesized that they might be beneficial in COVID-19 infection since it is a state of hyperinflammation with worse outcomes in people with atherosclerosis, obesity or T2DM. Short-term studies of patients in the ICU have shown that such medication is safe and effective for blood glucose management (134). However, data is not sufficient to recommend these agents in critically ill patients with T2DM and COVID-19. There is always the risk of gastrointestinal side effects, such as nausea and vomiting and the risk of aspiration in such patients (106).

Metformin has already been found to have anti-inflammatory properties and to reduce inflammatory biomarkers, such as Il-6 and TNF-a in people with T2DM, as well as in an ARDS model (135–137). Since exacerbated inflammation due to cytokine storm has been recognized as a major key of bad prognosis in COVID-19, it could be hypothesized that metformin might have a beneficial role. Still though, the immunomodulatory actions of metformin in the context of COVID-19 remain unclear. Evidence for other possible positive implications of metformin in COVID-19 such as reduction in insulin resistance and inhibition of the virus entry through adenosine monophosphate-activated protein kinase (AMPK) activation and phosphorylation of ACE2 are also scant. There are few retrospective studies that have shown that metformin may have a positive effect on prognosis of hospitalized patients with T2DM and COVID-19 and especially on reduction of mortality, even though with a degree of heterogeneity (138, 139). In addition, a recent cohort study in the United Kingdom showed that metformin was not associated with the risk of COVID-19 or COVID-19-related mortality, indicating that continuation of metformin is safe in adults with diabetes (140). Randomized controlled trials (RCTs) are needed to draw more robust conclusions.

Sulfonylureas should be avoided in patients with DM and COVID-19 because of the risk of hypoglycemia, especially if oral intake is poor or with simultaneous use of chloroquine or hydroxychloroquine (66).

Insulin has been the first choice of treatment for glucose control in critically ill patients. In accordance, available evidence suggests that it is also the most appropriate glucose lowering therapy for hospitalized patients with DM and severe COVID-19 (64, 66, 106). Furthermore, it has been shown to have anti-inflammatory properties in acute illness, a fact that has also been observed in hospitalized patients with COVID-19 (141, 142). Recent studies have also shown that in many severe cases with new-onset or pre-existing DM with COVID-19, high doses of intravenous insulin infusion are needed to achieve glycaemic control (67–71) Fortunately, continuous glucose monitoring during hospitalization has contributed to achieve such glucose management with minimizing the risk of hypoglycemia. More than this, it has achieved improvement of glycaemic control in ICU hospitalized patients and offers the advantage of remote monitoring (143–146).

On regards to direct comparison of different medications, even though there are few data suggesting that insulin treatment in hospitalized diabetic patients with COVID-19 has worse clinical outcomes compared with other agents such as metformin, we should keep in mind that such an observation could reflect a more advanced stage of diabetes with accompanying comorbidities not allowing the use of other hypoglycemic medication (133, 147, 148). Similarly, a recent nationwide observational cohort study in England showed that T2DM patients prescribed metformin, SGLT2is and sulfonylureas were at a lower risk of COVID-19-related mortality than those who were not prescribed these drugs. The risk was higher in those prescribed insulin and DPP4is. However, since the differences in risk were small and due to confounding rather than direct drug effects, no evidence supports a change in prescription of glucose-lowering drugs in people with T2DM in the context of COVID-19 pandemic (149).

Hence, to make sense of available evidence, we suggest discontinuation of SGLT2is in patients who are severely affected by COVID-19 and who are at risk for dehydration (66, 106). Thiazolidinediones should be discontinued in hemodynamically unstable patients with cardiac or hepatic dysfunction. Their use in COVID-19 patients with DM is controversial and further studies are needed (64, 65). GLP-1 RA, until more detailed trials are available, should only be recommended in patients with mild or moderate COVID-19. Focusing on metformin, we should highlight that it should be stopped in cases of severe gastrointestinal symptoms. It should also be avoided in patients with severe COVID-19, hemodynamically unstable patients with hypoxia, hepatic, renal or heart failure because of the risk of lactic acidosis (66, 106). Current data support the use of DPP4is to be limited to mild or moderate COVID-19 cases in either inpatient or outpatient settings, but insulin should continue to remain the cornerstone of treatment in severely and critically ill patients (64, 66, 106).

DM POST COVID-19

In addition to pancreatic and liver effects, damage of endocrine organs during the infection may contribute to the development of glucose and metabolic abnormalities in survivors of COVID-19 (10). People with ARDS and other critical conditions admitted to ICUs exhibit post-traumatic stress disorder with cognitive impairment, depression, impaired sensing of hunger and satiety, increased fat accumulation and increased risk of cardiovascular abnormalities (150). Furthermore, decreased exercise capacity and deranged lean muscle mass have been reported to diminish insulin sensitivity in survivors of ARDS and sepsis. Similarly, cachexia and muscle weakness are probable in severe and critical cases of COVID-19 (151, 152). Finally, rhabdomyolysis, which might contribute to long-term metabolic abnormalities, has been reported during the infection (153). In a study from China, subjects with SARS -CoV infection presented with metabolic disturbances including hyperlipidemia, cardiovascular abnormalities, abnormal glucose metabolism, such as hyperglycemia, hyperinsulinemia, insulin resistance, T1DM or T2DM twelve years after recovery (154). While the pandemic evolves over time, a cross-sectional study of 543 COVID survivors 1 year after hospital discharge, reports new-onset diabetes at 1% of them. Moreover, from the 109 people with diabetes alive after one year (from a total of 189 at discharge), 10% reported impaired glycemic control, 9,2% had to intensify oral therapy, 4,6% required new prescription of insulin (155).

DISCUSSION

The contribution of diabetes -as a risk factor- in the pathophysiology of COVID-19, 2 years after the pandemic outbreak, is undoubtable. Among diabetes chronic complications and comorbidities such as aging, and obesity, new evidence has put the endothelium in the spotlight. Chronic endothelial dysfunction -seen in DM- predisposes to severe COVID-19 infection by inducing alterations to the glycocalyx and endothelial cells. This leads to increases in leucocyte adhesion, which in turn promotes a procoagulant and antifibrinolytic state. Chronic endothelial dysfunction due to DM together with the direct damage of endothelial cells by SARS-CoV-2 result in further impairment of the microcirculation contributing to the pathogenesis of acute respiratory syndrome and multi-organ failure.

But the cycle is vicious. COVID-19 can cause severe derangements in glucose homeostasis. Glucotoxicity with its consequences, in conjunction with the inflammatory cytokine storm of COVID-19, express increased oxidative stress. Oxidative stress deranges the immune system further and damages the endothelial cells, resulting to metabolic complications -such as increased risk of thromboembolism and multiorgan damage- in individuals with DM (64–66).

The effects of Covid-19 infection on glucose homeostasis are multifactorial, enabling both insulin resistance and β-cell dysfunction. Uncommon requirements of insulin to maintain glycemic control have been observed in all studies, along with extreme fluctuations of glucose. This glucose storm has imposed an emerging interest in research on β-cell invasion, and more specifically in the ability of SARS-CoV-2 to invade and destroy islets through its identified receptors. Besides ACE2, various other receptors have emerged as alternative means of SARS-CoV-2 to enter into cells, that remain to be characterized and further investigated. However, even if SARS-CoV-2 enters β-cells conditionally, it can indirectly affect their function. This is where the endothelium plays an important role because it may connect all COVID-19 target organs, and could explain the β-cell dysfunction, as pericytes and microvasculature are prerequisites for intact β-cell function.

The wealth of existing knowledge about these mechanisms has prompted the scientific community to look into the effect of several antidiabetic medications to COVID-19 outcomes. As expected, DPP4i are of particular and promising interest, not only due to their safety profile in hospitalized patients but also due to the mechanistic knowledge that involves DPP4 as an alternative entry receptor for SARS-CoV-2. Newer agents -namely SGLT-2is and GLP-1 RA- may contribute with their antiinflammatory properties. However, to date, no robust evidence exists to inform practice.

Given the fact that COVID-19 came into being quite recently, it is still unclear whether the dysregulation of glucose metabolism during severe COVID-19 is permanent after recovery or whether SARS-CoV-2 can induce T1DM or T2DM or even a new type of diabetes. Long-term follow up studies are needed to evaluate whether the virus has a diabetogenic impact on individuals with a higher risk for DM or whether it can stimulate a new type of DM.

AUTHOR CONTRIBUTIONS

PK wrote the manuscript. SA, AM, and VL edited the manuscript. VL, II, IK, and AM generated the hypothesis and guided the literature review, based on their clinical and research experience in COVID-19 wards and ICU. All authors reviewed the literature, discussed the findings, and reviewed the manuscript. All authors contributed to the article and approved the submitted version.

REFERENCES

1. Li B, Yang J, Zhao F, Zhi L, Wang X, Liu L, et al. Prevalence and Impact of Cardiovascular Metabolic Diseases on COVID-19 in China. *Clin Res Cardiol* (2020) 109(5):531–8. doi: 10.1007/s00392-020-01626-9
2. Hill MA, Mantzoros C, Sowers JR. Commentary: COVID-19 in Patients With Diabetes. *Metab Clin Exp* (2020) 107:154217. doi: 10.1016/j.metabol.2020.154217
3. Klonoff DC, Umpierrez GE. Letter to the Editor: COVID-19 in Patients With Diabetes: Risk Factors That Increase Morbidity. *Metab Clin Exp* (2020) 108:154224. doi: 10.1016/j.metabol.2020.154224

4. Chow N, Fleming-Dutra K, Gierke R, Hall A, Hughes M, Pilishvili T, et al. Preliminary Estimates of the Prevalence of Selected Underlying Health Conditions Among Patients With COVID-19 - US, February 12-March 28, 2020. *MMWR Morb Mortal Wkly Rep* (2020) 69(13):382–6. doi: 10.15585/mmwr.mm6913e2
5. Wu Z, McGoogan JM. Characteristics of and Important Lessons From the Coronavirus Disease 2019 (COVID-19) Outbreak in China: Summary of a Report of 72 314 Cases From the Chinese Center for Disease Control and Prevention. *JAMA* (2020) 323(13):1239–42. doi: 10.1001/jama.2020.2648
6. Yang X, Yu Y, Xu J, Shu H, Xia J, Liu H, et al. Clinical Course and Outcomes of Critically Ill Patients With SARS-CoV-2 Pneumonia in Wuhan, China: A Single-Centered, Retrospective, Observational Study. *Lancet Respir Med* (2020) 8(5):475–81. doi: 10.1016/S2213-2600(20)30079-5
7. Richardson S, Hirsch JS, Narasimhan M, Crawford JM, McGinn T, Davidson KW, et al. Presenting Characteristics, Comorbidities, and Outcomes Among 5700 Patients Hospitalized With COVID-19 in the New York City Area. *JAMA* (2020) 323(20):2052–9. doi: 10.1001/jama.2020.6775
8. Barron E, Bakhai C, Kar P, Weaver A, Bradley D, Ismail H, et al. Associations of Type 1 and Type 2 Diabetes With COVID-19-Related Mortality in England: A Whole-Population Study. *Lancet Diabetes Endocrinol* (2020) 8(10):813–22. doi: 10.1016/S2213-8587(20)30272-2
9. Williamson EJ, Walker AJ, Bhaskaran K, Bacon S, Bates C, Morton CE, et al. Factors Associated With COVID-19-Related Death Using OpenSAFELY. *Nature* (2020) 584(7821):430–6. doi: 10.1038/s41586-020-2521-4
10. Kazakou P, Paschou SA, Psaltopoulou T, Gavriatopoulou M, Korompoki E, Stefanaki K, et al. Early and Late Endocrine Complications of COVID-19. *Endocr Connect* (2021) 10(9):R229–39. doi: 10.1530/EC-21-0184
11. Holman N, Knighton P, Kar P, O'Keefe J, Curley M, Weaver A, et al. Risk Factors for COVID-19-Related Mortality in People With Type 1 and Type 2 Diabetes in England: A Population-Based Cohort Study. *Lancet Diabetes Endocrinol* (2020) 8(10):823–33. doi: 10.1016/S2213-8587(20)30271-0
12. Cariou B, Hadjadj S, Wargny M, Pichelin M, Al-Salameh A, Allix I, et al. Phenotypic Characteristics and Prognosis of Inpatients With COVID-19 and Diabetes: The CORONADO Study. *Diabetologia* (2020) 63(8):1500–15. doi: 10.1007/s00125-020-05180-x
13. McGurnaghan SJ, Weir A, Bishop J, Kennedy S, Blackbourn LAK, McAllister DA, et al. Risks of and Risk Factors for COVID-19 Disease in People With Diabetes: A Cohort Study of the Total Population of Scotland. *Lancet Diabetes Endocrinol* (2021) 9(2):82–93. doi: 10.1016/S2213-8587(20)30405-8
14. Schrijvers BF, de Vriese AS, Flyvbjerg A. From Hyperglycemia to Diabetic Kidney Disease: The Role of Metabolic, Hemodynamic, Intracellular Factors and Growth Factors/Cytokines. *Endocr Rev* (2004) 25(6):971–1010. doi: 10.1210/er.2003-0018
15. Kreutmair S, Unger S, Núñez NG, Ingelfinger F, Alberti C, de Feo D, et al. Distinct Immunological Signatures Discriminate Severe COVID-19 From Non-SARS-CoV-2-Driven Critical Pneumonia. *Immunity* (2021) 54 (7):1578–93.e5. doi: 10.1016/j.immuni.2021.05.002
16. Schechter AN, Gladwin MT. Hemoglobin and the Paracrine and Endocrine Functions of Nitric Oxide. *N Engl J Med* (2003) 348(15):1483–5. doi: 10.1056/NEJMcibr023045
17. Furchgott RF, Zawadzki JV. The Obligatory Role of Endothelial Cells in the Relaxation of Arterial Smooth Muscle by Acetylcholine. *Nature* (1980) 288 (5789):373–6. doi: 10.1038/288373a0
18. Deanfield JE, Halcox JP, Rabelink TJ. Endothelial Function and Dysfunction: Testing and Clinical Relevance. *Circulation* (2007) 115(10):1285–95. doi: 10.1161/CIRCULATIONAHA.106.652859
19. VanTeeffelen JW, Brands J, Stroes ES, Vink H. Endothelial Glycocalyx: Sweet Shield of Blood Vessels. *Trends Cardiovasc Med* (2007) 17:101–5. doi: 10.1016/j.tcm.2007.02.002
20. Perrin RM, Harper SJ, Bates DO. A Role for the Endothelial Glycocalyx in Regulating Microvascular Permeability in Diabetes Mellitus. *Cell Biochem Biophys* (2007) 49(2):65–72. doi: 10.1007/s12013-007-0041-6
21. Onat D, Brillon D, Colombo PC, Schmidt AM. Human Vascular Endothelial Cells: A Model System for Studying Vascular Inflammation in Diabetes and Atherosclerosis. *Curr Diabetes Rep* (2011) 11(3):193–202. doi: 10.1007/s11892-011-0182-2
22. Lemkes BA, Nieuwdorp M, Hoekstra JBL, Holleman F. The Glycocalyx and Cardiovascular Disease in Diabetes: Should We Judge the Endothelium by Its Cover? *Diabetes Technol Ther* (2012) 14(SUPPL. 1):S3–10. doi: 10.1089/dia.2012.0011
23. Nieuwdorp M, van Haeften TW, Gouverneur MCLG, Mooij HL, van Lieshout MHP, Levi M, et al. Loss of Endothelial Glycocalyx During Acute Hyperglycemia Coincides With Endothelial Dysfunction and Coagulation Activation *In Vivo*. *Diabetes* (2006) 55(2):480–6. doi: 10.2337/diabetes.55.02.06.db05-1103
24. van den Oever IAM, Raterman HG, Nurmohamed MT, Simsek S. Endothelial Dysfunction, Inflammation, and Apoptosis in Diabetes Mellitus. *Mediators Inflamm* (2010) 2010:792393. doi: 10.1155/2010/792393
25. Lambadiari V, Pavlidis G, Kousathana F, Maratou E, Georgiou D, Andreadou I, et al. Effects of Different Antidiabetic Medications on Endothelial Glycocalyx, Myocardial Function, and Vascular Function in Type 2 Diabetic Patients: One Year Follow–Up Study. *J Clin Med* (2019) 8 (7):983. doi: 10.3390/jcm8070983
26. Ikonomidis I, Pavlidis G, Lambadiari V, Kousathana F, Varoudi M, Spanoudi F, et al. Early Detection of Left Ventricular Dysfunction in First-Degree Relatives of Diabetic Patients by Myocardial Deformation Imaging: The Role of Endothelial Glycocalyx Damage. *Int J Cardiol* (2017) 233:105–12. doi: 10.1016/j.ijcard.2017.01.056
27. Donath MY, Shoelson SE. Type 2 Diabetes as an Inflammatory Disease. *Nat Rev Immunol* (2011) 11(2):98–107. doi: 10.1038/nri2925
28. Knapp S. Diabetes and Infection: Is There a Link? - A Mini-Review. *Gerontology* (2013) 59(2):99–104. doi: 10.1159/000345107
29. Grossmann V, Schmitt VH, Zeller T, Panova-Noeva M, Schulz A, Laubert-Reh D, et al. Profile of the Immune and Inflammatory Response in Individuals With Prediabetes and Type 2 Diabetes. *Diabetes Care* (2015) 38(7):1356–64. doi: 10.2337/dc14-3008
30. Casqueiro J, Casqueiro J, Alves C. Infections in Patients With Diabetes Mellitus: A Review of Pathogenesis. *Indian J Endocrinol Metab* (2012) 16 Suppl 1(7):S27–36. doi: 10.4103/2230-8210.94253
31. Kim JH, Park K, Lee SB, Kang S, Park JS, Ahn CW, et al. Relationship Between Natural Killer Cell Activity and Glucose Control in Patients With Type 2 Diabetes and Prediabetes. *J Diabetes Invest* (2019) 10(5):1223–8. doi: 10.1111/jdi.13002
32. Wang S, Ma P, Zhang S, Song S, Wang Z, Ma Y, et al. Fasting Blood Glucose at Admission Is an Independent Predictor for 28-Day Mortality in Patients With COVID-19 Without Previous Diagnosis of Diabetes: A Multi-Centre Retrospective Study. *Diabetologia* (2020) 63(10):2102–11. doi: 10.1007/s00125-020-05209-1
33. Wu J, Huang J, Zhu G, Wang Q, Lv Q, Huang Y, et al. Elevation of Blood Glucose Level Predicts Worse Outcomes in Hospitalized Patients With COVID-19: A Retrospective Cohort Study. *BMJ Open Diabetes Res Care* (2020) 8(1):e001476. doi: 10.1136/bmjdrc-2020-001476
34. Bode B, Garrett V, Messler J, McFarland R, Crowe J, Booth R, et al. Glycemic Characteristics and Clinical Outcomes of COVID-19 Patients Hospitalized in the United States. *J Diabetes Sci Technol* (2020) 14(4):813–21. doi: 10.1177/1932296820924469
35. Lazarus G, Audrey J, Wangsaputra VK, Tamara A, Tahapary DL. High Admission Blood Glucose Independently Predicts Poor Prognosis in COVID-19 Patients: A Systematic Review and Dose-Response Meta-Analysis. *Diabetes Res Clin Pract* (2021) 171:108561. doi: 10.1016/j.diabres.2020.108561
36. Guo W, Li M, Dong Y, Zhou H, Zhang Z, Tian C, et al. Diabetes is a Risk Factor for the Progression and Prognosis of COVID-19. *Diabetes Metab Res Rev* (2020) 36(7):e3319. doi: 10.1002/dmrr.3319
37. Zeng Z, Yu H, Chen H, Qi W, Chen L, Chen G, et al. Longitudinal Changes of Inflammatory Parameters and Their Correlation With Disease Severity and Outcomes in Patients With COVID-19 From Wuhan, China. *Crit Care (London England)* (2020) 24(1):525. doi: 10.1186/s13054-020-03255-0
38. Codo AC, Davanzo GG, Monteiro L de B, de Souza GF, Muraro SP, Virgilio-da-Silva JV, et al. Elevated Glucose Levels Favor SARS-CoV-2 Infection and Monocyte Response Through a HIF-1α/Glycolysis-Dependent Axis. *Cell Metab* (2020) 32(3):437–446.e5. doi: 10.1016/j.cmet.2020.07.007
39. Marfella R, Paolisso P, Sardu C, Bergamaschi L, D'Angelo EC, Barbieri M, et al. Negative Impact of Hyperglycaemia on Tocilizumab Therapy in Covid-

19 Patients. *Diabetes Metab* (2020) 46(5):403–5. doi: 10.1016/j.diabet.2020.05.005

40. Yang JK, Feng Y, Yuan MY, Yuan SY, Fu HJ, Wu BY, et al. Plasma Glucose Levels and Diabetes are Independent Predictors for Mortality and Morbidity in Patients With SARS. *Diabetic Med* (2006) 23(6):623–8. doi: 10.1111/j.1464-5491.2006.01861.x
41. Yang J-K, Lin S-S, Ji X-J, Guo L-M. Binding of SARS Coronavirus to Its Receptor Damages Islets and Causes Acute Diabetes. *Acta Diabetol* (2010) 47 (3):193–9. doi: 10.1007/s00592-009-0109-4
42. Hamming I, Timens W, Bulthuis M, Lely A, Navis G, van Goor H. Tissue Distribution of ACE2 Protein, the Functional Receptor for SARS Coronavirus. A First Step in Understanding SARS Pathogenesis. *J Pathol* (2004) 203(2):631–7. doi: 10.1002/path.1570
43. Oudit GY, Kassiri Z, Jiang C, Liu PP, Poutanen SM, Penninger JM, et al. SARS-Coronavirus Modulation of Myocardial ACE2 Expression and Inflammation in Patients With SARS. *Eur J Clin Invest* (2009) 39(7):618–25. doi: 10.1111/j.1365-2362.2009.02153.x
44. Chen L, Li X, Chen M, Feng Y, Xiong C. The ACE2 Expression in Human Heart Indicates New Potential Mechanism of Heart Injury Among Patients Infected With SARS-CoV-2. *Cardiovasc Res* (2020) 116(6):1097–100. doi: 10.1093/cvr/cvaa078
45. Lambadiari V, Kousathana F, Raptis A, Katogiannis K, Kokkinos A, Ikonomidis I. Pre-Existing Cytokine and NLRP3 Inflammasome Activation and Increased Vascular Permeability in Diabetes: A Possible Fatal Link With Worst COVID-19 Infection Outcomes? *Front Immunol* (2020) 11:557235/full(November). doi: 10.3389/fimmu.2020.557235/full
46. Chen G, Wu D, Guo W, Cao Y, Huang D, Wang H, et al. Clinical and Immunological Features of Severe and Moderate Coronavirus Disease 2019. *J Clin Invest* (2020) 130(5):2620–9. doi: 10.1172/JCI137244
47. Szotowski B, Antoniak S, Poller W, Schultheiss H-P, Rauch U. Procoagulant Soluble Tissue Factor Is Released From Endothelial Cells in Response to Inflammatory Cytokines. *Circ Res* (2005) 96(12):1233–9. doi: 10.1161/01.RES.0000171805.24799.fa
48. Wassmann S, Stumpf M, Strehlow K, Schmid A, Schieffer B, Böhm M, et al. Interleukin-6 Induces Oxidative Stress and Endothelial Dysfunction by Overexpression of the Angiotensin II Type 1 Receptor. *Circ Res* (2004) 94 (4):534–41. doi: 10.1161/01.RES.0000115557.25127.8D
49. Chelazzi C, Villa G, Mancinelli P, de Gaudio AR, Adembri C. Glycocalyx and Sepsis-Induced Alterations in Vascular Permeability. *Crit Care* (2015) 19(1):26. doi: 10.1186/s13054-015-0741-z
50. Lambadiari V, Mitrakou A, Kountouri A, Thymis J, Katogiannis K, Korakas E, et al. Association of COVID-19 With Impaired Endothelial Glycocalyx, Vascular Function and Myocardial Deformation 4 Months After Infection. *Eur J Heart Fail* (2021) 23(11):1916–26. doi: 10.1002/ejhf.2326
51. Giamarellos-Bourboulis EJ, Netea MG, Rovina N, Akinosoglou K, Antoniadou A, Antonakos N, et al. Complex Immune Dysregulation in COVID-19 Patients With Severe Respiratory Failure. *Cell Host Microbe* (2020) 27(6):992–1000.e3. doi: 10.1016/j.chom.2020.04.009
52. Salama C, Han J, Yau L, Reiss WG, Kramer B, Neidhart JD, et al. Tocilizumab in Patients Hospitalized With Covid-19 Pneumonia. *N Engl J Med* (2021) 384(1):20–30. doi: 10.1056/NEJMoa2030340
53. He L, Ding Y, Zhang Q, Che X, He Y, Shen H, et al. Expression of Elevated Levels of Pro-Inflammatory Cytokines in SARS-CoV-Infected ACE2 + Cells in SARS Patients: Relation to the Acute Lung Injury and Pathogenesis of SARS. *J Pathol* (2006) 210(3):288–97. doi: 10.1002/path.2067
54. Varga Z, Flammer AJ, Steiger P, Haberecker M, Andermatt R, Zinkernagel AS, et al. Endothelial Cell Infection and Endotheliitis in COVID-19. *Lancet* (2020) 395(10234):1417–8. doi: 10.1016/S0140-6736(20)30937-5
55. Toki S, Goleniewska K, Reiss S, Zhang J, Bloodworth MH, Stier MT, et al. Glucagon-Like Peptide 1 Signaling Inhibits Allergen-Induced Lung IL-33 Release and Reduces Group 2 Innate Lymphoid Cell Cytokine Production In Vivo. *J Allergy Clin Immunol* (2018) 142(5):1515–28.e8. doi: 10.1016/j.jaci.2017.11.043
56. Copin M-C, Parmentier E, Duburcq T, Poissy J, Mathieu D. Time to Consider Histologic Pattern of Lung Injury to Treat Critically Ill Patients With COVID-19 Infection. *Intensive Care Med* (2020) 46(6):1124–6. doi: 10.1007/s00134-020-06057-8
57. Dungan KM, Braithwaite SS, Preiser J-C. Stress Hyperglycaemia. *Lancet (London England)* (2009) 373(9677):1798–807. doi: 10.1016/S0140-6736(09)60553-5
58. Mifsud S, Schembri EL, Gruppetta M. Stress-Induced Hyperglycaemia. *Br J Hosp Med* (2018) 79(11):634–9. doi: 10.12968/hmed.2018.79.11.634
59. Šestan M, Marinović S, Kavazović I, Cekinović Đ, Wueest S, Turk Wensveen T, et al. Virus-Induced Interferon-γ Causes Insulin Resistance in Skeletal Muscle and Derails Glycemic Control in Obesity. *Immunity* (2018) 49 (1):164–77.e6. doi: 10.1016/j.immuni.2018.05.005
60. Channappanavar R, Perlman S. Pathogenic Human Coronavirus Infections: Causes and Consequences of Cytokine Storm and Immunopathology. *Semin Immunopathol* (2017) 39(5):529–39. doi: 10.1007/s00281-017-0629-x
61. Groop LC, Bonadonna RC, DelPrato S, Ratheiser K, Zyck K, Ferrannini E, et al. Glucose and Free Fatty Acid Metabolism in Non-Insulin-Dependent Diabetes Mellitus. Evidence for Multiple Sites of Insulin Resistance. *J Clin Invest* (1989) 84(1):205–13. doi: 10.1172/JCI114142
62. Korytkowski M, Antinori-Lent K, Drincic A, Hirsch IB, McDonnell ME, Rushakoff R, et al. A Pragmatic Approach to Inpatient Diabetes Management During the COVID-19 Pandemic. *J Clin Endocrinol Metab* (2020) 105(9):3076–87. doi: 10.1210/clinem/dgaa342
63. Pal R, Banerjee M. COVID-19 and the Endocrine System: Exploring the Unexplored. *J Endocrinol Invest* (2020) 43(7):1027–31. doi: 10.1007/s40618-020-01276-8
64. Lim S, Bae JH, Kwon H-S, Nauck MA. COVID-19 and Diabetes Mellitus: From Pathophysiology to Clinical Management. *Nat Rev Endocrinol* (2021) 17(1):11–30. doi: 10.1038/s41574-020-00435-4
65. Apicella M, Campopiano MC, Mantuano M, Mazoni L, Coppelli A, del Prato S. COVID-19 in People With Diabetes: Understanding the Reasons for Worse Outcomes. *Lancet Diabetes Endocrinol* (2020) 8(9):782–92. doi: 10.1016/S2213-8587(20)30238-2
66. Drucker DJ. Coronavirus Infections and Type 2 Diabetes—Shared Pathways With Therapeutic Implications. *Endocr Rev* (2020) 41(3):457–70. doi: 10.1210/endrev/bnaa011
67. Rubino F, Amiel SA, Zimmet P, Alberti G, Bornstein S, Eckel RH, et al. New-Onset Diabetes in Covid-19. *N Engl J Med* (2020) 383(8):789–90. doi: 10.1056/NEJMc2018688
68. Li H, Tian S, Chen T, Cui Z, Shi N, Zhong X, et al. Newly Diagnosed Diabetes is Associated With a Higher Risk of Mortality Than Known Diabetes in Hospitalized Patients With COVID -19. *Diabetes Obes Metab* (2020) 22(10):1897–906. doi: 10.1111/dom.14099
69. Chee YJ, Ng SJH, Yeoh E. Diabetic Ketoacidosis Precipitated by Covid-19 in a Patient With Newly Diagnosed Diabetes Mellitus. *Diabetes Res Clin Pract* (2020) 164:108166. doi: 10.1016/j.diabres.2020.108166
70. Rayman G, Lumb A, Kennon B, Cottrell C, Nagi D, Page E, et al. Guidance on the Management of Diabetic Ketoacidosis in the Exceptional Circumstances of the COVID-19 Pandemic. *Diabetic Med* (2020) 37 (7):1214–6. doi: 10.1111/dme.14328
71. Li J, Wang X, Chen J, Zuo X, Zhang H, Deng A. COVID -19 Infection may Cause Ketosis and Ketoacidosis. *Diabetes Obes Metab* (2020) 22(10):1935–41. doi: 10.1111/dom.14057
72. Sathish T, Kapoor N, Cao Y, Tapp RJ, Zimmet P. Proportion of Newly Diagnosed Diabetes in COVID-19 Patients: A Systematic Review and Meta-Analysis. *Diabetes Obes Metab* (2021) 23(3):870–4. doi: 10.1111/dom.14269
73. Kim NY, Ha E, Moon JS, Lee YH, Choi EY. Acute Hyperglycemic Crises With Coronavirus Disease-19: Case Reports. *Diabetes Metab J* (2020) 44 (2):349–53. doi: 10.4093/dmj.2020.0091
74. Zhu L, She ZG, Cheng X, Qin JJ, Zhang XJ, Cai J, et al. Association of Blood Glucose Control and Outcomes in Patients With COVID-19 and Pre-Existing Type 2 Diabetes. *Cell Metab* (2020) 31(6):1068–77.e3. doi: 10.1016/j.cmet.2020.04.021
75. Kamrath C, Mönkemöller K, Biester T, Rohrer TR, Warncke K, Hammersen J, et al. Ketoacidosis in Children and Adolescents With Newly Diagnosed Type 1 Diabetes During the COVID-19 Pandemic in Germany. *JAMA* (2020) 324(8):801. doi: 10.1001/jama.2020.13445
76. Rabbone I, Schiaffini R, Cherubini V, Maffeis C, Scaramuzza A. Has COVID-19 Delayed the Diagnosis and Worsened the Presentation of Type 1 Diabetes in Children? *Diabetes Care* (2020) 43(11):2870–2. doi: 10.2337/dc20-1321

77. Tittel SR, Rosenbauer J, Kamrath C, Ziegler J, Reschke F, Hammersen J, et al. Did the COVID-19 Lockdown Affect the Incidence of Pediatric Type 1 Diabetes in Germany? *Diabetes Care* (2020) 43(11):e172–3. doi: 10.2337/dc20-1633
78. Lazzerini M, Barbi E, Apicella A, Marchetti F, Cardinale F, Trobia G. Delayed Access or Provision of Care in Italy Resulting From Fear of COVID-19. *Lancet Child Adolesc Health* (2020) 4(5):e10–1. doi: 10.1016/S2352-4642(20)30108-5
79. Unsworth R, Wallace S, Oliver NS, Yeung S, Kshirsagar A, Naidu H, et al. New-Onset Type 1 Diabetes in Children During COVID-19: Multicenter Regional Findings in the U.K. *Diabetes Care* (2020) 43(11):e170–1. doi: 10.2337/dc20-1551
80. Hollstein T, Schulte DM, Schulz J, Glück A, Ziegler AG, Bonifacio E, et al. Autoantibody-Negative Insulin-Dependent Diabetes Mellitus After SARS-CoV-2 Infection: A Case Report. *Nat Metab* (2020) 2(10):1021–4. doi: 10.1038/s42255-020-00281-8
81. Ekpebegh C, Longo-Mbenza B, Blanco-Blanco E. Glycosylated Haemoglobin I Markedly Elevated in New and Known Diabetes Patients With Hyperglycaemic Ketoacidosis. *Afr Health Sci* (2014) 14(3):526. doi: 10.4314/ahs.v14i3.5
82. Li M-Y, Li L, Zhang Y, Wang X. Expression of the SARS-CoV-2 Cell Receptor Gene ACE2 in a Wide Variety of Human Tissues. *Infect Dis Poverty* (2020) 9(1):45. doi: 10.1186/s40249-020-00662-x
83. Letko M, Marzi A, Munster V. Functional Assessment of Cell Entry and Receptor Usage for SARS-CoV-2 and Other Lineage B Betacoronaviruses. *Nat Microbiol* (2020) 5(4):562–9. doi: 10.1038/s41564-020-0688-y
84. Bao L, Deng W, Huang B, Gao H, Liu J, Ren L, et al. The Pathogenicity of SARS-CoV-2 in Hace2 Transgenic Mice. *Nature* (2020) 583(7818):830–3. doi: 10.1038/s41586-020-2312-y
85. Hoffmann M, Kleine-Weber H, Schroeder S, Krüger N, Herrler T, Erichsen S, et al. SARS-CoV-2 Cell Entry Depends on ACE2 and TMPRSS2 and Is Blocked by a Clinically Proven Protease Inhibitor. *Cell* (2020) 181(2):271–80.e8. doi: 10.1016/j.cell.2020.02.052
86. Hikmet F, Méar L, Edvinsson Å, Micke P, Uhlén M, Lindskog C. The Protein Expression Profile of ACE2 in Human Tissues. *Mol Syst Biol* (2020) 16(7): e9610. doi: 10.15252/msb.20209610
87. Ayres JS. A Metabolic Handbook for the COVID-19 Pandemic. *Nat Metab* (2020) 2(7):572–85. doi: 10.1038/s42255-020-0237-2
88. Liu F, Long X, Zhang B, Zhang W, Chen X, Zhang Z. ACE2 Expression in Pancreas May Cause Pancreatic Damage After SARS-CoV-2 Infection. *Clin Gastroenterol Hepatol* (2020) 18(9):2128–30.e2. doi: 10.1016/j.cgh.2020.04.040
89. Akarsu C, Karabulut M, Aydin H, Sahbaz NA, Dural AC, Yegul D, et al. Association Between Acute Pancreatitis and COVID-19: Could Pancreatitis Be the Missing Piece of the Puzzle About Increased Mortality Rates? *J Invest Surg* (2020) 35(1):119–25. doi: 10.1080/08941939.2020.1833263
90. Yang L, Han Y, Nilsson-Payant BE, Gupta V, Wang P, Duan X, et al. A Human Pluripotent Stem Cell-Based Platform to Study SARS-CoV-2 Tropism and Model Virus Infection in Human Cells and Organoids. *Cell Stem Cell* (2020) 27(1):125–36.e7. doi: 10.1016/j.stem.2020.06.015
91. Müller JA, Groß R, Conzelmann C, Krüger J, Merle U, Steinhart J, et al. SARS-CoV-2 Infects and Replicates in Cells of the Human Endocrine and Exocrine Pancreas. *Nat Metab* (2021) 3(2):149–65. doi: 10.1038/s42255-021-00347-1
92. Wu C-T, Lidsky PV, Xiao Y, Lee IT, Cheng R, Nakayama T, et al. SARS-CoV-2 Infects Human Pancreatic β Cells and Elicits β Cell Impairment. *Cell Metab* (2021) 33(8):1565–76.e5. doi: 10.1016/j.cmet.2021.05.013
93. Tang X, Uhl S, Zhang T, Xue D, Li B, Vandana JJ, et al. SARS-CoV-2 Infection Induces Beta Cell Transdifferentiation. *Cell Metab* (2021) 33 (8):1577–91.e7. doi: 10.1016/j.cmet.2021.05.015
94. Roca-Ho H, Palau V, Gimeno J, Pascual J, Soler MJ, Riera M. Angiotensin-Converting Enzyme 2 Influences Pancreatic and Renal Function in Diabetic Mice. *Lab Invest* (2020) 100(9):1169–83. doi: 10.1038/s41374-020-0440-5
95. Xuan X, Gao F, Ma X, Huang C, Wang Y, Deng H, et al. Activation of ACE2/angiotensin (1–7) Attenuates Pancreatic β Cell Dedifferentiation in a High-Fat-Diet Mouse Model. *Metab Clin Exp* (2018) 81:83–96. doi: 10.1016/j.metabol.2017.12.003
96. Shoemaker R, Yiannikouris F, Thatcher S, Cassis L. ACE2 Deficiency Reduces β-Cell Mass and Impairs β-Cell Proliferation in Obese C57BL/6 Mice. *Am J Physiol Endocrinol Metab* (2015) 309(7):E621–31. doi: 10.1152/ajpendo.00054.2015
97. Lu C-L, Wang Y, Yuan L, Li Y, Li X-Y. The Angiotensin-Converting Enzyme 2/Angiotensin (1-7)/Mas Axis Protects the Function of Pancreatic β Cells by Improving the Function of Islet Microvascular Endothelial Cells. *Int J Mol Med* (2014) 34(5):1293–300. doi: 10.3892/ijmm.2014.1917
98. Kusmartseva I, Wu W, Syed F, van der Heide V, Jorgensen M, Joseph P, et al. Expression of SARS-CoV-2 Entry Factors in the Pancreas of Normal Organ Donors and Individuals With COVID-19. *Cell Metab* (2020) 32(6):1041–51.e6. doi: 10.1016/j.cmet.2020.11.005
99. Coate KC, Cha J, Shrestha S, Wang W, Gonçalves LM, Almaça J, et al. SARS-CoV-2 Cell Entry Factors ACE2 and TMPRSS2 Are Expressed in the Microvasculature and Ducts of Human Pancreas But Are Not Enriched in β Cells. *Cell Metab* (2020) 32(6):1028–40.e4. doi: 10.1016/j.cmet.2020.11.006
100. Fignani D, Licata G, Brusco N, Nigi L, Grieco GE, Marselli L, et al. SARS-CoV-2 Receptor Angiotensin I-Converting Enzyme Type 2 (ACE2) Is Expressed in Human Pancreatic β-Cells and in the Human Pancreas Microvasculature. *Front Endocrinol* (2020) 11(November):1–19. doi: 10.3389/fendo.2020.596898
101. Steenblock C, Richter S, Berger I, Barovic M, Schmid J, Schubert U, et al. Viral Infiltration of Pancreatic Islets in Patients With COVID-19. *Nat Commun* (2021) 12(1):3534. doi: 10.1038/s41467-021-23886-3
102. Wei J, Alfajaro MM, DeWeirdt PC, Hanna RE, Lu-Culligan WJ, Cai WL, et al. Genome-Wide CRISPR Screens Reveal Host Factors Critical for SARS-CoV-2 Infection. *Cell* (2021) 184(1):76–91.e13. doi: 10.1016/j.cell.2020.10.028
103. Cantuti-Castelvetri L, Ojha R, Pedro LD, Djannatian M, Franz J, Kuivanen S, et al. Neuropilin-1 Facilitates SARS-CoV-2 Cell Entry and Infectivity. *Science* (2020) 370(6518):856–60. doi: 10.1126/science.abd2985
104. Liang Y, Deng H, Bi S, Cui Z, A L, Zheng D, et al. Urinary Angiotensin Converting Enzyme 2 Increases in Patients With Type 2 Diabetic Mellitus. *Kidney Blood Pressure Res* (2015) 40(2):101–10. doi: 10.1159/000368486
105. Cherney DZI, Xiao F, Zimpelmann J, Har RLH, Lai V, Scholey JW, et al. Urinary ACE2 in Healthy Adults and Patients With Uncomplicated Type 1 Diabetes. *Can J Physiol Pharmacol* (2014) 92(8):703–6. doi: 10.1139/cjpp-2014-0065
106. Bornstein SR, Rubino F, Khunti K, Mingrone G, Hopkins D, Birkenfeld AL, et al. Practical Recommendations for the Management of Diabetes in Patients With COVID-19. *Lancet Diabetes Endocrinol* (2020) 8:546–50. Lancet Publishing Group doi: 10.1016/S2213-8587(20)30152-2
107. Pal R, Bhansali A. COVID-19, Diabetes Mellitus and ACE2: The Conundrum. *Diabetes Res Clin Pract* (2020) 162:108132. doi: 10.1016/j.diabres.2020.108132
108. Drucker DJ. The Biology of Incretin Hormones. *Cell Metab* (2006) 3(3):153–65. doi: 10.1016/j.cmet.2006.01.004
109. Raj VS, Mou H, Smits SL, Dekkers DHW, Müller MA, Dijkman R, et al. Dipeptidyl Peptidase 4 Is a Functional Receptor for the Emerging Human Coronavirus-EMC. *Nature* (2013) 495(7440):251–4. doi: 10.1038/nature12005
110. Shirato K, Kawase M, Matsuyama S. Middle East Respiratory Syndrome Coronavirus Infection Mediated by the Transmembrane Serine Protease TMPRSS2. *J Virol* (2013) 87(23):12552–61. doi: 10.1128/JVI.01890-13
111. Vankadari N, Wilce JA. Emerging COVID-19 Coronavirus: Glycan Shield and Structure Prediction of Spike Glycoprotein and Its Interaction With Human CD26. *Emerg Microbes Infect* (2020) 9(1):601–4. doi: 10.1080/22221751.2020.1739565
112. Li Y, Zhang Z, Yang L, Lian X, Xie Y, Li S, et al. The MERS-CoV Receptor DPP4 as a Candidate Binding Target of the SARS-CoV-2 Spike. *iScience* (2020) 23(6):101160. doi: 10.1016/j.isci.2020.101160
113. Bonnet F, Scheen AJ. Effects of SGLT2 Inhibitors on Systemic and Tissue Low-Grade Inflammation: The Potential Contribution to Diabetes Complications and Cardiovascular Disease. *Diabetes Metab* (2018) 44 (6):457–64. doi: 10.1016/j.diabet.2018.09.005
114. Meyer EJ, Gabb G, Jesudason D. SGLT2 Inhibitor-Associated Euglycemic Diabetic Ketoacidosis: A South Australian Clinical Case Series and Australian Spontaneous Adverse Event Notifications. *Diabetes Care* (2018) 41(4):e47–9. doi: 10.2337/dc17-1721
115. Hahn K, Ejaz AA, Kanbay M, Lanaspa MA, Johnson RJ. Acute Kidney Injury From SGLT2 Inhibitors: Potential Mechanisms. *Nat Rev Nephrol* (2016) 12 (12):711–2. doi: 10.1038/nrneph.2016.159

116. Vitale RJ, Valtis YK, McDonnell ME, Palermo NE, Fisher NDL. Euglycemic Diabetic Ketoacidosis With COVID-19 Infection in Patients With Type 2 Diabetes Taking SGLT2 Inhibitors. *AACE Clin Case Rep* (2021) 7(1):10–3. doi: 10.1016/j.aace.2020.11.019
117. Palermo NE, Sadhu AR, McDonnell ME. Diabetic Ketoacidosis in COVID-19: Unique Concerns and Considerations. *J Clin Endocrinol Metab* (2020) 105(8):2819–29. doi: 10.1210/clinem/dgaa360
118. Kosiborod MN, Esterline R, Furtado RHM, Oscarsson J, Gasparyan SB, Koch GG, et al. Dapagliflozin in Patients With Cardiometabolic Risk Factors Hospitalised With COVID-19 (DARE-19): A Randomised, Double-Blind, Placebo-Controlled, Phase 3 Trial. *Lancet Diabetes Endocrinol* (2021) 9 (9):586–94. doi: 10.1016/S2213-8587(21)00180-7
119. Yki-Järvinen H. Thiazolidinediones. *N Engl J Med* (2004) 351(11):1106–18. doi: 10.1177/1461444810365020
120. Li AC, Brown KK, Silvestre MJ, Willson TM, Palinski W, Glass CK. Peroxisome Proliferator-Activated Receptor γ Ligands Inhibit Development of Atherosclerosis in LDL Receptor-Deficient Mice. *J Clin Invest* (2000) 106(4):523–31. doi: 10.1172/JCI10370
121. Kernan WN, Viscoli CM, Furie KL, Young LH, Inzucchi SE, Gorman M, et al. Pioglitazone After Ischemic Stroke or Transient Ischemic Attack. *N Engl J Med* (2016) 374(14):1321–31. doi: 10.1056/NEJMoa1506930
122. Mulvihill EE, Drucker DJ. Pharmacology, Physiology, and Mechanisms of Action of Dipeptidyl Peptidase-4 Inhibitors. *Endocr Rev* (2014) 35(6):992–1019. doi: 10.1210/er.2014-1035
123. Iacobellis G. COVID-19 and Diabetes: Can DPP4 Inhibition Play a Role? *Diabetes Res Clin Pract* (2020) 162:108125. doi: 10.1016/j.diabres.2020.108125
124. Kulcsar KA, Coleman CM, Beck SE, Frieman MB. Comorbid Diabetes Results in Immune Dysregulation and Enhanced Disease Severity Following MERS-CoV Infection. *JCI Insight* (2019) 4(20):e131774. doi: 10.1172/jci.insight.131774
125. Kawasaki T, Chen W, Htwe YM, Tatsumi K, Dudek SM. DPP4 Inhibition by Sitagliptin Attenuates LPS-Induced Lung Injury in Mice. *Am J Physiol Lung Cell Mol Physiol* (2018) 315(5):L834–45. doi: 10.1152/ajplung.00031.2018
126. Inn K-S, Kim Y, Aigerim A, Park U, Hwang E-S, Choi M-S, et al. Reduction of Soluble Dipeptidyl Peptidase 4 Levels in Plasma of Patients Infected With Middle East Respiratory Syndrome Coronavirus. *Virology* (2018) 518 (January):324–7. doi: 10.1016/j.virol.2018.03.015
127. Raj VS, Smits SL, Provacia LB, van den Brand JMA, Wiersma L, Ouwendijk WJD, et al. Adenosine Deaminase Acts as a Natural Antagonist for Dipeptidyl Peptidase 4-Mediated Entry of the Middle East Respiratory Syndrome Coronavirus. *J Virol* (2014) 88(3):1834–8. doi: 10.1128/JVI.02935-13
128. Solerte SB, D'Addio F, Trevisan R, Lovati E, Rossi A, Pastore I, et al. Sitagliptin Treatment at the Time of Hospitalization Was Associated With Reduced Mortality in Patients With Type 2 Diabetes and COVID-19: A Multicenter, Case-Control, Retrospective, Observational Study. *Diabetes Care* (2020) 43(12):2999–3006. doi: 10.2337/dc20-1521
129. Mirani M, Favacchio G, Carrone F, Betella N, Biamonte E, Morenghi E, et al. Impact of Comorbidities and Glycemia at Admission and Dipeptidyl Peptidase 4 Inhibitors in Patients With Type 2 Diabetes With COVID-19: A Case Series From an Academic Hospital in Lombardy, Italy. *Diabetes Care* (2020) 43(12):3042–9. doi: 10.2337/dc20-1340
130. Dalan R, Ang LW, Tan WYT, Fong S-W, Tay WC, Chan Y-H, et al. The Association of Hypertension and Diabetes Pharmacotherapy With COVID-19 Severity and Immune Signatures: An Observational Study. *Eur Heart J Cardiovasc Pharmacother* (2021) 7(3):e48–51. doi: 10.1093/ehjcvp/pvaa098
131. Lim S, Oh TJ, Dawson J, Sattar N. Diabetes Drugs and Stroke Risk: Intensive Versus Conventional Glucose-Lowering Strategies, and Implications of Recent Cardiovascular Outcome Trials. *Diabetes Obes Metab* (2020) 22 (1):6–15. doi: 10.1111/dom.13850
132. Lim S, Lee GY, Park HS, Lee D-H, Tae Jung O, Kyoung Min K, et al. Attenuation of Carotid Neointimal Formation After Direct Delivery of a Recombinant Adenovirus Expressing Glucagon-Like Peptide-1 in Diabetic Rats. *Cardiovasc Res* (2017) 113(2):183–94. doi: 10.1093/cvr/cvw213
133. Drucker DJ. Mechanisms of Action and Therapeutic Application of Glucagon-Like Peptide-1. *Cell Metab* (2018) 27(4):740–56. doi: 10.1016/j.cmet.2018.03.001
134. Hulst AH, Plummer MP, Hollmann MW, DeVries JH, Preckel B, Deane AM, et al. Systematic Review of Incretin Therapy During Peri-Operative and Intensive Care. *Crit Care (London England)* (2018) 22(1):299. doi: 10.1186/s13054-018-2197-4
135. Yu LL, Zhu M, Huang Y, Zhao YM, Wen JJ, Yang XJ, et al. Metformin Relieves Acute Respiratory Distress Syndrome by Reducing miR-138 Expression. *Eur Rev Med Pharmacol Sci* (2018) 22(16):5355–63. doi: 10.26355/eurrev_201808_15737
136. Cameron AR, Morrison VL, Levin D, Mohan M, Forteath C, Beall C, et al. Anti-Inflammatory Effects of Metformin Irrespective of Diabetes Status. *Circ Res* (2016) 119(5):652–65. doi: 10.1161/CIRCRESAHA.116.308445
137. Pernicova I, Kelly S, Ajodha S, Sahdev A, Bestwick JP, Gabrovska P, et al. Metformin to Reduce Metabolic Complications and Inflammation in Patients on Systemic Glucocorticoid Therapy: A Randomised, Double-Blind, Placebo-Controlled, Proof-of-Concept, Phase 2 Trial. *Lancet Diabetes Endocrinol* (2020) 8(4):278–91. doi: 10.1016/S2213-8587(20) 30021-8
138. Crouse A, Grimes T, Li P, Might M, Ovalle F, Shalev A. Metformin Use Is Associated With Reduced Mortality in a Diverse Population With COVID-19 and Diabetes. *medRxiv Preprint Server Health Sci* (2020) 11:600439/full (January). doi: 10.3389/fendo.2020.600439/full
139. Scheen AJ. Metformin and COVID-19: From Cellular Mechanisms to Reduced Mortality. *Diabetes Metab* (2020) 46(6):423–6. doi: 10.1016/j.diabet.2020.07.006
140. Wang J, Cooper JM, Gokhale K, Acosta-Mena D, Dhalla S, Byne N, et al. Association of Metformin With Susceptibility to COVID-19 in People With Type 2 Diabetes. *J Clin Endocrinol Metab* (2021) 106(5):1255–68. doi: 10.1210/clinem/dgab067
141. Sardu C, D'Onofrio N, Balestrieri ML, Barbieri M, Rizzo MR, Messina V, et al. Outcomes in Patients With Hyperglycemia Affected by COVID-19: Can We Do More on Glycemic Control? *Diabetes Care* (2020) 43(7):1408–15. doi: 10.2337/dc20-0723
142. Hansen TK, Thiel S, Wouters PJ, Christiansen JS, van den Berghe G. Intensive Insulin Therapy Exerts Antiinflammatory Effects in Critically Ill Patients and Counteracts the Adverse Effect of Low Mannose-Binding Lectin Levels. *J Clin Endocrinol Metab* (2003) 88(3):1082–8. https://academic.oup.com/jcem/article/88/3/1082/2845194. doi: 10.1210/jc.2002-021478
143. Galindo RJ, Aleppo G, Klonoff DC, Spanakis EK, Agarwal S, Vellanki P, et al. Implementation of Continuous Glucose Monitoring in the Hospital: Emergent Considerations for Remote Glucose Monitoring During the COVID-19 Pandemic. *J Diabetes Sci Technol* (2020) 14(4):822–32. doi: 10.1177/1932296820932903
144. Davis GM, Faulds E, Walker T, Vigliotti D, Rabinovich M, Hester J, et al. Remote Continuous Glucose Monitoring With a Computerized Insulin Infusion Protocol for Critically Ill Patients in a COVID-19 Medical ICU: Proof of Concept. *Diabetes Care* (2021) 44(4):1055–8. doi: 10.2337/dc20-2085
145. Agarwal S, Mathew J, Davis GM, Shephardson A, Levine A, Louard R, et al. Continuous Glucose Monitoring in the Intensive Care Unit During the COVID-19 Pandemic. *Diabetes Care* (2021) 44(3):847–9. doi: 10.2337/dc20-2219
146. Davis GM, Galindo RJ, Migdal AL, Umpierrez GE. Diabetes Technology in the Inpatient Setting for Management of Hyperglycemia. *Endocrinol Metab Clinics North Am* (2020) 49(1):79–93. doi: 10.1016/j.ecl.2019.11.002
147. Cariou B, Hadjadj S, Wargny M, Pichelin M, Gourdy P. Comment on Chen Et al. Clinical Characteristics and Outcomes of Patients With Diabetes and COVID-19 in Association With Glucose-Lowering Medication. Diabetes Care 2020;43:1399–1407. *Diabetes Care* (2020) 43(10):e163–4. doi: 10.2337/dc20-1205
148. Chen Y, Yang D, Cheng B, Chen J, Peng A, Yang C, et al. Clinical Characteristics and Outcomes of Patients With Diabetes and COVID-19 in Association With Glucose-Lowering Medication. *Diabetes Care* (2020) 43 (7):1399–407. doi: 10.2337/dc20-0660
149. Khunti K, Knighton P, Zaccardi F, Bakhai C, Barron E, Holman N, et al. Prescription of Glucose-Lowering Therapies and Risk of COVID-19 Mortality in People With Type 2 Diabetes: A Nationwide Observational Study in England. *Lancet Diabetes Endocrinol* (2021) 9(5):293–303. doi: 10.1016/S2213-8587(21)00050-4
150. Huang M, Parker AM, Bienvenu OJ, Dinglas VD, Colantuoni E, Hopkins RO, et al. Psychiatric Symptoms in Acute Respiratory Distress Syndrome Survivors: A 1-Year National Multicenter Study. *Crit Care Med* (2016) 44 (5):954–65. doi: 10.1097/CCM.0000000000001621

151. Pfoh ER, Wozniak AW, Colantuoni E, Dinglas VD, Mendez-Tellez PA, Shanholtz C, et al. Physical Declines Occurring After Hospital Discharge in ARDS Survivors: A 5-Year Longitudinal Study. *Intensive Care Med* (2016) 42 (10):1557–66. doi: 10.1007/s00134-016-4530-1

152. Rocheteau P, Chatre L, Briand D, Mebarki M, Jouvion G, Bardon J, et al. Sepsis Induces Long-Term Metabolic and Mitochondrial Muscle Stem Cell Dysfunction Amenable by Mesenchymal Stem Cell Therapy. *Nat Commun* (2015) 6(May):1–12. doi: 10.1038/ncomms10145

153. Chan KH, Slim J. Rhabdomyolysis as Potential Late Complication Associated With COVID-19. *Emerg Infect Dis* (2020) 26(10):2535–5. doi: 10.3201/eid2610.202225

154. Wu Q, Zhou L, Sun X, Yan Z, Hu C, Wu J, et al. Altered Lipid Metabolism in Recovered SARS Patients Twelve Years After Infection. *Sci Rep* (2017) 7 (1):9110. doi: 10.1038/s41598-017-09536-z

155. Maestre-Muñiz MM, Arias Á, Mata-Vázquez E, Martín-Toledano M, López-Larramona G, Ruiz-Chicote AM, et al. Long-Term Outcomes of Patients With Coronavirus Disease 2019 at One Year After Hospital Discharge. *J Clin Med* (2021) 10(13):2945. doi: 10.3390/jcm10132945

24

Interaction of Severe Acute Respiratory Syndrome Coronavirus 2 and Diabetes

Shiying Shao [1,2], Qin Yang[3], Ruping Pan[4], Xuefeng Yu [1,2] and Yong Chen [1,2]*

[1] *Division of Endocrinology, Tongji Hospital, Huazhong University of Science and Technology, Wuhan, China,* [2] *Branch of National Clinical Research Center for Metabolic Diseases, Hubei, China,* [3] *Division of Pathology, Tongji Hospital, Huazhong University of Science and Technology, Wuhan, China,* [4] *Department of Nuclear Medicine, Tongji Hospital, Huazhong University of Science and Technology, Wuhan, China*

Correspondence:
Yong Chen
tj.y.chen@vip.163.com

Severe acute respiratory syndrome coronavirus 2 (SARS-CoV-2) is causing a worldwide epidemic. It spreads very fast and hits people of all ages, especially patients with underlying diseases such as diabetes. In this review, we focus on the influences of diabetes on the outcome of SARS-CoV-2 infection and the involved mechanisms including lung dysfunction, immune disorder, abnormal expression of angiotensin-converting enzyme 2 (ACE2), overactivation of mechanistic target of rapamycin (mTOR) signaling pathway, and increased furin level. On the other hand, SARS-CoV-2 may trigger the development of diabetes. It causes the damage of pancreatic β cells, which is probably mediated by ACE2 protein in the islets. Furthermore, SARS-CoV-2 may aggravate insulin resistance through attacking other metabolic organs. Of note, certain anti-diabetic drugs (OADs), such as peroxisome proliferator-activated receptor γ(PPARγ) activator and glucagon-like peptide 1 receptor (GLP-1R) agonist, have been shown to upregulate ACE2 in animal models, which may increase the risk of SARS-CoV-2 infection. However, Metformin, as a first-line medicine for the treatment of type 2 diabetes mellitus (T2DM), may be a potential drug benefiting diabetic patients with SARS-CoV-2 infection, probably *via* a suppression of mTOR signaling together with its anti-inflammatory and anti-fibrosis function in lung. Remarkably, another kind of OADs, dipeptidyl Peptidase 4 (DPP4) inhibitor, may also exert beneficial effects in this respect, probably *via* a prevention of SARS-CoV-2 binding to cells. Thus, it is of significant to identify appropriate OADs for the treatment of diabetes in the context of SARS-CoV-2 infections.

Keywords: SARS-CoV-2 (2019-nCoV), COVID – 19, diabetes - quality of life, OADs, immunocellular response

1 INTRODUCTION

Coronavirus disease 2019 (COVID-19), caused by severe acute respiratory syndrome coronavirus 2 (SARS-CoV-2)-a novel β-coronavirus, has influenced over 100 million people. This SARS-CoV-2 strain has become the third most lethal pathogenic human coronavirus since SARS-CoV-1, which was responsible for severe acute respiratory syndrome (SARS) in 2002 (1), and Middle-East respiratory syndrome coronavirus (MERS-CoV), which was responsible for MERS in 2012 (2).

The coronavirus belongs to a large family of single-stranded, enveloped RNA viruses, which can be divided into four genera: α-, β-, γ- and δ- coronavirus (3). All of the above 3 viruses belong to the β-genus (1, 2, 4), sharing a structural analogy (4, 5). Although the pathophysiological mechanisms and clinical invasiveness of SARS-CoV-2 have not yet been fully investigated, it probably, at least in part resembles SARS-CoV-1 and MERS-CoV.

There are more and more studies demonstrating the association between COVID-19 and diabetes, disclosing that these two diseases appear to be bi-directional. Diabetes may magnify the pathogenicity of SARS-CoV-2 because part of pathological mechanisms of diabetes overlaps with COVID-19, resulting in an increase in susceptibility and severity of COVID-19 among diabetic patients. Investigation of the underlying mechanisms would contribute to improve the clinic outcomes of these patients. On the other hand, SARS-CoV-2 infection may induce new onset diabetes, which could be possibly overlooked by nonendocrinologists. Thus, this review focuses on the bi-directional interaction between SARS-CoV-2 and diabetes and the possible mechanisms. Moreover, some glucose lowering agents may provide extra benefits for COVID-19 treatment, which may disclose some new clues for the treatment of non-diabetic patients with SARS-CoV-2 infection.

2 IMPACT OF PRE-EXISTING DIABETES ON COVID-19 PROGRESSION

Emerging data indicates that patients with diabetes are at a higher risk of SARS-CoV-2 infection. In one SARS-CoV-2 study, which includes 1,099 patients from 552 hospitals in China, the rate of diabetes was around 15%, including children and adults (6). Diabetes was reported in 34.6% of the subjects with a composite endpoint including intensive care unit admission, requirement for ventilation, and death (7). Moreover, a study with 5700 patients in New York City, USA, identified that one of the most common comorbidities caused by SARS-CoV-2 was diabetes, with a rate of 33.8% (8). Stokes et al. reported that, as of May 30, 2020, in a population of about 1.3 million patients with SARS-CoV-2 infection in the USA, around 30% of whom have been suffering from diabetes (9). Of note, the exact rates of type 2 diabetes mellitus (T2DM) in patients with SARS-CoV-2 infection vary. The inconsistent rate can be attributed to the diagnosis of both conditions, which depends on the testing methods of SARS-CoV-2 (nasal test or pharyngeal test, nucleic acids or antibodies), enrolled population (out-patient or hospitalized patients), the severity of illness (mild or severe symptom), sample sizes, and different locations.

In addition, diabetic patients are associated with a more severe course of COVID-19, who account for a higher proportion of intensive care unit (ICU)-admitted cases. A retrospective cohort study of 7,337 patients with SARS-CoV-2 infection in China showed that subjects with T2DM had a significantly higher mortality and morbidity of multiple organ injury than the non-diabetic individuals (10). The authors further demonstrated that the in-hospital death rate was significantly lower in the well-controlled blood glucose group relative to the poorly controlled group (10). An analysis of a randomly selected subset of fatal SARS-CoV-2 cases in Italy revealed a high prevalence of diabetes, with a rate as high as 35.5% (11). A COVID-19 study in Pisa, Italy identified that the mortality of SARS-CoV-2 patients was greater in hyperglycemia subjects (about 39.4%) than in patients with normal glycemia (about 16.8%) (12). The authors concluded that hyperglycemia acts as an independent factor associated with severe prognosis in hospitalized patients with SARS-CoV-2 infection (12). Lately, a large study relevant to diabetic patients from the Chinese Center for Disease Control and Prevention with 72,314 SARS-CoV-2 cases across the Mainland China also showed a higher fatality rate in diabetic patients (7.3% vs. 2.3% overall) than regular patients, second only to patients with cardiovascular diseases (13). A meta-analysis based on six published clinical studies further confirmed the negative influence of diabetes on SARS-CoV-2 infection, that diabetic patients displayed 2.95-fold higher risk of fatality after SARS-CoV-2 infection, compared to those without diabetes (14). However, most of these studies did not indicate whether the included patients were type 1 diabetes mellitus (T1DM) or T2DM. In addition, stratified analyses according to Hemoglobin A1c (HbA1c), insulin sensitivity, β cell function, and c peptide level were limited.

Likewise, patients with SARS-CoV-2 infection display increased risk of ketosis and hyperglycaemic emergencies. One observation retrieved from the Chinese population described that 42 (6.4%) out of 658 patients with SARS-CoV-2 infection presented with ketosis on admission with no obvious fever or diarrhea, and 3 (20.0%) out of the 15 COVID-19 cases with diabetic ketosis developed acidosis (15). Of note, there was only one T1DM among these included patients, indicating that it was T2DM rather than T1DM tended to develop ketosis under the context of COVID-19. A recent retrospective analysis characterized 35 T1DM and T2DM patients with hyperglycaemic emergencies including diabetic ketoacidosis (DKA), hyperosmolar hyperglycaemic state (HHS), and hyperglycaemic ketosis in the context of SARS-CoV-2 from three hospitals in north London in UK. They concluded that SARS-CoV-2 is associated with the occurrence of hyperglycemia emergencies with overrepresentation of T2DM in patients presenting with DKA and long-lasting ketosis (16). Accordingly, ketone monitoring becomes very important among diabetic patients in the COVID-19 epidemics, especially in T2DM patients. Howbeit, the sample size of these studies was relatively small. Larger study population and longer observation were needed.

3 POTENTIAL MECHANISMS OF DIABETES ON COVID-19 PROGRESSION

The reasons for increased risk of coronaviral infection in diabetic patients are not fully identified. Multifarious mechanisms are possibly involved in the disease susceptibility and progression. Particularly, previous investigations on SARS-CoV-1 and MERS-CoV may provide evidence on the pathophysiology of SARS-CoV-2 infection in patients with diabetes.

3.1 Diabetes and Lung Dysfunction

Diabetes is associated with a change in lung physiology and structure. It has been reported an increase of extracellular matrix synthesis in the pulmonary alveolar wall in diabetic rat model, resulting in a reduction of lung elasticity and a decrease in alveolar space (17). Furthermore, Weynand et al. identified that alveolar epithelial basal lamina in diabetic patients was significantly thicker than that in healthy subjects. This result reveals that hyperglycemia leads to the thickening of the pulmonary microvascular wall (18), which potentially participates in the damage of alveolar-capillary membrane, and in turn, reduces the gas diffusion rate in diabetic patients (19).

The above structure changes in lung result in abnormalities of pulmonary function including lung volume, pulmonary diffusing capacity, pulmonary ventilation, bronchomotor tone, and neuroadrenergic bronchial innervation (20). A prospective study of 125 patients with T2DM revealed that absolute and percentage-predicted lung function measures including forced vital capacity (FVC), forced expiratory volume in 1 s (FEV1), vital capacity (VC), and peak expiratory flow (PEF) were significantly reduced after 7-year follow-up (21).

Accordingly, the impaired pulmonary function in patients with pre-existing diabetes may partly explain the susceptibility and poor outcomes of diabetic patients after SARS-CoV-2 infection (**Figure 1**).

3.2 Diabetes and Immune Dysfunction

Diabetes, even a short-term hyperglycemia, has been shown to impair the balance of immune system (22). Although the immunologic mechanisms induced by SARS-CoV-2 are not fully elucidated, existing data derived from the close counterparts SARS-CoV and MERS-CoV may bring some enlightenment. Part of mechanisms of immune dysfunction between diabetes and COVID-19 may cross, including impaired neutrophil function, pro-inflammatory inclination and T cell imbalance under hyperglycemia.

3.2.1 Diabetes and Impaired Neutrophil Function

In the innate immune response, neutrophils play a crucial role in chemotaxis and phagocytosis. Under hyperglycemia, neutrophil dysfunction has been observed in both humans and rodents (23). Possibly, acute hyperglycemia impairs the respiratory burst capacity of neutrophils, the process by which immune cells release toxic chemicals and kill pathogensr (24). Moreover, hyperglycemia reduced neutrophil degranulation (25) and impaired superoxide production from activated neutrophils (26).

Thus, impaired neutrophil function leads to an increase in risk and severity of infections (**Figure 1**), suggesting that glucose homeostasis in patients with SARS-CoV-2 infection may help to stabilize the ability of neutrophils for a proper innate immune response. Interestingly, a significant increase in neutrophil counts was observed in patients with both diabetes and SARS-CoV-2 infection (10, 12). Howbeit, few literature have described the function of neutrophils under the context of SARS-CoV-2 infection, which requires further investigation.

3.2.2 Diabetes and Pro-Inflammatory State

It has been known that both diabetes and obesity cause a low grade pro-inflammatory state in the body with increased secretion of cytokines including interleukin (IL)-1, IL-6, IL-8 and tumor necrosis factor-α (TNF-α) (23). In diabetic and obese patients, excess cytokines in circulation keep the immune system in "threat" mode.

This hypercytokinemia seems to play a crucial role in the development of pulmonary fibrosis (27, 28). Evidences show that cytokine storm, also known as cytokine release syndrome (CRS),

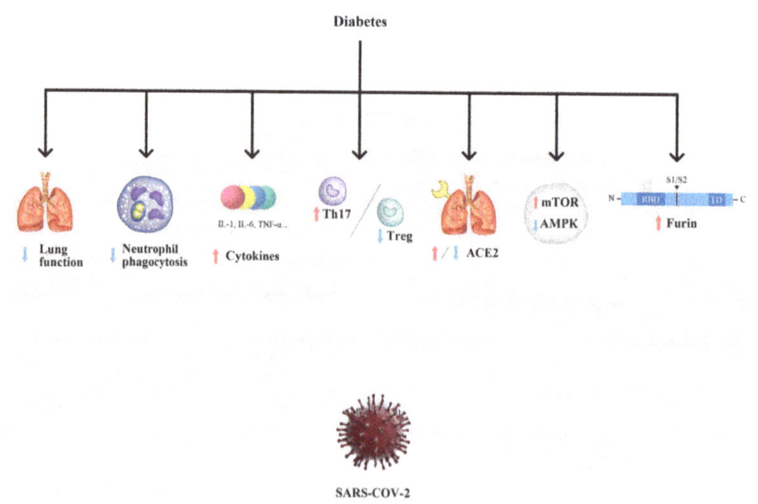

FIGURE 1 | Potential mechanism of diabetes on the susceptibility and severity of COVID-19. ACE2, Angiotensin-converting enzyme 2; AMPK, Adenosine 5'-monophosphate-activated protein kinase; IL, interleukin; mTOR, mechanistic target of rapamycin; RBD, receptor binding domain; SARS-CoV-2, severe acute respiratory syndrome coronavirus 2; TD, transmembrane domain; Th17, T helper 17; TNF-α, tumor necrosis factor-α; Treg, regulatory T.

might be involved in lung injury and increased mortality, thus playing a major role in severe COVID-19 cases. Inflammatory cytokines and chemokines, including IL-1β, IL-2, IL-4, IL-6, IL-7, IL-10, IL-12, IL-17, TNF-α, interferon- γ (IFNγ), interferon gamma-induced protein 10 (IP10) and monocyte chemoattractant protein-1 (MCP-1), were significantly elevated in COVID-19 patients (29–34), some of which overlap with the cytokine panel in diabetes.

Among those overlapped cytokines, IL-6 is of particular interest and appears to be closely related to the occurrence of severe SARS-CoV-2 infection. It is an important pleiotropic cytokine, which is involved in acute inflammatory response and lung injury (35). In addition, elevated levels of IL-6 were observed in patients with SARS in 2004 and, in particular, were positively correlated to disease severity (36). A retrospective, multicentre cohort study in Wuhan in this epidemic found that IL-6 levels were closely associated with the mortality in patients with SARS-CoV-2 infection (34). Likewise, ICU patients with severe pneumonia in another study also showed a significant elevation in plasma level of IL-6 (37).

Importantly, serum levels of IL-6 in patients with diabetes and SARS-CoV-2 infection were significantly higher than those in non-diabetic patients (10, 38). This might be explained by that the increased cytokine baseline level and pro-inflammatory state observed in diabetic patients are further amplified by SARS-CoV-2 infection (**Figure 1**), resulting in an aggressive inflammatory response, even CRS.

3.2.3 Diabetes and T Cell Imbalance

It has been demonstrated that in patients with either T1DM or T2DM, some "helpful" immune cells including certain subsets of $CD4^+$ and $CD8^+$ T cells are decreased, while some proinflammatory immune cells, such as T helper 17 (Th17) cells, are increased (39). Data supports the concept that Th17/regulatory T (Treg) cell mediated immune responses are involved in the pathogenesis in obesity-related T2DM (39).

A previous evidence demonstrated that acute intracellular bacterial infection in the diabetic host was associated with the Th17/Treg-mediated immune imbalance, resulting in exaggerated inflammatory cascades (40). In 2019, Kulcsar et al. created a diabetic mouse model with the expression of human dipeptidyl peptidase 4 (DPP4), which is identified as the cellular binding site for MERS-CoV (41). These mice developed severe infection and displayed a more prominent Th17 response with increased levels of IL-17. Due to the viral homology between SARS-CoV-2 and MERS-CoV, it is speculated that Th17/Treg-mediated immune responses may play an essential role in the aggravation of SARS-CoV-2 infection in diabetic patients.

It has been revealed that the pathological characteristics of COVID-19 observed by postmortem pathology greatly resemble those observed in SARS-CoV-1 and MERS-CoV infection (42). In this SARS-CoV-2 case, pro-inflammatory T cells were overactivated, manifested by increase of $CCR4^+CCR6^+$ Th17 cells and high cytotoxicity of $CD8^+$ T cells (42). Notably, an extensive multi-omics dataset demonstrated that the frequencies of $CD4^+$ T cells that can secrete Th17 cytokines, including IL17-A and IL17-F, are increased in SARS-CoV-2 infected patients (43). Moreover, Pacha et al. indicated that the severity of disease is positively correlated with plasma levels of IL-17 and other Th17 cell-related cytokines (33). Specifically, Qin et al. identified that patients with SARS-CoV-2 infection also show lower levels of Treg cells, which are even lower in severe cases (44).

Thus, SARS-CoV-2 may affect circulating immune cells and exacerbate the uncoordination of the innate immune system, which are previously present in diabetic patients, and therefore, resulting in a deluge of inflammatory cytokines and a further damage of the organs (**Figure 1**).

3.3 Diabetes and mTOR Signaling

During the progression of T2DM, Adenosine 5'-monophosphate (AMP)-activated protein kinase (AMPK) is inactivated, leading to a chronic overactivation of mechanistic target of rapamycin (mTOR) C1 (45), which has been associated with insulin resistance and progression of diabetes-induced complications (46).

Increasing evidences also highlight mTOR as a key factor in regulating the replication of viruses. Rapamycin, which is a mTOR inhibitor, was found to be a potent inhibitor for the RNA replication of hepatitis C virus (HCV) (47) and MERS-CoV (48). In patients with severe H1N1 pneumonia, early adjuvant treatment with corticosteroids and mTOR inhibitor effectively blocked the expression of viral protein and the release of virion, and therefore, significantly improved the prognosis of disease (49). These findings disclose a potential anti-viral treatment for the patients with SARS-CoV-2 infection through an inhibition of the metabolic sensor mTOR.

It is known that stress-induced Regulated in Development and DNA Damage Responses 1 (REDD1) negatively regulates mTOR activity (50). Interestingly, IL-6, which is closely related to the progression and severity of COVID-19, directly enhances the activation of mTOR by reducing the expression of REDD1 (50). On the contrary, IL-37 performs its immunosuppressive activity by targeting mTOR as well, suggesting that IL-37 administration may be a possible therapeutic strategy for SARS-CoV-2 treatment (51). More importantly, a recent study tested 16 repurposable anti-human coronavirus (HCoV) drugs, that may provide a synergistic effect for the treatment of SARS-CoV-2, by analyzing their drug-gene signatures and HCoV-induced transcriptomics in human cell lines. Among these candidates, Sirolimus, which consists of an mTOR inhibitor and dactinomycin, may be a potential drug for COVID-19 treatment (52).

Thus, these findings suggest that the dysregulation of AMPK/mTOR signaling in the setting of T2DM may be a plausible explanation for the increased susceptibility of diabetic patients to COVID-19 (**Figure 1**).

3.4 Diabetes and ACE2

Angiotensin-converting enzyme 2 (ACE2) is a transmembrane glycoprotein which is expressed in organs throughout the whole human body, mainly in lung, intestine, kidney, blood vessels, and pancreas. The renin-angiotensin system (RAS) signaling pathway comprises both ACE, which metabolizes angiotensin I (Ang I) into angiotensin II (Ang II), and ACE2, which degrades Ang II to Ang 1-7 peptide (53). It has been reported that both

SARS-CoV-1 and SARS-CoV-2 bind and gain entry to infected cells through ACE2 (4, 54), so that increased expression of ACE2 may contribute to increased chances of SARS-CoV-2 infection.

However, the role of ACE2 in the crosstalk between COVID-19 and diabetes is still a matter of debate, which may be largely attributed to the inconsistent expression of ACE2 in different tissues and stages of diabetes (**Figure 1**). The effect of hyperglycemia on the expression of ACE2 in different organs was investigated in non-obese diabetes (NOD) mouse models with the increased expression of ACE2 in the serum, liver, and pancreas (55). In rats with streptozotocin-induced diabetes, there also showed an upregulation of ACE2 in isolated jejunal enterocytes (56). In addition, in adipocytes from obese and diabetic patients, an increased expression of ACE2 was also observed, suggesting that adipose tissue is a viral reservoir and could be a potential target for antiviral treatment (57). Recently, a phenome-wide Mendelian randomization study has explored and identified T2DM as a disease causally associated with increased expression of ACE2 (58).

Surprisingly, Roca-Ho et al. has reported that the activity ratio of ACE2/ACE in the lung was significantly decreased in the late-stage of diabetes in NOD Mouse (55). Although a study from Wysocki et al. has concluded that ACE2 expression was increased at the posttranscriptional level in the renal cortex in diabetic mice (59), ACE2 expression was shown to be decreased in the tubules in individuals with overt diabetic nephropathy (60).

Remarkably, it remains controversial whether an increased expression of ACE2 is responsible for the increased infectivity and severity of COVID-19. Some authors even consider that ACE2 plays a beneficial role in patients with COVID-19 (61, 62). It was demonstrated that ACE2 protects murine lungs from acute respiratory distress syndrome (ARDS) by decreasing inflammation and vascular permeability (63, 64). Previous studies have shown that the transmembrane spike (S) glycoprotein of SARS-CoV-1 downregulates ACE2 by shedding its ectodomain, an enzymatically active domain, and transforming it to soluble ACE2 (sACE2) (65–68). The biological function of sACE2 remains poorly investigated. However, it is assumed that sACE2 may act as a competitive interceptor for SARS-CoV-2 by inhibiting the binding of the S protein to ACE2 (69). A recent study has shown that treatment with clinical-grade human recombinant soluble ACE2 (hrsACE2) *in vitro* significantly inhibited the growth of SARS-CoV-2 in the monkey kidney cells (70), indicating that sACE2 potentially prevents SARS-CoV-2 infection. Howbeit, whether sACE2 plays a role in the disease progress in diabetic patients with SARS-CoV-2 infection remains unknown.

Taken together, ACE2 not only serves as a portal entry for SARS-CoV-2, but also plays a protective role against lung injury in its soluble form. The contradictory function of ACE2, especially, its role in the state with both diabetes and SARS-CoV-2 requires further investigations.

3.5 Diabetes and Furin

Afore mentioned transmembrane S protein of coronavirus is composed of two functional subunits: S1 region, which is responsible for its binding to the host cell ACE2 receptor, and S2 region, which is responsible for fusion of the viral RNA and cellular membranes. The S1 region could be cut and released by proteases, following by the entry of virus into the cells (71). It was previously discovered that MERS-CoV S protein can be activated by furin, a common protease responsible for membrane fusion (72). Likewise, it has been identified a furin cleavage site at the S1/S2 boundary of SARS-CoV-2 (73), indicating that furin could also cleave SARS-CoV-2 S protein (74) and possibly promote the viral entry.

Interestingly, diabetic patients show increased levels of furin (75). It may be driven by osteopontin, which is a cytokine-like matrix-associated phosphoglycoprotein and is shown to be elevated in diabetes (76). In addition, both T1DM and T2DM are associated with higher levels of plasmin(ogen), a protease enzyme that can cleave S protein of SARS-CoV-2 at furin site (77, 78). Thus, increased levels of furin and plasmin may aggravate the viral infection through assisting their entry, fusion, duplication, and release in cells.

4 COVID-19 MAY TRIGGER/WORSEN THE DEVELOPMENT OF DIABETES

As described above, diabetes worsens SARS-CoV-2 infection through mechanisms including impairing the pulmonary structure and function, disturbing the immune function, enhancing the expression of ACE2, overactivating the mTOR signaling, and inducing the furin levels. However, interplay between diabetes and COVID-19 appears to be bi-directional, as new onset diabetes has been observed in patients with SARS-CoV-2 infection (79). Multicenter regional data from North West London reported that thirty children, aged 23 months to 16.8 years, displayed new onset T1DM in this season. In comparison with the data from a typical year, it represents an additional 12-15 new T1DM cases with an increase rate of 80% during the COVID-19 pandemic (80).

These observations revealed a potential diabetogenic effect of COVID-19. The so induced diabetes may be different from the well-recognized notion of hyperglycemia induced by severe illness-associated stress response. To address the issues about the frequency, phenotype, and pathophysiology of SARS-CoV-2-induced new onset diabetes, an international group of leading diabetes researchers participating in the CoviDIAB Project have established a global registry of patients with SARS-CoV-2-related diabetes (covidiab.e-dendrite.com) (81).

The theoretical basis of new onset diabetes induced by SARS-CoV-2 could be supported by the findings of ACE2 expression in both exocrine and endocrine pancreas (islet cells) (82). In addition to lung, SARS-CoV-2 also attacks other organs and tissues including liver, brain, cardiovascular system, gastrointestinal system and pancreas, largely because of the wide distribution of ACE2 in those organs. Interestingly, the expression of ACE2 on the mRNA level in pancreas is slightly higher than that in the lung (82). Thus, SARS-CoV-2 probably causes the damage of pancreatic islets *via* ACE2 in pancreas (**Table 1**).

SARS-CoV-2 infection may not only worsen the preexisting diabetes but also cause new cases of diabetes in non-diabetic subjects through a direct pancreatic damage and a resultant impairment of insulin secretion from β-cells. This can be partly proved by the study from Wang and colleagues (83). It was found that 9 out of 52 hospitalized patients with SARS-CoV-2-associated pneumonia in China displayed a pancreatic injury, which was determined by the plasma levels of amylase and lipase. Of note, 6/9 of these subjects exhibited moderate increases in plasma glucose (83). This phenomenon is in accordance with what is observed in patients after SARS-CoV-1 infection at the beginning of this century. Yang et al. reported that patients with SARS-CoV-1 infection, who had never received glucocorticoids, presented significantly higher levels of fasting plasma glucose compared to patients with non-SARS pneumonia (87). They supposed that SARS-CoV-1 may mediate the damage of pancreatic β-cells and resulted in a development of 'acute diabetes' in patients with SARS (87). In fact, SARS-CoV-1 has been identified in the pancreas of the patients who died of SARS by means of immunohistochemistry and *in situ* hybridization (88). Thus, coronavirus, SARS-CoV-1 as well as SARS-CoV-2, could be one of the pathogens and trigger the development of diabetes.

Apart from direct pancreatic β-cell damage, abnormal immune response such as inflammatory storm and T cell imbalance could also be another explanation for the new onset diabetes caused by SARS-CoV-2 (**Table 1**). As described previously, cytokines including IL-1β, IL-6, IL-17, TNF-α, and IFNγ were significantly elevated in patients with SARS-CoV-2 infection (29–34). Interestingly, the prospective population-based European Prospective Investigation into Cancer and Nutrition (EPIC)-Potsdam study revealed that a combined elevation of IL-1β and IL-6 has been shown to independently increase the risk of the development of T2DM (84). Th17 cytokine profile, which plays a major role in the regulation of inflammation and hyperglycemia, could mathematically predict T2DM in obese people (89). These findings further suggest that SARS-CoV-2 might trigger the development of new onset diabetes through an overactivation of the immune system.

Moreover, SARS-CoV-2 could worsen the insulin resistance in patients with pre-existing T2DM. As ACE2 expression is particularly amplified in key metabolic organs such as the liver, adipose tissue, and the small intestine (55–57), SARS-CoV-2 may attack these organs, resulting in insulin insensitivity and an exacerbation of hyperglycemia. In addition, it has been reported that acute viral infection by murine cytomegalovirus (MCMV) could induce a rapid development of transient insulin resistance through a specifical downregulation of the insulin receptors in skeletal muscle in rodents (90). Whether SARS-CoV-2 enhances the progression of systemic insulin resistance and its mechanisms still require further investigations.

Notably, glucocorticoid, which is an essential medication to control CRS in COVID-19, impairs insulin sensitivity and result in hyperglycemia too. Human immunodeficiency virus (HIV) protease inhibitors (PIs), such as Lopinavir-ritonavir, are used for the treatment of COVID-19. However, it is reported that HIV PIs may acutely and reversibly inhibit the insulin-responsive glucose transporter 4, leading to peripheral insulin resistance and impaired glucose tolerance (85). In a cross-sectional study recruited 710 HIV-infected patients, lopinavir/ritonavir was found to be significantly associated with some metabolic syndromes after adjustment for age and BMI (86). Thus, some medications, such as glucocorticoid and HIV PIs, which are used for SARS-CoV-2 treatment, should be further evaluated, particularly in SARS-CoV-2 infected patients with pre-existing diabetes or at high risk of diabetes (**Table 1**).

5 TREATMENT OF COVID-19 IN PATIENTS WITH DIABETES

In concerning to an optimized treatment of patients with coexistent diabetes and COVID-19, a glycemic control seems to be very urgent (10, 91). However, there are still several cautions need to be taken to achieve the appropriate therapeutic strategies, especially in T2DM patients.

5.1 Metformin

As mentioned above, SARS-CoV-2 infection might worsen the prognosis of diabetes by dysregulating the AMPK/mTOR signaling (**Figure 1**) (45, 46, 51, 52). Observations suggest that activating AMPK and/or inhibiting mTOR-mediated signaling could be novel therapeutic intervention strategies for COVID-19 treatment (51, 52). Of note, dimethylbiguanide metformin is so far a first-line medication for the treatment of T2DM, which works as an AMPK activator (92). To a certain extent, this molecular mechanism makes the classical medication possible as antivirals in patients with COVID-19.

Interestingly, although a hypoglycemic effect of metformin was discovered in the 1920s, it was disregarded until 1940s when biguanide was reinvestigated in the search for antimalarial agents and repurposed to treat influenza (93). Another biguanide, which is so-called flumamine, is still in use as an anti-influenza and anti-malarial medication in the Philippines (94). As

TABLE 1 | Potential mechanisms of SARS-CoV-2 that triggers and worsens the development of diabetes.

Potential mechanism	Reference
SARS-CoV-2 causes the direct damage of pancreatic islets, partly *via* ACE2 in pancreas	(82, 83)
SARS-CoV-2 causes abnormal immune response such as inflammatory storm and T cell imbalance	(84)
SARS-CoV-2 worsens the insulin resistance through attacking key metabolic organs such as the liver, adipose tissue, and the small intestine	(55–57)
Medications for SARS-CoV-2 treatment, such as glucocorticoid and HIV PIs, impairs insulin sensitivity	(85, 86)

ACE2, Angiotensin-converting enzyme 2; HIV, Human immunodeficiency virus; PI, protease inhibitor; SARS-CoV-2, severe acute respiratory syndrome coronavirus 2; T2DM, type 2 diabetes mellitus.

antivirals, biguanides do not cause lung toxicity. Thus, when inhaled, it may deliver more predictable amount of biguanide to the lung than oral dosing and limit the risk of systemic side-effects (95).

Moreover, metformin exerts anti-inflammatory actions by decreasing the circulating biomarkers of inflammation in people with or without T2DM (96). Metformin can also modulate the immune response and restore immune homeostasis in T cells (97), and more in particular, a reciprocal balance between Th17 and Treg cells *in vitro* and *in vivo* (98). In a cohort of 1,213 hospitalized patients with COVID-19 and pre-existing T2DM, Cheng et al. show that the dynamic trajectories of serum inflammatory factors, including IL-6, IL-2, and TNF-a, all showed lower degrees of elevation in the metformin group than in the non-metformin group, particularly compared to the subgroup of individuals with severe COVID-19 (99). This consists with the findings from Chen et al. that metformin applicants showed overall lower levels of IL-6 on admission compared to ordinary patients (100).

Lately, it was identified that metformin exerts potent antifibrotic effects in the lung by inhibiting transforming growth factor (TGF)-β1 action, suppressing collagen formation, activating peroxisome proliferator-activated receptor γ (PPARγ) signaling and inducing lipogenic differentiation in lung fibroblasts (101). However, there is scant information about the antifibrotic actions of metformin in the context of coronavirus infection.

In this respect, metformin may have the potential to benefit diabetic patients with SARS-CoV-2 infection in some ways (**Figure 2**). Interestingly, two observational studies also identified its application resulted in a decrease in the mortality of patients with COVID-19 and T2DM (102, 103). More extensive studies are necessitated to estimate the effectiveness of metformin in COVID-19. Howbeit, metformin-associated acidosis in these patients, particularly in cases with severe COVID19 needs to be noted (99). Regular monitoring of lactic acid levels is recommended after metformin administration in certain patients.

5.2 DPP4 Inhibitor

DPP4 inhibitors act selectively to inhibit the catalytic activity of DPP4, and are widely used in clinic for the treatment of T2DM (104). A recent retrospective study identified that the use of DPP4 inhibitors was significantly and independently associated with a lower mortality (Hazard ratio 0.13) and a less severe pneumonia among diabetic patients with SARS-CoV-2 infection (105). Consistent results were reported by Solerte and colleagues, that treatment with sitagliptin, a highly selective DPP4 inhibitor, at the time of hospitalization resulted in an improved clinical outcomes and a greater number of hospital discharges (106).

Interestingly, membrane-associated human DPP4 acts as a functional coronavirus receptor (107). Transgenic mice engineered to express human DPP4 (hDPP4) became susceptible to MERS-CoV (108). Moreover, DPP4 also acts as a functional receptor for hCoV-Erasmus Medical Center (hCoV-EMC), another member of coronavirus family, which was identified to cause severe and sometimes lethal lower respiratory tract infection (107). Furthermore, it was identified that the S1 domain of SARS-CoV-2 spike glycoprotein potentially interacts with the human DPP4 by means of a computational model based selective docking (109).

Although above findings revealed that DPP4 serves as a potential co-receptor for coronaviruses, few data have been shown whether DPP4 inhibitors interfere the binding of SARS-CoV-2 to DPP4. Available evidences were mostly derived from studies on MERS-CoV. Anti-DPP4 antibodies blocked acute MERS-CoV infection in susceptible bat cells in a dose-dependent manner (110). Administration of two human anti-DPP4 antibodies (REGN3051 and REGN3048) could interrupt the interaction between MERS-CoV spike protein and hDPP4, and lead to a mitigated lung pathology in mice with experimental MERS-CoV infection (111). Similarly, Tang et al. also reported that human neutralizing antibodies directed against the receptor-binding domain (RBD) of the MERS-CoV spike protein, which blocked the viral binding to hDPP4 (112).

Our previous review has proposed that DPP4 inhibition also presents potential modulatory functions in the immune system (113), which may contributes to a reduction in inflammatory response in patients with SARS-CoV-2 infection (**Figure 2**). DPP4, originally known as the lymphocyte cell surface protein CD26, is widely expressed in many types of immune cells including $CD4^+$ and $CD8^+$ T cells, B cells, natural killer (NK) cells, dendritic cells, and macrophages; and plays a role in the regulation of cell function (113). Enzymatic activity inhibition of DPP4 leads to an upregulation of Treg lymphocytes, downregulation of Th17 cells, and suppression on the secretion of pro-inflammatory cytokines, such as IL-1, 6 and 10 (113). Thus, when applied in T2DM patients with SARS-CoV-2 infection, it would be significant to monitor DPP4 inhibitor-induced alterations in immune indexes.

5.3 PPARγ Activator and GLP-1R Agonist

Certain anti-diabetic drugs like PPARγ activators have been shown to upregulate ACE2 in animal models (114). Treatment of diabetic rats with liraglutide, a glucagon-like peptide 1 receptor (GLP-1R) agonist, also provoked a strong elevation in pulmonary ACE and ACE2 expression on mRNA levels (115). As such, it is speculated that treatment for diabetes with pioglitazone/liraglutide may increase the risk of severe and fatal COVID-19 development (**Figure 2**).

On the other hand, pulmonary lipofibroblasts located in the alveolar interstitium displayed an ability to differentiate into myofibroblasts, which play an integral role in pulmonary fibrosis (57) and are potentially involved in the exacerbation of pneumonia in patients with SARS-CoV-2 infection. Yet, PPARγ activators are able to stabilize lipofibroblasts in their "inactive" state, preventing the transition of the cells into myofibroblasts, so that they inhibit the development of pulmonary fibrosis (116). The therapeutic effect of rosiglitazone in the murine models of bleomycin-induced pulmonary fibrosis is well determined (117, 118). However, the putative pathophysiological significance of these findings in the context of experimental coronavirus infection has not been fully explored.

GLP-1R agonists exert broad anti-inflammatory actions in humans with T2DM as well as in obese individuals (119). It was

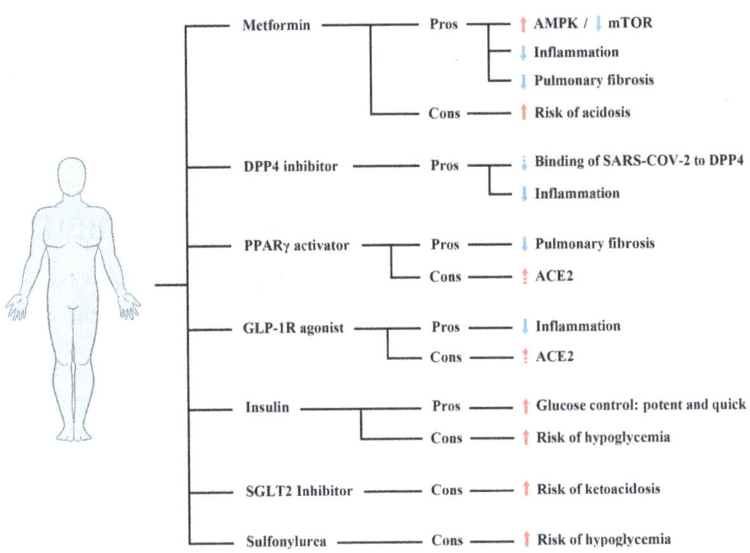

FIGURE 2 | Pros and cons of glycemic lowering agents in diabetic patients with SARS-CoV-2 infection. Dashed arrow represents the assumption requiring further verification. ACE2, Angiotensin-converting enzyme 2; AMPK, Adenosine 5'-monophosphate-activated protein kinase; mTOR, mechanistic target of rapamycin; DPP4, dipeptidyl Peptidase 4; GLP-1R, glucagon-like peptide 1 receptor; PPARγ, peroxisome proliferator-activated receptor γ; SARS-CoV-2, severe acute respiratory syndrome coronavirus 2; SGLT2, sodium-glucose cotransporter 2.

revealed that GLP-1 agonists contribute to a reduction in plasma levels of pro-inflammatory cytokines including TNF-α, IL-1β and IL-6, and an increase in plasma levels of adiponectin, which belongs to the anti-inflammatory adipokines, in T2DM patients (120). Moreover, multiple preclinical studies have demonstrated that GLP-1R agonists attenuate pulmonary inflammation and even preserve lung function in rodent models with experimental lung injury (121–124).

So far, the safety about continuous administration of PPARγ activators and GLP-1R agonists in patients with SARS-CoV-2 infection are not stated. Further studies are needed to clarify whether the administration of these two medicines is suitable for diabetic patients with SARS-CoV-2 infection.

5.4 Insulin, SGLT2 Inhibitor, and Sulfonylurea

Insulin has been extensively used for decades to control blood glucose in critically ill patients with diabetes (125, 126). Accordingly, insulin therapy has been recommended by many experts for the treatment of diabetic patients with SARS-CoV-2 infection (127, 128). However, in a study with 120 patients with COVID-19 and T2DM by Chen et al., the insulin and non-insulin groups showed no significant difference in the percentages of severe and critical illness on admission (100). Surprisingly, a retrospective analysis of 689 patients with COVID-19 and T2DM revealed a markedly increased mortality in patients with insulin treatment (129). Hypoglycemia may be one of the important drivers causing insulin-associated higher mortality. Accordingly, frequent glucose monitoring, even the application of continuous glucose monitoring may lower the rates of hypoglycemia emergence and improve the clinical outcomes.

Sodium-glucose cotransporter 2 (SGLT2) inhibitors are a novel class of anti-diabetic drugs (OADs) which inhibit the reabsorption of sodium and glucose in urine (130). It has been reported that this kind of OAD could increase ketone accumulation and may induce euglycemic ketoacidosis (euDKA) (130). Besides, SARS-CoV-2 infection may be associated with anorexia, dehydration, and rapid deterioration in clinical status. Although SGLT2 inhibitors are generally well tolerated in the outpatient setting, it may still increase the risk of volume depletion and euDKA in symptomatic individuals with T2DM and acute SARS-CoV-2 infection (131). Accordingly, the use of SGLT2 inhibitors should be cautiously re-evaluated in patients with severe SARS-CoV-2 infection, particularly in patients suffering from dehydration. Furthermore, sulfonylureas should be avoided to use in T2DM patients with gastrointestinal symptoms such as diarrhea and nausea, owing to its hypoglycemia side effect.

5.5 Non-Hypoglycemic Agents

ACE inhibitors (ACEIs) and angiotensin II type-I receptor blockers (ARBs) are frequently taken by individuals with diabetes. However, it was found that ACEI and ARB treatment in T1DM and T2DM cause a substantially raise of ACE2 expression in the renal, duodenal, and cardiovascular systems (132–134). Yet, an elevation of ACE2 levels in the respiratory system after ACE/ARBs application has not been reported. Clinical outcomes of patients with SARS-CoV-2 infection who took RAS inhibitors were comparable with those of patients without ACEI/ARB administration (100, 135). Nevertheless, whether these medicines are safe for the treatment of patients with SARS-CoV-2 infection requires more experimental and clinical evidences.

6 CONCLUSIONS

In this review, the relationship of diabetes and COVID-19 were discussed. However, most of the existing studies failed to distinguish the potential difference of type 1 and type 2 diabetes among COVID-19 subjects. Furthermore, we describe the potential mechanisms which are involved in the regulation of an increased susceptibility and illness severity of diabetic patients to COVID-19. On the other hand, SARS-CoV-2 infection may also trigger the new onset diabetes. The rapid increase in new experimental information stemming from the SARS-CoV-2 epidemic requires careful evaluation to help understand the pathology of COVID-19, especially for the treatment of patients with both diabetes and COVID-19. All medications used in diabetes displayed advantages and disadvantages. Physicians should estimate the status of patients individually, especially the risk of hypoglycemia, acidosis and gastrointestinal symptoms, to optimize the therapeutic strategies for glycemic control in patients with SARS-CoV-2 infection.

AUTHOR CONTRIBUTIONS

SS and YC wrote the manuscript. RP and QY edited the manuscript. XY edited the revised manuscript. All authors contributed to the article and approved the submited version.

REFERENCES

1. Drosten C, Gunther S, Preiser W, van der Werf S, Brodt HR, Becker S, et al. Identification of a Novel Coronavirus in Patients With Severe Acute Respiratory Syndrome. *N Engl J Med* (2003) 348(20):1967–76. doi: 10.1056/NEJMoa030747
2. Arabi YM, Balkhy HH, Hayden FG, Bouchama A, Luke T, Baillie JK, et al. Middle East Respiratory Syndrome. *N Engl J Med* (2017) 376(6):584–94. doi: 10.1056/NEJMsr1408795
3. Perlman S, Netland J. Coronaviruses Post-SARS: Update on Replication and Pathogenesis. *Nat Rev Microbiol* (2009) 7(6):439–50. doi: 10.1038/nrmicro2147
4. Lu R, Zhao X, Li J, Niu P, Yang B, Wu H, et al. Genomic Characterisation and Epidemiology of 2019 Novel Coronavirus: Implications for Virus Origins and Receptor Binding. *Lancet* (2020) 395(10224):565–74. doi: 10.1016/S0140-6736(20)30251-8
5. Li F. Structure, Function, and Evolution of Coronavirus Spike Proteins. *Annu Rev Virol* (2016) 3(1):237–61. doi: 10.1146/annurev-virology-110615-042301
6. Guan WJ, Ni ZY, Hu Y, Liang WH, Ou CQ, He JX, et al. Clinical Characteristics of Coronavirus Disease 2019 in China. *N Engl J Med* (2020) 382(18):1708–20. doi: 10.1056/NEJMoa2002032
7. Guan WJ, Liang WH, Zhao Y, Liang HR, Chen ZS, Li YM, et al. Comorbidity and Its Impact on 1590 Patients With COVID-19 in China: A Nationwide Analysis. *Eur Respir J* (2020) 55(5):2000547. doi: 10.1183/13993003.01227-2020
8. Richardson S, Hirsch JS, Narasimhan M, Crawford JM, McGinn T, Davidson KW, et al. Presenting Characteristics, Comorbidities, and Outcomes Among 5700 Patients Hospitalized With COVID-19 in the New York City Area. *JAMA* (2020) 323(20):2052–9. doi: 10.1001/jama.2020.6775
9. Stokes EK, Zambrano LD, Anderson KN, Marder EP, Raz KM, El Burai Felix S, et al. Coronavirus Disease 2019 Case Surveillance - United States, January 22-May 30, 2020. *MMWR Morb Mortal Wkly Rep* (2020) 69(24):759–65. doi: 10.15585/mmwr.mm6924e2
10. Zhu L, She ZG, Cheng X, Qin JJ, Zhang XJ, Cai J, et al. Association of Blood Glucose Control and Outcomes in Patients With COVID-19 and Pre-Existing Type 2 Diabetes. *Cell Metab* (2020) 31(6):1068–77.e1063. doi: 10.1016/j.cmet.2020.04.021
11. Onder G, Rezza G, Brusaferro S. Case-Fatality Rate and Characteristics of Patients Dying in Relation to COVID-19 in Italy. *JAMA* (2020) 323 (18):1775–6. doi: 10.1001/jama.2020.4683
12. Coppelli A, Giannarelli R, Aragona M, Penno G, Falcone M, Tiseo G, et al. Hyperglycemia at Hospital Admission Is Associated With Severity of the Prognosis in Patients Hospitalized for COVID-19: The Pisa COVID-19 Study. *Diabetes Care* (2020) 43(10):2345–8. doi: 10.2337/dc20-1380
13. Wu Z, McGoogan JM. Characteristics of and Important Lessons From the Coronavirus Disease 2019 (COVID-19) Outbreak in China: Summary of a Report of 72314 Cases From the Chinese Center for Disease Control and Prevention. *JAMA* (2020) 323(13):1239–42. doi: 10.1001/jama.2020.2648
14. Wu J, Zhang J, Sun X, Wang L, Xu Y, Zhang Y, et al. Influence of Diabetes Mellitus on the Severity and Fatality of SARS-CoV-2 (COVID-19) Infection. *Diabetes Obes Metab* (2020) 22(10):1907–14. doi: 10.1111/dom.14105
15. Li J, Wang X, Chen J, Zuo X, Zhang H, Deng A. COVID-19 Infection may Cause Ketosis and Ketoacidosis. *Diabetes Obes Metab Oct* (2020) 22 (10):1935–41. doi: 10.1111/dom.14057
16. Armeni E, Aziz U, Qamar S, Nasir S, Nethaji C, Negus R, et al. Protracted Ketonaemia in Hyperglycaemic Emergencies in COVID-19: A Retrospective Case Series. *Lancet Diabetes Endocrinol* (2020) 8(8):660–3. doi: 10.1016/S2213-8587(20)30221-7
17. Kida K, Utsuyama M, Takizawa T, Thurlbeck WM. Changes in Lung Morphologic Features and Elasticity Caused by Streptozotocin-Induced Diabetes Mellitus in Growing Rats. *Am Rev Respir Dis* (1983) 128(1):125–31. doi: 10.1164/arrd.1983.128.1.125
18. Weynand B, Jonckheere A, Frans A, Rahier J. Diabetes Mellitus Induces a Thickening of the Pulmonary Basal Lamina. *Respiration* (1999) 66(1):14–9. doi: 10.1159/000029331
19. Guazzi M, Brambilla R, De Vita S, Guazzi MD. Diabetes Worsens Pulmonary Diffusion in Heart Failure, and Insulin Counteracts This Effect. *Am J Respir Crit Care Med* (2002) 166(7):978–82. doi: 10.1164/rccm.200203-234OC
20. Fuso L, Pitocco D, Antonelli-Incalzi R. Diabetic Lung, an Underrated Complication From Restrictive Functional Pattern to Pulmonary Hypertension. *Diabetes Metab Res Rev* (2019) 35(6):e3159. doi: 10.1002/dmrr.3159
21. Davis WA, Knuiman M, Kendall P, Grange V, Davis TM, Fremantle Diabetes S. Glycemic Exposure Is Associated With Reduced Pulmonary Function in Type 2 Diabetes: The Fremantle Diabetes Study. *Diabetes Care* (2004) 27(3):752–7. doi: 10.2337/diacare.27.3.752
22. Jafar N, Edriss H, Nugent K. The Effect of Short-Term Hyperglycemia on the Innate Immune System. *Am J Med Sci* (2016) 351(2):201–11. doi: 10.1016/j.amjms.2015.11.011
23. Geerlings SE, Hoepelman AI. Immune Dysfunction in Patients With Diabetes Mellitus (DM). *FEMS Immunol Med Microbiol* (1999) 26(3-4):259–65. doi: 10.1111/j.1574-695X.1999.tb01397.x
24. Nielson CP, Hindson DA. Inhibition of Polymorphonuclear Leukocyte Respiratory Burst by Elevated Glucose Concentrations *In Vitro*. *Diabetes* (1989) 38(8):1031–5. doi: 10.2337/diabetes.38.8.1031
25. Stegenga ME, van der Crabben SN, Blumer RM, Levi M, Meijers JC, Serlie MJ, et al. Hyperglycemia Enhances Coagulation and Reduces Neutrophil Degranulation, Whereas Hyperinsulinemia Inhibits Fibrinolysis During Human Endotoxemia. *Blood* (2008) 112(1):82–9. doi: 10.1182/blood-2007-11-121723
26. Perner A, Nielsen SE, Rask-Madsen J. High Glucose Impairs Superoxide Production From Isolated Blood Neutrophils. *Intensive Care Med* (2003) 29 (4):642–5. doi: 10.1007/s00134-002-1628-4
27. Sun L, Louie MC, Vannella KM, Wilke CA, LeVine AM, Moore BB, et al. New Concepts of IL-10-Induced Lung Fibrosis: Fibrocyte Recruitment and

M2 Activation in a CCL2/CCR2 Axis. *Am J Physiol Lung Cell Mol Physiol* (2011) 300(3):L341–353. doi: 10.1152/ajplung.00122.2010
28. Yang Y, Shen C, Li J, Yuan J, Wei J, Huang F, et al. Plasma IP-10 and MCP-3 Levels Are Highly Associated With Disease Severity and Predict the Progression of COVID-19. *J Allergy Clin Immunol* (2020) 146(1):119–27.e114. doi: 10.1016/j.jaci.2020.04.027
29. Huang C, Wang Y, Li X, Ren L, Zhao J, Hu Y, et al. Clinical Features of Patients Infected With 2019 Novel Coronavirus in Wuhan, China. *Lancet* (2020) 395(10223):497–506. doi: 10.1016/S0140-6736(20)30183-5
30. Liu B, Li M, Zhou Z, Guan X, Xiang Y. Can We Use Interleukin-6 (IL-6) Blockade for Coronavirus Disease 2019 (COVID-19)-Induced Cytokine Release Syndrome (CRS)? *J Autoimmun* (2020) 111:102452. doi: 10.1016/j.jaut.2020.102452
31. Maddaloni E, Buzzetti R. Covid-19 and Diabetes Mellitus: Unveiling the Interaction of Two Pandemics. *Diabetes Metab Res Rev* (2020) 31: e33213321. doi: 10.1002/dmrr.3321
32. Mehta P, McAuley DF, Brown M, Sanchez E, Tattersall RS, Manson JJ, et al. COVID-19: Consider Cytokine Storm Syndromes and Immunosuppression. *Lancet* (2020) 395(10229):1033–4. doi: 10.1016/S0140-6736(20)30628-0
33. Pacha O, Sallman MA, Evans SE. COVID-19: A Case for Inhibiting IL-17? *Nat Rev Immunol* (2020) 20(6):345–6. doi: 10.1038/s41577-020-0328-z
34. Zhou F, Yu T, Du R, Fan G, Liu Y, Liu Z, et al. Clinical Course and Risk Factors for Mortality of Adult Inpatients With COVID-19 in Wuhan, China: A Retrospective Cohort Study. *Lancet* (2020) 395(10229):1054–62. doi: 10.1016/S0140-6736(20)30566-3
35. Le TT, Karmouty-Quintana H, Melicoff E, Le TT, Weng T, Chen NY, et al. Blockade of IL-6 Trans Signaling Attenuates Pulmonary Fibrosis. *J Immunol* (2014) 193(7):3755–68. doi: 10.4049/jimmunol.1302470
36. Zhang Y, Li J, Zhan Y, Wu L, Yu X, Zhang W, et al. Analysis of Serum Cytokines in Patients With Severe Acute Respiratory Syndrome. *Infect Immun* (2004) 72(8):4410–5. doi: 10.1128/IAI.72.8.4410-4415.2004
37. Chen G, Wu D, Guo W, Cao Y, Huang D, Wang H, et al. Clinical and Immunological Features of Severe and Moderate Coronavirus Disease 2019. *J Clin Invest* (2020) 130(5):2620–9. doi: 10.1172/JCI137244
38. Guo W, Li M, Dong Y, Zhou H, Zhang Z, Tian C, et al. Diabetes Is a Risk Factor for the Progression and Prognosis of COVID-19. *Diabetes Metab Res Rev* (2020) 31:e3319. doi: 10.1002/dmrr.3319
39. Wang M, Chen F, Wang J, Zeng Z, Yang Q, Shao S. Th17 and Treg Lymphocytes in Obesity and Type 2 Diabetic Patients. *Clin Immunol* (2018) 197:77–85. doi: 10.1016/j.clim.2018.09.005
40. Hodgson K, Morris J, Bridson T, Govan B, Rush C, Ketheesan N. Immunological Mechanisms Contributing to the Double Burden of Diabetes and Intracellular Bacterial Infections. *Immunology* (2015) 144 (2):171–85. doi: 10.1111/imm.12394
41. Kulcsar KA, Coleman CM, Beck SE, Frieman MB. Comorbid Diabetes Results in Immune Dysregulation and Enhanced Disease Severity Following MERS-CoV Infection. *JCI Insight* (2019) 4(20):e131774. doi: 10.1172/jci.insight.131774
42. Xu Z, Shi L, Wang Y, Zhang J, Huang L, Zhang C, et al. Pathological Findings of COVID-19 Associated With Acute Respiratory Distress Syndrome. *Lancet Respir Med* (2020) 8(4):420–2. doi: 10.1016/S2213-2600 (20)30076-X
43. Su Y, Chen D, Yuan D, Lausted C, Choi J, Dai CL, et al. Multi-Omics Resolves a Sharp Disease-State Shift Between Mild and Moderate COVID-19. *Cell* (2020) 183(6):1479–95. doi: 10.1016/j.cell.2020.10.037
44. Qin C, Zhou L, Hu Z, Zhang S, Yang S, Tao Y, et al. Dysregulation of Immune Response in Patients With Coronavirus 2019 (COVID-19) in Wuhan, China. *Clin Infect Dis* (2020) 71(15):762–8. doi: 10.1093/cid/ciaa248
45. Ruderman N, Prentki M. AMP Kinase and Malonyl-CoA: Targets for Therapy of the Metabolic Syndrome. *Nat Rev Drug Discov* (2004) 3 (4):340–51. doi: 10.1038/nrd1344
46. Korsheninnikova E, van der Zon GC, Voshol PJ, Janssen GM, Havekes LM, Grefhorst A, et al. Sustained Activation of the Mammalian Target of Rapamycin Nutrient Sensing Pathway Is Associated With Hepatic Insulin Resistance, But Not With Steatosis, in Mice. *Diabetologia* (2006) 49 (12):3049–57. doi: 10.1007/s00125-006-0439-5
47. Stohr S, Costa R, Sandmann L, Westhaus S, Pfaender S, Anggakusuma, et al. Host Cell Mtorc1 Is Required for HCV RNA Replication. *Gut* (2016) 65 (12):2017–28. doi: 10.1136/gutjnl-2014-308971
48. Kindrachuk J, Ork B, Hart BJ, Mazur S, Holbrook MR, Frieman MB, et al. Antiviral Potential of ERK/MAPK and PI3K/AKT/mTOR Signaling Modulation for Middle East Respiratory Syndrome Coronavirus Infection as Identified by Temporal Kinome Analysis. *Antimicrob Agents Chemother* (2015) 59(2):1088–99. doi: 10.1128/AAC.03659-14
49. Wang CH, Chung FT, Lin SM, Huang SY, Chou CL, Lee KY, et al. Adjuvant Treatment With a Mammalian Target of Rapamycin Inhibitor, Sirolimus, and Steroids Improves Outcomes in Patients With Severe H1N1 Pneumonia and Acute Respiratory Failure. *Crit Care Med* (2014) 42(2):313–21. doi: 10.1097/CCM.0b013e3182a2727d
50. Pinno J, Bongartz H, Klepsch O, Wundrack N, Poli V, Schaper F, et al. Interleukin-6 Influences Stress-Signalling by Reducing the Expression of the mTOR-Inhibitor REDD1 in a STAT3-Dependent Manner. *Cell Signal* (2016) 28(8):907–16. doi: 10.1016/j.cellsig.2016.04.004
51. Conti P, Ronconi G, Caraffa A, Gallenga CE, Ross R, Frydas I, et al. Induction of Pro-Inflammatory Cytokines (IL-1 and IL-6) and Lung Inflammation by Coronavirus-19 (COVI-19 or SARS-CoV-2): Anti-Inflammatory Strategies. *J Biol Regul Homeost Agents* (2020) 34(2):327–31. doi: 10.23812/CONTI-E
52. Zhou Y, Hou Y, Shen J, Huang Y, Martin W, Cheng F. Network-Based Drug Repurposing for Novel Coronavirus 2019-Ncov/SARS-CoV-2. *Cell Discovery* (2020) 6:14. doi: 10.1038/s41421-020-0153-3
53. Tikellis C, Thomas MC. Angiotensin-Converting Enzyme 2 (ACE2) Is a Key Modulator of the Renin Angiotensin System in Health and Disease. *Int J Pept* (2012) 2012:256294. doi: 10.1155/2012/256294
54. Hoffmann M, Kleine-Weber H, Schroeder S, Kruger N, Herrler T, Erichsen S, et al. SARS-CoV-2 Cell Entry Depends on ACE2 and TMPRSS2 and Is Blocked by a Clinically Proven Protease Inhibitor. *Cell* (2020) 181(2):271–80.e278. doi: 10.1016/j.cell.2020.02.052
55. Roca-Ho H, Riera M, Palau V, Pascual J, Soler MJ. Characterization of ACE and ACE2 Expression Within Different Organs of the NOD Mouse. *Int J Mol Sci* (2017) 18(3):563. doi: 10.3390/ijms18030563
56. Wong TP, Ho KY, Ng EK, Debnam ES, Leung PS. Upregulation of ACE2-ANG-(1-7)-Mas Axis in Jejunal Enterocytes of Type 1 Diabetic Rats: Implications for Glucose Transport. *Am J Physiol Endocrinol Metab* (2012) 303(5):E669–81. doi: 10.1152/ajpendo.00562.2011
57. Kruglikov IL, Scherer PE. The Role of Adipocytes and Adipocyte-Like Cells in the Severity of COVID-19 Infections. *Obes (Silver Spring)* (2020) 28 (7):1187–90. doi: 10.1002/oby.22856
58. Rao S, Lau A, So HC. Exploring Diseases/Traits and Blood Proteins Causally Related to Expression of ACE2, the Putative Receptor of SARS-CoV-2: A Mendelian Randomization Analysis Highlights Tentative Relevance of Diabetes-Related Traits. *Diabetes Care* (2020) 43(7):1416–26. doi: 10.2337/dc20-0643
59. Wysocki J, Ye M, Soler MJ, Gurley SB, Xiao HD, Bernstein KE, et al. ACE and ACE2 Activity in Diabetic Mice. *Diabetes* (2006) 55(7):2132–9. doi: 10.2337/db06-0033
60. Mizuiri S, Hemmi H, Arita M, Ohashi Y, Tanaka Y, Miyagi M, et al. Expression of ACE and ACE2 in Individuals With Diabetic Kidney Disease and Healthy Controls. *Am J Kidney Dis* (2008) 51(4):613–23. doi: 10.1053/j.ajkd.2007.11.022
61. Gurwitz D. Angiotensin Receptor Blockers as Tentative SARS-CoV-2 Therapeutics. *Drug Dev Res* (2020) 81(5):537–40. doi: 10.1002/ddr.21656
62. Zhang H, Penninger JM, Li Y, Zhong N, Slutsky AS. Angiotensin-Converting Enzyme 2 (ACE2) as a SARS-CoV-2 Receptor: Molecular Mechanisms and Potential Therapeutic Target. *Intensive Care Med* (2020) 46(4):586–90. doi: 10.1007/s00134-020-05985-9
63. Kuba K, Imai Y, Penninger JM. Angiotensin-Converting Enzyme 2 in Lung Diseases. *Curr Opin Pharmacol* (2006) 6(3):271–6. doi: 10.1016/j.coph.2006.03.001
64. Imai Y, Kuba K, Penninger JM. The Discovery of Angiotensin-Converting Enzyme 2 and Its Role in Acute Lung Injury in Mice. *Exp Physiol* (2008) 93 (5):543–8. doi: 10.1113/expphysiol.2007.040048

65. Jia HP, Look DC, Tan P, Shi L, Hickey M, Gakhar L, et al. Ectodomain Shedding of Angiotensin Converting Enzyme 2 in Human Airway Epithelia. *Am J Physiol Lung Cell Mol Physiol* (2009) 297(1):L84–96. doi: 10.1152/ajplung.00071.2009
66. Haga S, Yamamoto N, Nakai-Murakami C, Osawa Y, Tokunaga K, Sata T, et al. Modulation of TNF-Alpha-Converting Enzyme by the Spike Protein of SARS-CoV and ACE2 Induces TNF-Alpha Production and Facilitates Viral Entry. *Proc Natl Acad Sci USA* (2008) 105(22):7809–14. doi: 10.1073/pnas.0711241105
67. Lambert DW, Yarski M, Warner FJ, Thornhill P, Parkin ET, Smith AI, et al. Tumor Necrosis Factor-Alpha Convertase (ADAM17) Mediates Regulated Ectodomain Shedding of the Severe-Acute Respiratory Syndrome-Coronavirus (SARS-CoV) Receptor, Angiotensin-Converting Enzyme-2 (ACE2). *J Biol Chem* (2005) 280(34):30113–9. doi: 10.1074/jbc.M505111200
68. Kuba K, Imai Y, Rao S, Gao H, Guo F, Guan B, et al. A Crucial Role of Angiotensin Converting Enzyme 2 (ACE2) in SARS Coronavirus-Induced Lung Injury. *Nat Med* (2005) 11(8):875–9. doi: 10.1038/nm1267
69. Batlle D, Wysocki J, Satchell K. Soluble Angiotensin-Converting Enzyme 2: A Potential Approach for Coronavirus Infection Therapy? *Clin Sci (Lond)* (2020) 134(5):543–5. doi: 10.1042/CS20200163
70. Monteil V, Kwon H, Prado P, Hagelkruys A, Wimmer RA, Stahl M, et al. Inhibition of SARS-CoV-2 Infections in Engineered Human Tissues Using Clinical-Grade Soluble Human Ace2. *Cell* (2020) 181(4):905–13.e907. doi: 10.1016/j.molcel.2020.04.022
71. Belouzard S, Chu VC, Whittaker GR. Activation of the SARS Coronavirus Spike Protein *via* Sequential Proteolytic Cleavage at Two Distinct Sites. *Proc Natl Acad Sci USA* (2009) 106(14):5871–6. doi: 10.1073/pnas.0809524106
72. Millet JK, Whittaker GR. Host Cell Entry of Middle East Respiratory Syndrome Coronavirus After Two-Step, Furin-Mediated Activation of the Spike Protein. *Proc Natl Acad Sci USA* (2014) 111(42):15214–9. doi: 10.1073/pnas.1407087111
73. Walls AC, Park YJ, Tortorici MA, Wall A, McGuire AT, Veesler D. Structure, Function, and Antigenicity of the SARS-CoV-2 Spike Glycoprotein. *Cell* (2020) 181(2):281–92.e286. doi: 10.1016/j.cell.2020.02.058
74. Hoffmann M, Kleine-Weber H, Pohlmann S. A Multibasic Cleavage Site in the Spike Protein of SARS-CoV-2 Is Essential for Infection of Human Lung Cells. *Mol Cell* (2020) 78(4):779–84.e775. doi: 10.1016/j.molcel.2020.04.022
75. Fernandez C, Rysa J, Almgren P, Nilsson J, Engstrom G, Orho-Melander M, et al. Plasma Levels of the Proprotein Convertase Furin and Incidence of Diabetes and Mortality. *J Intern Med* (2018) 284(4):377–87. doi: 10.1111/joim.12783
76. Adu-Agyeiwaah Y, Grant MB, Obukhov AG. The Potential Role of Osteopontin and Furin in Worsening Disease Outcomes in COVID-19 Patients With Pre-Existing Diabetes. *Cells* (2020) 9(11):2528. doi: 10.3390/cells9112528
77. Buhl KB, Oxlund CS, Friis UG, Svenningsen P, Bistrup C, Jacobsen IA, et al. Plasmin in Urine From Patients With Type 2 Diabetes and Treatment-Resistant Hypertension Activates ENaC *In Vitro*. *J Hypertens* (2014) 32 (8):1672–1677; discussion 1677. doi: 10.1097/HJH.0000000000000216
78. Ray EC, Miller RG, Demko JE, Costacou T, Kinlough CL, Demko CL, et al. Urinary Plasmin(ogen) as a Prognostic Factor for Hypertension. *Kidney Int Rep* (2018) 3(6):1434–42. doi: 10.1016/j.ekir.2018.06.007
79. Chee YJ, Ng SJH, Yeoh E. Diabetic Ketoacidosis Precipitated by Covid-19 in a Patient With Newly Diagnosed Diabetes Mellitus. *Diabetes Res Clin Pract* (2020) 164:108166. doi: 10.1016/j.diabres.2020.108166
80. Unsworth R, Wallace S, Oliver NS, Yeung S, Kshirsagar A, Naidu H, et al. New-Onset Type 1 Diabetes in Children During COVID-19: Multicenter Regional Findings in the U.K. *Diabetes Care* (2020) 43(11):e170–1. doi: 10.2337/dc20-1551
81. Rubino F, Amiel SA, Zimmet P, Alberti G, Bornstein S, Eckel RH, et al. New-Onset Diabetes in Covid-19. *N Engl J Med* (2020) 383(8):789–90. doi: 10.1056/NEJMc2018688
82. Liu F, Long X, Zhang B, Zhang W, Chen X, Zhang Z. ACE2 Expression in Pancreas May Cause Pancreatic Damage After SARS-CoV-2 Infection. *Clin Gastroenterol Hepatol* (2020) 18(9):2128–2130 e2122. doi: 10.1016/j.cgh.2020.04.040
83. Wang F, Wang H, Fan J, Zhang Y, Wang H, Zhao Q. Pancreatic Injury Patterns in Patients With Coronavirus Disease 19 Pneumonia. *Gastroenterology* (2020) 159(1):367–70. doi: 10.1053/j.gastro.2020.03.055
84. Spranger J, Kroke A, Mohlig M, Hoffmann K, Bergmann MM, Ristow M, et al. Inflammatory Cytokines and the Risk to Develop Type 2 Diabetes: Results of the Prospective Population-Based European Prospective Investigation Into Cancer and Nutrition (EPIC)-Potsdam Study. *Diabetes* (2003) 52(3):812–7. doi: 10.2337/diabetes.52.3.812
85. Koster JC, Remedi MS, Qiu H, Nichols CG, Hruz PW. HIV Protease Inhibitors Acutely Impair Glucose-Stimulated Insulin Release. *Diabetes* (2003) 52(7):1695–700. doi: 10.2337/diabetes.52.7.1695
86. Jerico C, Knobel H, Montero M, Ordonez-Llanos J, Guelar A, Gimeno JL, et al. Metabolic Syndrome Among HIV-Infected Patients: Prevalence, Characteristics, and Related Factors. *Diabetes Care* (2005) 28(1):132–7. doi: 10.2337/diacare.28.1.132
87. Yang JK, Lin SS, Ji XJ, Guo LM. Binding of SARS Coronavirus to Its Receptor Damages Islets and Causes Acute Diabetes. *Acta Diabetol* (2010) 47(3):193–9. doi: 10.1007/s00592-009-0109-4
88. Ding Y, He L, Zhang Q, Huang Z, Che X, Hou J, et al. Organ Distribution of Severe Acute Respiratory Syndrome (SARS) Associated Coronavirus (SARS-CoV) in SARS Patients: Implications for Pathogenesis and Virus Transmission Pathways. *J Pathol* (2004) 203(2):622–30. doi: 10.1002/path.1560
89. Ip B, Cilfone NA, Belkina AC, DeFuria J, Jagannathan-Bogdan M, Zhu M, et al. Th17 Cytokines Differentiate Obesity From Obesity-Associated Type 2 Diabetes and Promote TNFalpha Production. *Obes (Silver Spring)* (2016) 24 (1):102–12. doi: 10.1002/oby.21243
90. Sestan M, Marinovic S, Kavazovic I, Cekinovic D, Wueest S, Turk Wensveen T, et al. Virus-Induced Interferon-Gamma Causes Insulin Resistance in Skeletal Muscle and Derails Glycemic Control in Obesity. *Immunity* (2018) 49(1):164–77.e166. doi: 10.2337/diacare.28.1.132
91. Holman N, Knighton P, Kar P, O'Keefe J, Curley M, Weaver A, et al. Risk Factors for COVID-19-Related Mortality in People With Type 1 and Type 2 Diabetes in England: A Population-Based Cohort Study. *Lancet Diabetes Endocrinol* (2020) 8(10):823–33. doi: 10.1016/S2213-8587(20)30271-0
92. Zhou G, Myers R, Li Y, Chen Y, Shen X, Fenyk-Melody J, et al. Role of AMP-Activated Protein Kinase in Mechanism of Metformin Action. *J Clin Invest* (2001) 108(8):1167–74. doi: 10.1172/JCI13505
93. Bailey CJ. Metformin: Historical Overview. *Diabetologia* (2017) 60(9):1566–76. doi: 10.1007/s00125-017-4318-z
94. Garcia EY. Flumamine, a New Synthetic Analgesic and Anti-Flu Drug. *J Philipp Med Assoc* (1950) 26(7):287–93.
95. Lehrer S. Inhaled Biguanides and mTOR Inhibition for Influenza and Coronavirus (Review). *World Acad Sci J* (2020) 2(3):1. doi: 10.3892/wasj.2020.42
96. Cameron AR, Morrison VL, Levin D, Mohan M, Forteath C, Beall C, et al. Anti-Inflammatory Effects of Metformin Irrespective of Diabetes Status. *Circ Res* (2016) 119(5):652–65. doi: 10.1161/CIRCRESAHA.116.308445
97. Pollak M. The Effects of Metformin on Gut Microbiota and the Immune System as Research Frontiers. *Diabetologia* (2017) 60(9):1662–7. doi: 10.1007/s00125-017-4352-x
98. Kim EK, Lee SH, Lee SY, Kim JK, Jhun JY, Na HS, et al. Metformin Ameliorates Experimental-Obesity-Associated Autoimmune Arthritis by Inducing FGF21 Expression and Brown Adipocyte Differentiation. *Exp Mol Med* (2018) 50(1):e432. doi: 10.1038/emm.2017.245
99. Cheng X, Liu YM, Li H, Zhang X, Lei F, Qin JJ, et al. Metformin Is Associated With Higher Incidence of Acidosis, But Not Mortality, in Individuals With COVID-19 and Pre-Existing Type 2 Diabetes. *Cell Metab* (2020) 32(4):537–47.e533. doi: 10.1016/j.cmet.2020.08.013
100. Chen Y, Yang D, Cheng B, Chen J, Peng A, Yang C, et al. Clinical Characteristics and Outcomes of Patients With Diabetes and COVID-19 in Association With Glucose-Lowering Medication. *Diabetes Care* (2020) 43 (7):1399–407. doi: 10.2337/dc20-0660
101. Kheirollahi V, Wasnick RM, Biasin V, Vazquez-Armendariz AI, Chu X, Moiseenko A, et al. Metformin Induces Lipogenic Differentiation in Myofibroblasts to Reverse Lung Fibrosis. *Nat Commun* (2019) 10(1):2987. doi: 10.1038/s41467-019-10839-0

102. Bramante C, Ingraham N, Murray T, Marmor S, Hoversten S, Gronski J, et al. Observational Study of Metformin and Risk of Mortality in Patients Hospitalized With Covid-19. *medRxiv* (2020) 28:2020.06.19.20135095. doi: 10.1101/2020.06.19.20135095
103. Luo P, Qiu L, Liu Y, Liu XL, Zheng JL, Xue HY, et al. Metformin Treatment Was Associated With Decreased Mortality in COVID-19 Patients With Diabetes in a Retrospective Analysis. *Am J Trop Med Hyg* (2020) 103(1):69–72. doi: 10.4269/ajtmh.20-0375
104. Bergman AJ, Stevens C, Zhou Y, Yi B, Laethem M, De Smet M, et al. Pharmacokinetic and Pharmacodynamic Properties of Multiple Oral Doses of Sitagliptin, a Dipeptidyl Peptidase-IV Inhibitor: A Double-Blind, Randomized, Placebo-Controlled Study in Healthy Male Volunteers. *Clin Ther* (2006) 28(1):55–72. doi: 10.1016/j.clinthera.2006.01.015
105. Mirani M, Favacchio G, Carrone F, Betella N, Biamonte E, Morenghi E, et al. Impact of Comorbidities and Glycemia at Admission and Dipeptidyl Peptidase 4 Inhibitors in Patients With Type 2 Diabetes With COVID-19: A Case Series From an Academic Hospital in Lombardy, Italy. *Diabetes Care* (2020) 43(12):3042–9. doi: 10.2337/dc20-1340
106. Solerte SB, D'Addio F, Trevisan R, Lovati E, Rossi A, Pastore I, et al. Sitagliptin Treatment at the Time of Hospitalization Was Associated With Reduced Mortality in Patients With Type 2 Diabetes and COVID-19: A Multicenter, Case-Control, Retrospective, Observational Study. *Diabetes Care* (2020) 43(12):2999–3006. doi: 10.2337/dc20-1521
107. Raj VS, Mou H, Smits SL, Dekkers DH, Muller MA, Dijkman R, et al. Dipeptidyl Peptidase 4 Is a Functional Receptor for the Emerging Human Coronavirus-EMC. *Nature* (2013) 495(7440):251–4. doi: 10.1038/nature12005
108. Li K, Wohlford-Lenane C, Perlman S, Zhao J, Jewell AK, Reznikov LR, et al. Middle East Respiratory Syndrome Coronavirus Causes Multiple Organ Damage and Lethal Disease in Mice Transgenic for Human Dipeptidyl Peptidase 4. *J Infect Dis* (2016) 213(5):712–22. doi: 10.1093/infdis/jiv499
109. Vankadari N, Wilce JA. Emerging WuHan (COVID-19) Coronavirus: Glycan Shield and Structure Prediction of Spike Glycoprotein and Its Interaction With Human CD26. *Emerg Microbes Infect* (2020) 9(1):601–4. doi: 10.1080/22221751.2020.1739565
110. Cai Y, Yu SQ, Postnikova EN, Mazur S, Bernbaum JG, Burk R, et al. CD26/DPP4 Cell-Surface Expression in Bat Cells Correlates With Bat Cell Susceptibility to Middle East Respiratory Syndrome Coronavirus (MERS-CoV) Infection and Evolution of Persistent Infection. *PloS One* (2014) 9(11): e112060. doi: 10.1371/journal.pone.0112060
111. Pascal KE, Coleman CM, Mujica AO, Kamat V, Badithe A, Fairhurst J, et al. Pre- and Postexposure Efficacy of Fully Human Antibodies Against Spike Protein in a Novel Humanized Mouse Model of MERS-CoV Infection. *Proc Natl Acad Sci USA* (2015) 112(28):8738–43. doi: 10.1073/pnas.1510830112
112. Tang XC, Agnihothram SS, Jiao Y, Stanhope J, Graham RL, Peterson EC, et al. Identification of Human Neutralizing Antibodies Against MERS-CoV and Their Role in Virus Adaptive Evolution. *Proc Natl Acad Sci USA* (2014) 111(19):E2018–26. doi: 10.1073/pnas.1402074111
113. Shao S, Xu Q, Yu X, Pan R, Chen Y. Dipeptidyl Peptidase 4 Inhibitors and Their Potential Immune Modulatory Functions. *Pharmacol Ther* (2020) 209:107503. doi: 10.1016/j.pharmthera.2020.107503
114. Zhang W, Xu YZ, Liu B, Wu R, Yang YY, Xiao XQ, et al. Pioglitazone Upregulates Angiotensin Converting Enzyme 2 Expression in Insulin-Sensitive Tissues in Rats With High-Fat Diet-Induced Nonalcoholic Steatohepatitis. *Scientific World J* (2014) 2014:603409. doi: 10.1155/2014/603409
115. Romani-Perez M, Outeirino-Iglesias V, Moya CM, Santisteban P, Gonzalez-Matias LC, Vigo E, et al. Activation of the GLP-1 Receptor by Liraglutide Increases ACE2 Expression, Reversing Right Ventricle Hypertrophy, and Improving the Production of SP-A and SP-B in the Lungs of Type 1 Diabetes Rats. *Endocrinology* (2015) 156(10):3559–69. doi: 10.1210/en.2014-1685
116. Rehan VK, Torday JS. PPARgamma Signaling Mediates the Evolution, Development, Homeostasis, and Repair of the Lung. *PPAR Res* (2012) 2012:289867. doi: 10.1155/2012/289867
117. Genovese T, Cuzzocrea S, Di Paola R, Mazzon E, Mastruzzo C, Catalano P, et al. Effect of Rosiglitazone and 15-Deoxy-Delta12,14-Prostaglandin J2 on Bleomycin-Induced Lung Injury. *Eur Respir J* (2005) 25(2):225–34. doi: 10.1183/09031936.05.00049704
118. Burgess HA, Daugherty LE, Thatcher TH, Lakatos HF, Ray DM, Redonnet M, et al. PPARgamma Agonists Inhibit TGF-Beta Induced Pulmonary Myofibroblast Differentiation and Collagen Production: Implications for Therapy of Lung Fibrosis. *Am J Physiol Lung Cell Mol Physiol* (2005) 288 (6):L1146–1153. doi: 10.1152/ajplung.00383.2004
119. Drucker DJ. Mechanisms of Action and Therapeutic Application of Glucagon-Like Peptide-1. *Cell Metab* (2018) 27(4):740–56. doi: 10.1016/j.cmet.2018.03.001
120. Hogan AE, Gaoatswe G, Lynch L, Corrigan MA, Woods C, O'Connell J, et al. Glucagon-Like Peptide 1 Analogue Therapy Directly Modulates Innate Immune-Mediated Inflammation in Individuals With Type 2 Diabetes Mellitus. *Diabetologia* (2014) 57(4):781–4. doi: 10.1007/s00125-013-3145-0
121. Viby NE, Isidor MS, Buggeskov KB, Poulsen SS, Hansen JB, Kissow H. Glucagon-Like Peptide-1 (GLP-1) Reduces Mortality and Improves Lung Function in a Model of Experimental Obstructive Lung Disease in Female Mice. *Endocrinology* (2013) 154(12):4503–11. doi: 10.1210/en.2013-1666
122. Toki S, Goleniewska K, Reiss S, Zhang J, Bloodworth MH, Stier MT, et al. Glucagon-Like Peptide 1 Signaling Inhibits Allergen-Induced Lung IL-33 Release and Reduces Group 2 Innate Lymphoid Cell Cytokine Production *In Vivo*. *J Allergy Clin Immunol* (2018) 142(5):1515–28.e1518. doi: 10.1016/j.jaci.2017.11.043
123. Zhou F, Zhang Y, Chen J, Hu X, Xu Y. Liraglutide Attenuates Lipopolysaccharide-Induced Acute Lung Injury in Mice. *Eur J Pharmacol* (2016) 791:735–40. doi: 10.1016/j.ejphar.2016.10.016
124. Bloodworth MH, Rusznak M, Pfister CC, Zhang J, Bastarache L, Calvillo SA, et al. Glucagon-Like Peptide 1 Receptor Signaling Attenuates Respiratory Syncytial Virus-Induced Type 2 Responses and Immunopathology. *J Allergy Clin Immunol* (2018) 142(2):683–7.e612. doi: 10.1016/j.jaci.2018.01.053
125. Clayton SB, Mazur JE, Condren S, Hermayer KL, Strange C. Evaluation of an Intensive Insulin Protocol for Septic Patients in a Medical Intensive Care Unit. *Crit Care Med* (2006) 34(12):2974–8. doi: 10.1097/01.CCM.0000248906.10399.CF
126. Patkova A, Joskova V, Havel E, Kovarik M, Kucharova M, Zadak Z, et al. Energy, Protein, Carbohydrate, and Lipid Intakes and Their Effects on Morbidity and Mortality in Critically Ill Adult Patients: A Systematic Review. *Adv Nutr* (2017) 8(4):624–34. doi: 10.3945/an.117.015172
127. Bornstein SR, Rubino F, Khunti K, Mingrone G, Hopkins D, Birkenfeld AL, et al. Practical Recommendations for the Management of Diabetes in Patients With COVID-19. *Lancet Diabetes Endocrinol* (2020) 8(6):546–50. doi: 10.1016/S2213-8587(20)30152-2
128. Gupta R, Ghosh A, Singh AK, Misra A. Clinical Considerations for Patients With Diabetes in Times of COVID-19 Epidemic. *Diabetes Metab Syndr* (2020) 14(3):211–2. doi: 10.1016/j.dsx.2020.03.002
129. Yu B, Li C, Sun Y, Wang DW. Insulin Treatment Is Associated With Increased Mortality in Patients With COVID-19 and Type 2 Diabetes. *Cell Metab* (2020) 33(1):65–77.e2. doi: 10.1016/j.cmet.2020.11.014
130. Peters AL, Buschur EO, Buse JB, Cohan P, Diner JC, Hirsch IB. Euglycemic Diabetic Ketoacidosis: A Potential Complication of Treatment With Sodium-Glucose Cotransporter 2 Inhibition. *Diabetes Care* (2015) 38 (9):1687–93. doi: 10.2337/dc15-0843
131. Hamblin PS, Wong R, Ekinci EI, Fourlanos S, Shah S, Jones AR, et al. SGLT2 Inhibitors Increase the Risk of Diabetic Ketoacidosis Developing in the Community and During Hospital Admission. *J Clin Endocrinol Metab* (2019) 104(8):3077–87. doi: 10.1210/jc.2019-00139
132. Ferrario CM, Jessup J, Chappell MC, Averill DB, Brosnihan KB, Tallant EA, et al. Effect of Angiotensin-Converting Enzyme Inhibition and Angiotensin II Receptor Blockers on Cardiac Angiotensin-Converting Enzyme 2. *Circulation* (2005) 111(20):2605–10. doi: 10.1161/CIRCULATIONAHA.104.510461
133. Vuille-dit-Bille RN, Camargo SM, Emmenegger L, Sasse T, Kummer E, Jando J, et al. Human Intestine Luminal ACE2 and Amino Acid Transporter Expression Increased by ACE-Inhibitors. *Amino Acids* (2015) 47(4):693–705. doi: 10.1007/s00726-014-1889-6
134. Ishiyama Y, Gallagher PE, Averill DB, Tallant EA, Brosnihan KB, Ferrario CM. Upregulation of Angiotensin-Converting Enzyme 2 After Myocardial Infarction by Blockade of Angiotensin II Receptors. *Hypertension* (2004) 43 (5):970–6. doi: 10.1161/01.HYP.0000124667.34652.1a
135. Bean DM, Kraljevic Z, Searle T, Bendayan R, Kevin O, Pickles A, et al. Angiotensin-Converting Enzyme Inhibitors and Angiotensin II Receptor Blockers Are Not Associated With Severe COVID-19 Infection in a Multi-Site UK Acute Hospital Trust. *Eur J Heart Fail* (2020) 22(6):967–74. doi: 10.1002/ejhf.1924

25

Interleukin-37: A Link Between COVID-19, Diabetes and the Black Fungus

Sima Tokajian[1], Georgi Merhi[1], Charbel Al Khoury[1] and Georges Nemer[2,3]*

[1] *Department of Natural Sciences, School of Arts and Sciences, Lebanese American University, Byblos, Lebanon,*
[2] *Department of Biochemistry and Molecular Genetics, Faculty of Medicine, American University of Beirut, Beirut, Lebanon,*
[3] *Division of Genomics and Translational Biomedicine, College of Health and Life Sciences, Hamad Bin Khalifa University, Doha, Qatar*

Correspondence:
Sima Tokajian
stokajian@lau.edu.lb

The COVID-19 pandemic involved millions of people and diabetes was identified as an associated comorbidity. Initiation of systemic corticosteroids in patients suffering from severe COVID-19 was associated with lower mortality. A surge of invasive fungal infections of the maxillofacial region, namely mucormycosis, was linked to a deadly infection known as black fungus. Black fungus, diabetes, corticosteroids, and coronavirus disease 2019 (COVID-19) all have a dysregulated immune response in common, which partly could also be attributed to interleukin 37 (IL-37). IL-37, a new cytokine of the IL-1 family, known for broadly reducing innate inflammation as well as acquired immune responses. The use of corticosteroids in diabetic COVID-19 patients, crowded hospitals, and lack of medical oxygen should be carefully considered to reduce COVID-associated secondary infections.

Keywords: COVID-19, T2D, corticosteroids, mucormycosis, IL-37

INTRODUCTION

In early December 2019, the first pneumonia cases of unknown origin were identified in Wuhan caused by severe acute respiratory syndrome coronavirus 2 (SARS-CoV-2). The disease is known as coronavirus disease 2019 (COVID-19) with severity ranging from mild to lethal. Symptoms of COVID-19, include, but are not limited to, fever, cough, shortness of breath, muscle aches, anosmia, fatigue, and diarrhea (Molteni et al., 2021). The pandemic involved millions of people with some chronic conditions being associated with severe outcomes. People with preexisting conditions such as diabetes, hyperglycemia, cardiovascular diseases, hypertension, and obesity were linked to higher hospitalization and mortality rates (Rawshani et al., 2018; Corrao et al., 2021). The global diabetes prevalence in 2019 was estimated to be 9.3% (463 million people), with half a billion people suffering (Colagiuri et al., 2019) from diabetes worldwide, and the number was estimated to increase by 25% in 2030. Untreated chronic hyperglycemia imposes damage on numerous cell types and is strongly correlated with limb amputations, kidney failure, and cardiovascular diseases (World Health Organization, 2019). To add a new level of complexity to an already challenging situation, diabetic patients present a high-risk factor for COVID-19 infection. It was pointed out that abnormally high concentrations of glucose in the blood, a feature of diabetes mellitus, may increase the virulence of some pathogens (Joshi et al., 1999; Casqueiro et al., 2012). People with type 2 diabetes (T2D) do not exhibit increased susceptibility to SARS-CoV-2 infection. However, they had more than twice the likelihood for COVID-19-related hospitalization and intensive care admission with a dramatic increase in mortality (Roberts et al., 2020). Guan et al. (2020) showed that 16.2% of the SARS-CoV-2-infected patients that manifested severe symptoms had diabetes. Moreover, results obtained by Zhang et al. (2020) provided further evidence that diabetes was

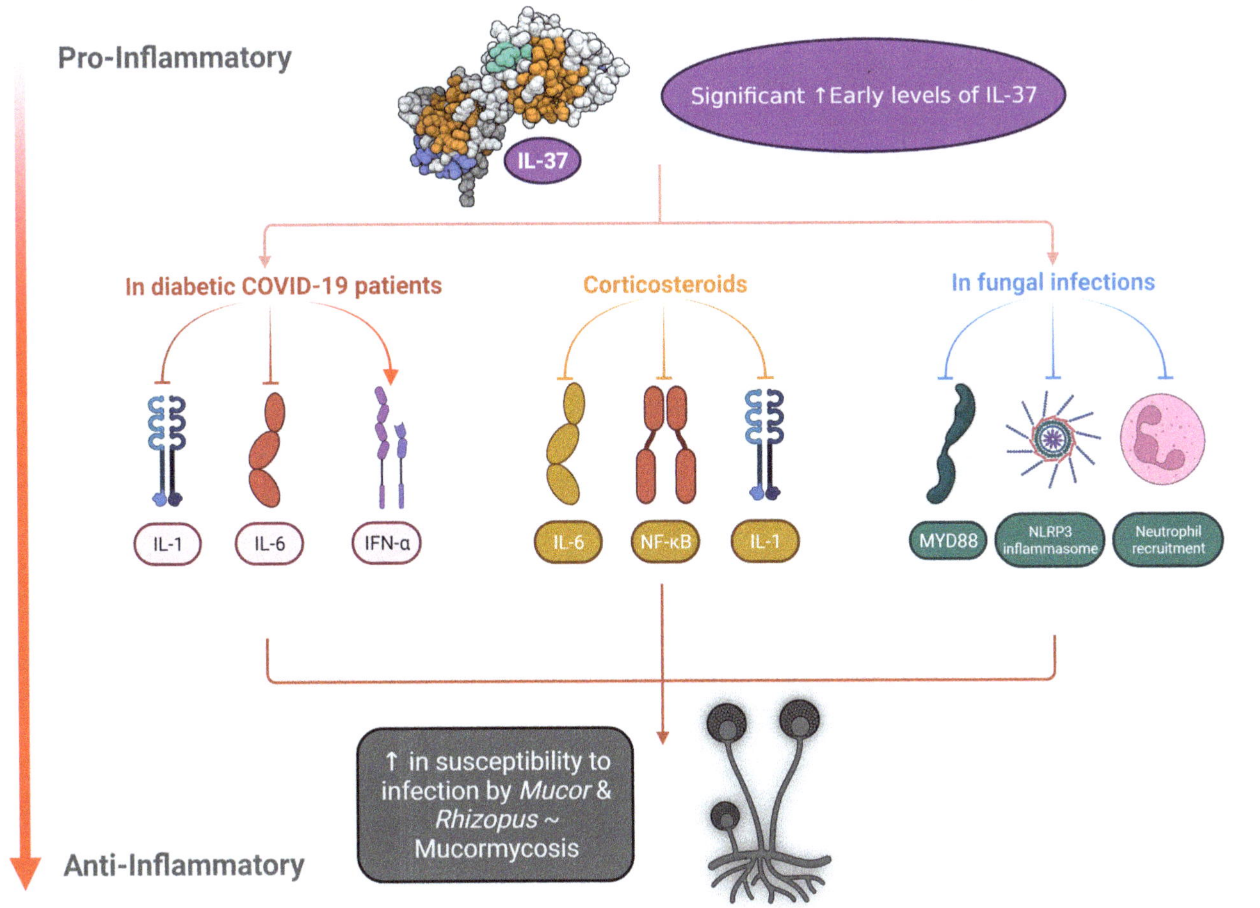

GRAPHICAL ABSTRACT |

among the most common comorbidities seen (Kayina et al., 2020) among COVID-19 patients. Higher blood glucose levels were also detected in COVID-19 patients. In diabetic this can be attributable to (i) interference of macrophages and T-cell cytokines release diminishing neutrophil recruitment (Delamaire et al., 1997) (ii) reduction of interferon-α (IFN-α) production by blood dendritic cells (Summers et al., 2006) and (iii) disruption of innate immune responses (Zykova et al., 2000). Additionally, the virus surface spike protein facilitates its entry through (Hoffmann et al., 2020) attaching to the human angiotensin-converting enzyme 2 (ACE2) *via* its receptor-binding domain, and targeting ACE2 in the endocrine tissues of the pancreas leading as a result to islets damage (Yang et al., 2010). Liu et al. (2020) revealed the significant pancreatic damage that could occur in patients infected with SARS-CoV-2. The authors expressed mounting concern about the long-term effects of SARS-CoV-2 infection on patients that may be due to its increased infectivity and affinity relative to the other coronaviruses. Here, we review and highlight the interrelationship between T2D and severe clinical course and outcomes of COVID-19 patients.

TYPE 2 DIABETES PATHOGENESIS AND THE ROLE INTERLEUKIN 37

Obesity leads to adipose tissue dysfunction that was directly linked to the development of health hazards such as diabetes mellitus and cardiovascular diseases. The adipose tissue expansion occurs through hypertrophy (increase in existing adipocyte size) and hyperplasia (increase in adipocyte number) (Greenberg and Obin, 2006). The fat tissue was recognized as a highly active endocrine organ mainly producing inflammatory mediators known as adipokines (Kershaw and Flier, 2004). Adipokines are a family of hormones having anti- or pro-inflammatory effects (Tilg and Moschen, 2006). In the event of obesity, more pro-inflammatory cytokines were produced when compared to the anti-inflammatory ones (Shibata et al., 2017). For that, T2D is associated with low-grade chronic inflammation linked to excessive visceral adipose tissue, affecting homeostatic glucose regulation and peripheral insulin sensitivity (Iacobellis, 2020). Tumor necrosis factor α (TNF-α), resistin, and interleukin-6 (IL-6) were linked previously to insulin resistance, while adiponectin was found to enhance insulin

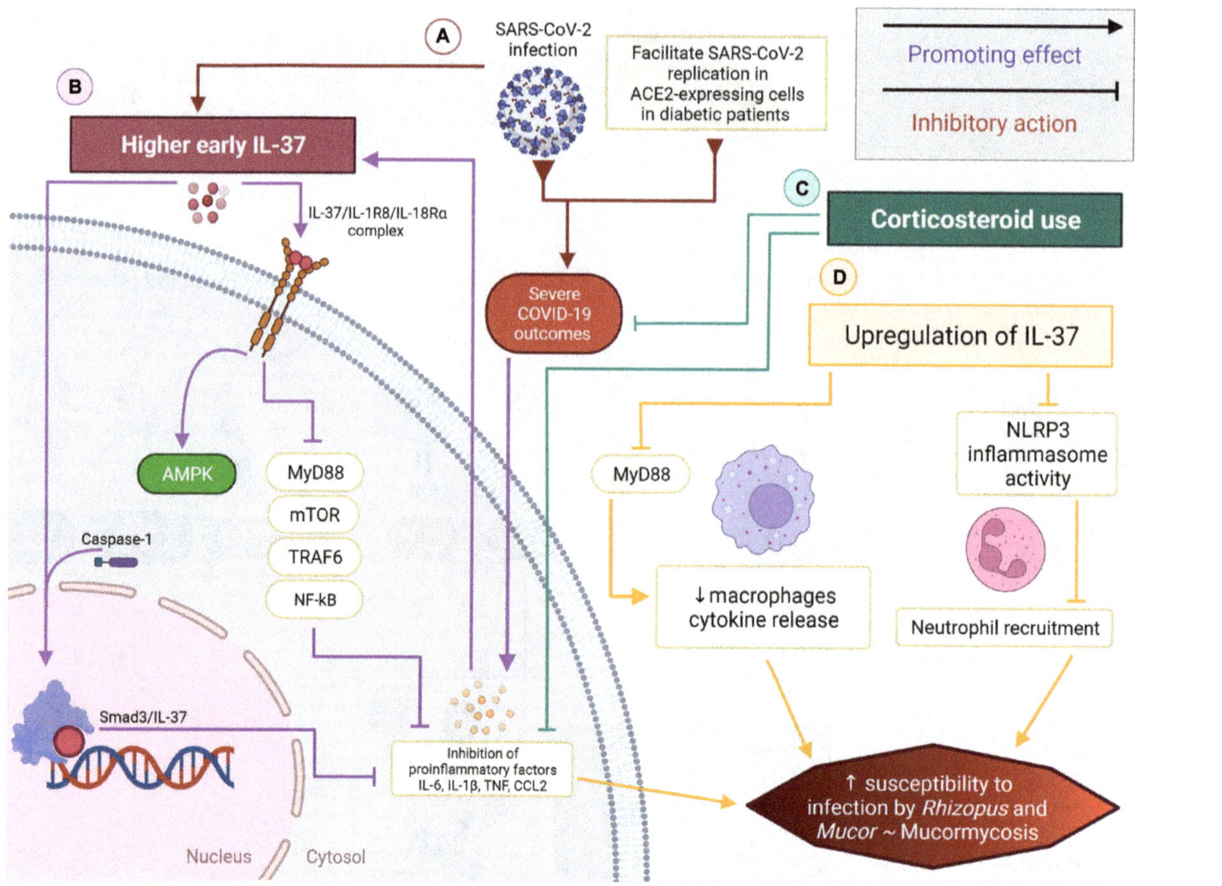

FIGURE 1 | The role of IL-37 and corticosteroids in diabetic COVID-19 patients and their association with the black fungus infection. **(A)** SARS-CoV-2 infection in hyperglycemic patients promotes a dysregulated pro-inflammatory cytokine storm while also promoting higher early expression of IL-37 **(B)** IL-37/IL-1R8/IL-18Rα complex inhibits the mobilization of MyD88, mTOR, TRAF6, NF-κB, subsequently impeding the secretion of pro-inflammatory cytokines. IL-37 could be directly processed by caspase-1, intracellularly, and associates with SMAD3 in the nucleus. **(C)** Corticosteroids and the loss of immune homeostasis linked partly to IL-37, coupled with diabetes, can increase the risk of black fungus infection/mucormycosis. **(D)** Higher early IL-37 and corticosteroid use in diabetic COVID-19 patients inhibit proinflammatory signals. The upregulation of IL-37 interferes with the innate immune system driven inflammation by promoting the decrease of macrophage cytokine release, reducing the NLRP3 inflammasome activity and inhibiting neutrophil recruitment. These factors, when combined, significantly elevate the risk and susceptibility to mucormycosis.

sensitivity, increase glucose transepithelial transport, lower glucose synthesis in the liver, and suppress IL-6 and TNF-α (Yamauchi and Kadowaki, 2008).

Inflammation has an active role in the pathogenesis of hyperglycemia (Gianchandani et al., 2020), and acute viral respiratory infection by SARS-CoV was linked to transient insulin resistance and hyperglycemia induced by a temporary inflammation of the pancreas' islet cells (Yang et al., 2010). Stress hyperglycemia, which is a temporary increase in blood sugar, may have a negative impact in acute illness (Corrao et al., 2021). Chronic hyperglycemia and inflammation can cause an abnormal and ineffective immune response with the combined elevated levels of interleukin-1β (IL-1β), IL-6, and C-reactive protein (CRP) being predictive of T2D (Manson et al., 2001; **Figure 1**). Hypoxia and cell death of expanding adipose tissue, activation of the nuclear factor-κB (NF-κB) and JUN *N*-terminal kinase (JNK) pathway, activation of interleukin-1β (IL-1β), and recruitment and activation of immune cells were all linked to the inflammatory state in T2D (Donath and Shoelson, 2011; Gianchandani et al., 2020). IL-1 family cytokines play a crucial role in immune homeostasis. Strikingly, most proinflammatory factors present at high levels in the blood of patients with T2D were IL-1 dependent, with IL-37 adjusting obesity-induced inflammation and insulin resistance (Ballak et al., 2014; **Table 1**). IL-37 plays an important role in metabolic and autoimmune diseases as well as infections. The development in the *in silico* research of human databases has led to the discovery of IL-37 by several independent groups (Boraschi et al., 2011). Fragments of mRNA sequence encoding an IL-1-like molecule were expressed in human databases (accession number AI014548) and characterized by having five different isoforms (IL-37a-e) (Busfield et al., 2000; Kumar et al., 2000; Pan et al., 2001). IL-37, which can be produced in intra- and extracellular domains, was linked to anti-inflammatory actions through inhibiting innate responses (Dinarello and Bufler, 2013) and detected in the nucleus affecting gene transcription. The

TABLE 1 | The role of IL-37 and its biological functions in infectious and metabolic syndrome associated diseases.

Biological function/Role of IL-37 in infectious diseases and metabolic syndrome and associated diseases	Mechanism of function	References
Protective against Gram-negative LPS induced septic shock	Downregulating the expression of proinflammatory cytokines IL-6, INF-γ, IL-1β, IL-17 and attenuating the action of DCs.	Nold et al., 2010
Inhibits HIV replication	Significant increase in IL-37 mRNA transcription.	Su and Tao, 2021
Potent anti-inflammatory agent in viral-mediated myocarditis	Lowers IL-6 and IL-17A levels. Increases IL-10 expression. Modulates Th17 and Treg cells functions.	An et al., 2017
Linked to significant increase in liver tissue damage in chronic Hepatitis B patients	Not well understood	Li et al., 2013
Higher early IL-37 responses linked to positive COVID-19 prognosis	Blocking IL-1 related cytokine storm. Lowers levels of IL-6 and IL-8. Increases levels of IFN-α.	Su and Tao, 2021
Disseminated candidiasis	Inhibits TNF-α expression and neutrophil recruitment.	van de Veerdonk et al., 2015
Limits inflammatory response mediated by *Aspergillus* infection-protective for lung tissues.	Lowers NLRP3 dependent neutrophil recruitment and inflammasome activity. Decrease in IL-1β secretion.	Allam et al., 2020
Poor prognosis of Eumycetoma which is driven by infection with *Madurella mycetomatis*.	Diminished levels of IL-1β.	Abushouk et al., 2019
Reduces pro-inflammatory cytokine secretion in adipose tissue ameliorating metabolic syndrome associated diseases- obesity and type 2 diabetes (T2D)	Reduction in lipid buildup in the liver Boosts insulin-dependent response and decreases macrophage permeability to adipose tissue Increase in the release of adiponectin coupled with the decrease of leptin in adipose tissue	Cavalli and Dinarello, 2018, Su and Tao, 2021
Athero-protective in atherogenesis Sustains plaque stability in COVID-19 patients	Lessens oxidized low-density lipoprotein (oxLDL) buildup. Downregulates Treg activation, with a reduction in IL-1β, IL-6 and IL-12 expression.	Law et al., 2021

expression levels of TNF, IL-1, IL-6, and chemokine MIP-2 were significantly decreased in lipopolysaccharide (LPS)-stimulated macrophages transfected with human IL-37 when compared to those transfected with an empty plasmid (Nold et al., 2010). Sharma et al. (2008) showed that efficient caspase-1 inhibitors can reduce IL-37 entry to the nucleus, and hence caspase-1 processing could be fundamental for IL-37 translocation. Translocation to the nucleus, after caspase-1 processing, involves SMAD3, which is part of TGF-β anti-inflammatory signaling pathway (**Figure 1**). Investigations were conducted to confirm the functional interaction of SMAD3 with IL-37. Nold et al. (2010) observed the formation of IL-37-SMAD3 complex in perinuclear and cytosolic regions in IL-37-transfacted A549 cells. This correlated favorably with the results obtained previously (Bar et al., 2004) and which demonstrated that the inhibition of SMAD3 could be accountable in reversing the inhibition of IL-6 and IL-1 expression in cells transfected with IL-37. Furthermore, it was exhibited that the potential for IL-37 to reduce the production of IL-1, IL-9, IL-6 and TNF decreased after introducing short hairpin RNA (shRNA) into human macrophages and which inhibited SMAD3 expression (Nold et al., 2010). IL-37 exerts inhibitory properties on the innate inflammatory and acquired immune responses and has a dualfunction with both intra- and extracellular mechanisms of action (Bulau et al., 2014). IL-18 induces activation of IL-1 receptor-associated kinase and tumor necrosis factor (TNF) receptor-associated factor 6 (TRAF-6), with the net outcome of activating the kinases being the translocation of NF-κB (Matsumoto et al., 1997). IL-37 may also inhibit IL-18 dependent pro-inflammatory cytokine production (Ballak et al., 2014). IL-37b and IL-18 are phylogenetically related, and both have two symmetric key structural amino acid residues (Glu-35 and Lys-124) (Dinarello and Bufler, 2013). IL-37 could also interact and bind, but with low affinity, to IL-18 receptor α subunit (IL-18Rα) (Dinarello and Bufler, 2013). IL-37, however, binds to the IL-18 binding protein (IL-18BP), the natural inhibitor of IL-18, and forms a complex reducing IL-18's activity. IL-37b is the receptor antagonist of IL-18, it binds to the IL-18 binding protein (IL-18BP) followed by binding to the IL-18Rα, recruiting IL-1R8, and forming the IL-37/IL-1R8/IL-18Rα complex (Donath and Shoelson, 2011).

CORRELATION BETWEEN INTERLEUKIN 37 AND COVID-19

The potential involvement of IL-37 in suppressing the cytokine storm that contributes to poor prognosis and mortality in COVID-19 patients was studied (Ragab et al., 2020). The mass release of pro-inflammatory cytokines causes acute respiratory distress syndrome and multiple organ failure (Ragab et al., 2020). Controlling the cytokine storm is critical in preventing the progression of the disease and saving patients' lives. A noteworthy strategy that comes into play are anti-inflammatory factors, such as IL-37, that can maintain biochemical homeostasis. Since IL-37 is considered as the natural inhibitor of IL-1, the main modulator of pro-inflammatory cytokines and inflammatory responses, it is safe to assume that IL-37 could provide relief in systemic inflammation that occurs after COVID-19 infection (**Table 1**). Recently, the correlation between IL-37 production, pro-inflammatory cytokines level, and clinical outcomes in SARS-CoV-2 infection was revealed (Li et al., 2021). An enzyme linked immunosorbent assay demonstrated significantly higher concentrations of IL-37 in the plasma of SARS-CoV-2-infected subjects when compared to healthy ones. Li et al. (2021), showed that mild and severe clinical outcomes are directly associated with reduced and elevated plasma levels of IL-37, respectively. Given the fact that high early IL-37 responses were accompanied with speedy recovery among hospitalized patients (earlier viral clearance, chest tomographic improvement, and cough relief) (**Table 1**), the authors suggested that IL-37 administration may be used to maintain a balanced inflammatory response (Li et al., 2021). Moreover, Ahmed and Ad'hiah (2021a) revealed the role of IL-37 in the virus-mediated pathogenesis. In a case-control study involving 200 patients, the sequencing of the *IL37* gene (Gene ID: 27178) identified a couple of single nucleotide polymorphisms (SNPs) that were directly linked with the susceptibility to COVID-19. The two variants of *IL*37 gene with rs3811046 and rs3811047 SNPs, may increase the risk of developing COVID-19 by 2.55 and 2.02-fold. The authors showed a significant correlation between the presence of these polymorphisms and increased incidence of severe COVID-19. The data revealed that SNP rs3811046 detection was significantly higher in patients (61%) when compared to controls (38.0%), which was also the case with SNP rs3811047 (patients 39% vs. controls 24%). In contrast to the previous findings, a more recent study showed that IL-37 expression was suppressed in COVID-19 patients but was prominent in obese patients (Ahmed and Ad'hiah, 2021b). Therefore, it is evident that low IL-37 plasma levels could be used as COVID-19 severity marker. IL-37 was also found to ameliorate influenza pneumonia *in vivo* (Qi et al., 2019). Interestingly, treatment of H1N1-infected mice using IL-37 reduced (by 2 days) the body weight recovery time. The body weights of mice treated with oseltamivir phosphate in combination with IL-37 and oseltamivir phosphate alone began to increase at 7- and 9-days post-inoculation, respectively. The intravenous IL-37 administration improved the survival rates in H1N1- infected mice with a total of 71% of the mice surviving, compared to 57% survival when using a single dose of oseltamivir phosphate. IL-37 additionally relieved H1N1-induced lung tissue damage. The correlation between IL-37 and severity of viral infection was noteworthy. IL-37 treatment modulates (suppresses) the immune response by shifting the cytokine equilibrium away from excess inflammation. Qi et al. (2019) also demonstrated that IL-37 can reduce the levels of pro-inflammatory modulators in mice infected with respiratory viruses. Using RT-qPCR as well as Cytometric Beads Array, they showed that IL-37 treatment significantly reduced the excessive production of IL-6, TNF-α, MCP-1, IL-1α, IL-1β, MIP-1α, MIP-1β, IP-10, MIG, RANTES, IFN-γ and IL-10 in the lung tissues of infected mice.

DIABETES AND COVID-19

Diabetes has been identified as comorbidity associated with COVID-19 severity. Higher risks of COVID-19-related mortality was linked to cardiovascular and renal complications associated with diabetes, glycemic control, and body mass index (BMI) (Holman et al., 2020). Blood glucose level was revealed to be a key mediator of severe symptoms in COVID-19. Persistent inflammation is associated with a compensatory anti-inflammatory response. T2D-related immunosuppression may facilitate SARS-CoV-2 replication in ACE2-expressing cells, promoting cytokine storms and inducing immune dysregulation, partly explaining the more severe COVID-19 outcomes in patients with diabetes (Roberts et al., 2020). IL-37 performs its immunosuppressive activity by acting on mTOR and increasing the adenosine monophosphate (AMP) kinase. It inhibits class II histocompatibility complex (MHC) molecules and inflammation in inflammatory diseases by suppressing MyD88 and subsequently IL-1β, IL-6, TNF, and CCL2 (Conti et al., 2020; **Figure 1**). Li et al. (2019) revealed the association between IL-37 and T2D. The authors showed an overexpression of IL-37 in the peripheral blood monocyte cells of T2D patients when compared to healthy controls. A significant difference was detected using ELISA between the serum level of IL-37 in T2D vs. control subjects. Additionally, the study showed that gut microbiota dysbiosis significantly contributed to the development of T2D and that a better response to insulin therapy was seen in patients with higher IL-37 levels (Ballak et al., 2014; Li et al., 2019). Furthermore, a mouse model receiving high-fat diet treatment provided further evidence on the link between IL-37 and T2D. IL-37 increases insulin sensitivity and reduces gut microbiota dysbiosis.

CORTICOSTEROIDS AND THE BLACK FUNGUS

Numerous therapeutic options to modulate the inflammatory response against SARS-CoV-2-infection were considered. It is widely known that corticosteroids administration successfully prohibits extensive immune responses and accordingly used in controlling hyperinflammation and acute respiratory distress syndrome (Barnes, 2006). During the COVID-19 pandemic, an alarmingly high prevalence of self-medication was reported (Quispe-Cañari et al., 2021), with the corticosteroids being one of the most drugs used due to their high affordability and accessibility (Chaudhry et al., 2021). The RECOVERY Collaborative Group demonstrated that the incidence of death was lower in patients treated with dexamethasone (29.3%) when compared to those who received usual care (41.4%) (Recovery Collaborative Group, 2021). The World Health Organization (WHO) has recommended against using corticosteroids for COVID-19 treatment, but this recommendation was later reversed (World Health Organization, 2020). Corticosteroids regulate inflammation and can block the function of transcription factors mediating inflammatory responses, such as NF-κB and activator protein 1 (AP-1) and inhibit the production of proinflammatory cytokines (IL-1, TNFα, IL-6) (Cain and Cidlowski, 2017). However, the utilization of corticosteroids appears to be a double-edged sword against COVID-19. Their use in respiratory viral infection was linked to an increased risk of secondary opportunistic bacterial or fungal infections (Conti et al., 2020). A surge of invasive fungal infections (IFI) of the maxillofacial region, namely mucormycosis, was reported in India and linked to a rare and possibly deadly infection known as black fungus. Mucormycosis, previously known as zygomycosis, is rare, though increasingly prevalent, and a dangerous angio-invasive infection caused by mucormycetes

(Skiada et al., 2020). The most common causative agents of the disease are *Rhizopus* and *Mucor* (Roden et al., 2005). These ubiquitous fungi can be found particularly in the soil in association with decaying leaves, compost piles, and rotten wood (Sridhara et al., 2005). Mucormycetes infections occur more frequently in summer and fall compared to the winter and spring and affect the sinuses and the lungs after inhaling fungal conidia (Sugar, 1990). The fungus can also be introduced through a break in the skin such as a cut, burn, or other types of skin injury (Roden et al., 2005). The mucormycetes invade blood vessels which may reduce the blood and nutrient flow to downstream organs consequently leading to necrosis (Skiada et al., 2020). Hosts susceptible to mucormycosis include diabetics, those on systemic corticosteroid use, and immunocompromised individuals. Healthcare-associated mucormycosis is a matter of concern and was previously linked to the use of contaminated devices or environmental reservoirs (Rammaert et al., 2012b).

Opportunistic fungal infections, such as the black fungus commonly seen in diabetics, hyperglycemia, COVID-19 patients, and linked to corticosteroids have all in common a dysregulated immune response that partly could also be attributed to IL-37 (Rammaert et al., 2012a; van Paassen et al., 2020; Kumar et al., 2021). A significant correlation exists between well-controlled blood glucose and lower serum levels of inflammatory markers such as IL-6, high sensitivity c-reactive protein (CRP), and lactate dehydrogenase in COVID-19 patients (Gianchandani et al., 2020). Corticosteroids, on the other hand, can downregulate the expression of IL-37, which plays an essential regulatory role in innate and adaptive immunity. Its expression in human adipose tissue was associated with enhanced insulin sensitivity and reduced adipose tissue inflammation (**Table 1**; Ballak et al., 2014). IL-37 exerts significant anti-inflammatory and metaboregulatory effects, dramatically reducing cytokine secretion in macrophages and dendritic cells, with higher early IL-37 responses in COVID-19 patients leading to earlier viral RNA negative conversion (Wang et al., 2018; Yi et al., 2020). It protects the body by inhibiting excessive immune response. Still, it could also lead to increased infection and mortality caused by some pathogens, possibly due to its inhibitory effects on the immune response. The regulatory role it plays could explain the link between the severity of COVID-19 in some diabetic patients being treated with corticosteroids and their potential to additionally acquire black fungus disease in poorly maintained critical care units.

INTERLEUKIN 37 AND ITS CENTRAL ROLE IN COVID-19, DIABETES, AND MUCORMYCOSIS

Most serious fungal disease arises from poorly cleared infection or disrupted barrier integrity (Rautemaa-Richardson and Richardson, 2021). Mucormycosis is an invasive and potentially life-threatening opportunistic fungal infection. The predisposing conditions vary geographically with diabetes mellitus being the most common risk factor in Asia (Hoang et al., 2020). Different subtypes of monocytes and macrophages play a pivotal role in the production of pro-inflammatory mediators and initiation of an inflammatory response. Previously Waldorf et al. (1984) showed that bronchoalveolar macrophages formed part of an efficient defense against *Rhizopus oryzae* by inhibiting germination and interfering with the conversion of *R. oryzae* to its tissue invasive phase. Neutrophils and monocytes are critical components of the host response to mucormycosis which efficiently eliminate fungal spores and hyphae by oxidative and non-oxidative killing mechanisms (Diamond et al., 1982; Waldorf et al., 1984). Enhanced susceptibility to mucormycosis was observed in human diabetics. Hyperglycemia and acidosis are known to impair chemotaxis and the killing activity of phagocytic cells against Mucorales by weakening oxidative and non-oxidative mechanisms (Chinn and Diamond, 1982). Corticosteroids, on the other hand, act on monocytes and macrophages, induce anti-inflammatory mediators and differentiation of anti-inflammatory phenotypes, and limit T-cell activation (Ehrchen et al., 2019).

IL-37, as mentioned above, is also an inhibitor of innate immunity through the caspase-1-dependent nuclear translocation or by the extracellular mechanism engaging the IL-18 receptor (**Figure 1** and **Table 1**; Bulau et al., 2014). The timing of IL-37 expression at the site of inflammation is critical. IL-37 based anti-inflammatory strategies could have a negative impact on susceptibility to infections by inhibiting host defenses or be beneficial for the outcome of the host. Higher early IL-37 responses were correlated with earlier viral RNA negative conversion, chest computed tomographic improvement, and cough relief in COVID-19 patients (Li et al., 2021). In contrast, IL-37 interfered with the innate protective anti-*Candida* host response by reducing the production of proinflammatory cytokines and suppressing neutrophil recruitment in response to *Candida* (**Table 1**), resulting in an increased susceptibility to disseminated candidiasis (van de Veerdonk et al., 2015).

CONCLUSION

There are several measures that can be employed to minimize COVID-19 mortalities and reduce the risk of mucormycosis in people with diabetes. Maintaining and monitoring the glucose level is essential to improve outcomes and reduce secondary infections, renal dysfunction, ICU stay, and ventilator dependence. The pro-inflammatory metabolic state in diabetic patients could promote a virus-linked inflammatory surge leading to insulin resistance and severe hyperglycemia. People with diabetes and COVID-19 should be monitored for inflammatory and prothrombotic markers (Gianchandani et al., 2020). CRP is a good inflammatory marker revealing the association between diabetes and adverse COVID-19 outcomes, including the need for ICU admission, dyspnea, and length of stay (Koh et al., 2021), whereas fibrinogen for coagulation dysfunction (Varikasuvu et al., 2021). The use of corticosteroids can modulate the risk when used prudently. Limitations to their use associated with corticosteroid-mediated inhibition of glucose uptake and reductions in insulin sensitivity in COVID-19 patients and their role in increasing the susceptibility to acquire other infections are among the major concerns. IL-37 is a cytokine that exerts anti-inflammatory effects both intracellularly and extracellularly and is a therapeutic approach that should be considered and further studied. Finally, epidemiological observations combined with molecular epidemiology and experimental data are needed to understand and uncover risk factors related to the host, the pathogen, and variants of concern.

AUTHOR CONTRIBUTIONS

ST: conceptualization. ST, GM, CA, and GN: investigation, writing—original draft, and writing—review and editing. ST and GN: validation. All authors contributed to the article and approved the submitted version.

ACKNOWLEDGMENTS

We would like to thank the insightful comments of the reviewers of this article.

REFERENCES

1. Abushouk, A., Nasr, A., Masuadi, E., Allam, G., Siddig, E. E., and Fahal, A. H. (2019). The Role of Interleukin-1 cytokine family (IL-1β, IL-37) and interleukin-12 cytokine family (IL-12, IL-35) in eumycetoma infection pathogenesis. *PLoS Negl. Trop. Dis.* 13:e0007098. doi: 10.1371/journal.pntd.000 7098
2. Ahmed, A. A., and Ad'hiah, A. H. (2021a). Interleukin-37 gene polymorphism and susceptibility to coronavirus disease 19 among Iraqi patients. *Meta Gene* 31:100989. doi: 10.1016/j.mgene.2021.100989
3. Ahmed, A. A., and Ad'hiah, A. H. (2021b). Interleukin-37 is down-regulated in serum of patients with severe coronavirus disease 2019 (COVID-19). *Cytokine* 148:155702. doi: 10.1016/j.cyto.2021.155702
4. Allam, G., Gaber, A. M., Othman, S. I., and Abdel-Moneim, A. (2020). The potential role of interleukin-37 in infectious diseases: role of IL-37 in HIV-1, viral myocarditis, HCV, HBV, tuberculosis, leprosy, pneumonia, listeria, aspergillosis, candidiasis, and eumycetoma infection. *Int. Rev. Immunol.* 39, 3–10. doi: 10.1080/08830185.2019.1677644
5. An, B., Liu, X., Li, G., and Yuan, H. (2017). IL-37 ameliorates coxsackievirus B3- induced viral myocarditis by modulating the Th17/Treg immune response. *J. Cardiovasc. Pharmacol.* 69, 305–313.
6. Ballak, D. B., Van Diepen, J. A., Moschen, A. R., Jansen, H. J., Hijmans, A., Groenhof, G., et al. (2014). IL-37 protects against obesity-induced inflammation and insulin resistance. *Nat. Commun.* 5, 1–13.
7. Bar, D., Apte, R. N., Voronov, E., Dinarello, C. A., and Cohen, S. (2004). A continuous delivery system of IL-1 receptor antagonist reduces angiogenesis and inhibits tumor development. *FASEB J.* 18, 161–163. doi: 10.1096/fj.03- 0483fje
8. Barnes, P. J. (2006). How corticosteroids control inflammation: quintiles prize lecture 2005. *Br. J. Pharmacol.* 148, 245–254. doi: 10.1038/sj.bjp.0706736
9. Boraschi, D., Lucchesi, D., Hainzl, S., Leitner, M., Maier, E., Mangelberger, D., et al. (2011). IL-37: a new anti-inflammatory cytokine of the IL-1 family. *Eur. Cytokine Netw.* 22, 127–147. doi: 10.1684/ecn.2011.0288
10. Bulau, A., Nold, M. F., Li, S., Nold-Petry, C. A., Fink, M., Mansell, A., et al. (2014). Role of caspase-1 in nuclear translocation of IL-37, release of the cytokine, and IL-37 inhibition of innate immune responses. *Proc. Natl. Acad. Sci. U.S.A.* 111, 2650–2655. doi: 10.1073/pnas.1324140111
11. Busfield, S. J., Comrack, C. A., Yu, G., Chickering, T. W., Smutko, J. S., Zhou, H., et al. (2000). Identification and gene organization of three novel members of the IL-1 family on human chromosome 2. *Genomics* 66, 213–216. doi: 10.1006/ geno.2000.6184
12. Cain, D. W., and Cidlowski, J. A. (2017). Immune regulation by corticosteroids. *Nat. Rev. Immunol.* 17, 233–247.
13. Casqueiro, J., Casqueiro, J., and Alves, C. (2012). Infections in patients with diabetes mellitus: a review of pathogenesis. *Indian J. Endocrinol. Metab.* 16:S27. doi: 10.4103/2230-8210.94253
14. Cavalli, G., and Dinarello, C. A. (2018). Suppression of inflammation and acquired immunity by IL-37. *Immunol. Rev.* 281, 179–190. doi: 10.1111/imr. 12605
15. Chaudhry, Z., Shawe-Taylor, M., Rampling, T., Cutfield, T., Bidwell, G., Chan, X. H. S., et al. (2021). Short durations of corticosteroids for hospitalised COVID-19 patients are associated with a high readmission rate. *J. Infect.* 82, 276–316. doi: 10.1016/j.jinf.2021.03.002
16. Chinn, R. Y., and Diamond, R. D. (1982). Generation of chemotactic factors by *Rhizopus oryzae* in the presence and absence of serum: relationship to hyphal damage mediated by human neutrophils and effects of hyperglycemia and ketoacidosis. *Infect. Immun.* 38, 1123–1129. doi: 10.1128/iai.38.3.1123-1129. 1982
17. Colagiuri, S., Guariguata, L., Motala, A. A., and Ogurtsova, K. (2019). Global and regional diabetes prevalence estimates for 2019 and projections for 2030 and 2045: results from the international diabetes federation diabetes atlas, 9 (th) edition. *Diabetes Res. Clin. Pract.* 157:107843. doi: 10.1016/j.diabres.2019. 107843
18. Conti, P., Ronconi, G., and Caraffa, A. (2020). Induction of pro-inflammatory cytokines (Interleukin-1 and Interleukin-6) and lung inflammation by Coronavirus-19 (COVI-19 or SARS-CoV-2): anti-inflammatory strategies. *J. Biol. Regul. Homeost. Agents* 34:327–331. doi: 10.23812/CONTI-E
19. Corrao, S., Pinelli, K., Vacca, M., Raspanti, M., and Argano, C. (2021). Type 2 diabetes mellitus and COVID-19: a narrative review. *Front. Endocrinol.* 12:609470. doi: 10.3389/fendo.2021.609470
20. Delamaire, M., Maugendre, D., Moreno, M., Le Goff, M., Allannic, H., and Genetet, B. (1997). Impaired leucocyte functions in diabetic patients. *Diabetic Med.* 14, 29–34. doi: 10.1002/(SICI)1096-9136(199701)14:1<29::AID-DIA300>3.0. CO;2-V
21. Diamond, R. D., Haudenschild, C. C., and Erickson, N. F. III (1982). Monocyte- mediated damage to *Rhizopus oryzae* hyphae in vitro. *Infect. Immun.* 38, 292–297.
22. Dinarello, C. A., and Bufler, P. (2013). Interleukin-37. *Semin. Immunol.* 25, 466– 468.
23. Donath, M. Y., and Shoelson, S. E. (2011). Type 2 diabetes as an inflammatory disease. *Nat. Rev. Immunol.* 11, 98–107.
24. Ehrchen, J. M., Roth, J., and Barczyk-Kahlert, K. (2019). More than suppression: glucocorticoid action on monocytes and macrophages. *Front. Immunol.* 10:2028. doi: 10.3389/fimmu.2019.02028
25. Gianchandani, R., Esfandiari, N. H., Ang, L., Iyengar, J., Knotts, S., Choksi, P., et al. (2020). Managing hyperglycemia in the COVID-19 inflammatory storm. *Diabetes* 69, 2048–2053. doi: 10.2337/dbi20-0022
26. Greenberg, A. S., and Obin, M. S. (2006). Obesity and the role of adipose tissue in inflammation and metabolism. *Am. J. Clin. Nutr.* 83, 461S–465S. doi: 10.1093/ ajcn/83.2.461S
27. Guan, W., Ni, Z., Hu, Y., Liang, W., Ou, C., He, J., et al. (2020). Clinical characteristics of coronavirus disease 2019 in China. *N. Engl. J. Med.* 382, 1708–1720.
28. Hoang, K., Abdo, T., Reinersman, J. M., Lu, R., and Higuita, N. I. A. (2020). A case of invasive pulmonary mucormycosis resulting from short courses of corticosteroids in a well-controlled diabetic patient. *Med. Mycol. Case Rep.* 29, 22–24. doi: 10.1016/j.mmcr.2020.05.008
29. Hoffmann, M., Kleine-Weber, H., Schroeder, S., Krüger, N., Herrler, T., Erichsen, S., et al. (2020). SARS-CoV-2 cell entry depends on ACE2 and TMPRSS2 and is blocked by a clinically proven protease inhibitor. *Cell* 181, 271–280. e8.
30. Holman, N., Knighton, P., Kar, P., O'Keefe, J., Curley, M., Weaver, A., et al. (2020). Risk factors for COVID-19-related mortality in people with type 1 and type 2 diabetes in England: a population-based cohort study. *Lancet Diabetes Endocrinol.* 8, 823–833. doi: 10.1016/S2213-8587(20)30271-0
31. Iacobellis, G. (2020). COVID-19 and diabetes: can DPP4 inhibition play a role? *Diabetes Res. Clin. Pract.* 162:108125.
32. Joshi, N., Caputo, G. M., Weitekamp, M. R., and Karchmer, A. W. (1999). Infections in patients with diabetes mellitus. *N. Engl. J. Med.* 341, 1906–1912.
33. Kayina, C. A., Maitra, S., Anand, R. K., Ray, B. R., Baidya, D. K., and Subramaniam, R. (2020). Sars-cov-2 infection presenting with hyperglycemia and ketosis: a case series of three diabetic patients. *Indian J. Crit. Care Med.* 24:1141. doi: 10.5005/jp-journals-10071-23595

34. Kershaw, E. E., and Flier, J. S. (2004). Adipose tissue as an endocrine organ. *J. Clin. Endocrinol. Metab.* 89, 2548–2556.
35. Koh, H., Moh, A. M. C., Yeoh, E., Lin, Y., Low, S. K. M., Ooi, S. T., et al. (2021). Diabetes predicts severity of COVID-19 infection in a retrospective cohort: a mediatory role of the inflammatory biomarker C-reactive protein. *J. Med. Virol.* 93, 3023–3032. doi: 10.1002/jmv.26837
36. Kumar, M., Sarma, D. K., Shubham, S., Kumawat, M., Verma, V., Singh, B., et al. (2021). Mucormycosis in COVID-19 pandemic: risk factors and linkages. *Curr. Res. Microb. Sci.* 2:100057. doi: 10.1016/j.crmicr.2021.100057
37. Kumar, S., McDonnell, P. C., Lehr, R., Tierney, L., Tzimas, M. N., Griswold, D. E., et al. (2000). Identification and initial characterization of four novel members of the interleukin-1 family. *J. Biol. Chem.* 275, 10308–10314. doi: 10.1074/jbc. 275.14.10308
38. Law, C. C., Puranik, R., Fan, J., Fei, J., Hambly, B. D., and Bao, S. (2021). Clinical implications of IL-32, IL-34 and IL-37 in atherosclerosis: speculative role in cardiovascular manifestations of COVID-19. *Front. Cardiovasc. Med.* 8:882. doi: 10.3389/fcvm.2021.630767
39. Li, A., Ling, Y., Song, Z., Cheng, X., Ding, L., Jiang, R., et al. (2021). Correlation between early plasma interleukin 37 responses with low inflammatory cytokine levels and benign clinical outcomes in severe acute respiratory syndrome coronavirus 2 infection. *J. Infect. Dis.* 223, 568–580. doi: 10.1093/infdis/jiaa713
40. Li, C., Ji, H., Cai, Y., Ayana, D. A., Lv, P., Liu, M., et al. (2013). Serum interleukin- 37 concentrations and HBeAg seroconversion in chronic HBV patients during telbivudine treatment. *J. Interferon Cytokine Res.* 33, 612–618. doi: 10.1089/jir. 2013.0001
41. Li, T., Li, H., Li, W., Chen, S., Feng, T., Jiao, W., et al. (2019). Interleukin-37 sensitize the elderly type 2 diabetic patients to insulin therapy through suppressing the gut microbiota dysbiosis. *Mol. Immunol.* 112, 322–329. doi: 10.1016/j.molimm.2019.06.008
42. Liu, F., Long, X., Zhang, B., Zhang, W., Chen, X., and Zhang, Z. (2020). ACE2 expression in pancreas may cause pancreatic damage after SARS-CoV-2 infection. *Clin. Gastroenterol. Hepatol.* 18:2128. doi: 10.1016/j.cgh.2020.04.040 Manson, J. E., Rifai, N., Buring, J. E., and Ridker, P. M. (2001). C-reactive protein, interleukin 6, and risk of developing type 2 diabetes mellitus. *JAMA* 286, 327–334. doi: 10.1001/jama.286.3.327
43. Matsumoto, S., Tsuji-Takayama, K., Aizawa, Y., Koide, K., Takeuchi, M., Ohta, T., et al. (1997). Interleukin-18 activates NF-κB in murine T helper type 1 cells. *Biochem. Biophys. Res. Commun.* 234, 454–457. doi: 10.1006/bbrc.1997.6665
44. Molteni, E., Astley, C. M., Ma, W., Sudre, C. H., Magee, L. A., Murray, B., et al. (2021). Symptoms and syndromes associated with SARS-CoV-2 infection and severity in pregnant women from two community cohorts. *Sci. Rep.* 11, 1–11. doi: 10.1038/s41598-021-86452-3
45. Nold, M. F., Nold-Petry, C. A., Zepp, J. A., Palmer, B. E., Bufler, P., and Dinarello, C. A. (2010). IL-37 is a fundamental inhibitor of innate immunity. *Nat. Immunol.* 11, 1014–1022.
46. Pan, G., Risser, P., Mao, W., Baldwin, D. T., Zhong, A. W., Filvaroff, E., et al. (2001). IL-1H, an interleukin 1-related protein that binds IL-18 receptor/IL-1Rrp. *Cytokine.* 13, 1–7. doi: 10.1006/cyto.2000.0799
47. Qi, F., Liu, M., Li, F., Lv, Q., Wang, G., Gong, S., et al. (2019). Interleukin-37 ameliorates influenza pneumonia by attenuating macrophage cytokine production in a MAPK-dependent manner. *Front. Microbiol.* 10:2482. doi: 10. 3389/fmicb.2019.02482
48. Quispe-Cañari, J. F., Fidel-Rosales, E., Manrique, D., Mascaró-Zan, J., Huamán- Castillón, K. M., Chamorro-Espinoza, S. E., et al. (2021). Self-medication practices during the COVID-19 pandemic among the adult population in Peru: a cross-sectional survey. *Saudi Pharm. J.* 29, 1–11. doi: 10.1016/j.jsps.2020.12. 001
49. Ragab, D., Salah Eldin, H., Taeimah, M., Khattab, R., and Salem, R. (2020). The COVID-19 cytokine storm; what we know so far. *Front. Immunol.* 11:1446. doi: 10.3389/fimmu.2020.01446
50. Rammaert, B., Lanternier, F., Zahar, J., Dannaoui, E., Bougnoux, M., Lecuit, M., et al. (2012b). Healthcare-associated mucormycosis. *Clin. Infect. Dis.* 54, S44–S54.
51. Rammaert, B., Lanternier, F., Poirée, S., Kania, R., and Lortholary, O. (2012a). Diabetes and mucormycosis: a complex interplay. *Diabetes Metab.* 38, 193–204. doi: 10.1016/j.diabet.2012.01.002
52. Rautemaa-Richardson, R., and Richardson, M. D. (2021). Systemic fungal infections. *Medicine* 45, 757–762.
53. Rawshani, A., Rawshani, A., Franzén, S., Sattar, N., Eliasson, B., Svensson, A., et al. (2018). Risk factors, mortality, and cardiovascular outcomes in patients with type 2 diabetes. *N. Engl. J. Med.* 379, 633–644. doi: 10.1056/NEJMoa1800256
54. Recovery Collaborative Group (2021). Dexamethasone in hospitalized patients with Covid-19. *N. Engl. J. Med.* 384, 693–704.
55. Roberts, J., Pritchard, A. L., Treweeke, A. T., Rossi, A. G., Brace, N., Cahill, P., et al. (2020). Why is COVID-19 more severe in patients with diabetes? The role of angiotensin-converting enzyme 2, endothelial dysfunction and the immunoinflammatory system. *Front. Cardiovasc. Med.* 7:629933. doi: 10.3389/fcvm.2020.629933
56. Roden, M. M., Zaoutis, T. E., Buchanan, W. L., Knudsen, T. A., Sarkisova, T. A., Schaufele, R. L., et al. (2005). Epidemiology and outcome of zygomycosis: a review of 929 reported cases. *Clin. Infect. Dis.* 41, 634–653. doi: 10.1086/432579 Sharma, S., Kulk, N., Nold, M. F., Gräf, R., Kim, S., Reinhardt, D., et al. (2008). The IL-1 family member 7b translocates to the nucleus and down- regulates proinflammatory cytokines. *J. Immunol.* 180, 5477–5482. doi: 10. 4049/jimmunol.180.8.5477
57. Shibata, R., Ouchi, N., Ohashi, K., and Murohara, T. (2017). The role of adipokines in cardiovascular disease. *J. Cardiol.* 70, 329–334.
58. Skiada, A., Pavleas, I., and Drogari-Apiranthitou, M. (2020). Epidemiology and diagnosis of mucormycosis: an update. *J. Fungi* 6:265. doi: 10.3390/jof6040265 Sridhara, S. R., Paragache, G., Panda, N. K., and Chakrabarti, A. (2005). Mucormycosis in immunocompetent individuals: an increasing trend. *J. Otolaryngol.* 34, 402–406.
59. Su, Z., and Tao, X. (2021). Current understanding of IL-37 in human health and disease. *Front. Immunol.* 12:2562. doi: 10.3389/fimmu.2021.696605
60. Sugar, A. M. (1990). "Agents of mucormycosis and related species," in *Principles And Practice Of Infectious Diseases*, eds G. L. Mandell, R. G. Douglas Jr., and J. E. Bennett (Boston, MA: Department of Medicine, Boston University School of Medicine), 1962–1972.
61. Summers, K. L., Marleau, A. M., Mahon, J. L., McManus, R., Hramiak, I., and Singh, B. (2006). Reduced IFN-α secretion by blood dendritic cells in human diabetes. *Clin. Immunol.* 121, 81–89. doi: 10.1016/j.clim.2006.05.015
62. Tilg, H., and Moschen, A. R. (2006). Adipocytokines: mediators linking adipose tissue, inflammation and immunity. *Nat. Rev. Immunol.* 6, 772–783. doi: 10. 1038/nri1937
63. van de Veerdonk, F. L., Gresnigt, M. S., Oosting, M., van der Meer, J. W., Joosten, L. A., Netea, M. G., et al. (2015). Protective host defense against disseminated candidiasis is impaired in mice expressing human interleukin-37. *Front. Microbiol.* 7:762. doi: 10.3389/fmicb.2014.00762
64. van Paassen, J., Vos, J. S., Hoekstra, E. M., Neumann, K. M., Boot, P. C., and Arbous, S. M. (2020). Corticosteroid use in COVID-19 patients: a systematic review and meta-analysis on clinical outcomes. *Crit. Care* 24, 1–22. doi: 10. 1186/s13054-020-03400-9
65. Varikasuvu, S. R., Varshney, S., and Dutt, N. (2021). Markers of coagulation dysfunction and inflammation in diabetic and non-diabetic COVID-19. *J. Thromb. Thrombolysis* 51, 941–946. doi: 10.1007/s11239-020-02270-w
66. Waldorf, A. R., Ruderman, N., and Diamond, R. D. (1984). Specific susceptibility to mucormycosis in murine diabetes and bronchoalveolar macrophage defense against Rhizopus. *J. Clin. Invest.* 74, 150–160. doi: 10.1172/JCI11 1395
67. Wang, L., Quan, Y., Yue, Y., Heng, X., and Che, F. (2018). Interleukin-37: a crucial cytokine with multiple roles in disease and potentially clinical therapy. *Oncol. Lett.* 15, 4711–4719. doi: 10.3892/ol.2018.7982
68. World Health Organization (2019). *Classification Of Diabetes Mellitus.* Geneva: World Health Organization. World Health Organization (2020). *No Title: Corticosteroids for COVID-19: Living Guidance, 2 September 2020.* Geneva: World Health Organization.
69. Yamauchi, T., and Kadowaki, T. (2008). Physiological and pathophysiological roles of adiponectin and adiponectin receptors in the integrated regulation of metabolic and cardiovascular diseases. *Int. J. Obes.* 32, S13–S18. doi: 10.1038/ijo.2008.233
70. Yang, J., Lin, S., Ji, X., and Guo, L. (2010). Binding of SARS coronavirus to its receptor damages islets and causes acute diabetes. *Acta Diabetol.* 47, 193–199. doi: 10.1007/s00592-009-0109-4
71. Yi, Y., Lagniton, P. N., Ye, S., Li, E., and Xu, R. (2020). COVID-19: what has been learned and to be learned about the novel coronavirus disease. *Int. J. Biol. Sci.* 16:1753. doi: 10.7150/ijbs.45134

72. Zhang, J., Dong, X., Cao, Y., Yuan, Y., Yang, Y., Yan, Y., et al. (2020). Clinical characteristics of 140 patients infected with SARS- CoV-2 in Wuhan, China. *Allergy* 75, 1730–1741. doi: 10.1111/all. 14238

73. Zykova, S. N., Jenssen, T. G., Berdal, M., Olsen, R., Myklebust, R., and Seljelid, R. (2000). Altered cytokine and nitric oxide secretion in vitro by macrophages from diabetic type II-like db/db mice. *Diabetes* 49, 1451–1458. doi: 10.2337/diabetes.49.9.1451

Permissions

All chapters in this book were first published Frontiers; hereby published with permission under the Creative Commons Attribution License or equivalent. Every chapter published in this book has been scrutinized by our experts. Their significance has been extensively debated. The topics covered herein carry significant findings which will fuel the growth of the discipline. They may even be implemented as practical applications or may be referred to as a beginning point for another development.

The contributors of this book come from diverse backgrounds, making this book a truly international effort. This book will bring forth new frontiers with its revolutionizing research information and detailed analysis of the nascent developments around the world.

We would like to thank all the contributing authors for lending their expertise to make the book truly unique. They have played a crucial role in the development of this book. Without their invaluable contributions this book wouldn't have been possible. They have made vital efforts to compile up to date information on the varied aspects of this subject to make this book a valuable addition to the collection of many professionals and students.

This book was conceptualized with the vision of imparting up-to-date information and advanced data in this field. To ensure the same, a matchless editorial board was set up. Every individual on the board went through rigorous rounds of assessment to prove their worth. After which they invested a large part of their time researching and compiling the most relevant data for our readers.

The editorial board has been involved in producing this book since its inception. They have spent rigorous hours researching and exploring the diverse topics which have resulted in the successful publishing of this book. They have passed on their knowledge of decades through this book. To expedite this challenging task, the publisher supported the team at every step. A small team of assistant editors was also appointed to further simplify the editing procedure and attain best results for the readers.

Apart from the editorial board, the designing team has also invested a significant amount of their time in understanding the subject and creating the most relevant covers. They scrutinized every image to scout for the most suitable representation of the subject and create an appropriate cover for the book.

The publishing team has been an ardent support to the editorial, designing and production team. Their endless efforts to recruit the best for this project, has resulted in the accomplishment of this book. They are a veteran in the field of academics and their pool of knowledge is as vast as their experience in printing. Their expertise and guidance has proved useful at every step. Their uncompromising quality standards have made this book an exceptional effort. Their encouragement from time to time has been an inspiration for everyone.

The publisher and the editorial board hope that this book will prove to be a valuable piece of knowledge for researchers, students, practitioners and scholars across the globe.

List of Contributors

Jiaoyue Zhang, Wen Kong, Hanyu Wang, Huiqing Li, Juan Zheng, Wenfang Xia, Geng Liu, Xueyu Zhong, Kangli Qiu, Han Wang, Yuxiu Wang, Xiaoli Song, Hua Liu, Zhenhai Cui, Lulu Chen and Tianshu Zeng
Department of Endocrinology, Union Hospital, Tongji Medical College, Huazhong University of Science and Technology, Wuhan, China
Hubei Provincial Clinical Research Center for Diabetes and Metabolic Disorders, Wuhan, China

Hui Sun
Department of Endocrinology, Union Hospital, Tongji Medical College, Huazhong University of Science and Technology, Wuhan, China
Hubei Provincial Clinical Research Center for Diabetes and Metabolic Disorders, Wuhan, China
SenseTime Research, Beijing, China

Pengfei Xia and An Pan
Department of Epidemiology and Biostatistics, School of Public Health, Tongji Medical College, Huazhong University of Science and Technology, Wuhan, China

Ying Xu and Si Xiong
Department of Endocrinology, The Fifth Hospital of Wuhan, Wuhan, China

Li Li and Yan Li
Department of Endocrinology, Wuhan Wuchang Hospital, Wuchang Hospital Affiliated to Wuhan University of Science and Technology, Wuhan, China

Qin Li
Department of Endocrinology, General Hospital of the Yangtze River Shipping, Wuhan, China

Li Yang
Department of Endocrinology, Hankou Hospital of Wuhan City, Wuhan, China

Qi Wei
Department of Endocrinology, Red Cross Hospital of Wuhan City, Wuhan, China

Yu Hu
Institute of Hematology, Union Hospital, Tongji Medical College, Huazhong University of Science and Technology, Wuhan, China
Hubei Clinical and Research Centre of Thrombosis and Haemostasis, Wuhan, China

Andrew B. Crouse and Matthew Might
Hugh Kaul Precision Medicine Institute, University of Alabama at Birmingham, Birmingham, AL, United States

Tiffany Grimes, Fernando Ovalle and Anath Shalev
Comprehensive Diabetes Center, Department of Medicine, Division of Endocrinology, Diabetes and Metabolism, University of Alabama at Birmingham, Birmingham, AL, United States

Peng Li
School of Nursing, University of Alabama at Birmingham, Birmingham, AL, United States

Nan Zhang, Lu-Lu Chen, Miao-Miao Peng and Kang Li Qiu
Department of Endocrinology, Union Hospital, Tongji Medical College, Huazhong University of Science and Technology, Wuhan, China

Cheng Wang and Feng Zhu
Department of Cardiology, Union Hospital, Tongji Medical College, Huazhong University of Science and Technology, Wuhan, China

Hong Mao and Na Li
Department of Endocrinology, Tongji Medical College, Central Hospital of Wuhan, Huazhong University of Science and Technology, Wuhan, China

Peng Bai and Yixuan Wang
Department of Cardiovascular Surgery, Union Hospital, Tongji Medical College, Huazhong University of Science and Technology, Wuhan, China

Muqing Yu, Shuyun Xu, Jianping Zhao and Min Zhou
Department of Pulmonary and Critical Care Medicine, Tongji Hospital, Tongji Medical College, Huazhong University of Science and Technology, Wuhan, China
Key Laboratory of Respiratory Diseases, National Ministry of Health of the People's Republic of China and National Clinical Research Center for Respiratory Disease, Wuhan, China

Louis Y. Tee, Sharifah Munirah Alhamid, Jeriel L. Tan, Theik Di Oo, Primavera Galinato and Barbara Helen Rosario
Department of Geriatric Medicine, Changi General Hospital, Singapore

Jaime Chien, Seow Yen Tan, Shafi Humaira and Raymond Kok Choon Fong
Department of Infectious Diseases, Changi General Hospital, Singapore

Troy H. Puar, Wann Jia Loh and Joan Khoo
Department of Endocrinology, Changi General Hospital, Singapore

Anindita Santosa
Department of Rheumatology, Changi General Hospital, Singapore

Nasim Rahmani-Kukia
Department of Biochemistry, School of Medicine, Shiraz University of Medical Sciences, Shiraz, Iran

Ardeshir Abbasi
Department of Immunology, Faculty of Medical Sciences, Tarbiat Modares University, Tehran, Iran

Maria Ida Maiorino, Giuseppe Bellastella, Miriam Longo, Paola Caruso and Katherine Esposito
Department of Advanced Medical and Surgical Sciences, University of Campania "Luigi Vanvitelli", Naples, Italy

Li-Chi Huang
Department of Endocrinology and Metabolism, Cathay General Hospital, Taipei, Taiwan

Ching-Ling Lin
Department of Endocrinology and Metabolism, Cathay General Hospital, Taipei, Taiwan
Department of Internal Medicine, School of Medicine, College of Medicine, Taipei Medical University, Taipei, Taiwan

Yao-Tsung Chang and Ruey-Yu Chen
School of Public Health, Taipei Medical University, Taipei, Taiwan

Shwu-Huey Yang
School of Nutrition and Health Sciences, Taipei Medical University, Taipei, Taiwan
Nutrition Research Center, Taipei Medical University Hospital, Taipei, Taiwan
Research Center of Geriatric Nutrition, College of Nutrition, Taipei Medical University, Taipei, Taiwan

Meifang Han, Ke Ma, Xiaojing Wang, Weiming Yan, Hongwu Wang, Jie You, Huilong Chen, Wei Guo, Tao Chen and Qin Ning
Department and Institute of Infectious Disease, Tongji Hospital of Tongji Medical College, Huazhong University of Science and Technology, Wuhan, China

Qiuxia Wang
Department of Radiology, Tongji Hospital, Tongji Medical College, Huazhong University of Science and Technology, Wuhan, China

Xiaoping Luo
Department of Pediatrics, Center for the Diagnosis of Genetic Metabolic Diseases, Tongji Hospital, Tongji Medical College, Huazhong University of Science and Technology, Wuhan, China

Juan Chen and Jiangyi Yu
Department of Endocrinology, Jiangsu Province Hospital of Chinese Medicine, Affiliated Hospital of Nanjing University of Chinese Medicine, Nanjing, China

Chunhua Wu
Department of General Practice, Zhongda Hospital, Medical School, Southeast University, Nanjing, China

Xiaohang Wang and Zilin Sun
Department of Endocrinology, Zhongda Hospital, Institute of Diabetes, Medical School, Southeast University, Nanjing, China

Lei Yang, Bolin Li and Xiaopu Zheng
Department of Cardiology, The First Affiliated Hospital of Xi'an Jiaotong University, Xi'an, China

Dou Xu and Zhongyu Li
School of Software Engineering, Xi'an Jiaotong University, Xi'an, China

Yiqing Tan
Department of Radiology, Wuhan Third Hospital, Tongren Hospital of Wuhan University, Wuhan, China

Dan Zhu, Jingbo Wang and Ling Zhu
Department of Radiology, Shanghai Ninth People's Hospital Affiliated to JiaoTong University School of Medicine, Shanghai, China

Xinglong Liu
SenseTime Research, Beijing, China

Hermine Muniangi-Muhitu and Elina Akalestou
Section of Cell Biology and Functional Genomics, Division of Diabetes, Endocrinology and Metabolism, Department of Metabolism, Digestion and Reproduction, Imperial College London, London, United Kingdom

Victoria Salem
Section of Endocrinology, Division of Diabetes, Endocrinology and Metabolism, Department of Metabolism, Digestion and Reproduction, Imperial College London, London, United Kingdom

Shivani Misra and Nicholas S. Oliver
Section of Metabolic Medicine, Division of Diabetes, Endocrinology and Metabolism, Department of Metabolism, Digestion and Reproduction, Imperial College London, London, United Kingdom

Guy A. Rutter
Section of Cell Biology and Functional Genomics, Division of Diabetes, Endocrinology and Metabolism, Department of Metabolism, Digestion and Reproduction, Imperial College London, London, United Kingdom
Lee Kong Chian School of Medicine, Nan Yang Technological University, Singapore

Moein Zangiabadian, Seyed Aria Nejadghaderi and Mohammad Mahdi Zahmatkesh
Student Research Committee, School of Medicine, Shahid Beheshti University of Medical Sciences, Tehran, Iran

Bahareh Hajikhani and Mohammad Javad Nasiri
Department of Microbiology, School of Medicine, Shahid Beheshti University of Medical Sciences, Tehran, Iran

Mehdi Mirsaeidi
Department of Medicine, Division of Pulmonary, Critical Care, Sleep and Allergy, University of Miami, Coral Gables, FL, United States

Ernestina M. De Francesco, Veronica Vella and Antonino Belfiore
Department of Clinical and Experimental Medicine, University of Catania, and ARNAS Garibaldi, P.O. Garibaldi-Nesima, Catania, Italy

Isabela Roque Marçal, Bianca Fernandes, Ariane Aparecida Viana and Emmanuel Gomes Ciolac
Exercise and Chronic Disease Research Laboratory (ECDR), Department of Physical Education, School of Sciences, Campus Bauru (UNESP), São Paulo State University, Bauru, Brazil

Karen Pinelli, Martina Vacca, Massimo Raspanti and Christiano Argano
Department of Internal Medicine, National Relevance and High Specialization Hospital Trust ARNAS Civico, Di Cristina, Benfratelli, Palermo, Italy

Salvatore Corrao
Department of Internal Medicine, National Relevance and High Specialization Hospital Trust ARNAS Civico, Di Cristina, Benfratelli, Palermo, Italy
Dipartimento di Promozione della Salute, Materno Infantile, Medicina Interna e Specialistica di Eccellenza "G. D'Alessandro", PROMISE, University of Palermo, Palermo, Italy

Jeff M. P. Holly, Kalina Biernacka, Nick Maskell and Claire M. Perks
Faculty of Medicine, School of Translational Health Science, Southmead Hospital, University of Bristol, Bristol, United Kingdom

Siwei Song, Shujing Zhang, Sufei Wang, Yanling Ma, Pei Ma and Yang Jin
Department of Respiratory and Critical Care Medicine, NHC Key Laboratory of Pulmonary Diseases, Union Hospital, Tongji Medical College, Huazhong University of Science and Technology, Wuhan, China

Zhihui Wang
Department of Scientific Research, Union Hospital, Tongji Medical College, Huazhong University of Science and Technology, Wuhan, China

Huilin Luo
Department of Anesthesia, Wuhan Red Cross Hospital, Wuhan, China

Mengyuan Wang
Department of Endocrinology, Union Hospital, Tongji Medical College, Huazhong University of Science and Technology, Wuhan, China

Zeming Liu, Jianglong Huang, Liang Guo and Yihui Huang
Department of Plastic Surgery, Zhongnan Hospital of Wuhan University, Wuhan, China

Jinpeng Li
Department of Thyroid and Breast Surgery, Zhongnan Hospital of Wuhan University, Wuhan, China

Rongfen Gao
Department of Rheumatology and Immunology, Tongji Medical College, Tongji Hospital, Huazhong University of Science and Technology, Wuhan, China

Kuan Luo
Department of Neurosurgery, Wuhan Puren Hospital, Wuhan, China

Guang Zeng
Department of Urology, Zhongnan Hospital of Wuhan University, Wuhan, China

Tingbao Zhang, Jincao Chen and Xiaohui Wu
Department of Neurosurgery, Zhongnan Hospital of Wuhan University, Wuhan, China

Meilin Yi
Department of Burn and Plastic Surgery, College of Traditional Chinese Medicine, Three Gorges University, Yichang Hospital of Traditional Chinese Medicine, Yichang, China

Yibin Yang
Department of Respiratory and Critical Care Medicine, Zhongnan Hospital of Wuhan University, Wuhan, China

Shi Jin
Department of Endocrinology, The Fourth Affiliated Hospital of China Medical University, Shenyang, China

Weina Hu
Department of Cardiology, The Fourth Affiliated Hospital of China Medical University, Shenyang, China

Mohamed Abu-Farha, Sina Kavalakatt and Jehad Abubaker
Department of Biochemistry and Molecular Biology, Dasman Diabetes Institute, Dasman, Kuwait

Fahd Al-Mulla and Thangavel Alphonse Thanaraj
Department of Genetics and Bioinformatics, Dasman Diabetes Institute, Dasman, Kuwait

Hamad Ali
Department of Genetics and Bioinformatics, Dasman Diabetes Institute, Dasman, Kuwait
Department of Medical Laboratory Sciences, Faculty of Allied Health Sciences, Health Sciences Center, Kuwait University, Jabriya, Kuwait

Mohammed Abdul Ghani
Diabetes Division, University of Texas Health Science Center at San Antonio, San Antonio, TX, United States

Amany Magdy Beshbishy
National Research Center for Protozoan Diseases, Obihiro University of Agriculture and Veterinary Medicine, Obihiro, Japan

Victor B. Oti
Department of Microbiology, Nasarawa State University, Keffi, Nigeria

Diaa E. Hussein
Researcher, Department of Food Hygiene, Agricultural Research Center, Animal Health Research Institute, Port of Alexandria, Egypt

Ibrahim F. Rehan
Department of Husbandry and Development of Animal Wealth, Faculty of Veterinary Medicine, Menofa University, Shebin Alkom, Egypt

Oluyomi S. Adeyemi
Medicinal Biochemistry, Infectious Diseases, Nanomedicine & Toxicology Laboratory, Department of Biochemistry, Landmark University, Omu-Aran, Nigeria

Nallely Rivero-Perez and Adrian Zaragoza-Bastida
Área Académica de Medicina Veterinaria y Zootecnia, Instituto de Ciencias Agropecuaria, Universidad Autónoma del Estado de Hidalgo, Tulancingo, Mexico

Muhammad Ajmal Shah
Department of Pharmacognosy, Faculty of Pharmaceutical Sciences, Government College University, Faisalabad, Pakistan

Khaled Abouelezz and Helal F. Hetta
Department of Medical Microbiology and Immunology, Faculty of Medicine, Assiut University, Assiut, Egypt

Natália Cruz-Martins
Faculty of Medicine, University of Porto, Porto, Portugal
Institute for Research and Innovation in Health (i3S), University of Porto, Porto, Portugal
Laboratory of Neuropsychophysiology, Faculty of Psychology and Education Sciences, University of Porto, Porto, Portugal

Gaber El-Saber Batiha
Department of Pharmacology and Therapeutics, Faculty of Veterinary Medicine, Damanhour University, Damanhour, Egypt

Yan Yang, Zixin Cai and Jingjing Zhang
National Clinical Research Center for Metabolic Diseases, Metabolic Syndrome Research Center, Key Laboratory of Diabetes Immunology, Ministry of Education, and Department of Metabolism and Endocrinology, The Second Xiangya Hospital of Central South University, Changsha, China

Paraskevi Kazakou, Georgios Panagopoulos, Stavros Athanasopoulos and Asimina Mitrakou
Diabetes Centre, Department of Clinical Therapeutics, Alexandra Hospital, School of Medicine, National and Kapodistrian University of Athens, Athens, Greece

Vaia Lambadiari and Aikaterini Kountouri
Second Department of Internal Medicine, Attikon University Hospital, National and Kapodistrian University of Athens, Medical School, Athens, Greece

Ignatios Ikonomidis
Laboratory of Preventive Cardiology, Second Cardiology Department, Attikon University Hospital National and Kapodistrian University of Athens, Medical School, Athens, Greece

Eleni Korompoki
Department of Clinical Therapeutics, Alexandra Hospital, School of Medicine, National and Kapodistrian University of Athens, Athens, Greece

Ioannis Kalomenidis
1st Department of Intensive Care, Evangelismos Hospital, National and Kapodistrian University of Athens, Medical School, Athens, Greece

Meletios A. Dimopoulos
Unit of Hematology and Oncology, Department of Clinical Therapeutics, Alexandra Hospital, School of Medicine, National and Kapodistrian University of Athens, Athens, Greece

Shiying Shao, Xuefeng Yu and Yong Chen
Division of Endocrinology, Tongji Hospital, Huazhong University of Science and Technology, Wuhan, China
Branch of National Clinical Research Center for Metabolic Diseases, Hubei, China

Qin Yang
Division of Pathology, Tongji Hospital, Huazhong University of Science and Technology, Wuhan, China

Ruping Pan
Department of Nuclear Medicine, Tongji Hospital, Huazhong University of Science and Technology, Wuhan, China

Sima Tokajian, Georgi Merhi and Charbel Al Khoury
Department of Natural Sciences, School of Arts and Sciences, Lebanese American University, Byblos, Lebanon

Georges Nemer
Department of Biochemistry and Molecular Genetics, Faculty of Medicine, American University of Beirut, Beirut, Lebanon
Division of Genomics and Translational Biomedicine, College of Health and Life Sciences, Hamad Bin Khalifa University, Doha, Qatar

Index